HANDBOOK ON LONGEVITY: GENETICS, DIET AND DISEASE

HANDBOOK ON LONGEVITY: GENETICS, DIET AND DISEASE

JENNIFER V. BENTELY
AND
MARY ANN KELLER
EDITORS

Nova Biomedical Books
New York

Library of Congress Cataloging-in-Publication Data

Handbook on longevity : genetics, diet, and disease / [edited by] Jennifer V. Bentely and Mary Ann Keller.
    p. ; cm.
  Includes bibliographical references and index.
  ISBN 978-1-60741-075-1 (hardcover : alk. paper)
  1. Longevity. 2. Longevity--Genetic aspects. 3. Longevity--Nutritional aspects. I. Bentely, Jennifer V. II. Keller, Mary Ann.
  [DNLM: 1. Longevity--genetics. 2. Aging--physiology. 3. Diet. WT 116 H236 2009]
  QP85.H26 2009
  612.6'8--dc22
                    2009008022

Published by Nova Science Publishers, Inc. ✦ *New York*

Contents

Preface   **vii**

Chapter I   Introducing New Definition of Elderly in Japan   **1**
                    Yasuharu Tokuda

Chapter II   Aging Puzzle   **5**
                    Mladen Davidovic, Dragoslav P. Milosevic, Nebojsa Despotovic,
                    Jelena Vukcevic and Predrag Erceg

Chapter III   Toward the Mitigation of Glycation: A Practical Protocol   **23**
                    Nūn Sava-Siva Amen-Ra

Chapter IV   Prospects of a Longer Life Span beyond the Beneficial Effects of a
                    Healthy Lifestyle   **35**
                    Giacinto Libertini

Chapter V   Stress Resistance and Aging in Long-Lived Rodent Models   **97**
                    James M. Harper and Adam B. Salmon

Chapter VI   Longevity-Associated Mitochondrial DNA 5178 C/A
                    Polymorphism Modifies the Effect of Coffee Consumption on
                    Glucose Tolerance in Middle-Aged Japanese Men   **139**
                    Akatsuki Kokaze, Mamoru Ishikawa, Naomi Matsunaga,
                    Kanae Karita, Masao Yoshida, Tadahiro Ohtsu,
                    Takako Shirasawa, Yahiro Haseba, Masao Satoh, Koji Teruya,
                    Hiromi Hoshino and Yutaka Takashima

Chapter VII   Pesticides and Longevity   **161**
                    Sáenz de Cabezón Irigaray, Francisco Javier; Carvajal Montoya,
                    Luz Dary and Moreno Grijalba, Fernando

Chapter VIII   The Optimal Human Diet: Theoretical Foundations of the Amen
                    Protocol   **177**
                    Nūn Sava-Siva Amen-Ra

Chapter IX   Protective Effect of Calorie Restriction on Age-Induced Fibrosis   **241**
                     E. Chiarpotto, L. Castello, E. Bergamini, and G. Poli

Chapter X   Engineered Natural Longevity-Enhancing Interventions   **255**
                     Arkadi F. Prokopov and Tamara N.Voronina

Chapter XI   Be Young in Mind - Against Aging and Alzheimer's Disease   **291**
                     Kun Zou

Chapter XII   Understanding Aging: Prejudices and Misconceptions   **303**
                     Carles Zafon

Chapter XIII   Longevity: Genetics, Diet and Disease   **309**
                     E. Naumova, I. Atanasova, M. Ivanova and G. Pawelec

Chapter XIV   Effects of Chewing Ability on Longevity   **337**
                     Toshihiro Ansai, Yutaka Takata and Tadamichi Takehara

Chapter XV   Research on Aging and Longevity in the Parthenogenetic Marbled
                     Crayfish, with Special Emphasis on Stochastic Developmental
                     Variation, Allocation of Metabolic Resources, Regeneration, and
                     Social Stress   **353**
                     Günter Vogt

Chapter XVI   Genetic Background for Longevity in Livestock Species: A Review   **373**
                     Joaquim Casellas

Chapter XVII   Genetic and Environmental Factors Affecting Inflammatory
                     Responses to Infection   **397**
                     C.C. Blackwell, S.M. Moscovis, S.T. Hall, J. Stuart,
                     C.J. Ashhurst-Smith, J. Roberts-Thomson, D. Yarnold and R.J. Scott

Chapter XVIII   Mammalian Cell Sporulation – A Possible Link to Disease
                     and Aging   **429**
                     Yonnie Wu, Kyle Heim and Erick Vasquez

Index   **453**

Preface

The word longevity is sometimes used as a synonym for "life expectancy" in demography. Aging is the accumulation of changes in an organism or object over time. Aging in humans refers to a multidimensional process of physical, psychological, and social change. Some dimensions of aging grow and expand over time, while others decline. Reaction time, for example, may slow with age, while knowledge of world events and wisdom may expand. Research shows that even late in life potential exists for physical, mental, and social growth and development. Aging is an important part of all human societies reflecting the biological changes that occur, but also reflecting cultural and societal conventions. Age is usually measured in full years ¡ª and months for young children. At present, the biological basis of aging is unknown. This new book presents the latest research in this dynamic field.

Chapter 1 - Japan is currently developing into an extraordinarily rapidly-aging society. The current official definition of elderly in Japan is "age of 65 years or older" and this aged population has exceeded beyond 20% in 2006. In addition, because of the lowest birth rate ever in Japan, the proportion of the younger aged group is also shrinking. These population dynamics in Japan can cause soaring healthcare costs, shrinking work forces, and possible collapsing pension programs. Since many of the Japanese elderly, around the age of 65-75 years, are still able to actively work and contribute to society and the average remaining life expectancy of Japanese at age 65 is about 23 years for females and 18 years for males, the authorshave recently proposed re-defining elderly to "aged 75 or older". Older workers can remain productive and stay healthy longer. Work participation among seniors is beneficial for maintaining autonomy and quality of later life. The revised definition of elderly could make a huge and important impact in terms of maintaining the social and economic integrity in this country and many senior workers would remain active, stay healthier and are integrated in a rewarding social network.

Chapter 2 - In the past couple of centuries, scientists proposed great number of aging theories, but neither of them was completely satisfactory.

In the statistical sense scientists are faced with an even greater dilemma because of the presence of a large array of factors that affect ageing. Although most of these factors are well known at this point, just the fact of their innumerability complicates scientists approach to the issue at hand. These factors in the positive sense involve: starvation, Mediterranean diet, the life styles, activity and so on. In the negative sense scientists are talking about unhealthy habits, including the omission of the positive life styles listed above.

If the authors tried to sum up everything we know today about ageing into two sentences, as much as such simplifications can be dangerous, they would probably come up with the following two sentences or basic observations:

- First, caloric restriction diet does prolong life and secondly,
- Delay of the reproductive processes also prolongs life.
- Most recently it appears that high-predation risk in one group the guppies also prolong reproduction life span as life span in general.
- More and more authors are trying to explain the unknowns in the understanding of these observations about ageing, by adding the statement that there are two subgroups in the general population. Such statement is in no contradiction with the basic observations listed here. This acknowledgement of two subpopulations explains why there are numerous cases that can not be explained or defined or fitted in these basic observations about caloric restrictions and the delay of reproduction.

The two known options for the prolongation of life, that are listed here as basic observations about ageing, are applicable to the majority of the general population. The rest of the population, as much as it might seem awkward, can be considered as privileged. The primary groups, i.e., the majority of the population, are those that have evolved successfully, in other words there would be no evolution, if there wasn't for this group. The privileged group, "the selfish ones", are those that are genetically more stable. If the privileged group was the majority, human race would not have gone down the same evolutionary road.

Chapter 3 - The purpose of this chapter is to establish the theoretical and practical efficacy of a dietary/lifestyle regimen in reducing glycative damage and, by so doing, improving health and longevity. Known as the Amen Optimal Health Protocol, the regimen seeks to synergistically combine established experimental interventions with efficacy in lengthening lifespan or modulating physiological processes known to be operative in aging. Chief among such processes is glycation. Glycation is a chemical process wherein the carbonyl moieties of reducing sugars such as glucose or its metabolites react covalently with nitrogenous constituents of amino acids, proteins, or certain lipids. Through a series of complex chemical conversions various sugar-protein and sugar-lipid adducts eventuate in so-called advanced glycation endproducts (AGEs). It is these multifarious endproducts of glycation that have been determined to be deleterious to health and longevity.

Chapter 4 - Life span is limited by the effects of diseases and ageing. For the aim of a longer life span, it is indispensable that a rational analysis of the primary causes of these phenomena is not limited to the description of their physio-pathological mechanisms. If Dobzhansky's statement that "nothing in biology makes sense, except in the light of evolution" is true, it appears logical to maintain that evolution theory must be the main tool for such analysis.

From an evolutionary point of view, diseases are the predictable consequence of: 1) defects in the maintenance and transmission of genetic information; 2) alterations of the ecological niche to which the species is adapted (in particular, for our species, due to civilisation); 3) interactions with other species (bacteria, viruses, fungi, protozoa, parasitic worms, etc.); and 4) conditions for which the species is not adapted.

Moreover, evolution theory allows the paradoxical prediction that, in particular ecological conditions, kin selection favours a progressive fitness decline, usually, in its more evident manifestations, referred to as ageing and that must not be classified as a disease. This decline is genetically determined and regulated and is obtained with a progressive limitation of cell turnover through a sophisticated modulation of the telomere-telomerase system.

A lifestyle compatible with the ecological niche to which our species is adapted and good medical treatment permit the attainment of the highest life span defined by the genetic program of our species (within the limits of individual genetic peculiarities) but do not allow the overcoming of the maximal values of longevity defined by the same program.

To increase these values, it is indispensable to modify the genetic planning of ageing, with a different modulation of the telomere-telomerase system.

In principle, granted that this will be considered ethically acceptable, it is possible to propose a modification of that part of the genetic program that modulates ageing so that an unlimited survival is obtained, similar to the so-called "negligible senescence" observed for many animal and plant species.

A possible schedule to achieve this aim and the effects on human civilisation are outlined.

Chapter 5 - The aging process affects nearly every biochemical and physical system measured to date. Nevertheless, the mechanism(s) responsible for modulating the rate of aging have yet to be identified. A number of mechanistic theories have predicted that the accumulation of damage to cellular macromolecules could be key determinants of the rate of aging and the progression of age-related disease. These theories also predict that aging may be slowed by the attenuation of damage accumulation, a process that may be accomplished by enhanced resistance to stress.

Treatments that extend lifespan, for example the restriction of caloric intake, are known to reduce the accumulation of cellular damage, including oxidation and DNA mutation, as well as increase the resistance to numerous stressors such as oxidative stress, DNA damage and heat. In addition, genetic mutations that extend murine lifespan have consistently shown a corresponding increase in resistance to multiple types of stress. For instance, dwarf mutations, like the Snell and Ames dwarf, have been shown to extend lifespan by 40-60% while delaying multiple age-related pathologies. Dwarf mice also show an increased resistance to oxidative stress *in vivo*, as well as cellular resistance to multiple cytotoxic and metabolic insults.

In addition to these well-characterized mutant mouse models, wild-derived and free-living rodent populations are a virtually untapped resource in the context of stress resistance, aging and disease. Recent studies have shown that wild-derived mouse stocks are very different physiologically from laboratory mouse stocks and that they exhibit significant differences in life span. Work in these underutilized strains and other long-lived rodent models, has suggested that they also exhibit enhanced stress resistance, and especially an enhanced resistance to oxidative stress. Hence, it may be that among models of extended longevity, resistance to stress plays an important role in the maintenance of cellular homeostasis, thereby preserving cell and tissue function and delaying the progression of age-related phenotypes.

Chapter 6 - Mitochondrial DNA 5178 C/A (Mt5178 C/A), NADH dehydrogenase subunit-2 237 leucine/methionine (ND2-237 Leu/Met), polymorphism is reported to be associated with longevity, blood pressure, serum lipid levels, fasting plasma glucose levels, glucose tolerance, serum uric acid levels, pulmonary function, hematological parameters, intraocular pressure, serum electrolyte levels, and serum protein fraction levels in the Japanese population. Mt5178A (ND2-237lMet) genotype reportedly provides resistance to diabetes and atherosclerotic diseases, such as myocardial infarction and cerebrovascular diseases. Several epidemiological studies have shown that habitual coffee consumption exerts a protective effect against abnormal glucose tolerance in a Japanese population. This study investigated whether longevity-associated Mt5178 C/A (ND2-237 Leu/Met) polymorphism modifies the effects of coffee consumption on the risk of abnormal glucose tolerance in middle-aged Japanese men. A total of 332 male subjects (age, 52.8 ± 7.8 years; mean $\pm$ SD) were selected from individuals visiting the hospital for regular medical check-ups. After adjustment, the odds ratio (OR) for abnormal glucose tolerance was significantly lower in subjects with Mt5178C (ND2-237Leu) who consume more than four cups of coffee daily compared with those who consume less than one cup of coffee daily (OR = 0.245; 95% CI: 0.066 - 0.914). On the other hand, the association between Mt5178A genotype and risk for abnormal glucose tolerance did not depend on coffee consumption. These results suggest that longevity-associated Mt5178 C/A (ND2-237 Leu/Met) polymorphism modifies the effects of coffee consumption on reduced abnormal glucose tolerance risk in middle-aged Japanese men. This novel diet-gene interaction may contribute to the individualized prevention of lifestyle-related adult-onset diseases and allow for healthy aging and longevity.

Chapter 7 - Most common and effective way of a pesticide to take effect is through direct ingestion via food, water or air. Once the active ingredient is inside the body of the target (pest) or non-target organism (humans, environment, wild and domesticated fauna), it can either affect vital processes killing the organism, or display single or multiple side effects that can have serious effects on other life processes affecting the longevity of the organism. After more than 7 decades depending on heavy use of chemical in agriculture, the rise of concern about how these active ingredients affect the physiology of different organisms, have developed ways to analyze and to describe the deleterious effects of pesticides on human and environmental health. In this chapter, the authors will discuss the interaction of pesticides, with target and non target physiological systems, giving emphasis on secondary effects (hormonal, developmental, genetic, general homeostatic changes) that can impair not only the life (longevity) of the affected organism but can have effects on successive generations. In this way, the authors will obtain an idea of how pesticide exposure can have various effects on human health, those effects can interact, synergize and lead to chronic damage at various physiological systems and organizational levels, as a result, if damages are important enough to impair or interfere with metabolic, homeostatic or/and functional responses, the target can view its lifespan, including reproductive outcomes, reduced.

Chapter 8 - The purpose of this chapter is to explicate the central elements of a theoretically optimal human diet. Such a diet is herein defined as one that is plausibly capable of increasing human longevity, decreasing disease susceptibility, augmenting mental acuity and generally facilitating the attainment and maintenance of an aesthetic ideal encompassing muscularity, leanness and juvenescence. The main parameters pertinent to the conceptualization of this theoretical diet are temporal, quantitative and qualitative. That is, consideration is given to the frequency with which food is to be ingested and the time at which it should be ingested, the amount of calories that should be consumed and the composition of the food so consumed. This chapter will review and analyze scientific studies and fundamental physiological principles that form the theoretical and empirical bases of the diet. Caloric restriction and cyclic fasting—experimental interventions known to increase maximum mammalian lifespan—are the empirical cornerstones of the theoretically formulated regimen. As to the qualitative component of the diet, consideration is given to foods whose chemical constituents are known to influence the same physiological processes modulated by caloric restriction and cyclic fasting. Such processes include facilitation of detoxification, augmentation of antioxidant defense, attenuation of inflammation and oxidative damage, inhibition of glycation and maintenance of membrane, protein and genomic integrity. Thus, a major tenet of my theoretical complex is what I herein term *selective synergism*. In the context of this treatise, selective synergism entails ascertainment of the mechanisms involved in lifespan prolongation and disease diminution secondary to caloric restriction and attempting to augment these effects dietetically. Finally, consideration shall be given to psychological factors influencing compliance with such a restrictive protocol, including experiential insights gleaned from the author's own self-imposed adoption of the protocol in question spanning a period of four years.

Chapter 9 - Starting from research by McCay et al., several studies have demonstrated that controlled calorie restriction (CR) exerts an anti-ageing effect in different organisms, from invertebrates to mammals. Observational studies suggest that CR also has beneficial effects on human longevity. However, the anti-aging mechanisms of CR are still not clearly understood. One mechanism might be protection against the age-associated increase of oxidative stress and consequent cellular damage.

In parallel, a role of oxidative stress in fibrosis induction and progression has been demonstrated in many human diseases, such as pneumoconiosis, interstitial pulmonary fibrosis, cystic fibrosis, cirrhosis, neurodegenerative diseases and atherosclerosis.

In fibrosis, fibroblasts or fibroblast-like cells are activated by various cytokines, among which transforming growth factor β1 (TGFβ1) is prominent, to proliferate and produce high levels of extracellular matrix and collagen. High TGFβ1 levels have been found in human diseases of different organs all characterized by excessive ECM deposition and marked fibrosis (cirrhosis, chronic hepatitis, glomerulonephritis, diabetic nephropathy, atherosclerosis, sclerodermia, pulmonary fibrosis). Fibrosis is also a constant distinctive feature in tissue aging.

TGFβ1 exerts its multiple biological activities through interaction with type I and type II receptors. Signaling to the nucleus is principally through cytoplasmic proteins of the Smad family, but in various cell types TGFβ1 also activates mitogen activated protein kinase (MAPK) pathways, i.e. extracellular regulated kinase 1 and 2 (ERK1/2), c-Jun N-terminal kinase (JNK) and p38, leading to collagen type I synthesis through activation of the transcription factor activator protein 1 (AP-1).

In this context, it is of interest to study the possible protective effect of CR against the onset of fibrosis in the frame of tissue and soma aging.

In this connection, our group has shown that, with aging, there is an increase of oxidative stress in rat aorta, with a progressive hoarding of biologically-active end-products, in particular 4-hydroxy-2,3-nonenal (HNE). Moreover, the increase of oxidative stress with aging is accompanied by increased fibrosis in terms of TGFβ1 and collagen levels. CR protects against both phenomena.

With regard to possible protective mechanisms of CR against fibrosclerosis, we believe they may be closely connected to the reduction of oxidative stress: by decreasing HNE levels in older rat aortae, CR significantly decreases JNK and p38 activity. Since JNK is central for AP-1 activation, by negatively modulating JNK, CR also prevents AP-1 activation and consequently down-regulates transcription of AP-1-dependent genes, including TGFβ1, vimentin and collagen.

The possibility of controlling the fibrogenesis process by modifying dietary habits opens new nutritional horizons in the prevention and treatment of several pathological processes characterized by excessive fibrosis. However, since it seems difficult to transpose animal CR model as such to man, interest in natural and/or pharmacological CR mimetic molecules is increasing.

Chapter 10 - Currently developing engineered biogerontological interventions promise to radically extend healthy life span. Nevertheless, the exploration of natural strategies that underlie longevity and resistance to age-related diseases in exceptionally long-living mammals, such as the bowhead whale (BW, *Balena mysticetus*) and naked mole rat (NMR, *Heterocephalus glaber*) is also rational.

This paper is an attempt to analyze the advantages and limitations of these strategies, and to elucidate their existing derived applications, as well as to estimate their future prospects in the practice of biogerontology.

Two natural longevity-modulating strategies (intermittent calorie/nutrient restriction—ICR, and intermittent oxygen restriction—IOR) utilize the universal development-and adaptational genetic programs, evolutionary "preinstalled" in all aerobic organisms. ICR and IOR synergistically diminish the basal level of mitochondria-dependent oxidative stress that is supposed to be the key factor, modulating life span and resistance to age-related diseases in aerobes.

ICR and IOR employ a common mitochondria-rejuvenating pathway, *mitoptosis*—a selective elimination of excessively ROS-producing mitochondria in the cells. Mitoptosis is a natural process that maintains the "quality" of mitochondria in the female germinal cells during early embryogenesis, and can be stimulated and maintained by IOR and ICR also in the postmitotic cells of adult organisms. Behaviorally induced continuous mitoptosis seems to be the key mechanism responsible for exceptional longevity and resistance to age-related diseases in BW and NMR.

Additionally, ICR and IOR influence the longevity and tempo of development of age-related diseases via several mitochondria-independent pathways, such as suppressed protein glycation, enhanced DNA repair, accelerated protein turnover, stimulation of EPO, GH, HSP70 and other functional proteins. In addition, IOR distinctively intensifies stem-cell-dependent tissue repair.

The unified positive effect of IOR and ICR on the cells and organisms manifests in enhanced genome stability and increased non-specific resistance to multiple stressors.

Various forms of ICR and IOR have an impressively positive account of empiric and evidence-based use in the health-improving practices of various human cultures. Recently developed engineered techniques, such as short-termed, or alternate-day fasting (ADF, derivative of ICR) and intermittent hypoxic training/therapy (IHT, derivative of IOR) induce measurable mitochondrial and systemic rejuvenation.

The vitamin-nutriceutical supplementation synergistically enhances the efficiency of IOR and ICR.

Further development of engineered ICR and IOR protocols should facilitate their advanced clinical implementation and user-friendly, self-help applications.

Chapter 11 - Life expectancy around the world has increased steadily for nearly 200 years. The continuing increase in life expectancy has made us face age-related diseases that we overlooked in the nineteenth and early twentieth centuries. Age is by far the biggest risk factor for a wide range of clinical conditions that are prevalent today. Although cardiovascular diseases and cancers still remain the leading causes of death for both men and women among age-related diseases, Alzheimer's disease has been in the spotlight recently because the number of its patients is increasing at an unexpected speed. Onset of Alzheimer's disease begins with short-term memory loss in its early stage and gradually the sufferer loses minor, and then major bodily functions, until <u>death</u> occurs. Unlike cardiovascular diseases and cancers, current knowledge of the processes leading to Alzheimer's disease is still limited, and very few effective treatments are available. Many treatment strategies have reached the clinical trial stage and some hopeful clinical trials failed to improve the survival or the cognitive ability of Alzheimer's patients. Up to now, clinically validated treatments for Alzheimer's disease remain confined to symptomatic interventions and recent studies suggest that frequent cognitive activity in old age has been associated with reduced risk of Alzheimer's disease. Thus, preventive strategies have become important in our daily life against aging and Alzheimer's disease.

Chapter 12 - Current evolutionary biology has rejected any theory that supports a selective purpose for aging. However, recent findings have forced a reconsideration of this concept and an effort to update old statements that have been made. In accordance, several evolutionary propositions have been suggested to justify the broad presence of aging in the animal kingdom and the wide range of longevity. Nevertheless, many of these alternative hypotheses have been dismissed using a small set of arguments that have been systematically repeated without, in some cases, any compelling proof of evidence. Moreover, there exists a variety of preconceptions and biases that could hinder the progression in theoretical thought about aging and longevity. The aim of this "author comment" is to expose some of these preconceptions to generate a productive debate which can enrich the progress in the field of evolutionary biology of aging. In particular, the author will discuss three critical points that have not usually been considered in related papers. The first point is the "emotional bias" observed when authors argue the purpose of aging. The second point (When does aging begin?) pertains to the beginning of aging. The third topic (The old watchmaker) discusses the meaning of the aging process from an evolutionary perspective, and the evolutionary origin of the aging strategy.

Chapter 13 - The aging process is very complex. Human longevity is a multifactorial trait which is determined by genetic and environmental factors and the interaction of "disease" processes with "intrinsic" ageing processes. Twin and family studies imply that up to 25% of human lifespan is heritable and increases in long-lived people to 36-40%. Longevity is a complex phenotype associated with different genes and gene polymorphisms, some of which are involved in metabolic pathways and endocrine system functioning, which affect diet-related health risks. For example, about 10 loci in the human genome have now been found that seem to confer susceptibility to type 1 diabetes mellitus, where insulin deficiency is due to autoimmune beta cell destruction. Nutrition is one of the hypothetical disease-triggering factors and low and special carbohydrate diet is obligatory for disease control. The best studied longevity pathway involves the genes regulating insulin and insulin-like growth factor-1 (IGF-1) signaling, as well as environmental effects on gene expression. Some of these genes are responsible also for oxidative stress, inflammation and tumor suppression. Another conventional group of genes currently under intense investigation are those involved in innate and adaptive immune responses. The pathogenesis of some of the most frequent human age-related diseases, like metabolic syndrome, diabetes mellitus type 2, and atherosclerosis is associated with a change in the circulating levels of C-reactive protein, tumor necrosis factor-α, interleukin-6, leptin, resistin, adiponectin, omentin, visfatin, and expression of CD40, - CD40 ligand, E-selectin, ICAM-1, and VCAM-1. Some of these genes may be responsible for mediating the beneficial effects of caloric restriction by regulating energy balance as well as stress resistance and oxidative damage. Additionally, other genes such as those encoding TLR, CCR5, KIR and MBL2 have also been associated with different age-related diseases and therefore with human longevity.

There are rare monogenic human diseases which are models for accelerated aging and progeria. Others are caused by inborn errors of metabolism: inherited traits that are due to a mutation in a metabolic enzyme, mutations in regulatory proteins and in transport mechanisms. Some metabolic disorders are due to structural chromosome aberrations and genomic imprinting, such as life-threatening obesity in Prader-Willi and Angelman syndrome.

In conclusion, this review will summarize current information on genome-wide dietary target genes, regulatory pathways affecting human homeostasis and diseases, and the role of immune response genes and particularly genes of innate immunity with an impact on lifespan.

Chapter 14 - The oral cavity in humans has a variety of functions, such as eating, swallowing, and speaking, as well as chewing, which is one of its most important roles. Although the association of chronic periodontitis with systemic health has become an important issue, few studies have been conducted regarding the association between chewing ability and systemic health status. Recently, we conducted a population-based prospective study to determine the association between chewing ability and longevity in 697 (277 males, 420 females) community-dwelling elderly subjects in Japan, and herein present some of those results. Chewing ability was assessed based on the number of types of food each subject reported able to chew in answers to a questionnaire, which showed that individuals with higher chewing ability lived longer, after adjusting for various confounding factors (multivariate hazard ratio: 2.6; 95% confidence interval: 1.2-5.5). When the associations between causes of death and chewing ability were further analyzed, subjects reporting the lowest numbers of chewable foods were associated with a higher risk of mortality from cardiovascular disease (CVD) as compared with those able to chew all the types of food surveyed (multivariate hazard ratio: 5.1; 95% confidence interval: 1.1-23.8). On the other hand, there was no significant association between chewing ability and other causes of death including cancer. Our results indicate that maintenance of chewing ability in elderly individuals contributes to longevity. In addition, we discuss the significance of masticatory function in light of nutrition status.

Chapter 15 - This chapter presents first results on aging and longevity in the marbled crayfish, an isogenic invertebrate with indeterminate growth. The marbled crayfish is the only known parthenogenetic species of more than 10.000 decapod crustaceans and has a maximal life span of roughly 3.5 years. Its main advantages, aside from genetically identical offspring and lifelong growth, are the alternation of growth and reproduction phases, a high regeneration capacity and easy handling in the laboratory. In a group of seven genetically identical batch-mates life span varied from 437 to 910 days although the sibs were communally reared and fed ad libitum with the same pellet food. In the same group there was no clear-cut relationship between longevity and growth or reproduction frequency. However, the specimen with the lowest life span showed fast growth, early onset of reproduction, and short time intervals between reproduction cycles. Damages like loss of appendages were repaired and did not negatively affect longevity. Social stress, in contrast, shortened life expectancy. The biological peculiarities of the marbled crayfish and the data obtained so far argue for a more intense use of this animal in research on aging and longevity.

Chapter 16 - Longevity is a trait of major interest in livestock with important implications on both economic and animal welfare grounds. The relevance of longevity within the animal production framework was highlighted during the twentieth century with a plethora of studies focusing on environmental sources of variation. Although the specific molecular mechanisms involved in the longevity of domestic species remains unclear, recent studies have provided plenty of evidence of genetic determinism for aging-related traits in livestock. Indeed, longevity must be viewed as the final expression of a dynamic system governed by intrinsic (e.g. immunology, reproduction, and growth) and extrinsic determinants (e.g. temperature, food, and predators), in which every intrinsic determinant (and some extrinsic determinants, such as resistance to cold temperatures) is virtually modulated by genes. As the influence of genes is inextricably intertwined with longevity, it is virtually impossible to consider the broad determinants of longevity without a basic understanding of the underlying genetics.

Chapter 17 - The incidence of notifiable infectious diseases is higher in Indigenous Australians compared with the non-Indigenous population, and there are higher incidences of heart and kidney diseases for which infection and inflammation are thought to play important roles in their pathogenesis [Australian Bureau of Statistics, 2001]. These discrepancies in health have been attributed mainly to poor socioeconomic conditions in which many Indigenous families live. New evidence is emerging that indicates there are significant genetic differences which might contribute to susceptibility to or severity of infections. The objective of this review is to examine these differences in relation to classical risk factors to determine potential interactions between genetic background and environmental conditions that contribute to susceptibility to these diseases.

Chapter 18 - This chapter reviews the physiochemical properties of mammalian spores and straw cells, which develop in vitro from the transformation of normal mammalian cells exposed to desiccative conditions. We hypothesize that this transformation is directly linked with aging and aging related diseases. Unlike many of the current damage related aging theories involving damage to DNA and protein molecules (leading to improper gene expression and protein function), this transformation is an active process at the cellular level. The metamorphosis of a normal cell into a mammalian spore is an inherited survival mechanism that can cause the loss of the body's most basic life-sustaining unit, the cell.

Mammalian spores are extremely prevalent. It is estimated that a typical person currently possesses billions of spores in their blood; the amount of spores may fluctuate in a day, perhaps influenced by physiological conditions such as diet and exercise that affect the overall sporulation stress. These mammalian spores form long extensive and extremely hydrophilic filamentous network that could contribute to blood viscosity. Blood cholesterol level may be increased from sporulation of billions of cells per day.

The metamorphosis of a mammalian spore from a normal mammalian cell is marked by a variety of distinct physical changes. First, the nuclei is broken into many pieces and reassembled within a tiny tube shaped structure. Second, tubular walls are constructed. Finally, upon the reintroduction of water, mammalian spores revert to normal mammalian cells and begin to divide. The early steps of this transformation resemble the development of apoptotic bodies. However, instead of destroying itself, the cell enters a robust spore-like cell survival phase, allowing it to remain viable under severe external conditions. Mammalian spores construct a strong cell wall using sulfated-glucose polymers and glycosylated acidic proteins, allowing it to withstand harsh treatment such as UV-C radiation.

A direct inverse relationship is displayed between the number of mammalian spores present in the blood of 9 domestic animals and these animals' average lifespan. The number of mammalian spores present in the heart and lung tissues, as well as excreted in the urine, also increases with the age of the mammal. This increased production of mammalian spores may play a role in disrupting normal cell and organ function. The large number of mammalian spores produced by a variety of tissues makes this transformation appear to be a natural physiological process embedded within a cell's environmental response machinery. The universal nature of mammalian spores and their mobility within the bloodstream allow them to affect many parts of the body. The mobile character of these cells displays a potential link to longevity and the development of aging-related diseases, including the metastasis of various cancers.

Water is the most essential component for cell survival. Throughout evolution organisms have developed many novel adaptations for particular environmental deficiencies and conditions. The formation of spores may be an early form of environmental adaptation for single celled organisms. However, in multicellular organisms the mammalian spore survival mechanism may not be beneficial because the organism loses necessary functional cells. Inhibiting mammalian spore biogenesis would prevent the depletion of normal healthy cells, as well as the spread of potentially harmful cells, and therefore improve mammalian longevity. Intervention of sporulation using membrane interacting molecules is discussed.

Exogenous phosphotidylcholines (DOPC) significantly promote dehydration-induced sporulation while other phospholipids (DOPG, DOPE, DOPA, and DOPS) are ineffective.

In: Handbook on Longevity: Genetics, Diet and Disease   ISBN 978-1-60741-075-1
Editors: Jennifer V. Bentely and Mary Ann Keller   © 2009 Nova Science Publishers, Inc.

Chapter I

Introducing New Definition of Elderly in Japan

Yasuharu Tokuda[*]

Department of Medicine, St Luke's International Hospital
9-1 Akashi-cho, Chuo City, Tokyo 104-8560 Japan

Abstract

Japan is currently developing into an extraordinarily rapidly-aging society. The current official definition of elderly in Japan is "age of 65 years or older" and this aged population has exceeded beyond 20% in 2006. In addition, because of the lowest birth rate ever in Japan, the proportion of the younger aged group is also shrinking. These population dynamics in Japan can cause soaring healthcare costs, shrinking work forces, and possible collapsing pension programs. Since many of the Japanese elderly, around the age of 65-75 years, are still able to actively work and contribute to society and the average remaining life expectancy of Japanese at age 65 is about 23 years for females and 18 years for males, we have recently proposed re-defining elderly to "aged 75 or older". Older workers can remain productive and stay healthy longer. Work participation among seniors is beneficial for maintaining autonomy and quality of later life. The revised definition of elderly could make a huge and important impact in terms of maintaining the social and economic integrity in this country and many senior workers would remain active, stay healthier and are integrated in a rewarding social network.

Japan is now developing into an extraordinarily rapidly-aging society. The current official definition of elderly in Japan is "age of 65 years or older". Because of the baby boom after World War II, longer-living and healthier seniors, called "Dankai-sedai" in Japanese,

[*] Phone and FAX 81-(0)3-5550-2426
Email: tokuyasu@orange.ocn.ne.jp

are now reaching retirement age, around age of 60-65, in unprecedented numbers. At the same time, the birth rate in Japan has steadily kept dropping to the lowest on record. Since the mid-point of the twentieth century, the motto *"fewer children but better nurture"* has become popular and been widely accepted.[1] In addition, the birth rate decline has also been driven by underlying change of social values. In Japan, the important value changes affecting the birth rate in recent decades seem related to major educational and job gains by women, leading to greater economic independence and more emphasis on individualism and equality between the genders.[2] Because of high degree of ethnic and cultural homogeneity in Japan, values tend to be widely and quickly shared and thus the value change tends to occur in spurts.

These population dynamics will reduce the proportion of the younger aged group who are required to support the elderly through the national pension and insurance programs. The number of people between 15 and 64 is expected to decline by an average of about 750,000 each year for the next decade.[3] The potential consequences may include; soaring healthcare costs, shrinking work forces and collapsing pension programs. Although the notion of retirement at 65 seemed reasonable when those over 65 were tiny percentage of the population, it is unlikely to be acceptable as they approach over 20% (20.7% in Japan 2006).[4]

Recently, we have proposed new definition of elderly as "age of 75 or older".[5][6] Indeed, many of the Japanese elderly, around the age of 65-75 years, are still able to actively work and contribute to society. A recent survey shows that 78% of Japanese between the ages of 55 and 59 want to keep working beyond the traditional retirement age of around 60-65 years instead of being taken care of by the younger generations. Many Japanese corporations, including Mitsubishi and Canon, have started re-employment programs for their own retirees. Some other corporations have started similar programs, in which all employees who wish to work past retirement can be re-employed after 65 at more-flexible hours and payment, and often in a different work.[3]

The current definition of elderly as age of 65 years and older in Japan was determined about 45 years ago. At that time, the average life span of the Japanese was about 68 years. However, the health and longevity record of Japan is currently the best in the world.[7][8] Based on the life table data for 2004, the average life expectancy of Japanese newborns is 86 years for females and 79 for males. Moreover, the average remaining life expectancy of Japanese at age 65 is about 23 years for women and 18 years for men in 2004 (Table 1).

Older workers can remain productive and stay healthy longer in Japan. Some Japanese companies have introduced health counseling and ergonomic production programs that have resulted in less physical and mental strain. A recent ecological study in Japan indicated that a higher proportion of senior workers were significantly associated with longer disability-free life expectancy among several different prefectures.[9] Studies have also documented that work participation among seniors is beneficial for maintaining autonomy and quality of later life, and that active working among retirement-aged men was associated with a greater sense of subjective well-being.[10-13]

Table 1. Average remaining life expectancy of Japanese at age 65*

Year	Men	Women
1950	11.5 (year)	13.9 (year)
1955	11.8	14.1
1960	11.6	14.1
1965	11.9	14.6
1970	12.5	15.3
1975	13.7	16.6
1980	14.6	17.7
1985	15.5	18.9
1990	16.2	20.0
1995	16.5	20.9
2000	17.5	22.4
2004	18.2	23.3

*Based on data of Ministry of Health, Welfare and Labor.

A revised definition of elderly could make a huge and important impact in terms of maintaining the social and economic integrity of this country. Indeed, the Organization for Economic Cooperation and Development (OECD) suggested that the future prosperity of a member country depends on a growing contribution from the elderly. Furthermore, the 2006 World Economic Forum (an annual meeting of global political and business elites) in Davos, Switzerland, also indicated the issue of aging of the workforce and the accompanying skills shortage as top on the list of future challenges facing international business and economy.[3] If the new definition of elderly would be introduced and the retirement age would be reset in Japan, many senior workers would remain active, stay healthier, earn a greater income and be integrated in a rewarding social network and they would also enhance their life-satisfaction, self-esteem, morale, and happiness[14].

References

[1] Hiraizumi. W. (2000). Mass Longevity Transforms Our Society. *Proceedings, American Philosophical Society (vol. 144, no. 4, 2000)*; 144(4).

[2] Retherford, R.D., Ogawa, N. and Sakamoto, S. (1996). Values and Fertility Change in Japan. *Population Studies*; 50(1):5-25.

[3] Takayama, H., Nadeau, B., Barigazzi, J., and Lee, B. (2006). The New Old Age. *Newsweek*; Jan 30:20-23.

[4] Gawande A. (2007). The way we age now. *The Now Yorker*; April 30:50-59.

[5] Hinohara, S. (2006). *Living long, Living good*. Tokyo: IBC Publishing.

[6] Tokuda, Y. and Hinohara, S. (2008). Redefining the age of elderly in Japan. *J Am Geriatr Soc*. 56(3):573-4.

[7]   Mathers, C., Iburg, K., Salomon, J., Tandon, A., Chatterji, S., Ustun, B., et al. (2004). Global patterns of healthy life expectancy in the year 2002. *BMC Public Health*; 4(1):66.

[8]   Yoshinaga, K. and Une, H. (2005). Contributions of mortality changes by age group and selected causes of death to the increase in Japanese life expectancy at birth from 1950 to 2000. *European Journal of Epidemiology*, 20(1):49-57.

[9]   Kondo, N., Mizutani, T., Minai, J., Kazama, M., Imai, H., Takeda, Y., et al. (2005). Factors explaining disability-free life expectancy in Japan: the proportion of older workers, self-reported health status, and the number of public health nurses. *J Epidemiol.* 15(6):219-27.

[10] Miyata, N., Oomori, M., Mizuno, T., Inaba, R., and Iwata, H. (1997). [Health conditions and life styles of residential elderly. Part 1. Characteristics and factors related to being healthy elderly persons from a survey of health life style]. *Nippon Koshu Eisei Zasshi*;44(8):574-85.

[11] Kawamoto, R., Doi, T., Yamada, A., Okayama, M., Tsuruoka, K., Satho, M., et al. (1991). [Happiness and background factors in community-dwelling older persons]. *Nippon Ronen Igakkai Zasshi*;36(12):861-7.

[12] Tsutsui, Y., Hachisuka, K. and Matsuda, S. (2001). Items regarded as important for satisfaction in daily life by elderly residents in Kitakyushu, Japan. *J Uoeh.*23(3):245-54.

[13] Okamoto, K. (2006). Life expectancy at the age of 65 years and environmental factors: an ecological study in Japan. *Arch Gerontol Geriatr.*43(1):85-91.

[14] Tokuda, Y., Ohde, S., Takahashi, O., Shakudo, M., Yanai, H., Shimbo, T., et al. (2008). Relationships between Working Status and Health or Healthcare Utilization among Japanese Elderly. *Geriatrics & Gerontology International*;8(1):32.

In: Handbook on Longevity: Genetics, Diet and Disease   ISBN 978-1-60741-075-1
Editors: Jennifer V. Bentely and Mary Ann Keller   © 2009 Nova Science Publishers, Inc.

Chapter II

Aging Puzzle

Mladen Davidovic, Dragoslav P. Milosevic, Nebojsa Despotovic, Jelena Vukcevic and Predrag Erceg

Clinical Department for Geriatrics, "Zvezdara" University Hospital
Belgrade, Serbia

Abstract

In the past couple of centuries, scientists proposed great number of aging theories, but neither of them was completely satisfactory.

In the statistical sense we are faced with an even greater dilemma because of the presence of a large array of factors that affect ageing. Although most of these factors are well known to us at this point, just the fact of their innumerability complicates our approach to the issue at hand. These factors in the positive sense involve: starvation, Mediterranean diet, the life styles, activity and so on. In the negative sense we are talking about unhealthy habits, including the omission of the positive life styles listed above.

If we tried to sum up everything we know today about ageing into two sentences, as much as such simplifications can be dangerous, we would probably come up with the following two sentences or basic observations:

- First, caloric restriction diet does prolong life and secondly,
- Delay of the reproductive processes also prolongs life.
- Most recently it appears that high-predation risk in one group the guppies also prolong reproduction life span as life span in general.
- More and more authors are trying to explain the unknowns in the understanding of these observations about ageing, by adding the statement that there are two subgroups in the general population. Such statement is in no contradiction with the basic observations listed here. This acknowledgement of two subpopulations explains why there are numerous cases that can not be explained or defined or fitted in these basic observations about caloric restrictions and the delay of reproduction.

The two known options for the prolongation of life, that are listed here as basic observations about ageing, are applicable to the majority of the general population. The rest of the population, as much as it might seem awkward, can be considered as privileged. The primary groups, i.e. the majority of the population, are those that have evolved successfully, in other words there would be no evolution, if there wasn't for this group. The privileged group, "the selfish ones", are those that are genetically more stable. If the privileged group was the majority, human race would not have gone down the same evolutionary road.

Old Age, Old Problem

In the past couple of centuries, scientists proposed great number of aging theories, but neither of them was completely satisfactory. Changes in chromosomal structure or function are strongly associated with ageing, although scientific results cannot determine whether these changes are part of the cause or a consequence of ageing. The effects of ageing in humans appear to be a combination of influence of genetically programmed phenomena and exogenous environmental factors, and take place at the cellular level [1,2].

In the statistical sense we are faced with an even greater dilemma because of the presence of a large array of factors that affect ageing. Although most of these factors are well known to us at this point, just the fact of their innumerability complicates our approach to the issue at hand. These factors in the positive sense involve: starvation, Mediterranean diet, the life styles, activity and so on. In the negative sense we are talking about unhealthy habits, including the omission of the positive life styles listed above.

If we tried to sum up everything we know today about ageing into two sentences, as much as such simplifications can be dangerous, we would probably come up with the following two sentences or basic observations [3]:

- First, caloric restriction diet does prolong life and secondly,
- Delay of the reproductive processes also prolongs life [4].
- Most recently it's appear that high-predation risk in one group the guppies also prolong reproduction life span as life span in general [5].
- More and more authors are trying to explain the unknowns in the understanding of these observations about ageing, by adding the statement that there are two subgroups in the general population. Such statement is in no contradiction with the basic observations, listed here. This acknowledgement of two subpopulations explains why there are numerous cases that can not be explained or defined or fitted in these basic observations about caloric restrictions and the delay of reproduction.

The two known options for the prolongation of life, that are listed here as basic observations about ageing, are applicable to the majority of the general population. The rest of the population, as much as it might seem awkward, can be considered as privileged. The primary group, i.e. the majority of the population, are those that have evolved successfully, in other words there would be no evolution, if there wasn't for this group. The privileged group, "the selfish ones", are those that are genetically more stable. If the privileged group was the majority, human race would not have gone down the same evolutionary road [3,6].

For example, we could try to learn about the genetic stability of the privileged group and use that knowledge in an effort to increase the genetic stability of the normally ageing group [7, 8]. On the other hand, maybe we have already evolved sufficiently.

Are we a step from anti-aging vaccine?

I am certain that I do not need to start by saying that "Ageing is not an illness," but I am not so certain that I do not have to say that: "Ageing is a problem only for the human kind." I do not hold that we need to be searching for a cure for ageing or a way to reach immortality. The essential point is the progress and evolution of the species and that has to, therefore, be the start of our story. This being said, there are thousands of ways we can continue our story, but there is also insurmountable amount of time necessary to research all the possible endings. With the growing amount of references in the sciences, it is easy to support almost any claim in biology or medicine with at least 10 references. So, what is the only known way to prolong life, which we know of at this point?

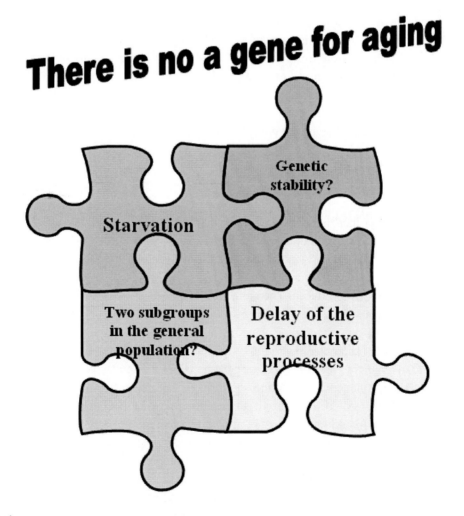

Figure 1.

By starvation we delay the essential goal, i.e. the reproduction and thus prolongation of the species

Aging Puzzle

Starvation seems to be the only known way. It is often said that the process of limited amount of caloric intake must start at an early age, but there are some who claim that even starting later in life can have beneficial effects for prolongation of life. Affirming this claim, we must ask ourselves: How does the limitation of the caloric intake prolong life? The mechanism behind this process seems to mirror the way the postponing of reproduction postpones ageing. When there is not a lot of food available, many animals, especially the desert animal postpone reproduction. With humans the case seems to be the same. It appears then that by starvation we delay the essential goal, i.e. the reproduction and thus prolongation of the species. This results in a "bonus" to the length of life for the purpose of getting another chance to reproduce.

The basic task is always simple. It is much more complicated to understand the mechanism towards the task. This mechanism is affected by many different factors, so much so that it is almost impossible to foresee all of them. Just like the gas engine burns gasoline and creates environmentally unsafe gases, the cellular motor burns oxygen and releases free radicals that are just as harmful for the body's environment. Free radicals can be induced by a large array of well-known environmental factors. It seems then that free radicals are the basic mechanism through which the ageing process takes place.

The Aging Process

The conclusion is that there is no gene for ageing. There is a large array of genes that have more then one function. In other words, in addition to their known function, many genes can for the purposes of the survival of the species also prolong life. By the removal of the free radical effects we can prevent certain illnesses, but we can also prolong life, but the process itself cannot be reproduced. The modification of the gene expression and their effects seem optimal. Currently there are a few successful ways.

Another relevant point regarding genetics is the genetic instability that allows us the basic evolutionary advantage compared to other species [7]. Primates have a similar genetic makeup, yet the reparation capability of our genome is twice as good. Would it be possible to return to the more stable genetic structure and through that make our species less susceptible to ageing and illness? All of the current advantages like vaccinations would play an even more important role. In addition, how sure are we that there is not a privileged group in our species which is more genetically stable? We should ask ourselves if the dolphins are truly inferior to us or, if they already knew this, and chose a simpler and better life.

Nature seems to be cyclical in its essence; it appears to act as a sum of births, existences and deaths of its parts. Human civilization seems to follow that same circle of existence. However just like the individuals in all other species every one of us is stained by our instinct for survival. Further, in human being, maybe due to our mental capacities, this survival instinct has translated into efforts to achieve longevity. The quest for longevity has been an integral part of our civilization; it has permited the way we think and act. Magic, medicine and religion have all played a role in this quest.

The way medicine has approached this issue has been to deal with symptoms. Cancers, strokes, heart attacks are still the number one cause of death, or low quality of life. We need to change the way we look at longevity, and old age. As long as humans have been around, we attempted to find a "cure" for old age, find some kind of fountain of youth, and although we have improved, our most meaningful accomplishments did not come from treating symptoms but from preventing illnesses. The introduction of vaccination has prolonged human life by 28 years in average. So would it be possible to find a "vaccine" for prevention of old age? [9,10]

We should consider the hypothesis that there are people with more and people with less stable genomes [3,7,11]. Identification of those two groups of individuals would allow us to "vaccinate" and through that act on the instable genomes and genes. By that we would be able to prevent the development of cancer. Working under the assumption that cancer will after enough chances for mutation sure to develop, than the two groups of individuals we are discussing are those with less stable genomes whose genes react faster to mutation, and those with more stable genomes whose genes react to mutation really late. If we were able to prevent or at least prolong the onset of malignant developments and cardio-vascular diseases, we would be able to prolong human life in a significant manner.

Thus, medical history has thought us that if we truly want to be effective we must not only treat symptoms, although at times that is the best we can do, but we must introduce preventive measures. Old age should be seen as something that can be prevented or postponed significantly as well.

The fact is that the knowledge we have now about aging, tell us that activity, healthy foods are all crucial for a healthy life. However, how many people do actually follow this prescription? The effect of these preventive measures is minimal today; however the effect of a "vaccine" would be broader and would cut across population lines. The whole human population could benefit from such an approach.

This attempt to deal with aging should not imply that old age can not be beautiful and meaningful but that prolonging the life can allow human beings to accomplish more and achieve that dream of longevity.

Critics might question to what extent is it up to us to prolong life, to what extent is it up to us to change the course of nature. And that is a reasonable concern, however, the concept of the "longevity vaccine" should be seen as a tool to improve quality of life not to alter it. Further, as of now we still do not have this tool, thus although it is reasonable to think about its ethical implications, we must also think about the ethical implications of not developing something that could improve the life of so many, without discrimination.

Further criticism might be directed at the far-reaching effects behind such an endeavor in terms of population growth and size. It is obvious that there are problems with the over-population of the planet, but in no way can we morally allow ourselves to attempt to deal with over-population by not offering the best medical services we can. Further, we should ask ourselves how would have this world looked like if .....lived longer.

Longevity and Genes

Aging is a complex phenomenon influenced by genetic and environmental factors. The evidence of a genetic involvement in human longevity first came from the studies on relatives using population genetics methods. The earliest report dates in 1899 when Beeton and Pearson [12] found lifespan correlation within families. From that time, numerous studies confirmed existence of transmittable familiar attributes which affects lifespan [13]. Furthermore, studies on twins confirmed genetic influence on survival, by separating the genetic from environmental factors [14]. Significant progress in identifying potential genes involved in aging process has been made in model organisms such as yeast, the nematode Caenorhabditis elegans, Drosophila melanogaster fruitflies, and mice [15]. These studies have revealed specific genes that regulate ageing, such as *age-1* and *clk-1* in nematodes, *sir-2* in yeasts, *Tor, mth* and *Indy* in flies and *klotho* in mice [16,17]. Recent studies in humans reported a number of genes with a potential role in longevity and disease. Good examples are "disease-protective alleles" as such as APOE and APOE2, APO C3, and some HLA variants, which have been described in higher frequency in centenarians [18].

With the accomplishment of the Human Genome Project and recent developments in genotyping techniques as well as in functional genomics, it is now possible to collect vast quantities of genetic data with the aim of deciphering the genetics of human complex traits [19]. Consequently, the amount of research on human ageing and longevity has been growing fast in recent years [13].

Classes of Genes that Might Have an Influence on Longevity

Previous genetic studies performed in model organisms such as yeast, nematodes, and mice discovered potential genes that either slows or accelerates aging. Richard Miller recently proposed a classification of longevity genes ranging from those hypothesized to either cause or accelerate aging to those that counteract it [20]. The proposed classes of longevity genes discussed below could help us to understand which kind of mechanisms may play a role in human aging.

1. Genes that Cause Aging

Studies in mice revealed that increased activity of P53 gene resulted in cancer prevention, but also accelerated aging in observed group. Mice with P53 mutation lived shorter than subjects in control group, but none of them developed cancer compared to the 45% of mice without mutation that developed malignancy [21]. This is in accordance with observation that aging in humans is associated with increased cancer prevalence. However, it is interesting to mention that two out of 217 mice with an inactive copy of P53 did not developed cancer and lived much longer than the wild type. This finding is consistent with the results from studies on centagenerians which reported lower cancer incidence among oldest-old [22].

2. Genes that Causes Diseases, which Resembles Accelerated Ageing

The progeroid syndromes, rare diseases that cause premature aging are good models for genetic research in human longevity. These syndromes are linked with mutations in single genes accelerating some, but not all, features of normal aging [23,24]. Werner's syndrome (WS) is the most common of the premature aging disorders, and it is caused by mutations of RecQ type DNA helicase [25]. At the molecular level, WS patients exhibits considerable genomic instability with chromosome breaks, translocations and large deletions [26]. Consequently, they accumulate DNA damage faster, which presumably leads to premature aging. WS patients demonstrate a large variety of clinical and biological manifestations in body systems (nervous, immune, connective tissue and endocrine-metabolic systems) early in life, which are comparable to normal aging. The chronological appearance of clinical and biological decline in body systems observed in WS suggests that the disorder is more than another rare syndrome; it could be the walkthrough for aging puzzle. A recent finding reported by Varela and colleagues suggests that combined treatment with statins and aminobisphosphonates extends longevity in a mouse model of human premature aging. This finding suggests new therapeutic strategies for human progeroid syndromes associated with nuclear-envelope abnormalities, such as Hutchinson-Gilford syndrome [27].

3. Genes that Affects or Cause Age-Related Disorders

Good example of age related disease associated with genetic influence is Alzheimer's disease (AD). Possession of an ApoE ε-4 allele increases the risk of developing AD [28]. It is interesting that Apolipoprotein E ε-4 allele is rare in centegenerians [29]. Hence, the centenarian genome may be a useful tool against which to compare the genomes of individuals with specific age-related diseases [22]. Genes that influence cardiovascular diseases are discussed separately in this chapter.

4. Genes that Extend Maximum Life Span

Studies made in experimental organisms such as yeasts, nematodes, fruit flies, and mice indicate that a few alleles can exert a strong influence on life span. Experiments made in C. elegans shows that specific mutations (daf-2, daf-16, daf-23, age-1 and clk-1) increase the nematode's life span three- to five-fold [30, 31]. The human homologue of daf-2 is the IGF-1-receptor [32]. Paradoxically, the homologous mutation of daf in humans leads to life-shortening insulin resistance, so its role in human longevity remains unclear [22]. Studies performed at yeast have revealed that sir-2 (silent information regulator-2) silences large regions of DNA and slows down aging [33]. In fruit flies, the Methuselah mutant of drosophila lives 35% longer than wild types Drosophila, [34]. In addition, over-expression of Cu/Zn super oxide dismutase increases the maximum life span of transgenic Drosophila up to 48% [35]. Studies have shown that super oxide dismutase plays a significant role in the scavenging of oxygen radicals [36]. Studies on transgenic mice have shown them to be useful models for human aging- and age-related diseases. Mutation in the mouse SHC gene (p66shc) is associated with a 30% longer life-span [37]. Ablation of this gene reduces the apoptotic response to oxidative stress damage, and consequently prolongs life of the mutant. Genotype-phenotype correlations in mouse models can provide important insights into basic mechanisms of aging that promote longevity [38].

5. Genetic Polymorphisms that Influence the Rate of Aging

Many quantitative trait loci have various influence on aging and age-related disorders. They play an important role in DNA repair and anti-oxidant defenses, gene expression, cell proliferation and senescence, maintenance of differential function, and signal transduction [22].

6. Genes that Influence Differences in Life Span among Species (Longevity Enabling Genes)

These genes may be relatively few in number because so many aging-related processes occur synchronously and with timing that is species-specific [20].

Recent progress in aging research is driven largely by the use of model systems, such as yeasts, nematodes, fruit flies, and mice. These models have discovered conservation in genetic pathways that balance energy production and its damaging byproducts with pathways that preserve somatic maintenance [38]. Maintaining genome stability is a major factor in longevity.

The Effects of Nutritional Factors on Lifespan

Ageing is a continual process of accumulation of changes in every organism that eventually leads to physical deterioration. Ageing is often viewed through the concept of primary and secondary aging [39]. Secondary aging represents the deterioration in tissue structure and biological function following the effects of numerous disease processes and harmful environmental factors, and the primary ageing is defined as the inevitable, progressive decline in biological function and tissue structure that occurs independently with age. Most of the achievements of modern civilization and medicine offer protection against secondary ageing, resulting in a constant increase of an average life expectancy, but without an effect on the maximal longevity which is thought to be primarily under the influence of primary ageing.

Since the desire for longevity is an immortal goal of mankind, the focus of the scientific attention is shifting to the factors behind primary ageing. Interestingly, out of many factors which play a role in primary ageing, there seams to be only one which is possibly correctable. This promising window for intervention is nutrition. Numerous studies over the past 70 years were conducted with an aim to determine the influence of nutritional factors of life longevity. Most of these studies examined the effect of feeding restriction in several vertebrate and non-vertebrate models including yeast, flies, worms, mice and rats. The most notable findings among these are ones performed on nematode worm *Caenorhabditis elegans* [40,41] and the fruit fly *Drosophila melanogaster* [42,43] demonstrating that caloric restriction (CR) slows the ageing process, prolongs the lifespan and has a beneficial influence on health. Most authors of these experiments agree that it is the total caloric content rather than specific nutritional composition that plays a role in life-span determination. In fact, CR is probably the only intervention that has consistently been shown to slow primary aging, as evidenced by an increase in maximal longevity. Regarding the importance of nutritional content on lifespan, generally viewed as less significant, there are some exceptions showing that in some cases reducing specific compounds (e.g. reducing methionine or tryptophan in rats [44] or reducing dietary sugar in Mediterranean fruit fly *Ceratitis capitata* [45]) can also extend life span.

Although the fundamental mechanisms of ageing are still unclear, a growing body of evidence points to the function of mitochondria and the continuous generation of free radicals at the mitochondrial inner membrane [46] as key players in the ageing process. This has inspired a number of investigators to propose a theory that the impact of CR on lifespan is in fact mediated by an effect on the mitochondrial free radical production. A lower mitochondrial free radical generation rate is observed in food-restricted animals compared with *ad libitum* fed animals [46,47]. Since it was proposed that CR decreases oxidative stress [46], several studies have shown that moderate caloric restriction leads to lower oxidative damage to cellular macromolecules. The effect of caloric restriction on oxidative damage to DNA and proteins has been extensively investigated in the last decades, as both macromolecules are viewed as the major factors in the aging process [48]. Mitochondria are the major consumers of cellular oxygen (about 85%) and the predominant production site of free radicals, a by-product of oxidative phosphorylation. Studies in mammals have shown that caloric restriction reduces the generation of free radicals by mitochondria, in parallel to reductions in mitochondrial proton leak [49] and whole-body energy efficiency (defined as oxidation or combustion of food and/or energy stores to meet the body's energy requirements) [49]. These data suggest that caloric restriction improves whole body energy efficiency by inducing the biogenesis of mitochondria that utilize less oxygen and produce less reactive oxygen species (ROS). Although antioxidants may decrease the oxidative damage, it is still uncertain whether antioxidant supplements have a beneficial effect on longevity. Some authors suggest that the use of carotene, vitamin A, and vitamin E may even increase mortality [50].

In addition to the most widely accepted theory involving the oxidative stress, further theories explaining the role of CR on lifespan have emerged. Some authors have focused on glucocorticoid pathways attenuating which plays the critical role in the body's stress response and therefore suspected as a cause of aging [51,52].

Yet another theory addressed the effect of CR on adipose deposits and body composition as the way in which it influences longevity [53]. The „decreased fat hypothesis" is based on the theory that adipocites are a source of humoral factors that promote aging. The reduction of adipose tissue promoted by CR would thus delay ageing [54].

A lot of attention was also brought to the „Hormesis Hypothesis of CR" which views the low caloric intake as a mildly stressful condition that provokes a survival response within the organism, helping its survival, contrary to the stressors of general nature, by altering metabolism and increasing the organism's defenses against the causes of aging, whatever they may be [55]. The proponents of this theory suggest that CR is the factor that provokes a survival response in the organism, which boosts resistance to stress and counteracts the causes of aging. The theory unites previously disparate observations about ROS defenses, apoptosis, metabolic changes, stress resistance, and hormonal changes and is rapidly becoming accepted as the best explanation for the effects of CR [54,55].

Results of recent studies have demonstrated that modifications and loss of functions of somatotropic, insulin or homologous signaling pathways on CR mice can extend the maximum life span in mice [46,56]. These data imply that somatotropic signaling is critically important in mediating the effects of CR on life span, as much as in the control of aging under conditions of unlimited food supply. The recent findings also support the concept that enhanced sensitivity to insulin plays prominent role in the actions of CR and growth hormone resistance on longevity [56].

While considerable data resulting from studies on animal models suggest possible mechanisms that are considered as relevant for humans, the only way to determine whether CR has an influence on our longevity is to study these relations in humans. Such studies are difficult to perform in the general population, and there is, therefore, still little information available on the effect of long-term CR in humans. An important principle of the CR hypothesis is that the diet must contain adequate amounts of protein, vitamins and minerals and only be deficient in energy. That is why the results of low calorie diets forced upon many populations throughout history by poverty, famine, war or other external circumstances are not relevant for these researches. The exception to this pattern is the older generation of Okinawans [57,58] whose centenarians have been cited as an evidence that mild form of prolonged CR may slow ageing in humans. Research in this area is further progressing to studies on healthy volunteers [59].

Longevity and Cardiovascular Diseases

Individuals with exceptional longevity have a lower incidence and/or significant delay in the onset of age-related disease, like cardiovascular disease [60]. There are two ways of successful ageing by avoiding cardiovascular diseases. The first one, although uncertain is nowadys only possible one- to correct those cardiovascular risk factors that could be changed. The second one is to have good genotype, which could protect us from cardiovascular disease even with positive one or more cardiovascular risk factors [3].

There were several studies concerning the incidence of young/middle-aged people without any of three most important cardiovascular (CV) risk factors (increased serum cholesterol, arterial hypertension and cigarette smoking) [61]. The Multiple Risk Factor Intervention Trial (16-year follow-up study) and the Chicago Heart Association Detection Project in Industry trial (16-year follow-up study) registered only 4.8-9.9% subjects without any of three main CV risk factors (low-risk was defined as serum cholesterol <200 mg/dl, BP≤120/80 mm Hg, currently non-smoking). Compared to others, low-risk persons had markedly lower all-cause mortality (40-58%) with estimated greater longevity (by 5.8-9.5 years). Among Framingham Heart Study participants who were free of CV disease at the age of 50, only 3.2% men and 4.5% women had all optimal factors (TC<180 mg/dl, BP<120/80 mm Hg, non-smoker and non-diabetic) [62].

Reducing salt intake could result in longer lifespan. Some of the largest studies such as NHANES and TOHP demonstrated significant benefit with restrict salt intake- the reduction of absolute risk over 10-20 years of 2-3% for protection from CV events [63]. The Mediterranean diet has benefits on risk factors for CV disease such as lipoprotein levels, endothelium vasodilatation, insulin resistance, the prevalence of metabolic syndrome, antioxidant capacity, incidence of acute myocardial infarction, CV mortality and even overall mortality [64]. The diet known as calorie restriction is the most reproducible way to extend the lifespan in mammals, increasing both mean and maximum lifespan. The life-long exercise, another way of extending the lifespan, increases only mean lifespan [65,66].

Nevertheless, the great importance for longevity has genotype itself. The knowledge about genotype which could reliably lead to long life without cardiovascular diseases is not reachable yet. Siblings of centenarians have an 8- fold (women) to 17-fold (men) higher probability to live more than 100 years [67]. The offspring of long-lived parents have an approximately 50% lower prevalence of hypertension, diabetes mellitus, myocardial infarction and stroke compared to aged-matched groups.

High levels of low-density lipoprotein (LDL) cholesterol and low levels of high-density lipoprotein (HDL) are correlated not only with CV disease, but may contribute to accelerated ageing through effects on vascular wall, cancer, or other mechanisms [60]. Not only the absolute levels of lipoproteins but also their size could be of importance. There are some data suggesting that there is particular longevity phenotype that is correlated with larger LDL and HDL particles and lower prevalence of hypertension, CV disease, metabolic syndrome and very old age. The marked heritability in the offspring could be explained with increased frequency of homozygosity for the codon 405 valine *CETP* allele. Cholesteryl ester transfer protein (*CETP*) is involved in the regulation of reverse cholesterol transport and HDL levels. Small LDL particles penetrate more readily into arterial tissue and are oxidized more rapidly than larger LDL particles that could result in endothelial dysfunction leading to CV disease. Small HDL particles as well have been reported in patients with CV disease; some lipid-lowering drugs may protect from CV disease by shifting the HDL particles to larger sizes. Therefore, large LDL and HDL particles may be important in protecting the vascular bed from age-related atherosclerosis and thus promoting exceptional longevity. Interestingly, LDL and HDL particle sizes are larger in women than in men, which could partly explain the lower incidence of CV disease and longer life expectancies in women. Insulin resistance and diabetes are also associated with lower LDL and HDL particle sizes [68].

The ε2, ε3, and ε4 alleles of the apolipoprotein E gene (apoE) encode three isoforms (apoe2, apoE3 and apoE4. ApoE is the main ligand for clearance of VLDL and chylomicron remnants changing the circulating levels of cholesterol and triglycerides. In a rare heritable deficiency of apoE, the hyperlipoproteinemia and consequently CV diseases happened. Two mechanisms are suggested to explain this effect. Firstly, high apoE levels reflect the presence of higher levels of lipoprotein classes such as LDL or VLDL or chylomicron levels, which ar proatherogenic. Secondly, apoE has proinflammatory properties. Nevertheless, in old age, high plasma apoE levels precede an increase of circulating CRP and strongly associates with mortality, independent of apoE genotype and plasma lipids [69].

Sirtuins are a conserved family of NAD$^+$-dependent deacetylases which overexpression in some species are reported to extend lifespan. They are suggested to play a role in lifespan extension induced by dietary restriction. The main function of sirtuin proteins might be to promote survival and stress resistance. There is suggestion that sirtuin 1 (Sirt1) could play a role in myocardial protection, since it was presented earlier as an essential endogenous apoptosis inhibitor in isolated cardiac myocites. The overexpression of Sirt1 could lead to high levels of Sirt1 and a consequently high NAD$^+$ consumption. The depletion of NAD$^+$ leads to deficiency of ATP, resulting in cellular dysfunction and cell death. As a stress response, Sirt1 is upregulated from normal 2.5-7.5 fold to 3-9 fold overexpression. A further increase in protein levels (12.5- or more-fold overexpression) augmented oxidative stress and cardiomyocyte damage [70].

Rosveratrol, a polyphenol found in red wine, is known to activate Sirt1. Overexpression of Sirt1 induced by rosveratrol, reduced angiotensin II type 1 receptor (AT1R) expression in the mouse aorta and blunted angiotensin II-induced arterial hypertension. The inhibition of rennin-angiotensin system may contribute to the rosveratrol-induced longevity and antiatherogenic effect of rosveratrol [71].

The overexpression of Sir 1 is partly the result of upregulation of catalase which prevents oxidative stress-induced cardiomyocyte damage. This upregulation of catalase is result of transcriptional activation of FoxO1a. Forkhead box O (FoxO) transcription factors are important in signaling pathway and crucial regulators of cell fate. They are regulated by a variety of different growth factors and hormones influencing in develop the different disease and ageing process [72].

Considering that the inflammation is very important in developing atherosclerosis and further CV disease shorting the lifespan, it is very important the hypothesis that there are people genetically predisposed to developing weak inflammatory activity. Those people seem to have fewer chances of developing CV diseases and live longer if they do not become affected by serious infections disease (usually in early years of life). Several authors support this hypothesis. The ASP299GLY allele of lipopolysaccaride TLR4, which initiates the immune response against gram-negative bacteria, is found in low frequency in patients with myocardial infarction, whereas the centenarians show the higher frequency of this form of TLR4 polymorphism. In the carriers bearing TLR4 mutations also the lower levels of IL-6 was found [73].

Different alleles at different cytokine genes coding for pro- (IL-6 or IFN-γ) or anti-inflammatory (IL-10) cytokines may affect individual lifespan expectancy by influencing the type and intensity of the immune-inflammatory against environmental stressors [74]. The increased serum level of circulating IL-8 and the low level of IL-6 is related to longevity [75]. Increased level of another inflammatory biomarker circulating CRP is reported to increase the risk of mortality and morbidity. In high-risk patients like acute coronary syndrome, decreasing the level of circulating CRP is as important as decreasing the serum level of LDL cholesterol [76].

IL-6 genotype is useful in assessing the genetic risk for atherothrombotic cerebral infarction and intracerebral hemorrhage. The -164G→C polymorphism f IL-6 was shown to be of importance for causing those diseases. Cytokines induce the production of matrix metalloproteinases which degrade the extracellular matrix around blood vessels and may damage the vascular wall. Another kind of polymorphism, -863C→A polymorphism of TNF, Gly243Asp polymorphism of PKD1-like and-55C→T polymorphism of UCP3 were found to be of importance for developing subarachnoid hemorrhage [77].

The polymorphism of CC-chemokine receptor-5 are found out to be of importance in developing acute myocardial infarction and have the importance for longevity. CCR5 is a β-chemokines receptor involved in the migration of monocytes, NK cells and some T cells to the inflammation cite. CCR532 variant seems to have a protective role against acute myocardial infarction and coronary heart diseases determining a slower progression of atherosclerotic lesion as a consequence of an attenuated inflammatory response [78].

References

[1]   Wojda, A. and Witt, M. (2003). Manifestations of ageing at the cytogenetic level. *J Appl Genet.* 44(3):383-99.

[2]   Wojda, A., Zietkiewicz, E., Mossakowska, M., Pawlowski, W., Skrzypczak, K., and Witt, M. (2006). Correlation between the level of cytogenetic aberrations in cultured human lymphocytes and the age and gender of donors. *J Gerontol A Biol Sci Med Sci.* 61(8):763-72.

[3]   Davidovic, M. (2004). Are we faced with two human species? *ScientificWorld Journal,* 4:943-7.

[4]   Nemoto, S. and Finkel, U. T. (2004). Ageing and the mystery at Arles. *Nature,* 429/13 149: 149-152.

[5]   Reznick1, D.N., Bryant, M.J., Roff1, D.,Ghalambor, C. K. and. Ghalambor, D.E (2004).Effect of extrinsic mortality on the evolution of senescence in guppies. *Nature,* 431 / 28 , 1095-1099.

[6]   Davidovic, M., Erceg, P., Trailov, D., Djurica, S., Milosevic, D., and Stevic, R. (2003). The privilege to be old. *Gerontology,* 49(5):335-9.

[7]   Davidović, M. (1999). Genetic stability: the key to longevity? *Med Hypotheses,* 53(4):329-32.

[8]   Davidovic, M. and Milosevic, D.P. (2006). Are all dilemmas in gerontology been swept under the carpet of intraindividual variability? *Med Hypotheses,* 66(2):432-6.

[9]   Davidovic, M., Milosevic, D.P. and Djurica, S. (2005). "Vaccine" against aging better than rejuvenation? *Med Hypotheses,* 65(2):415-6.

[10]   Davidovic, M., Milosevic, D.P., Despotovic, N., Sekularac, N., and Erceg, P. (2007). Is there such thing as "vaccine against aging"? *Adv Gerontol.* 20(2):56-9.

[11]   Erceg, P., Milosevic, D.P., Despotovic, N., and Davidovic, M. (2007). Chromosomal changes in ageing. *J Genet.* 86(3):277-8.

[12]   Beeton, M. and Pearson, K. Data for the problem of evolution in man, II, A first study of the inheritance of longevity and the selective death rate in man. Proceedings of the Royal Society of London. 1899;65: 290-305.

[13]   Tan, Q., Yashin, A.I., Christensen, K., Jeune, B., De Benedictis, G., Kruse, T.A., et al. (2004). Multidisciplinary Approaches in Genetic Studies of Human Aging and Longevity. *Curr Genomics,* 5:409-416.

[14]   Herskind, A.M,. McGue, M., Holm, N.V., et al. (1996).The heritability of human longevity, apopulation-based study of 2872 Danish twin pairs born 1870-1900. *Hum Genet.* 97: 319-23.

[15]   Guarente, L. and Kenyon, C. (2000). Genetic pathways that regulate ageing in model organisms. *Nature,* 408:255–62.

[16]   Christensen, K., Johnson, T.E. and Vaupel, J.W. (2006). The quest for genetic determinants of human longevity: challenges and insights. *Nat Rev Genet.* 7:436-48.

[17] Takahashi, Y., Kuro-o, M. and Ishikawa, F. (2000). Aging mechanisms. *Proc. Natl. Acad. Sci. U. S. A.* 97:12407-8.

[18] Lao, J.I., Montoriol, C., Morer, I., et al. (2005).Genetic contribution to aging: deleterious and helpful genes define life expectancy. *Ann NY Acad Sci.* 1057:50-63.

[19] Tan, Q., Kruse, T.A., and Christensen, K. (2006). Design and analysis in genetic studies of human ageing and longevity. *Ageing Res Rev.* 5(4):371-87.

[20] Miller, R.A. A Position Paper on Longevity genes. http://sageke.sciencemag.org/cgi/content/full/sageke;2001/9/vp6.

[21] Tyner, S.D., Venkatachalam, S., Choi, J., et al. (2002). p53 mutant mice that display early ageing-associated phenotypes. *Nature,* 415:45-53.

[22] Perls, T., Kunkel, L. and Puca, A. (2002). The genetics of aging. *Curr Opin Genet Dev.* 12(3):362-9.

[23] Kyng, K.J. and Bohr, V.A. (2005). Gene expression and DNA repair in progeroid syndromes and human aging. *Ageing Res Rev. Nov.* 4(4):579-602.

[24] Lans, H. and Hoeijmakers, J.H. (2006).Cell biology: ageing nucleus gets out of shape. *Nature,* 440(7080):32-4.

[25] Goto, M. (1997). Hierarchical deterioration of body systems in Werner's syndrome: implications for normal ageing. *Mech Ageing Dev.* 98(3):239-54.

[26] Yu, C.E., Oshima, J., Fu, Y.H., et al. (1996). Positional cloning of the Werner's syndrome gene. *Science,* 272:258-62.

[27] Varela, I., Pereira, S., Ugalde, A.P., et al. (2008).Combined treatment with statins and aminobisphosphonates extends longevity in a mouse model of human premature aging. *Nat Med.* 14(7):767-72.

[28] Hsiung, G.Y., Sadovnick, A.D. and Feldman, H. (2004).Apolipoprotein E epsilon 4 genotype as a risk factor for cognitive decline and dementia: data from the Canadian Study of Health and Aging. *CMAJ,* 171(8):863-7.

[29] Schächter, F., Faure-Delanef, L., Guenot, F., et al. (1994). Cohen: genetic associations with human longevity at the APOE and ACE loci. *Nat Genet.* 6:29-32.

[30] Van Voorhies, W.A. and Ward, S. (1999). Genetic and environmental conditions that increase longevity in Caenorhabditis elegans decrease metabolic rate. *Proc Natl Acad Sci USA,* 96:11399-11403.

[31] Van Voorhies, W.A., Curtsinger, J.W. and Rose, M.R. (2006). Do longevity mutants always show trade-offs? *Exp Gerontol.* 41(10):1055-8.

[32] Kimura, K.D., Tissenbaum, H.A., Liu, Y., et al. (1997). daf-2, an insulin receptor-like gene that regulates longevity and diapause in Caenorhabditis elegans. *Science,* 277:942-46.

[33] Vaziri, H., Dessain, S.K., Ng Eaton, E., et al. (2001). hSIR2 (SIRT1) functions as an NAD-dependent p53 deacetylase. *Cell,* 107:149-59.

[34] Lin, Y.J., Seroude, L. and Benzer, S. (1998). Extended life-span and stress resistance in the Drosophila mutant methuselah. *Science,* 282:943-46.

[35] Parkes, T.L., Elia, A.J., Dickinson, D., et al. (1998). Extension of Drosophila lifespan by overexpression of human SOD1 in motorneurons. *Nat Genet.* 19:171-4.

[36] Williams, M.D., Van Remmen, H., Conrad, C.C., et al. (1998).Increased oxidative damage is correlated to altered mitochondrial function in heterozygous manganese superoxide dismutase knockout mice. *J Biol Chem.* 273:28510-15.

[37] Migliaccio, E., Giorgio, M., Mele, S., et al. (1999). The p66shc adaptor protein controls oxidative stress response and life span in mammals. *Nature*, 402:309-13.

[38] Hasty, P., Campisi, J., Hoeijmakers, J., van Steeg, H., and Vijg, J. (2003). Aging and genome maintenance: lessons from the mouse? *Science*, 299(5611):1355-9.

[39] Holloszy, J.O. and Fontana, L. (2007). Caloric Restriction in Humans. *Exp Gerontol.* 42(8):709–12.

[40] Houthoofd, K. and Vanfleteren, J.R. (2006). The longevity effect of dietary restriction in Caenorhabditis elegans. *Exp gerontol.* 41(10):1026-31.

[41] Houthoofd, K., Braeckman, B.P., Lenaerts, I., Brys, K., De Vreese, A., Van Eygen, S., and Vanfleteren, J.R. (2002). Axenic growth up-regulates mass-specific metabolic rate, stress resistance, and extends life span in Caenorhabditis elegans. *Exp Gerontol.* 37:1371–1378.

[42] Mair, W., Goymer, P., Pletcher, S.D., and Partridge, L. (2003). Demography of dietary restriction and death in Drosophila. *Science,* 301:1731–1733.

[43] Partridge, L., Piper, M.D. and Mair, W. (2005). Dietary restriction in Drosophila. *Mech Ageing Dev.* 126:938–950.

[44] Masoro, E.J. (2006). Caloric restriction and aging: controversial issues. *J.Gerontol.* A *Biol. Sci. Med. Sci:* 14–19.

[45] Romanyukha, A., Carey, J., Karkach, A., and Yashin, A.I. (2004). The impact of diet switching on resource allocation to reproduction and longevity in Mediterranean fruitflies. *Proc. R. Soc. Lond. B Biol. Sci.* 1319–1324.

[46] Ricardo Gredilla and Gustavo Barja (1995). The Role of Oxidative Stress in Relation to Caloric Restriction and Longevity. *Endocrinology*, 146: 3713–3717.

[47] Sohal, R.S. and Weindruch, R. (1996). Oxidative stress, caloric restriction, and aging. *Science,* 273:59–63.

[48] Civitarese, A.., Carling, S..,Heilbronn, L., et al. (2007). Calorie Restriction Increases Muscle Mitochondrial Biogenesis in Healthy Humans. *PLOS Medicine,* (4) Issue 3| e76

[49] Bevilacqua, L., Ramsey, J.J., Hagopian, K., Weindruch, R., and Harper, ME. (2004). Effects of short- and medium-term calorie restriction on muscle mitochondrial proton leak and reactive oxygen species production. *Am J Physiol Endocrinol Metab.* 286:E852–861.

[50] Bjelakovic, G., Nikolova, D., Gluud, L.L., et al. (2007). Mortality in Randomized Trials of Antioxidant Supplements for Primary and Secondary Prevention. *JAMA.* 297:842-857.

[51] David A. Sinclair. (2005). Toward a unified theory of caloric restriction and longevity regulation .*Mechanisms of Ageing and Development,* (126): 987–1002.

[52] Nelson, K., Bergman, M.D. and Felicio, L.S. (1995). Neuroendocrine involvement in aging: evidence from studies of reproductive aging and caloric restriction. *Neurobiol. Aging*, (16): 837–84.

[53] Pamplona, R., Barja, G., and Portero-Otin. (2002). Membrane fatty acid unsaturation, protection against oxidative stress, and maximum life span: a homeoviscous longevity adaptation? *Ann NY Acad Sci.* 959:475–490.

[54] Barzilai, N. and Gabriely, I. (2001). The role of fat depletion in the biological benefits of caloric restriction. *J. Nutr.* 131: 903S–906S

[55] Anderson, R.M., Bitterman, K.J.,Wood, J.G., Medvedik, O., and Sinclair, D. (2003). Nicotinamide and Pncl govern lifespan extension by calorie restriction in S. cerevisiae. *Nature,* (423):181–185.

[56] Bonkowski, M.., Rocha, J., Masternak, M.., Regaiey, A. and Bartke A. (2006). Targeted disruption of growth hormone receptor interferes with the beneficial actions of calorie restriction. *PNAS,* 20(103):7901–05.

[57] Willcox, D., Bradley, J., and Willcox, Ć. (2006).Caloric restriction and human longevity: what can we learn from the Okinawans? *Biogerontology,* 7:173–177.

[58] Chan, Y.C., Suzuki, M. and Yamamoto, S. (1997). Dietary, anthropometric, hematological and biochemical assessment of the nutritional status of centenarians and elderly people in Okinawa, Japan. *J Am Coll Nutri..*16:229–235.

[59] Heilbronn, L.K. and Ravussin, E. (2003). Calorie restriction and ageing: review of the literature and implications for studies in humans. *Am J Clin Nutr.* 78:361–369.

[60] Barzilai, N., Atzmon, G., Schechter, C., Schaefer, E.J., Cupples, A.L., Lipton, R., Cheng, S., and Shuldiner, A.R. (2003). Unique lipoprotein phenotype and genotype associated with exceptional longevity. *JAMA,* 290:2030-40.

[61] Yamamoto, T., Nakamura, Y., Hozawa, A., Okamura, T., Kadowaki, T., Hayakawa, T., Murakami, Y., Kita, Y., Okayama, A., Abbott, R.D., and Ueshima, H. (2008). Low-risk profile for cardiovascular disease and mortality in Japanese. *Circ J.* 72:545-550.

[62] Stamler, J., Stamler, R., Neaton, J.D., Wentworth, D., Daviglus, M.L., Garside, D., Dyer, A.R., Kiang, L., and Greenland, P. (1999). Low risk-factor profile and long-term cardiovascular and noncardiovascular mortality and life expectancy. *JAMA,* 282:2012-2018.

[63] Walker, J., MacKenzie, A.D. and Dunning, J. (2007). Does reducing salt intake make you live longer? *Interact CardioVasc Thorac Surg.* 6:792-8.

[64] Roman, B., Carta, L., Martinez-Gonzalez, M..A., and Serra-Majem, L. (2008). Effectiveness of the Mediterranean diet in the elderly. *Clin Interv Aging,* 3(1):97-109.

[65] Sinclair, D.A. (2005). Toward a unified theory of caloric restriction and longevity regulation. *Mech Ageing Dev.* 126(9):987-1002.

[66] Carter, C.S., Hofer, T., Seo, A.Y., and Leeuwenburgh, C. (2007). Molecular mechanism of life- and health-span extension: role of calorie restriction and exercise intervention. *Appl Physiol Nutr Metab.* 32(5):954-66.

[67] Perls, T.T., Wilmoth, J., Levenson, R., Drinkwater, M., Cohen, M., Began, H., Joyce, E., Brewster, S., Kunkel, L., and Puca, A. (2002). Life-long sustained advantage of siblings of centenarians. *Proc NAtl Acad Sci U S A*; 99(12):8442-7.

[68] Asztalos, B.F., Horvath, K.V., McNamara, J.R., Roheim, P.S., Rubenstein, J.J., and Schaefer, E.J. (2002). Effects of atorvastatin on the HDL subpopulation profile of coronary heart disease patients. *J Lipid Res.* 43(10):1701-7.

[69] Mooijaart, S.P., Berbee, J.F., van Heemst, D., Havekes, L., de Craen, A.J.M., Slagboom, P.E., Rensen, P.C.N., and Westendorp, E.G.J. (2006). ApoE plasma levels and risk of cardiovascular mortality in old age. *PLoS Medicine*, 3(6):e176.

[70] Sedding, D. and Haendler, J. (2007). Do we age on Sirt1 expression? *Circulation Research*;100:1396.

[71] Miyazaki, R., Ichiki, T., Hashimoto, T., Inanaga, K., Imayama, I., Sadoshima, J., and Sunagawa, K. (2008). SIRT1, a longevity gene, downregulates angiotensin II type 1 receptor expression in vascular smooth muscle cells. *Arterioscler Thromb Vasc Biol.* 28(7):1263-9.

[72] Sedding, D.G. (2008). FoxO transcription factors in oxidative stress response and ageing – a new fork on the way of longevity? *Biol Chem.* 389(3):279-83.

[73] Candore, G., Aquino, A., Balistreri, C.R., Bulati, M., di Carlo, D., Grimaldi, M.P., Listi, F., Orlando, V., Vasto, S., Caruso, M., Colonna-Romano, G., Lio, D., and Caruso, C. (2006). Inflammation, longevity and cardiovascular diseases. *Ann N Y Acad Sci.* 1067:282-7.

[74] Caruso, C., Candore, G., Colonna-Romano, G., Lio, D., and Franceschi, C. (2005). Inflammation and life-span. *Science,* 307(5707):208-209.

[75] Wieczorowska,-Tobis, K., Niemir, Z.I., Podkowka, R., Korybalska, K., Mossakowska, M., and Breborowicz, A. (2006). Can an increased level of circulating IL-8 be a predictor of human longevity? *Med Sci Monit.* 12(3):CR118-121.

[76] Ridker, P.M. (2007) Inflammatory biomarkers and risks of myocardial infarction, stroke, and total mortality: implications and longevity. *Nutr Rev.* 65:S253-9.

[77] Yamada, Y., Metoki, N., Yoshida, H., Satoh, K., Ichihara, S., Kato, K., Kameyama, T., Yokoi, K., Matsuo, H., Segawa, T., Watanabe, S., and Nozawa, Y. (2006). Genetic risk for ischemic and hemorrhagic stroke. *Arterioscler Thromb Vasc Biol.* 26(8):1920-5.

[78] Balistreri, C.R., Candore, G., Caruso, M., Franceschi, C., and Caruso, C. (2008). Role of polymorphism of CC-chemokine receptor-5 gene in acute myocardial infarction and biological implications for longevity. *Haematologica*, 93(4):637-8.

In: Handbook on Longevity: Genetics, Diet and Disease   ISBN 978-1-60741-075-1
Editors: Jennifer V. Bentely and Mary Ann Keller   © 2009 Nova Science Publishers, Inc.

Chapter III

Toward the Mitigation of Glycation: A Practical Protocol

Nūn Sava-Siva Amen-Ra

Morgan State University, School of Community Health & Policy
Baltimore, Maryland

The purpose of this chapter is to establish the theoretical and practical efficacy of a dietary/lifestyle regimen in reducing glycative damage and, by so doing, improving health and longevity. Known as the Amen Optimal Health Protocol, the regimen seeks to synergistically combine established experimental interventions with efficacy in lengthening lifespan or modulating physiological processes known to be operative in aging. Chief among such processes is glycation. Glycation is a chemical process wherein the carbonyl moieties of reducing sugars such as glucose or its metabolites react covalently with nitrogenous constituents of amino acids, proteins, or certain lipids. Through a series of complex chemical conversions various sugar-protein and sugar-lipid adducts eventuate in so-called advanced glycation endproducts (AGEs). It is these multifarious endproducts of glycation that have been determined to be deleterious to health and longevity.

Experimental Approaches to AGE Diminution

Glycation occurs both endogenously and exogenously. Factors associated with elevated endogenous glycation include hyperglycemia, hyperphagia, obesity, chronological age and such conditions as diabetes and kidney disease (Boeing H et al. 2000; Van Liew JB et al. 1993). While a causal role for glycation in aging, diabetes, and renal failure cannot be clearly established upon the available evidence, several important investigations support the supposition that AGE exposure influences aging and disease susceptibility. Among these investigations, those concerning caloric restriction are arguably the most momentous. One of the earliest of these investigations was conducted by Edward J. Masoro and colleagues. Their study, published in a 1989 issue of the *Journal of Gerontology*, found that rats subjected to chronic caloric restriction exhibited substantial reductions in serum glucose concentration and significantly less hemoglobin glycation than their freely fed counterparts (Masoro EJ et al. 1989). Presumably, the difference in the degree of glycative damage to hemoglobin was a consequence of the hypoglycemic effect of caloric restriction. Several subsequent studies have confirmed the capacity of caloric restriction to substantially suppress glycation, corroborating the findings of Masoro and colleagues and lending support to what has been called the glycation hypothesis of aging (Iwashige K et al. 2004; Sell DR et al. 2003; Cefalu WT et al. 1995). Because caloric restriction consistently increases average and maximum lifespan in numerous animal models (Mattson MP 2008; Bishop & Guarente 2007; Spindler SR 2005), its influence on glycation naturally implicates AGEs in senescence.

In addition to quantitative caloric restriction, temporal caloric restriction has proven efficacious in the prolongation of maximum lifespan in animal models (Goodrick CL et al. 1982; Nelson & Halberg 1986). Temporal caloric restriction or, synonymously, cyclic fasting entails dietary deprivation of experimental subjects for defined periods of time (typically 1 full day or a substantial fraction thereof, say 20+ hours) while permitting them to feed freely or *ad libitum* otherwise. Interestingly, even in alternate day feeding studies wherein the energy intakes of intermittently restricted and freely fed subjects are equivalent, lifespan prolongation is still evident in the experimental group relative to controls (Goodrick CL et al. 1990). This implies that there is something about the fasted state as such that is conducive to heightened longevity (Bauer M et al. 2004). An investigation by Davis and colleagues would seem to suggest that glycation is among the factors at play. The study in question, published in the *Archives of Gerontology and Geriatrics*, found that while quantitative caloric restriction was most effective in reducing the age-associated rise in plasma protein glycation, alternate day feeding significantly attenuated glycative damage relative to controls fed *ad libitum* on a daily basis (Davis LJ et al. 1994). Thus, two dietary regimens know to promote lifespan extension—quantitative and temporal caloric restriction—also attenuate endogenous AGE formation.

A pharmacological measure may be added to the list of AGE-inhibiting, lifespan-extending interventions. Biguanides—a class of chemical compounds used in the treatment of diabetes—have been shown to extend mean and maximum lifespan in several studies using murine models (Anisimov VN et al. 2008; Anisimov VN et al. 2005; Anisimov VN et al. 2003). Biguanides generally exert their pharmacologic effects by suppressing serum glucose concentration and, consequently, curtailing glycation. More specifically, the compounds lower glycemia in the both the fasted and fed states, reduce uptake of glucose from the intestinal tract and augment insulin sensitivity as evidenced by enhanced glucose utilization on the part of peripheral tissues (e.g. skeletal muscle) (*Physician's Desk Reference*, 2007). As we shall see, the delineation of these specific mechanisms of action is of critical importance insofar as the elements of the present protocol are predicated upon modulating these same modalities.

Factors known to be associated with the formation of exogenous glycation endproducts include cooking and meat consumption (Henle T 2005; Goldberg T et al. 2004). Indeed, it is the pervasiveness of cooking that makes the threat posed by glycation particularly problematic and for meat-eaters moreover, cooking is altogether indispensable. Perhaps considering the triumvirate relationship between glycation, aging, and caloric restriction (quantitative and temporal), Weijing Cai and colleagues sought to determine the long-term effects of subsistence upon a diet markedly reduced in AGE content. By subjecting conventional rodent chow to less intense heat treatment, they consequently reduced its AGE content by half. They then fed this low-AGE chow to mice, affording them unlimited access thereto. Their findings were intriguing: animals exposed to the low-AGE diet exhibited less glycative damage to serum and tissue proteins, lower indices of oxidative stress, lower indices of renal impairment, higher antioxidant capacity, and, most momentously, higher average and maximum longevity (Cai W et al. 2007). Quite tellingly, there are now three distinct dietary protocols and one pharmacologic protocol that share the common features of inhibiting AGE formation and increasing longevity, thereby buttressing the notion that glycation plays an operative part in the aging process.

Considering the fact that caloric restriction has been justifiably considered to be the only conventional (non-genetic, non-invasive) means by which maximum lifespan can be substantially lengthened, a seminal study by the aforementioned Weijing Cai and colleagues warrants special attention (Cai W et al. 2008). As mentioned above, these insightful investigators had already determined that reducing the quantity of AGEs in the diets of experimental animals appreciably augmented lifespan relative to control subjects fed standard rodent diets. The researchers then reasoned that if reducing the AGE intake of animals resulted in increased longevity, the inherent attenuation of AGE ingestion that caloric restriction necessarily entails may partly explain its anti-aging efficacy. As such, they contrived two experimental groups of mice and one control group fed the standard laboratory diet *ad libitum*. Commencing at 4 months of age, the two experimental groups received diets deficient in calories (40% less than the control group). Additionally, one experimental group received rations elevated in AGE content by a factor of ~2 (relative to the control group). In contrast with their previous study, this elevation in AGEs was effectuated by *increasing* heat exposure—specifically, extending the heating interval by 15 minutes at a temperature of 120 °C. Expectedly, the animals subjected to conventional caloric restriction exhibited the customary increases in average and maximum longevity relative to the controls. Intriguingly, however, the animals who received the calorically restricted diet elevated in AGEs experienced no such extension in lifespan, despite consuming a quantity of calories equivalent to the conventional calorie-restricted group. Indeed, animals in the AGE-elevated calorie-restricted group had slightly shorter lifespans than even the control group. This investigation has several important implications, two of which bear explicit mention. First, caloric restriction may exert its anti-aging effect largely by reducing the quantity of AGEs in the diet. Secondly, it may be possible to simulate the longevity-enhancing effect of caloric restriction without necessarily restricting caloric intake—namely, by merely restricting the quantity of AGEs one ingests. Though this last point may be plausible, it is not conclusive. It is, in part, for this reason that the life-extension regimen presented in this chapter is multi-pronged, integrating multifarious independent interventions, each exhibiting some capacity to lengthen lifespan or influence physiological factors known to modulate longevity.

A Practical Approach to AGE Diminution

In the book, *Diet Therapy Research Trends*, I authored a chapter entitled "The Optimal Human Diet: Theoretical Foundations of the Amen Protocol" (Amen-Ra NS 2007). As the name implies, the purpose of the treatise was to delineate the theoretical foundations of a dietary regimen that I formulated with the express intent of ensuring optimal health and securing heightened longevity to the greatest extent practicable. Considering the centrality of glycation in the aging process (or more conservatively, its apparent correlation with aging) and its involvement in several chronic disease conditions, it is perhaps understandable why AGE attenuation factors so prominently in the protocol. It is the prominence of glycation in the theoretical Amen Protocol that led me to propose it as a practical, individualistic approach to addressing the problem of glycation. In fact, the protocol in question is theoretically based, experimentally based, and practically based. It is experimentally based insofar as I availed myself of scientific findings (largely though not exclusively in animals) related to lifespan prolongation, disease diminution, and glycation attenuation in order to craft a dietary/lifestyle regimen that, theoretically, should augment human health and longevity. The protocol is practical or experiential inasmuch as I, my spouse, and a close circle of collaborators and clients have dutifully adhered to it for the better part of a decade. Thus, it is sustainable over an appreciable period of time and therefore of practical value.

Elements of the Amen Protocol

There are three components of the protocol in question: a fasting component, a diet component and an exercise component. Moreover, one may conceive of three distinct domains or modalities of the regimen: quantitative, qualitative, and temporal. That is, consideration is given to the quantity of food that should ideally be ingested, the composition or quality of the food so ingested, and the frequency with which food should be ingested. My task shall be to explain the relevance of these factors to the mitigation of glycation and, by extension, the optimization of health and lifespan potential.

Briefly, the Amen Protocol centers upon cyclic fasting. The duration of the daily fast is approximately 23 hours, while the feeding period ensues over an hour interval. The caloric content of the daily meal ranges from 1000 to 1500 kilocalories depending on such factors as body size, sex, acclimation to the regimen, and the degree of dietary restriction desired. The composition of the diet is exclusively vegetal, an imperative upon which I shall elaborate below. Also, the diet is composed of several staple items, selected for their low AGE content. Moreover, certain components of, or ingredients in, the diet have exhibited experimental efficacy in lessening glycation *in vivo* or *ex vivo*. Finally, the exercise component of the protocol reinforces the overarching anti-AGE aim of the regimen as shall be explained subsequently.

The fasting component of the Amen Protocol is a measure aimed at inhibiting endogenous glycation. The reasoning is straightforward: the serum concentration of glucose increases appreciably after a meal. Prolonging the fasted state ensures that the body assumes the lowest level of glycemia practically attainable. This moderate hypoglycemia, in turn, lessens the amount of reactants available for glycation reactions *in vivo*. The fasting phase of the protocol ensues daily over a period of 23 hours, meaning that an adherent to the regimen spends roughly 95% of his/her time in a fasted state and less than 5% in a fully fed state. It requires a measure of discipline to maintain such a regimen consistently and I make no claims about its suitability for all individuals except to say that I and other healthy adults have subjected ourselves thereto for nearly a decade with no discernible detriments.

Throughout the fasting phase, no calorific commodities are consumed. However, tea and other aqueous agents are imbibed throughout the fast. Importantly, tea exhibits glycation-inhibiting effects, evidently attributable to its high catechin content. To cite one of several studies, Pon Babu and colleagues employed an animal model in which diabetes was experimentally induced. Upon oral administration of green tea extract for several weeks, the investigators analyzed its effects on AGE-mediated collagen cross-linkage and observed a significant reduction thereupon (Babu PV et al. 2006 A). [Similar studies by the same Indian investigators, using the same model of chemically-induced diabetes, revealed the capacity of green tea constituents to inhibit glycative damage in murine cardiac tissue as well (Babu PV et al. 2007; 2006 B).] Though the researchers did not determine the precise mechanism(s) by which green tea attenuated glycation, it is worth noting that serum glucose concentration in the experimental subjects was reportedly reduced by 50% (Babu PV et al. 2006 A). Induction of hypoglycemia (or more precisely, inhibition of postprandial hyperglycemia) is apparently one of the mechanisms by which ginseng, another element of the Amen Fast, inhibits AGE formation. Studies indicate that oral administration of ginseng (particularly the ground root of dried North American ginseng) reduces serum glucose concentration (Dascalu A et al 2007; Vuksan V et al. 2000). Glycemic reduction cannot be the sole mechanism by which ginseng inhibits glycation however, for it has been demonstrated that ginseng inhibits glycation *in vitro* as well (Bae & Lee 2004). This is an important point that has a bearing on the dietary component of the protocol as will be discussed below. On a typical day, I consume upwards of 2 liters of tea—about a liter of Pu-erh tea (aged black tea), .5 liter of ginseng, and .5-1liter of green or oolong tea. In addition, I consume *matcha* (powdered green tea) thrice daily—5 grams before and after my morning aerobic workout to enhance fat oxidation and offset the effects of glycolysis and an equivalent amount after the evening meal to mitigate the magnitude of glycemia.

As mentioned previously, the Amen Diet is thoroughly vegetal. In truth, this fact is fundamentally a matter of personal moral philosophy. Nevertheless, it incidentally comports with the anti-AGE agenda of the regimen insofar as meat is apparently a substantial source of glycotoxins, containing comparatively greater amounts of detectable AGE compounds than vegetal items (Goldberg T et al. 2004). Another important feature of the diet is its caloric paucity—1000-1500 kilocalories per day partaken in a single evening meal. As cited previously, several studies indicate that caloric restriction retards the formation of AGEs via known and unknown mechanisms. The quantity of calories ingested reflects an attempt on my part to ensure that the degree of dietary restriction is comparable to that designated in experimental animal studies, which ordinarily expose subjects to 30-50% dietary deficits relative to freely fed controls. As described in the Optimal Diet treatise, my goal is to attain a state of 50% caloric restriction. The question naturally arises, "Relative to what?". Relative to my estimated resting metabolic rate at the bodyweight I maintained when I initiated caloric restriction nearly a decade ago—roughly 100 kilograms. That is, a practical method of defining human caloric restriction is to compute (using any of several available metabolic rate equations) the amount of calories required to maintain energetic equilibrium upon initiation of the intervention and, therewith, consume a given fraction of this estimated quantity.

Not only is the Amen Diet devoid of meat and calorically sparse, it features staple foods selected specifically to offset or minimize glycation. These staple foods are oats, barley and bread. Among the oldest cultivated crops, barley (*Hordeum vulgare* L.) was chosen as the centerpiece of the diet primarily because it is amenable to preparation without cooking. To reiterate, cooking catalyzes the formation of AGEs, so subsistence upon a diet low in heat-treated foods should necessarily lessen one's ingestion of glycotoxins (Henle T 2005). Briefly, organic, non-hulled barley grains are misted with 3% hydrogen peroxide, rinsed, drained and incubated hydroponically for 24 hours in a sealed steel bowl containing 0.5% hydrogen peroxide. This solution is decanted after one day, replaced with purified water and allowed to germinate hydroponically for another day. After the 2-day germination period, the barley seedlings are blended in a base of germinated soymilk (i.e. an aqueous exudate of soy beans prepared in a manner similar to the barley and processed in a commercially available extractor). To this malted mixture is added matcha, which gives the preparation a pleasant, verdant visage. The resulting green gruel is sparingly sweetened and spiced with ground nutmeg and cinnamon, the bark of which exhibits antiglycation activity (Peng X et al. 2008). A feature of barley that bears mention is the presence of beta-glucans therein. Beta-glucans are a class of polysaccharides found in yeasts and various cereal grains. Of relevance to our present discussion is the effect of beta-glucans on glycemia. Several studies have demonstrated the capacity of beta-glucans to inhibit postprandial hyperglycemia (Mäkeläinen H et al. 2007; Casiraghi MC et al. 2006). Oats (*Avena sativa* L.) are also rich in beta-glucans and for this reason can be interchanged with barley if greater variety and simplicity are desired. [I suggest raw, rolled, organic oats served in a base of soymilk and topped with raw, unfiltered honey, dates, coconut and walnuts.] Finally, barley exhibits high antioxidant activity—higher than several comparable grains as assessed in one interesting study (Zdunczyk Z et al. 2006). Moreover, this inherently high antioxidant activity reportedly increases during the germination process (Lu J et al. 2007). Antioxidant capacity is an important consideration with respect to glycation inasmuch as free radical-mediated oxidation is operative in AGE propagation and vice versa (Selvaraj N et al. 2008; Osawa & Kato 2005). Thus, barley provides an ideal foundation for a low glycotoxin diet insofar as it is raw and therefore low in AGE, high in beta-glucans and therefore inhibitory toward hyperglycemia, and inherently high in antioxidants and therefore antagonistic toward AGE formation. Oats share these beneficial features. Indeed, oats contain unique antioxidant compounds called avenanthramides which exhibit anti-inflammatory and anti-atherogenic properties (Liu L et al. 2004). More importantly in the context of our present discussion is its demonstrated capacity to augment endogenous glutathione potency (Chen CY et al. 2007). The glutathione/glyoxalase antioxidant system is a principal mechanism by which the body detoxifies itself of AGEs (Di Loreto S et al. 2008). Avenanthramide-induced preservation of glutathione therefore makes oats an ideal staple of an anti-AGE diet. Lastly, both barley and oats contain glutathione and, as such, ostensibly contribute to the body's endogenous supply of the important anti-oxidant/anti-AGE pool (Zachariah VT et al. 2000; Patra & Panda 1988).

Bread comprises the other half of the standard Amen Meal. Bread is not a raw item, so some modifications must be made to render it suitable for inclusion in an ideal anti-AGE dietary regimen. These modifications are twofold: baking the bread rapidly (with added yeast) to minimize heat exposure and adding agents with demonstrated antiglycation activity. Briefly, the bread flour is comprised of three grain sources: barley, corn, and wheat. [The dough is mixed, and baked with the aid of a commercially available bread maker]. Seven agents are added to the dough prior to baking, each of which have exhibited anti-AGE activity in experimental investigations: powdered tea, powdered ginseng root, powdered turmeric root (Pari & Murugan 2007), thiamine, pyridoxine, pyridoxal-5-phosphate (Suji & Sivakami 2007) and L-carnitine (Rajasekar & Anuradha 2007). Conceivably, the interaction of these compounds with the carbohydrate-rich dough interferes with the exogenous process of glycation during the baking process, and, upon ingestion, may inhibit the formation of AGEs endogenously.

The third essential component of the Amen Protocol is the exercise regimen. Admittedly, the chief aim of the exercise regimen is not to thwart glycation, but as with the vegetarian nature of the diet, exercise of the sort prescribed by the protocol fortuitously facilitates AGE inhibition. First, the exercise regimen is bifurcated into two components: a morning aerobic session and an evening (pre-meal) resistance session. The main purpose of the aerobic session (ranging from 30-45 minutes) is to deplete stored glycogen and, therewith, promote the utilization of stored body fat throughout the day-long fast. Theoretically, promoting fatty acid oxidation over glycolysis as a means of energy production should lessen the generation of glycotoxins insofar as the carbonyl reactants in the glycolytic pathway promote AGE production (Gomes RA et al 2006; Hipkiss AR 2007 & 2006). Indeed, considering the fact that the exercise session is executed daily after an evening fasting interval of 6-8 hours, the vigorous aerobic activity ensures that glycogen levels remain chronically low, making fat oxidation the principal source of energy during the daily 23-hour fast.

Prior to the evening meal (~21st-22nd hour of the daily fast) the resistance session is executed. This rigorous weightlifting regimen has multifarious purposes—aesthetic, psychological, philosophical, and physiological. However, only the latter shall concern us presently, and only one aspect thereof. A major aim of the resistance regimen is to promote the preservation of lean muscle tissue and, concomitantly, avert the deposition of fat. Hence, muscularity is sought while adiposity is eschewed. The relevance of this aim to the topic before us is that muscle is more replete with insulin receptors than adipose tissue and plays a more prominent role in glucose disposal than does adipose (Evans DJ et al. 1984). Thus, promoting muscularity over adiposity should theoretically improve insulin sensitivity. The practical consequence of such improved insulin sensitivity should be to facilitate a more rapid influx and utilization of available glucose by cells, thus diminishing the duration of postprandial hyperglycemia. In keeping with our previous reasoning, reduced basal and postprandial glycemia should reduce the exposure of tissues to glucose and its glycolytic intermediaries and lessen the extent of glycation.

Summarily, I propose the Amen Protocol as a practical method by which glycation can be attenuated. Each aspect of the protocol comports with the aim of lessening glycative damage. To recapitulate: the fasting component ensures that serum glucose levels remain low throughout the day; the diet is restricted in calories and inclusive of foods that are low in AGEs and is inclusive of compounds that actively inhibit glycation; and the exercise component of the protocol preferentially promotes fat utilization over glycolysis, thereby lessening the formation of AGE precursors, and the exercise regimen potentially improves insulin sensitivity and by so doing inhibits glycation as a consequence of antagonizing hyperglycemia. To the extent that glycation is detrimental to health and longevity, the Amen Protocol should accordingly foster better health and greater longevity. The relevance of this proposition to public health is as follows: the "public" whose health the public health profession is predicated upon promoting is comprised of individuals. Lengthening the duration of healthy, productive life is a legitimate, laudable, attainable goal harbored by innumerable individuals. Therefore, interventions such as the Amen Protocol that are tailored to individuals and aimed at the augmentation of vitality and longevity should have a prominent place in the public health arena.

References

Amen-Ra, N.S. The Optimal Human Diet: Theoretical Foundation of the Amen Protocol, pp.177-240. In Robitaille, Francis P., editor. *Diet Therapy Research Trends*. New York: *Nova Biomedical Books*, 2007.

Anisimov, V.N., Semenchenko, A.V. and Yashin, A.I. (2003). Insulin and longevity: antidiabetic biguanides as geroprotectors. *Biogerontology*, 4(5):297-307.

Anisimov, V.N., Berstein, L.M., Egormin, P.A., Piskunova, T.S., Popovich, I.G., Zabezhinski, M.A., Kovalenko, I.G., Poroshina, T.E., Semenchenko, A.V., Provinciali, M., Re, F., and Franceschi, C. (2005). Effect of metformin on life span and on the development of spontaneous mammary tumors in HER-2/neu transgenic mice. *Exp Gerontol*. 40(8-9):685-93.

Anisimov, V.N., Berstein, L.M., Egormin, P.A., Piskunova, T.S., Popovich, I.G., Zabexhinski, M.A., Tyndyk, M.L., Yurova, M.V., Kovalenko, I.G., Poroshina, T.E., and Semenchenko, A.V. (2008). *Cell Cycle*, 7(17):2769-73.

Babu, P.V., Sabitha, K.E., Srinivasan, P., and Shyamaladevi, C.S. (2007). Green tea attenuates diabetes induced Maillar-type fluorescence and collagen cross-linking in the heart of streptozotocin diabetic rats. *Pharmacol Res*. 55(5):433-40.

Babu, P.V., Sabitha, K.E. and Shyamaladevi, C.S. (2006). Therapeutic effect of green tea extract on advanced glycation and cross-linking of collagen in the aorta of streptozotocin diabetic rats. *Clin Exp Parmacol Physiol*. A; 33(4):351-7.

Babu, P.V., Sabitha, K.E. and Shyamaladevi, C.S. (2006). Green tea impedes dyslipidemia, lipid peroxidation, protein glycation and ameliorates Ca2+ -ATPase activity in the heart of streptozotocin-diabetic rats. *Chem Biol Interact*. B; 25(162):157-64.

Bae, J.W. and Lee, M.H. (2004). Effect and putative mechanism of action of ginseng on the formation of glycated hemoglobin in vitro. *J Ethnopharmacol*. 91(1):137-40.

Bauer, M., Schorle, H., Pankratz, M.J., and Katzenberger, J.D. (2004). Starvation response in mouse liver shows strong correlation with life-span-prolonging processes. *Physiol Genomics*, 17(2):230-44.

Bishop, N.A. and Guarente, L. (2007). Genetic link between diet and lifespan: shared mechanisms from yeast to humans. *Nat Rev Genet*. 8(11):835-44.

Boeing, H., Weisgerber, Um, Jeckel, A., Rose, H.J., and Kroke, A. (2007). Association between glycated hemoglobin and diet and other lifestyle factors in a nondiabetic population: cross-sectional evaluation of dat from the Postdam cohort of the European Prospective Investigation into Cancer and Nutrition Study. *Am J Clin Nutr*. 71(5):1115-22.

Cai, W., He, J.C., Zhu, L., Chen, X., Striker, G.E., and Vlassara, H. (2008). Oral glycotoxins determine the effects of calorie restriction on oxidant stress, age-related diseases, and lifespan. *Am J Pathol*. 173(2):327-36.

Cai, W., He, J.C., Zhu, L., Chen, X., Wallenstein, S., Striker, G.E., and Vlassara, H. (2007). Reduced oxidant stress and extended lifespan in mice exposed to a low glycotoxin diet: association with increased AGER1 expression. *Am J Pathol*. 170(6):1893-902.

Casiraghi, M.C., Garsetti, M., Testolin, G., and Brigenti, F. (2006). Post-prandial responses to cereal products enriched with barley beta-glucan. *J Am Coll Nutr*. 25(4):313-20.

Cefalu, W.T., Bell-Farrow, A.D., Wang, Z.Q., Sonntag, W.E., Fu, M.X., Baynes, J.W., and Thorpe, S.R. (1995). Caloric restriction decreases age-dependent accumulation of the glycoxidation products, N epsilon-(carboxymethyl) lysine and pentosidine, in rat skin collagen. *J Gerontol A Biol Sci Med Sci*. 50(6):B337-41.

Chen, C.Y., Milbury, P.E., Collins, F.W., and Blumberg, J.B. (2007). Avenanthramides are bioavailable and have antioxidant activity in humans after acute consumption of and enriched mixture from oats. *J Nutr*. 137(6):1375-82.

Dascalu, A., Sievenpiper, J.L., Jenkins, A.L., Stavro, M.P., Leiter, L.A., Arnason, J.T., and Vuksan, V. (2007). Five batches representative of Ontario-grown American ginseng root produce comparable reductions of postprandial glycemia in healthy individuals. *Can J Physiol Pharmacol*. 85(9):856-64.

Di Loreto, S., Zimmitti, V., Sebastiani, P., Cervelli, C., Falone, S., and Amicarelli, F. (2008). Methylglyoxal causes strong weakening of detoxifying capacity and apoptotic cell death in rat hippocampal neurons. *Int J Biochem Cell Biol*. 40(2):245-57.

Evans, D.J., Murray, R. and Kissebah, A.H. (1984). Relationship between skeletal muscle insulin resistance, insulin-mediated glucose disposal, and insulin binding. Effects of obesity and body fat topography. *J Clin Invest*. 74(4):1515-25.

Goldberg, T., Cai, W., Peppa, M., Dardaine, V., Baliga, B.S., Uribarri, J., and Vlassara, H. (2004). Advanced glycoxidation end products in commonly consumed foods. *J Am Diet Assoc*. 104(8):1287-91.

Gomes, Ra., Miranda, H.V., Silva, M.S., Graca, G., Coelho, A.V., Ferreira, A.E., Cordeiro, C., and Freire, A.P. (2006). Yeast protein glycation in vivo by methylglyoxal. Molecular modification of glycolytic enzymes and heat shock proteins. *FEBS J*. 273(23):5273-87.

Goodrick, C.L., Ingram, D.K., Reynolds, M.A., Freeman, J.R., and Cider, N. (1990). Effects of intermittent feeding upon body weight and lifespan in inbred mice: interaction of genotype and age. *Mech Ageing Dev*. 55(1):69-87.

Goodrick, C.L., Ingram, D.K., Reynolds, M.A., Freeman, J.R., and Cider, N. (1982). Effects of intermittent feeding upon growth and life span in rats. *Gerontology,* 28(4):233-41.

Henle, T. (2005). Protein-bound andvanced glycation endproducts (AGEs) as bioactive amino acid derivatives in foods. *Amino Acids,* 29(4):313-22.

Hipkiss, A.R. (2007). Dietary restriction, glycolysis, hormesis and ageing. *Biogerontology,* 8(2):221-4.

Hipkiss, A.R. (2006). Does chronic glycolysis accelerate aging? Could this explain how dietary restriction works? *Ann N Y Acad Sci.* 1067:361-8.

Iwashige, K., Kouda, K., Kouda, M., Horiuchi, K., Takahashi, M., Nagano, A., Tanaka, T., and Takeuchi, H. (2004). Calorie restricted diet and urinary pentosidine in patients with rheumatoid arthritis. *J Physiol Anthropol Appl Human Sci.* 23(1):19-24.

Liu, L., Zubik, L., Collins, F.W., Marko, M., and Meydani, M. (2004). The antiatherogenic potential of oat phenolic compounds. *Atherosclerosis.* 175(1): 39-49.

Lu, J., Zhao, H., Chen, J., Fan, W., Dong, J., Kong, W., Sun, J., Cao, Y., and Cai, G. (2007). Evolution of phenolic compounds and antioxidant activity during malting. *J Agric Food Chem.* 55(26):10994-1001.

Makelainen, H., Anttila, H., Sihvonen, J., Hietanen, R.M., Tahvonen, R., Salminen, E., Mikola, M., and Sontag-Strohm, T. (2007). The effect of beta-glucan on the glycemic and insulin index. *Eur J Clin Nutr.* 61(6):779-85.

Masoro, E.J., Katz, M.S. and McMahan, C.A. (1989). Evidence for the glycation hypothesis of aging from the food-restricted rodent model. *J Gerontol.* 44(1):B20-22.

Mattson, M.P. (2008). Dietary factors, hormesis and health. *Ageing Res Rev.* 7(1):43-8.

Nelson, W. and Halberg, F. (1986). Meal-timing, circadian rhythms and life span of mice. *J Nutr.* 116(11):2244-53.

Osawa, T. and Kato, Y. (2005). Protective role of antioxidative food factors in oxidative stress caused by hyperglycemia. *Ann N Y Acad Sci.* 1043:440-51.

Pari, L. and Murugan, P. (2007). Influence of tetrahydrocurcumin on tail tendon collagen contents and its properties in rats with streptozotocin-nicotinamide-induced type 2 diabetes. *Fund Clin Pharmacol.* 21(6):665-71.

Patra, J. and Panda, B.B. (1998). A comparison of biochemical responses to oxidative and metal stress in seedlings of barley, Hordeum vulgare L. *Environ Pollut.* 101(1):99-105.

Peng, X., Ceng, K.W., Ma, J., Chen, B., Ho, C.T., Lo, C., Chen, F., and Wang, M. (2008). Cinnamon bark proanthocyanidins as reactive carbonyl scavenger to prevent the formation of advanced glycation endproducts. *J Agric Food Chem.* 56(6):1907-11.

Rajasekar, P. and Anuradha, C.V. (2007). L-carnitine inhibits protein glycation in vitro and in vivo: evidence for a role in diabetic management. *Acta Diabetol.* 44(2):83-90.

Physician's Desk Reference, 61st Edition. Montvale, NJ. Thomson PDR; 2007.

Rashid, I., van Reyk, D.M. and Davies, M.J. (2007). Carnosine and its constituents inhibit glycation of low-density lipoproteins that promotes foam cell formation in vitro. *FEBS Lett.* 581(5):1067-70.

Sell, D.R., Lane, M.A., Obrenovich, M.E., Mattison, J.A., Handy, A., Ingram, D.K., Cutler, R.G., Roth, G.S., and Monnier, V.M. (2003). The effect of caloric restriction on glycation and glycoxidation in skin collagen of nonhuman primates. *J Gerontol A Biol Sci Med Sci.* 58(6):508-16.

Selvaraj, N., Bobby, Z. and Sridhar, M.G. (2008). Increased glycation of hemoglobin in chronic renal failure: potential role of oxidative stress. *Arch Med Res*. 39(3):277-84.

Spindler, S.R. (2005). Rapid and reversible induction of the longevity, anticancer and genomic effects of caloric restriction. *Mech Ageing Dev*. 126(9):960-6.

Suji, G. and Sivakami, S. (2007). DNA damage during glycation of lysine by methylglyoxal: assessment of vitamins in preventing damage. *Amino Acids,* 33(4): 15-21.

Uribarri, J. and Tuttle, K.R. (2006). Advanced glycation end products and nephrotoxicity of high-protein diets. *Clin J Am Soc Nephrol*. 1(6):1293-9.

Van Liew, J.B., Davis, P.J., Davis, F.B., Bernardis, L.L., Deziel, M.R., Marinucci, L.N., and Kumar, D. (1993). Effects of aging, diet, and sex on plasma glucose, fructosamine, and lipid concentration in barrier-raised Fischer 344 rats. *J Gerontol*. 48(5):1115-22.

Vuksan, V., Stavro, M.P., Sievenpiper, J.L., Koo, V.Y., Wong, E., Beljan-Zdravkovic, U., Francis, T., Jenkins, A.L., Leiter, L.A., Josse, R.G., and Xu, Z. American ginseng improves glycemia in individuals with normal glucose tolerance: effect of dose and time escalation. *J Am Coll Nutr.* 200; 19(6):738-44.

Zachariah, V.T., Walsh-Sayles, N. and Singh, B.R. (2000).Isolation, purification, and characterization of glutathione S-transferase from oat (Avena sativa) seedlings. *J Protein Chem*. 19(6):425-30.

Zdunczyk, Z., Flis, M., Zielinski, H., Wroblewska, M., Antoszkiewicz, Z., and Juskiewicz, J. (2006). In vitro antioxidant activities of barley, husked oat, naked oat, tritcale, buckwheat wastes and their influence on the growth and biomarkers of antioxidant status in rats. *J Agric Food Chem*. 54(12):4168-75.

In: Handbook on Longevity: Genetics, Diet and Disease   ISBN 978-1-60741-075-1
Editors: Jennifer V. Bentely and Mary Ann Keller   © 2009 Nova Science Publishers, Inc.

Chapter IV

Prospects of a Longer Life Span beyond the Beneficial Effects of a Healthy Lifestyle

Giacinto Libertini

Naples, Italy

Azienda Sanitaria Locale NA3, giacinto.libertini@tin.it

Abstract

Life span is limited by the effects of diseases and ageing. For the aim of a longer life span, it is indispensable that a rational analysis of the primary causes of these phenomena is not limited to the description of their physio-pathological mechanisms. If Dobzhansky's statement that "nothing in biology makes sense, except in the light of evolution" is true, it appears logical to maintain that evolution theory must be the main tool for such analysis.

From an evolutionary point of view, diseases are the predictable consequence of: 1) defects in the maintenance and transmission of genetic information; 2) alterations of the ecological niche to which the species is adapted (in particular, for our species, due to civilisation); 3) interactions with other species (bacteria, viruses, fungi, protozoa, parasitic worms, etc.); and 4) conditions for which the species is not adapted.

Moreover, evolution theory allows the paradoxical prediction that, in particular ecological conditions, kin selection favours a progressive fitness decline, usually, in its more evident manifestations, referred to as ageing and that must not be classified as a disease. This decline is genetically determined and regulated and is obtained with a progressive limitation of cell turnover through a sophisticated modulation of the telomere-telomerase system.

A lifestyle compatible with the ecological niche to which our species is adapted and good medical treatment permit the attainment of the highest life span defined by the genetic program of our species (within the limits of individual genetic peculiarities) but do not allow the overcoming of the maximal values of longevity defined by the same program.

To increase these values, it is indispensable to modify the genetic planning of ageing, with a different modulation of the telomere-telomerase system.

In principle, granted that this will be considered ethically acceptable, it is possible to propose a modification of that part of the genetic program that modulates ageing so that an unlimited survival is obtained, similar to the so-called "negligible senescence" observed for many animal and plant species.

A possible schedule to achieve this aim and the effects on human civilisation are outlined.

Premise

Disease is usually defined as an alteration of physiological conditions. If it is true that evolutionary mechanisms are indispensable for the full understanding of any biologic phenomenon [1], it is necessary to investigate if and how diseases and other phenomena causing suffering, disability and/or death are explainable and classifiable in evolutionary terms and whether from this approach useful indications may be deduced.

This question is the object of so-called Darwinian or evolutionary medicine [2,3,4,5,6,7], proposed in 1991 [2] but with some known forerunners [8].

In fact, the main concept of evolutionary medicine, the "discordance" between the conditions to which our species is adapted and actual conditions of life as a very important cause of disease, was already clearly expressed and well documented before the term "Darwinian medicine" was formulated [9].

Another forerunner [10] stated many of the concepts expressed by Williams and Nesse [2,3] with a substantial difference. For current evolutionary medicine, in accordance with prevalent gerontological ideas [11], ageing is the result of insufficient selection for a greater longevity and, in particular, of a trade-off between better somatic maintenance and reproduction capacity versus greater longevity [12]. Alternatively, it was proposed that mechanisms underlying ageing are favoured by kin selection, in particular ecological conditions [10,13], and therefore age-related fitness decline should be considered a physiological function and not a set of unrelated pathological conditions insufficiently countered by natural selection. This paradoxical and heretical different interpretation of ageing, which is in accordance with the general hypothesis of ageing as adaptive phenomenon [14,15,16,17,18,19,20], has been reaffirmed recently with the support of empirical evidence that disproves the classic interpretation [21,22]. Moreover, regarding the possibility of drastic modifications of human longevity, ageing considered as "a specific biological function rather than the result of a disorder in complex living systems" [15] allows totally new perspectives, based both on theoretical arguments and on the extraordinary advances in the understanding of the telomere-telomerase system, apoptosis, cell turnover and related arguments.

The Basic Question

Anatomy, physiology and behaviour characterising each species, ours included, are modelled and influenced by natural selection which has acted for innumerable generations. As natural selection improves fitness and reproduction capacity, a logical prediction is that individuals of a species should have the best fitness and reproduction capacity, with the exception of rare particular cases.

Yet, individuals of our species suffer from many diseases or other disabling conditions, and death is a common end to many of these conditions (Figure 1).

The incredible complexity and the amazing capacities of the eyes, the brain, the metabolic pathways and innumerable other characteristics of living beings are a marvellous fruit of natural selection, but diseases and other disabling conditions are a clear challenge for our confidence in the power of natural selection [3].

In short, is the evolutionary design of our species, although complex and admirable, a partial failure because we are afflicted by many imperfections and severe defects? Alternatively, are these imperfections and severe defects intrinsic to the evolutionary process?

This question is particularly important for the understanding of the causes of diseases that torment our species.

The problem is not a useless theoretical disquisition [23]: a rational answer to this question is the basis for the comprehension of the primary causes of diseases and similar conditions, for elaborating correct strategies to limit morbidity and mortality and for enhancing life span (mean duration of life) and longevity (the greatest duration of life).

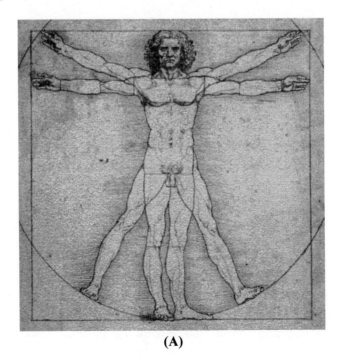

(A)

Figure 1 (Continued).

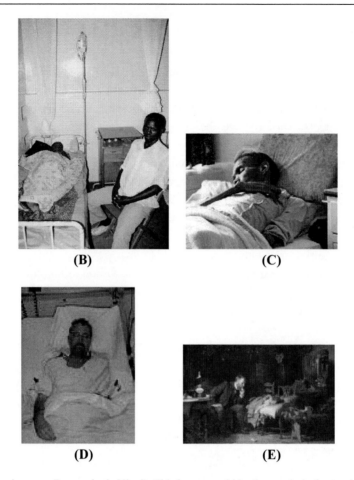

(B)   (C)

(D)   (E)

Figure 1. A) Vitruvian man (Leonardo da Vinci). This image could be the symbol of natural selection that shapes an organism without inappropriate imperfections. B) to E) Images illustrating some of the many conditions afflicting our species and that seem to indicate the failure of natural selection.

Evolutionary Classification of Diseases and Other Phenomena Causing Suffering, Disability and Death

1. Diseases Caused by Alterations of the Genotype

The preservation of genetic information and its transfer from a generation to the next is imperfect, a fact that is fundamental for the whole evolutionary theory as without genetic diversity selection would be impossible. Genetic information rules a sophisticated program that determines organism development and functions, both very complicated phenomena. A random modification in a very complex structure is, as more probable event if not neutral, an alteration that is a cause of dysfunction (Figure 2). Natural selection acts against the spreading of harmful alterations. Therefore, it is predictable that in a species there will be many alterations of genetic information, each with a low frequency by effect of natural selection.

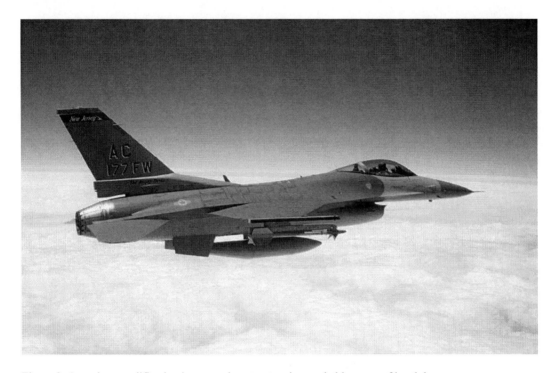

Figure 2. A random modification in a complex structure is a probable cause of breakdown.

The equilibrium frequency between the onset of new cases of genetic alterations and their elimination by natural selection is easily calculable. If the harmful gene C is recessive, its equilibrium frequency (C_e) will be:

$$C_e = \sqrt{-v/s} = \sqrt{v/[s]} \tag{1}$$

where v = mutation rate from an inactive allele (C'); -s = damage caused by C (the value is negative as C is harmful); [s] = absolute value of s (for the calculation of the formulas 1-7, see Appendix).

Using Hardy-Weinberg formula (CC + 2 CC' + C'C' = 1), the equilibrium frequency of the phenotype expressing the disadvantageous condition (P_e) will be:

$$P_e = C_e^2 = v/[s] \tag{2}$$

If C is dominant, its equilibrium frequency will be:

$$C_e = \frac{2\,s + 2\,\sqrt{s^2 + 3\,s\,v}}{6\,s} \approx 0.5\ v/[s] \tag{3}$$

and the equilibrium frequency of the phenotype expressing the disadvantageous condition (P_e) will be:

$$P_e = C_e^2 + 2\,C_e\,(1\text{-}C_e) = 2\,C_e - C_e^2 = \frac{(1 - \sqrt{1 + 3\,v/s})\,(5 + \sqrt{1 + 3\,v/s})}{9} \approx v/[s] \qquad (4)$$

These equilibrium frequencies are illustrated in Figure 3.

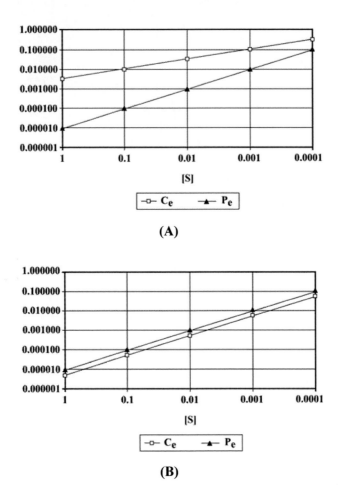

(A)

(B)

Figure 3. A) Equilibrium gene frequency (C_e) and phenotypic frequency (P_e) for a recessive harmful gene. B) Equilibrium gene frequency (C_e) and phenotypic frequency (P_e) for a dominant harmful gene.

For chromosome alterations, v can be interpreted as the frequency of the onset of a chromosome alteration and its equilibrium frequency, which coincides with its phenotypic frequency, is:

$$P_e = C_e = v/[s] \qquad (5)$$

as for a noxious gene in a haploid organism.

If n types of mutations, with a mean mutation rate v, can transform neutral alleles into C, the equilibrium phenotypic frequency of C will be:

$$P_e = n (v/[s])\qquad(6)$$

These formulas mean that with small values of v (e.g., v < 0.00001), if [s] is not very small, the predicted frequency of a disease (P_e) caused by particular alterations of the genotype is very small, that is harmful alleles are constantly and efficaciously removed by natural selection.

This is not true in two cases.

1) If the value of [s] is very small, e.g., in the case that the harmful expression of the gene is at ages when only a few individuals survive and their remaining expectation of life and therefore their reproductive value is minimal, P_e will be not small. This is an argument of the "mutation accumulation" theory of ageing (see later).

2) If C is disadvantageous in the homozygous state (s < 0) and advantageous in the heterozygote state (s' > 0), its equilibrium frequency will be:

$$C_e = - \frac{2\,s'}{s - 4\,s'} = \frac{2\,s'}{[s] + 4\,s'}\qquad(7)$$

and it is easy to calculate the equilibrium frequencies of homozygous and heterozygote conditions (if s > 0 and s' < 0, C_e=1). The high frequency of some types of genetically determined anaemias (sickle cell anaemia, thalassaemia, G6PD deficiency, etc.), which are mild in the heterozygote state and deadly in the homozygous state, is explained by their advantage against malaria in the heterozygote state [8].

However, disregarding these particular cases, the theoretical prediction is that in a species there will be many diseases caused by alterations of the genotype, each with a very low frequency (greater when many different mutations alter the same gene or the same metabolic pathway) but with an overall frequency not small.

2. Diseases Caused by Alterations of the Ecological Niche

A modification of the ecological conditions to which a species is adapted, is a change in a very complex and ordinate system. Therefore, a modification of the ecological niche will be, as more probable event if not neutral, a cause of physiological dysfunctions (Figure 4).

Evolution is a slow process. If a species has been for a long time (thousands of generations) in a particular ecological niche (climatic conditions, behavioural and nutritional habits, relations with other species, etc.), the species should be considered as well adapted.

If the ecological niche changes, the adaptation to the new conditions may require times very long for the human standards, e.g., thousands of generations, which means 20,000-30,000 years for each thousand of generations.

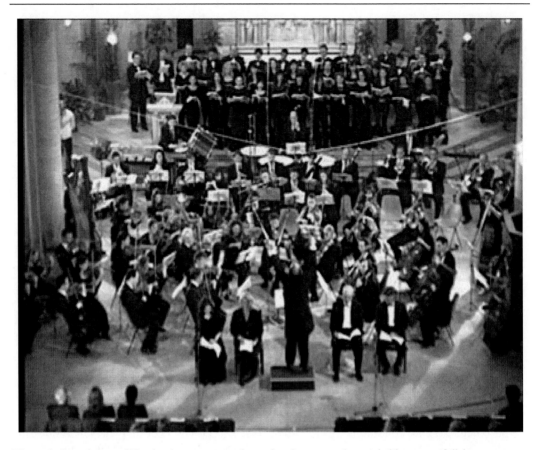

Figure 4. A random modification in a very complex ordered sequence is a probable cause of disharmony.

From the origins to about 10,000 years ago, our species lived in Palaeolithic conditions (Stone Age) and, presumably, was well adapted to this "ancestral condition". With the Neolithic revolution, agriculture and breeding modified strongly our ecological niche. Afterwards, the massive urbanisation, the huge increase in demographic density, technological innovations, the industrial revolution, etc., have caused even greater changes.

Only a partial adaptation to the new conditions is documented or plausible. For example, adult Stone Age men were unable to digest fresh milk after being weaned and the greater part of modern men have the same inability except some populations in Europe, western India and sub-Saharan Africa that, having reared cattle from thousands of years, have acquired the capacity to digest fresh milk in adulthood [24].

The radical modification of our conditions of life has strikingly worsened the mean health of modern men in comparison with populations living in Stone Age-like conditions (hunter-gatherers or foragers). Some years ago, there were a few remaining populations with these lifestyle (e.g., some Australian aborigines, Hadza in Tanzania, !Kung of Botswana, Ache of Paraguay, Efè of the Democratic Republic of the Congo, and Agta of the Philippines [8]) and they showed almost no dental caries [25], hypertension, diabetes, obesity, cardiovascular affections, cancer, psychological and emotional ailment [26], although more than 8% of the individuals exceeded 60 years of age [27].

Some examples of particular alterations of our ecological niche and the consequent diseases are listed in Table 1. A complete list with the discussion of the particular pathological mechanism for each disease would require a textbook.

Table 1.

Alterations of the ecological niche → Diseases
Excessive ingestion of salt → hypertension [9,28,29] (→ heart hypertrophy, congestive heart failure, arrhythmia and sudden death [30]) (Figure 5)
Excessive time spent focusing close up or in improper conditions of vision → myopia [31] (up to 70–90% of a population affected [32,33]), refractive defects (myopia, astigmatism, hyperopia) [34]
Excessive ingestion of unsaturated fats, caloric foods, meat with high fat content → obesity (→ renal cell carcinoma [35], heart hypertrophy, congestive heart failure, arrhythmia and sudden death [30]) (Figure 6), type 2-diabetes (Figure 7) and increased vascular risk (→ myocardial infarct, cerebral ischemia, infarcts in all the vascular districts, heart hypertrophy and failure, etc.) [9]
Occupational noise, smoking, high Body Mass Index → hearing loss [36]
Excessive exposure to noise → hearing loss [9,37]
Smoking and/or air pollution → chronic bronchitis [38], emphysema [39]
Smoking → coronary heart and other cardiovascular diseases, chronic respiratory diseases, pregnancy complications, and respiratory diseases in children [40], lung [40,41] / larynx [41,42] / bladder [41,43] / kidney [35] / pancreas [44] carcinoma, peptic ulcer [45,46]
Excessive ingestion of simple and refined carbohydrates (in particular sugar) and other dietary modifications → dental caries, pyorrhoea, crowded teeth [9,25] (Figure 8)
Scarce ingestion of fibre → constipation, colon diverticulosis, colon carcinoma, stomach carcinoma, type 2-diabetes, metabolic syndrome and cardiovascular diseases [47], appendicitis [48,49]
Scarce ingestion of calcium and reduced physical activity → osteoporosis [9,50], back pain [9]
Reduced exposure to natural allergens in the childhood → allergies [51]
Exposure to chemical substances artificially synthesised → allergic diseases [52]
Altered conditions of sociality, stress of civilised condition → mental and psychiatric disorders [3,9]
Various factors → increased incidence of various types of cancer [9,53]
Alcoholism → hepatic steatosis, steatohepatitis, cirrhosis [54], larynx carcinoma [42]

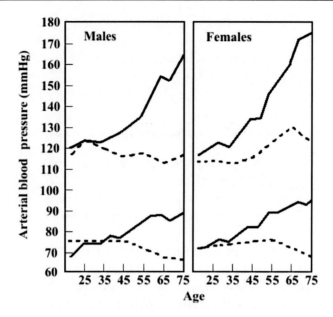

Figure 5. Arterial blood pressures in Kung individuals (dashed lines) and in London citizens (continuous lines) [55] (partially redrawn).

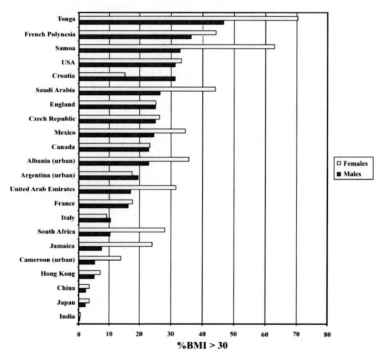

Data from International Obesity Task Force (from late 1990s to 2002; http://www.iotf.org/database/documents/GlobalPrevalenceofAdultObesityJuly08pdfv2.pdf).

Figure 6. Frequencies of Body Mass Index > 30 in some countries. Some years ago, for the few remaining hunter-gatherer populations, obesity was a rarity [26].

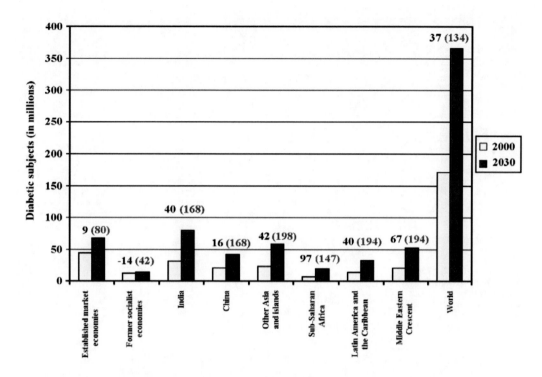

Figure 7. Estimated numbers (in millions) of people with diabetes by region for 2000 and 2030. Percentage of change in total population and (between brackets) percentage of change in population >65 years of age are also indicated [56]. Diabetes was a rarity in the few remaining hunter-gatherer populations [26].

It is essential a distinction between "proximate" and "evolutionary" causes of a disease [3]. Evolutionary (or ultimate or primary) causes explain "why" diseases happen. Proximate (or near) causes explain "how" diseases manifest themselves.

Genes making an individual vulnerable to a disease in particular conditions are the "proximate" causes, while the "evolutionary" cause is that an individual is exposed to ecological conditions to which the species is not adapted. For example, a "normal" modern diet includes an intake of salt more than ten times that estimated to be ingested in prehistoric times or in modern hunter-gatherer societies. Our body is not adapted to this "normal" intake of salt and, after years of excessive use of salt, "hypertension-predisposing" genes cause hypertension. The true cause of hypertension is the abnormal excessive intake of salt to which the organism is not adapted (evolutionary cause) and not the existence of "hypertension-predisposing" genes (proximate cause). The "normality" of modern diet is correct in its statistical meaning (average intake of salt in a modern population) as it is correct to say that blindness is statistically "normal" in a community of blind men. It should be stressed that "normal" modern diet is largely abnormal in evolutionary terms and that "hypertension-predisposing" genes are normal genes that in the modern harmful conditions of life cause hypertension. The pathological condition is the modern "normal" diet and not "hypertension-predisposing" genes and the attention should be focused on the real causes and their possible correction and not on proximate causes (Figure 9).

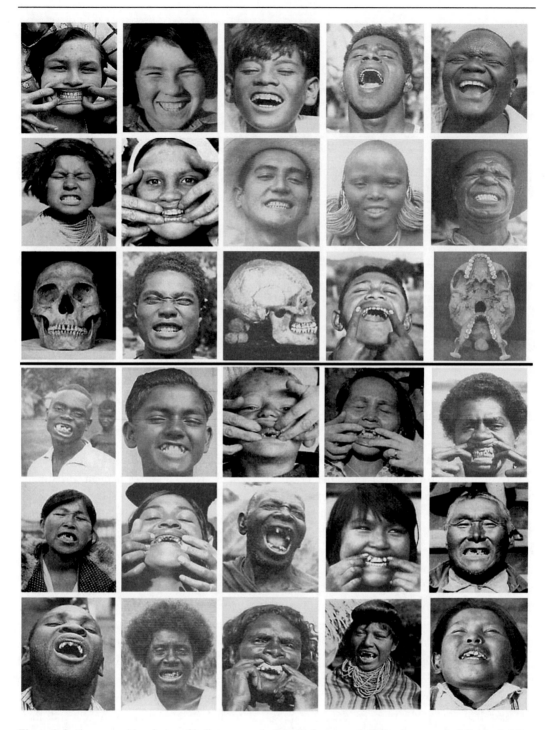

Figure 8. In the upper side: photos of indigenous and of skulls from people following ancestral dietary habits ("teeth ... excellent and free from dental caries"); in the lower side: photos of indigenous following modern diets (multiple dental caries, "crowding of the teeth", "changes in facial form", pyorrhoea) [25]. After about 70 years from publication, the evidence and the teaching of the extraordinary book of Price (called the "Charles Darwin of nutrition") is still perfectly topical and could be a symbol of the damages caused by thoughtless changes of the ecological niche.

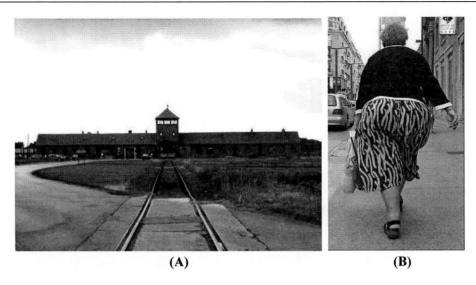

(A)   (B)

Figure 9. A) The victims of the Holocaust numbered in the millions (Hebrews, Roms, gays, political dissidents, etc.). Misleading interpretation (proximate cause): this was caused by their race, religious creed, etc. Correct interpretation (primary cause): this was caused by an insane and murderous ideology. B) The victims of diabetes, hypertension, atherosclerosis and their complications number in the tens of millions. Misleading interpretation (proximate cause): this is caused by their diabetes-, hypertension-, atherosclerosis-predisposing genes. Correct interpretation (primary cause): this is caused by alterations of the ecological niche (too many calories and unsaturated fats, too much salt, etc.) to which the organism is not adapted.

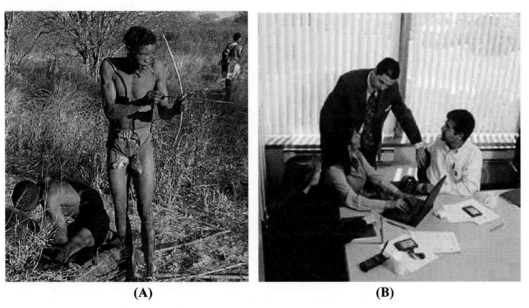

(A)   (B)

Figure 10. A) Bushmen tribes (!Kung San, Botswana), some years ago one of the few remaining hunter-gatherer populations, had a lifestyle analogous to Stone Age societies. They were quite well adapted to their ancient ecological niche and diseases such as hypertension, diabetes, obesity, cardiovascular affections, cancer, psychological and emotional ailments, dental caries, myopia, astigmatism, etc., were rare events for them;
B) Modern men. Their genes are practically the same of hunter-gatherer men but there is a noxious "discordance" between their habits and the ecological niche to which their genes are adapted: the above-mentioned affections, and many others, are the terrible consequence [9].

The mismatch between the ecological niche to which our genes are well adapted and the actual habits is the true ("primary") cause of large part of our ills ("Discordance Hypothesis") [9] (Figure 10).

3. Diseases Caused by Interactions with Other Species

As there is continuous competition among the species with conflictual evolutionary exigencies and, in particular, between an organism and its parasites (bacteria, viruses, fungi, protozoa, parasitic worms, etc.), a third general cause of disease is predictable.

The number of bacteria living in the gut of each man has been estimated to be ten times the number of his cells [57] and there are trillions of other bacteria living on our skin, mucosae and elsewhere on or in our body. Large part of these bacteria live with us without being harmful and often are useful, e.g., hindering settlement and attack of bacterial pathogenic species.

"The total set of over 1400 pathogen species breaks down into over 200 viruses, over 500 bacteria and rickettsia, over 300 fungi, over 50 protozoa, almost 300 helminths, and at least 2 kinds of prion" [58].

In this category of diseases, natural selection acts both on the side of the host and on the side of its parasites. The result must be a compromise between the competing exigencies to survive and propagate of both host and parasites.

The relationship between an organism and its parasites is analogous to that between a prey and its predators, and in it we have a troublesome position analogous to that of a prey. However, it is predictable that, in a similar way to what happens in the prey-predators case [59], to minimise disadvantages and maximise advantages both for host and parasite, parasites will damage more very young, sick and old individuals, with low reproductive potentiality, and less intermediate ages and healthy individuals with greater reproductive potentiality.

4. Diseases Caused by Conditions beyond Adaptation Range

Conditions beyond the adaptation range of the species (e.g., the fall of a man from an excessive height, the trauma of a violent car accident, etc.) are a sure cause of physiological dysfunctions or death.

5. Disease-Like Phenomena Caused by Natural Selection

Natural selection may determine disease-like phenomena, which may be apparently harmful or which are surely harmful in terms of individual fitness.

For this category of phenomena, which cannot be defined as diseases, a subdivision is necessary on the grounds of the selective mechanisms involved.

5.1. Phenomena That Are Defences against Harmful Agents

Natural selection favours physiological mechanisms that are defensive against infections and other harmful agents or conditions (e.g., fever, cough, sneezes, itch, inflammatory phenomena, nociceptive pain, diarrhoea, iron deficiency, morning sickness, emotions such as anxiety, fear, etc.) [2].

In particular: 1) iron deficiency, especially in pregnancy, appears an effective defence against infectious diseases [3,60] because: "Acquiring iron is a fundamental step in the development of a pathogen, and the complexity and redundancy of both host and pathogen mechanisms to acquire iron and control flux and availability illustrate the longstanding and ongoing battle for iron." [61]; 2) morning sickness of the pregnant woman protects the embryo from foods containing teratogen chemicals (e.g., natural toxic chemicals in vegetables) or potentially infected (e.g., meats, fish, poultry, and eggs) [62,63].

In certain cases, which must be considered as pathological noxious conditions of alteration of physiological and beneficial functions, the defensive mechanism is excessive or inappropriate or harmfully altered by a parasite to increase its propagation (e.g., diarrhoea in infections by *Vibrio cholerae* [64]).

5.2. Phenomena Damaging Other Individuals Genetically Related but Improving Overall Fitness of Progeny

Vertebrate immune system must discriminate between antigens of each host individual and those of the parasites, which try to overcome immunologic defences by using for their coverings proteins with the same antigenicity of the host (antigen mimicry). The defence of the host against antigen mimicry is to have the greatest inter-individual variability of antigen formulas so that a mimicry adapt to infect all the potential hosts is impossible [10]. The major histocompatibility complex (MHC) is the main tool by which the host organism obtains an extraordinary antigen variability. Differences between antigenic formulas of host and parasite give greater resistance to the infection while similarities cause susceptibility. Correlations between resistance or susceptibility to several infectious or infection-related diseases and specific human MHC alleles are well documented [65,66].

The best progeny is that with the greater antigen variability. This may be obtained through MHC-mediated mate choice and with post-copulatory selection. The first phenomenon has been observed in several vertebrate taxa and is widespread in nature [67]. MHC genes influence human mating preferences. Women college students rated the odours of MHC-dissimilar men as being 'more pleasant' than those of MHC-similar men [68,69]. In an isolate, ethnically homogenous community, significantly fewer couples was observed to match at a 16-locus MHC haplotype [70,71].

With the second phenomenon, also referred to as 'cryptic female choice' [72], miscarriage eliminates the production of offspring with lesser antigen variability having a future decreased fitness due to diminished disease potential resistance [73]. For animals, post-copulatory selection is well documented [74]. For humans, in a study, an excess of MHC-heterozygotes was found in newborn males [75]. A series of studies on an isolate and ethnically homogenous community have documented that couples with shared HLA-DR alleles in comparison with couples not sharing the same alleles have significantly less children [76], a greater interval between pregnancies [77] and a greater pregnancy loss rate [78].

In this sub-category, natural selection determines the death of healthy embryo individuals to optimise the survival potentiality of progeny. Infanticide or the abandonment of healthy new-born babies when the resources are insufficient are ancient and widespread behaviours [79], apparently determined by analogous evolutionary necessities of not giving place to progeny with reduced survival possibilities and that could subtract precious resources to kin individuals [9]. For animals, analogous behaviours are well known [59]. This sub-category indicates that natural selection may cause physiological events that could be interpreted as pathological or behaviours considered ethically unacceptable in our culture. This implicates that from an ethical point of view not all the effects of natural selection can be accepted uncritically or regarded in principle as not to be modified.

5.3. Phenomena Damaging the Individual but Favoured by Kin Selection

In the classic definition of natural selection, the variation of the frequency of a gene X between two generations (Δ_x) is depending on the advantage or disadvantage s caused by X, alias the variation of fitness, and of the reproductive value P of the individual in which X acts:

$$\Delta_x \propto s \cdot P \tag{8}$$

The definitions of inclusive fitness and kin selection have strongly modified this concept [59,80,81,82,83]. If a gene X, present in the individual I_1, determines effects on I_1 and on other individuals I_2, I_3, ... I_n genetically related (kins) to I_1, with coefficients of relationship (probability of genes in common) equal to r_2, r_3, ... r_n, respectively, and with reproductive values equals to P_1, P_2, P_3, ... P_n, respectively, to evaluate the spreading or decay of X within the species, the effects on the fitnesses of all individuals involved must be considered:

$$\Delta_x \propto \Sigma (s_z \cdot P_z \cdot r_z) \tag{9}$$

with z varying from 1 to n.

Only if no other individual than I_1 is involved in the action of X, formula (9) is transformed in the classic formula (8), as $r_1 = 1$.

This conceptual revolution allowed a convincing explanation of the social organisation of ants and bees and of many other otherwise inexplicable phenomena [59].

Inclusive fitness and kin selection are indispensable to understand the phenomena illustrated in this sub-category.

5.3.1. Altruistic Actions

For animals, behaviours or actions that damage or kill the individuals expressing them but increase the survival probabilities of kin individuals are well documented [59], e.g., the defence from predators of a drove of yellow baboons (*Papio cynocephalus*) [84] or of chacma baboons (*Papio ursinus*) [85] by the predominant males with great individual risk.

Actions damaging an individual and favouring kin individuals do not necessitate a wilful choice or even the existence of a nervous system. For example, apoptosis is a form of cell death genetically determined and highly regulated, for the first time described as phenomenon other than necrosis in normal liver epatocytes [86] and typical of eukaryotic organisms, even if monocellular [87]. In the yeast (*Saccharomyces cerevisiae*), the scarcity of nutrients triggers the apoptosis of older individuals enhancing "the chances of the rest of the population to survive and to sporulate, thus increasing the probability that the clone will survive" [88] and this is explained as "altruistic cell death" [88], alias as an "altruistic behaviour" [89] caused by kin selection.

For humans, behaviours and actions that reduce fitness or jeopardise health, and even life of individuals committing them, are well known and can be interpreted as altruistic behaviours determined by kin selection [90,91].

5.3.2. Ageing

For many species, ours included, an age-related fitness decline is well documented both in wild and in protected conditions [92,93,94,95,96,97,98,99,100]. This fitness decline is illustrated by the age-related continuous decline of athletic performances (Figure 11), which is mirrored in the age-related mortality increase: "No one would consider a man in his thirties senile, yet, according to athletic records and life tables, senescence is rampant during this decade" [101].

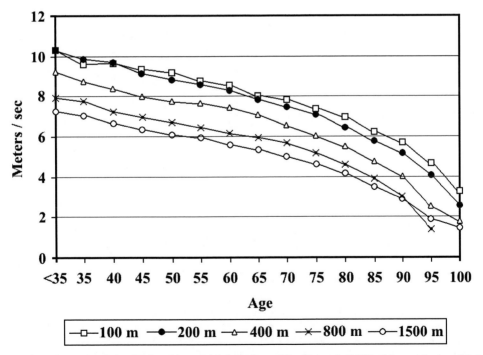

Source of data: for age group < 35 (world records), http://en.wikipedia.org/wiki/World_records_in_athletics; for other age groups, http://www.world-masters-athletics.org/records_output/rec_list_outdoor_m.php.
Figure 11. Age-related fitness decline.

In its more advanced manifestations, this phenomenon is universally known as ageing / senescence, but the use of these terms is scientifically tricky being often referred only to the more evident expressions of the fitness decline, rarely observable in the wild ("...there is scant evidence that senescence contributes significantly to mortality in the wild. ...As a rule wild animals simply do not live long enough to grow old" [11]). To avoid misunderstandings, other terms precisely describing the phenomenon as "increasing mortality with increasing chronological age in the wild" (IMICAW) [13] or "actuarial senescence in the wild" [99,100] or "age-related fitness decline in the wild", which do not refer to lower limits for the grade of fitness decline, are preferable.

A widespread opinion is that the age-related fitness decline in the wild is the result of insufficient selection at older ages against harmful mutations accumulated over evolutionary time (mutation accumulation theory) [102,103,104,105,106].

Against this hypothesis, it has been demonstrated that even with a great number of noxious gene expressing their harmful action at ages with a few survivors, natural selection reduces greatly frequencies and effects of the noxious genes so that life table is scarcely modified by their action (Figure 12). The conclusion, till now not falsified, is that mutation accumulation theory is untenable as explanation of age-related fitness decline in the wild [10,13,21].

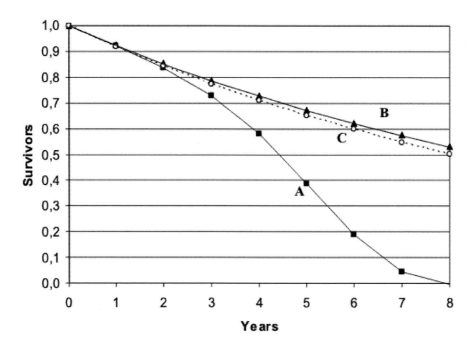

Figure 12. Curve A is the life table in the wild of a real species showing an age-related fitness decline. Curve B is a hypothetical life table of the same species with only the extrinsic mortality at its lowest value and without the age-related fitness decline. Curve C is a hypothetical life table with the same mortality of curve B plus the effects of a great number (n = 500 / year) of noxious genes acting at years t_1, t_2, ... Curve A is quite different from curve C and, therefore, it is unjustifiable as an effect of noxious genes insufficiently eliminated by natural selection [21].

To overcome the weakness of mutation accumulation theory, two new hypotheses were proposed. The first (antagonistic pleiotropy theory) suggested that fitness decline was determined by pleiotropic genes, beneficial at early ages and harmful at later ages [101,107]. The second (disposable soma theory) proposed that the causes of fitness decline were environmental or somatic and that at older ages natural selection was limited by physiological or environmental constraints, so that, in the subdivision of metabolic resources between reproduction and maintenance, reproduction was preferred [108,109].

However, "Few plausible candidates for antagonistically pleiotropic genes have been recognized, and the physiological mechanisms connecting opposing early and late effects on fitness are not well characterized ..." [100] and there is no proof of trade-off between greater reproduction and lesser longevity for primate and humans [110]. In an authoritative paper [11], no example of trade-off is reported for animals that show age-related fitness decline in the wild (documentation of trade-offs for animals that show age-related fitness decline in artificial conditions is reported, but this is a different phenomenon not subjected to natural selection [21,22]).

The common view of these three theories is that they consider age-related fitness decline as a nonadaptive phenomenon. Current gerontological theories reply to "Darwin's dilemma" [16,18] (Is ageing nonadaptive and therefore a great example of failure of natural selection or adaptive by being somehow evolutionarily advantageous?) maintaining that natural selection fails to make individuals very long-lived or not showing age-related fitness decline.

In clear contrast with this idea, age-related fitness decline has been explained as evolutionary advantageous in terms of kin selection in particular ecological conditions [10,13,21]. Afterwards, in accordance with the theoretical arguments but independently of them, empirical data in support of an adaptive meaning of fitness decline and against hypotheses interpreting age-related fitness decline as nonadaptive have been presented [22].

Indeed, only the heretical idea that age-related fitness decline is adaptive, hinted by various authors [13,14,15,20,21], allows to justify:

1) *the existence of species with no age-related fitness decline in the wild.* The individuals of many species survive in the wild till remarkable ages showing no detectable fitness decline (e.g., sturgeon, rockfish, turtles, bivalve mollusks, certain perennial trees, etc.; "animals with negligible senescence" [98]). For this phenomenon, truly strange for nonadaptive theories [111], particular variants of disposable soma theory have been developed [108,109], even to justify the case in which mortality rate decreases at greater ages [112]. However, these variants have the taste of adaptations *ad hoc* to justify data contrasting with theoretical predictions.

2) *the inverse relation of extrinsic and intrinsic mortality documented for some bird and mammal species in the wild* [100]. Current nonadaptive theories predict explicitly a direct relation and Ricklefs states clearly in his discussion that this prediction is confuted by empirical data [100]. On the contrary, adaptive theory predicts the inverse relation observed [10,13,21,22].

3) *the existence of sophisticated mechanisms, genetically determined and regulated, progressively limiting cell turnover and cell functionality.* The telomere-telomerase system limits cell duplication capacities (replicative senescence) and, consequently,

cell turnover and, moreover, causes a progressive decay of cell functionality (cell senescence) [113]. These mechanisms, genetically modulated and determined, which are a plausible cause of the progressive fitness decline [21,113], are not explained by nonadaptive hypothesis while are necessary for the validity of the adaptive hypothesis [22]. In particular, nonadaptive hypothesis tries to explain replicative senescence and cell senescence as a defence against malignant neoplasia [114,115], that is a terrible evolutionary trade-off between ageing and defence against cancer [116], but: a) old individuals of "animals with negligible senescence" such as rainbow trout and lobster show in the wild the same telomerase activity of young individuals [117,118] and no increase in cancer vulnerability, as their stable mortality rates prove; b) replicative senescence and cell senescence weaken the efficiency of immune system [113], a factor inversely related to cancer vulnerability and incidence [119]; c) shortened telomeres increases cancer probabilities because of dysfunctional telomere-induced instability [120,121]. Moreover, replicative senescence and cell senescence, although not caused by telomere shortening but by another unknown mechanism related to the number of duplications, are well documented in eukaryotic species such as yeast [122,123,124], which being unicellular species cannot be affected by cancer. However, these phenomena and others strictly associated [125,126] observed in yeast have been interpreted as adaptive [20,127,128,129,130,131] and they are consistent with the explanation that they determine a greater evolution rate and are favoured in conditions of K-selection [13].

Telomere-Telomerase System

It is known for many years that, in general, normal cells have a limited capacity of duplication (Hayflick limit) *in vitro* [132,133] and *in vivo* [134], documented for many types of cells [135,136,137], related to the life span of the species from which cells are derived [138], inversely related to the ages of donors of origin [139] and caused by something acting in the nucleus [140].

The cause of the Hayflick limit was hypothesised to be the progressive shortening of the DNA molecule at each duplication [141], as DNA polymerase cannot replicate a whole molecule of DNA and a little terminal portion of DNA would be ignored in replication [142].

One of the ends of DNA molecule (telomere) is constituted by a repetitive sequence, shown to be TTGGGG in a protozoan [143], and later for mammals, man included, to be only a little different (TTAGGG) [144] but common to many other species [145]. As hypothesised, telomere was proved to shorten at each duplication [146].

An enzyme, telomerase, capable to elongate telomere at each duplication, annulling DNA polymerase insufficiency, explained the existence of cells with unlimited duplication capacities, such as germ line cells [147]. It was shown that telomerase is present in immortal human cell lines [148] and repressed by regulatory proteins [149]. Its deactivation causes telomere shortening at each replication and the reduction of duplication capacity [150], while with its activation telomeres resulted elongated and cells acquired unlimited duplication capacities [151,152,153,154,155].

The final blockage of cell duplications (replicative senescence) is not an abrupt phenomenon but a progressive increase in the probability of blockage depending on telomere residual length [156,157]. Telomere is capped by particular protective nucleoproteins and oscillates between capped and uncapped states, with the duration of the capped state in direct relation to telomere length and with vulnerability for the passage to "noncycling state" (replicative senescence) in the uncapped state [158].

As stem cells, unlike germ cells, have levels of telomerase activity capable to restore only partially telomere length [159], *in vivo* stem cells even with partially shortened telomere, that is with a slight probability to pass to replicative senescence, could not duplicate unlimitedly [113].

The modulation of the telomere-telomerase function is likely different for each species [113] and this could explain why species with long telomeres [160] age precociously.

In correlation with telomere shortening, the overall cell functionality declines (cell senescence). This decay, as replicative senescence, is surely in correlation with the relative shortening of telomere (Fossel's "cell senescence limited model") [113]. In particular, experiments provoking telomerase activation reverse both replicative senescence and cell senescence [151,152,155]. The mechanism of cell senescence is likely a progressive repression of a subtelomeric DNA portion (transcriptional silencing), which regulates the overall cell functionality, caused by the progressive sliding of the protective nucleoproteins ("heterochromatin 'hood' ") of probable fixed length capping telomere and adjacent DNA in correlation with telomere shortening [113] (Figure 13).

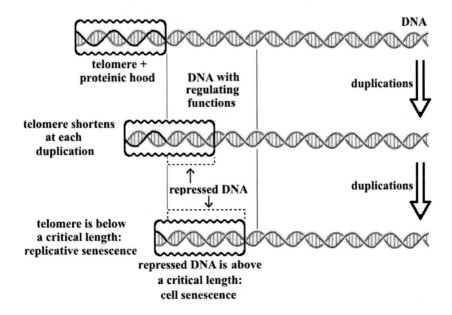

Figure 13. Telomere progressive shortening impairs the expression of many genes. It is likely the existence near to the telomere of a tract of DNA regulating overall cell functionality: with telomere shortening the proteinic "hood" capping the telomere slides down and alters this regulation.

The placing of a portion of DNA with essential regulatory activities in a position progressively impaired by telomere shortening is a strong element in support of the hypothesis that telomere-telomerase limits are adaptive.

In short, the limitation of cell duplication capacities and its modulation appear clearly to be not caused by insuperable physiological constraints but determined and regulated by genes specifically favoured by natural selection as adaptive.

Cell Turnover

Our body is composed of cells in continuous turnover with rates different for each cell type. It has been estimated that each year a mass of cell equal to our entire body weight is lost and substituted [161]. Even for some types of cells considered perennial, there is now evidence that they are subject to turnover (heart myocytes [162], muscle myocytes [163,164,165]). For other types of cells surely perennial, there is dependence on other cells with turnover, such as for the neurons on the gliocytes [113].

In normal conditions, cell elimination is the result of various forms of "programmed cell death" (PCD), such as removal by macrophages (red cells), keratinization and detaching from the somatic surface (skin) and apoptosis. In particular, apoptosis, an ordinate process of self-destruction with non-damaging disposal of cellular debris, was described for the first time as a phenomenon different from necrosis in a normal liver [86], is related to cell turnover in healthy adult organs [166,167,168] and is documented for many healthy tissues and organs [156,169,170,171,172,173,174,175,176,177,178,179,180].

The continuous elimination of cells by PCD must be balanced with the replication of appropriate stem cells and this cell turnover is limited by the genetic regulation of the telomere-telomerase system.

In short, for vertebrates but not for all animals (e.g., the adult stage of *Caenhorabditis elegans* has a fixed number of cells), three categories of cells are currently distinguished:

1) Those with high turnover: e.g., intestinal crypts cells [181];
2) Those with moderate turnover: e.g., cells of the deep layers of skin and endothelial cells [182], heart myocytes [162], muscle myocytes [163,164,165].
3) Those with no turnover, e.g., neurons, with a few possible exceptions [183] but always metabolically depending on gliocytes that are cells with turnover [113].

Atrophic Syndrome

The progressive shortening of telomeres, if we accept Fossel's cell senescence limited model [113], causes an "atrophic syndrome" characterised by:

a) increasing number of cells in replicative senescence (overall reduction of cell duplication capacities);
b) slowdown of the cell turnover;

c)   reduction of the overall number of cells (atrophy);
d)   hypertrophy of the remaining specific cells;
e)   possible substitution of the missing cells with nonspecific cells;
f)   increasing number of cell with altered functions (cell senescence);
g)   dysfunctional telomere-induced instability with consequent vulnerability to cancer [120].

A General Scheme for Ageing

It is easy to infer that cell turnover limitations caused by the telomere-telomerase system and linked or derived phenomena (cell senescence, atrophic syndrome, etc.) cause all the morphological and functional alterations that determine the fitness decline and, in their more advanced expression, the senile state (Fossel's cell senescence general model of ageing [21,113]) (Figure 14).

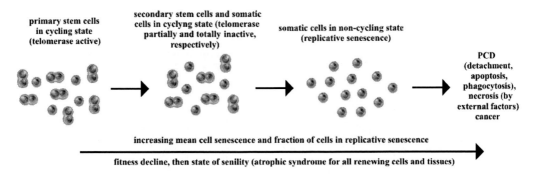

Figure 14. From primary stem cells with active telomerase, secondary stem cells and somatic cells with replicative capacity originate, but with telomerase partially and totally inactivated, respectively. From both types of cells, somatic cells in replicative senescence originate. Replicative senescence and cell senescence contribute to fitness decline that gradually becomes the senile state.

In support of this hypothesis:

1)   for mice, a factor inducing apoptosis and cell cycle arrest, provokes osteoporosis, a diminished stress tolerance, atrophy of all organs and a reduced longevity [184];

2)   in a rare human genetic disease (dyskeratosis congenita [185]), in which telomerase activity is low and telomeres are shorter than normal [186], tissues in which cells multiply rapidly (skin, nails, hair, gut and bone marrow, etc.) manifest precociously severe dysfunctions (alopecia, nail dystrophy, gut disorders, failure to produce blood cells, etc.) [182]. In this syndrome there is also a high cancer rate due to telomerase deficiency that cause unstable chromosomes [155,187].

3)   in another genetic disease, Werner syndrome, in which cell replication is impaired [188,189] and there is a limited replication capacity [139], tissues composed of cell with moderate turnover suffer from severe alterations (e.g., alterations in lens

epithelial cells, endothelial cells, Langherans β-cells, various types of derma cells provoke cataracts, atherosclerosis, type 2-diabetes, regional atrophy of subcutaneous tissue and skin atrophy, respectively) [190].

Examples of Normally Ageing Tissues

Intestinal Villi

In each intestinal crypt, there are four to six stem cells that with their intensive duplication activity renew continuously the epithelium of the small intestine [191]. In healthy old individuals, in comparison with young individuals the transit time for cells from crypts to villous tips decreases and villi become broader, shorter and with less cellularity [192] (Figure 15). These changes, surely due to a declining mitotic activity of crypt stem cells, as hypothesised from a long time [192], reduce intestinal functionality and, likely, overall fitness.

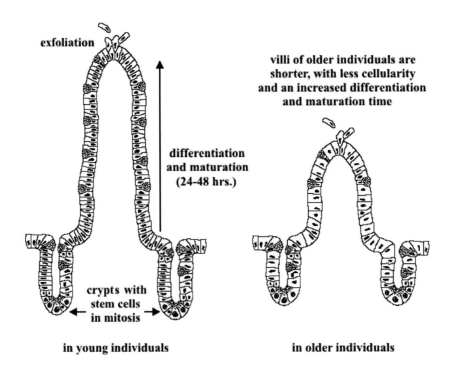

Figure 15. Intestinal villi in young and older individuals.

Endothelium

Endothelial cells manifest a continuous turnover assured by endothelial progenitor cells, derived by primary stem cells of bone marrow, and numerically in inverse relation with age [193]. A slackened turnover of endothelial cells increases the probability of endothelial dysfunction and, therefore, of diseases derived from altered blood circulation such as myocardial infarction and cerebral ischemia: indeed, the number of endothelial progenitor cells is a predictor of cardiovascular risk equal to or more significant than Framinghan risk score [193,194]. Diseases derived from compromised blood circulation are a common end to the life of healthy old individuals with no particular risk factor [195].

Epidermis

Human epidermis turnover is determined by stem cells located in the dermal-epidermal junction, a corrugated surface. In old subjects, dermal-epidermal junction is flattened, an indirect sign of the reduction of epidermis stem cells, and the rate of epidermal renewal is reduced [196]. In derma, as a likely consequence of the exhaustion of specific stem cells, a general reduction of all its components (melanocytes, Langerhans cells, dermal fibroblasts, capillaries, blood vessels within the reticular dermis, mast cells, eccrine glands, hair. etc.) is reported and nails grow more slowly [196].

Photoreceptor Cells

Photoreceptor cells (cones and rods) are highly differentiated nervous cells with no turnover, but metabolically depending from other cells with turnover, retina pigmented cells, which are highly differentiated gliocytes. Each day, with an extraordinary metabolic activity, every retina pigmented cell phagocytizes about 10% of the membranes with photopsin molecules of about 50 photoreceptor cells. With the age-related decline of retina pigmented cell turnover, the deficiency of their function kills the photoreceptors not served. This is above all manifested in the functionality of the more sensitive part of the retina, the macula, from which the name "age-related retina macular degeneration" (AMD) [197]. AMD affects 5%, 10% and 20% of subjects 60, 70 and 80 years old, respectively [198], and it is likely that a large proportion of older individuals suffer from AMD.

Neurons

Neurons are perennial cells but their vitality depends on other cells (e.g., microglia, a type of gliocytes) that show turnover. The hypothesis that Alzheimer Disease (AD) is caused by replicative senescence and cell senescence of microglia cells has been proposed [113,199].

Microglia cells degrade β-amyloid protein [200,201] and this function is known to be altered in AD [202] with the consequent noxious accumulation of the protein.

Telomeres have been shown to be significantly shorter in patients with probable AD than in apparently healthy control subjects [203]. AD could have, at least partially, a vascular aetiology due to age-related endothelial dysfunction [113] but "A cell senescence model might explain Alzheimer dementia without primary vascular involvement." [113]

An interesting comparison between AD and AMD is possible: both are probably determined by the death of cells with no turnover as a likely consequence of the age-related failure of cells with turnover (Figure 16). Moreover, AD frequency, as AMD, affects 1,5% of USA and Europe population at age 65 years and 30% at 80 [204] and a centenarian has a high probability of suffering from it.

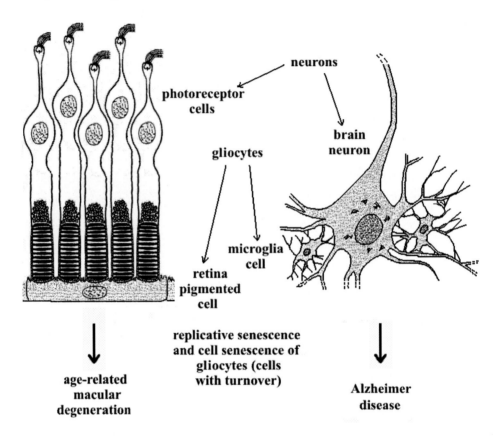

Figure 16. Schemes of retina photoreceptors and of a brain neuron (both neurons) served by two types of differentiated gliocytes, retina pigmented cells and microglia cells, respectively. Replicative senescence and cell senescence of retina pigmented cells and of microglia cells cause age-related macular degeneration and Alzheimer disease, respectively.

Other Organs/Tissues

In relation to the progressive failure of cell turnover, senescence in healthy subjects is also characterised by age-related: bone loss (→ osteoporosis), muscle atrophy (→ sarcopenia), reduction in the number and in the size of nephrons with consequent decline of renal function (→ renal insufficiency), atrophy of pulmonary alveoli (→ latent / manifest emphysema), decline of liver volume with increased size of the remaining epatocytes (→ latent / manifest hepatic insufficiency), loss of myocytes with hypertrophy of the remaining myocytes and enlargement of cardiac cavities (→ cardiac failure), reduction in the number of pacemaker cells in the sinus node (→ atrioventricular block and other arrhythmias), decline in the number and activity of pancreatic β-cells (→ latent / manifest diabetes mellitus), atrophy of gastric mucosa (→ atrophic gastritis), declining activity of lens epithelial cells (→ nuclear cataracts), atrophy of large intestine, atrophy of salivary glands, decrease of taste buds, thinning of the lingual epithelial, involution of red marrow with increasing decline of the number and activity of cells with hematological and immunological functions, etc. [195].

Moreover, telomere dysfunction in cells in replicative senescence, in particular those, mostly epithelial, with higher turnover, is a significant cause of cancer in older individuals [120].

Finally, we must consider the numberless complications for many organs deriving by the progressive impairment of endothelial, neuronal and immunological functions and, in general, by the interlacement of the decline of several functions [195].

Ageing in Short

The empirical evidence shows that an ageing individual suffers from a generalised atrophic syndrome and that death will be caused by the critical failure of one or several impaired functions. The atrophy of each tissue or organ is explained by the decline in cell turnover (Fossel's cell senescence general model of ageing [21,113]), which is caused by the limits of the telomere-telomerase system (Fossel's "cell senescence limited model" [113]).

The ageing phenomenon is therefore caused by limits genetically determined and regulated in a complex system [21] and these limits can be evolutionarily justified only accepting an adaptive meaning for fitness decline [16,18,21,22].

This conception is radically different from that currently accepted, which maintains:

1) *Ageing does not describe a distinct entity and is only an useful term to describe the numberless afflictions of the old age.* In fact, in the International Classification of Diseases (ICD-9-CM, http://icd9cm.chrisendres.com/), which has code numbers for each disease or physiological event needing medical advice (e.g., pregnancy, delivery, etc.), there is not a code for ageing / senescence but only a code for senility /old age (797) among "Symptoms, signs and ill-defined conditions". Likewise, in the ICD-10 (http://www.who.int/classifications/apps/icd/icd10online/) there is only a code for senility / old age (R54) in the chapter XVIII, titled "Symptoms, signs and abnormal clinical and laboratory findings, not elsewhere classified (R00-R99)", paragraph "General symptoms and signs (R50-R69)", and therefore not including distinct diseases or physiological events. In fact, for current medicine and in official classifications, ageing as a distinct entity is nonexistent and old individuals never die by ageing but, in general, by one or more diseases typical of old age.

2) *Old individuals have tissues and organs that have been progressively impaired by a lot of different damaging factors, in particular oxidizing agents.* This thesis appears to ignore cell turnover and the experiments where cells in replicative senescence and with all the manifestations of cell senescence are transformed by telomerase activation into cells with unlimited replication capacities and without signs of cell senescence [151,152,153,154,155]. "... there is something fundamental controlling the occurrence or accumulation of cellular free radical damage, something

controlling the balance between damage and homeostasis. Free radical damage accumulates in somatic cells, but homeostasis is a sufficient match in germ cell lines. Alteration in gene expression, modulated by telomere length, is a likely candidate for such control." [113] Oxidative damage becomes a problem when cell turnover slackens and cell senescence increases: limits in the telomere-telomerase system are the primary cause and oxidative damage only a consequence [113].

3) *Ageing, being the consequence of numberless and random factors, is in principle not likely controllable and strong efforts could obtain only a slowing down of an inevitable process.* This is contrast with the evidence of the telomere-telomerase system, cell turnover, atrophic syndrome caused by cell turnover decline, and experiments documenting that at cell level senescence is totally reversible and avoidable [113].

4) *Ageing is something intrinsic to the condition of the living being, in particular of multicellular organisms, and therefore it is inevitable.* This is in plain contrast with the existence of many species that in the wild show no increase in mortality (e.g., rockfish, sturgeon, turtles, bivalves, etc. [111]) and defined, if with considerable life spans, "animals with negligible senescence" [98] or "ageless animals" (http://www.agelessanimals.org/). There are even species with mortality decreasing with age, e.g., depending on an increasing body size [112]. On the contrary, individuals of some unicellular eukaryotic species age, that is the telomere-telomerase system allows only a limited number of duplications (replicative senescence) and, in relation to the previous number of duplications, causes a decline in the overall functionality of the cell (cell senescence) with an increasing sensibility to apoptotic stimuli [122,123,124].

5) *Age-related increasing mortality, alias fitness decline, cannot be adaptive because natural selection favours individuals with greater fitness.* Natural selection favours genes with positive inclusive fitness, even with negative individual fitness [59,80,81,82,83], and, therefore, in principle a gene causing age-related fitness decline, that is negative individual fitness, could be favoured by natural selection in particular ecological conditions [21]. The existence, in the wild, both of species with fitness decline and of species without fitness decline are a demonstration that unavoidable universal senescence-causing factors are unlikely and that both cases are somehow adaptive. It is remarkable that replicative senescence and cell senescence in yeast are weighed as adaptive [20,127,128,129,130,131] and the logical consequence would be to accept as possible that the effects of the telomere-telomerase system in multicellular organisms are adaptive too.

Weight of Ageing for Life Span and Longevity

The effects of fitness decline on life span (mean duration of life, ML) and longevity are huge and often underestimated. For a species with a fixed mortality rate (λ), survivors at time t (Y_t) are given by the formula:

$$Y_t = Y_0 (1 - \lambda)^t \tag{10}$$

With $Y_0 = 1$, life span (ML) is:

$$ML = {}_{t=0}[(1 - \lambda)^t]^{t=\infty} = - \frac{1}{Log_e(1 - \lambda)} \tag{11}$$

and the time t when Y_t individuals survive is:

$$t = \frac{Log(Y_t)}{Log(1 - \lambda)} \tag{12}$$

In USA, 2005 statistics say that for the total population the probability of dying between ages 20 to 25 and between ages 25 to 30 were 0.004869 and 0.004865, respectively, which is about 0.00097/year [205]. With $\lambda = 0.00097$, without the age-related mortality increase the life expectancy of 20-30 years old individuals (ML_{20-30}) would be about 1,030 years and 1% would be alive after 4,745 years.

Excluding accidents (unintentional injuries) and homicides, which caused in 2005 about half of the deaths for 20-30 years old individuals [205], that is roughly halving the value of λ to 0.0005, ML_{20-30} would be about 1,999 years and 1% would be alive after 9,208 years!

The same statistics say that the probability of dying between ages 55 to 60 was 0.036299, which is about 0.00726/year [205], 7.45 times the mortality of 20-25 and 25-30 years cohorts. With this value ML_{55-60} would be about 137 years and 1% would be alive after 632 years.

It must be underlined that an individual without an age-related increasing mortality rate would have an "unlimited longevity" but this should not be confused with the concept of "immortality" (infinite longevity and life span). In fact, an individual of a species with negligible senescence (ageless animal) or even of a species with age-related decreasing mortality (negative senescence [112]) dies by events that are mortal at any age (severe infections, accidents, predation, killing by other individuals of the same species, etc.; in short, extrinsic mortality) and, moreover, at ages when practically no individual survives in the wild for the extrinsic mortality and so there is no natural selection, if the individual survives because reared in protected conditions, it is possible the onset of unforeseeable and deadly internal imbalances. Therefore, a hypothetical man with no age-related increasing mortality should be in the condition of unlimited longevity but limited life span.

Interactions between Diseases of Different Categories and between Ageing and Diseases

Evolutionary interactions between diseases of different categories and between diseases and disease-like phenomena, in particular senescence, are important. For the sake of brevity, only some interactions will be outlined.

A. Interactions between Diseases Caused by Alterations of the Genotype (Category 1) and Ageing (Category 5.3.2)

Equilibrium frequency of a harmful gene C (C_e) and of its phenotypic expression (P_e) are both in inverse function of [s] (absolute value of the disadvantage s; see formulas 1-7), which is depending on the reproductive value of the individuals damaged by C. In species with age-related fitness decline, as older individual have a smaller expectation of life and, therefore, a smaller reproductive value, if C damages older individuals, C_e and P_e will be greater than for another harmful gene damaging younger individuals, that is a disease caused by an alteration of genotype that manifests itself at older ages (e.g., Huntington's disease) is expected to have higher frequency.

In numerical terms, if a dominant harmful gene C kills (s = -1) at an age when in the wild (or in the ancestral condition) only 1% of the population survives and the frequency of mutation into C from neutral alleles is 0.00001, the frequency of the diseases (P_e) is expected to be:

$$P_e \approx 0.00001 / [0.01 \cdot -1] = 0.001 \tag{13}$$

The opposite concept, the hypothesis that age-related fitness decline is caused by the combined effect of many harmful genes acting at older ages and insufficiently eliminated by natural selection (mutation accumulation theory) is untenable because contradicted by theoretical arguments [10,13,21] and unsupported by empirical evidence.

B. Interactions between Diseases Caused by Interactions with Other Species (Category 3) and Ageing (Category 5.3.2)

A parasite damaging an older individual of a host species with age-related fitness decline, causes a disadvantage lower than a parasite damaging a younger individual, as older individuals have less reproductive value. Therefore, it is expected that older individuals will suffer from the effects of parasite actions more severely that younger individuals as natural selection is less effective when the reproductive value is lower. For humans, the greater gravity of infections in older individuals is well known and documented [195].

C. Interactions between Diseases Caused by Alterations of the Ecological Niche (Category 2) and Diseases Caused by Interactions with Other Species (Category 3)

The huge and continuous modifications of human ecological niche caused by technological innovations, urbanisation, demographic growth, changes of lifestyle, foods, hygienic habits, etc., have greatly altered the conditions to which the species is adapted. Fragile and intricate evolutionary balances between the man and his numerous parasites, attained after thousands of human generations (and millions of parasite generations) have been crushed with catastrophic results, worse than for any other human disaster or calamitous event, war included. Some examples:

1) The extraordinary growth of human population and of its demographic density, its aggregation in urban crowds with water polluted and habitations infested by infected animals, the cohabitation or proximity with bred animals, dangerous hygienic habits, etc., have provoked from the ancient times dreadful epidemics (black death, bubonic plague, smallpox, typhus, cholera, influenza, hepatitis A, tuberculosis, HIV, etc.) with the deaths of hundreds of millions of men. From 1347 to 1640, Black Death, a disease probably different from bubonic plague [206] was the scourge of Europe and other parts of the world, with more than 100 millions of victims (Figure 17). In 1918-1920 a single epidemic of influenza (Spanish flu) killed perhaps 40-50 million people worldwide [207] or, according to current estimates, 50-100 millions [208], that is from 2 to 5 times the deaths caused by World War I in five years. When Europeans reached the America, they were selected, much more than American indigenous people, by centuries of terrible epidemics. The germs that they spread unintentionally in America were dangerous for them but very frequently lethal for indigenous populations, which were devastated by smallpox, measles, influenza and other diseases for which they had no evolutionary experience [209].

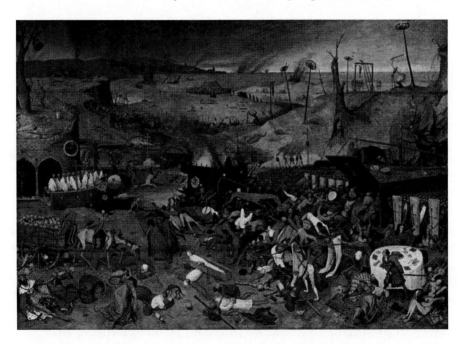

Figure 17. *The Triumph of Death* (black plague), a painting of Pieter Bruegel the Elder.

2) Statistical data show that alterations of the ecological niche and, on the other hand, corrections of these alterations are far more important of non-preventive medical treatment, antibiotics included. In fact, in USA infectious disease mortality rate has strongly declined before the introduction of sulphonamides and penicillin, and the usage of these drugs and of many new antibiotics has not changed sensibly the

decline of mortality by infections [210]. In recent years, mortality by infections is increasing because of HIV diffusion and, perhaps, of increasing antibiotic resistance (Figure 18).

Indeed, use and abuse of antibiotics and chemotherapeutic substances have selected antibiotic resistant bacteria with weighty consequences (about 90,000 U.S. residents die each year by nosocomial infections [211]). Even vaccines, a medical triumph, if not properly planned or used, can "provoke and even be overcome by pathogen evolution" [212].

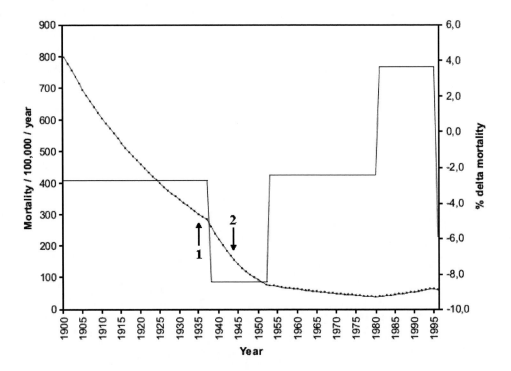

Figure 18. Overall trends in infectious disease mortality rate and per cent variation of mortality rate in USA from 1900 to 1996 [210]. The episodic strong increase in mortality due to 1918 influenza pandemic has been disregarded. Sulfonamids were released in 1935 (arrow 1) and the beginning of clinical use of penicillin was in 1943 (arrow 2) but there is no clear effect of their use on mortality rates.

3) Hygienic or iper-hygienic habits restrict and delay the first exposure to microbes and parasitic worms or make impossible infections or infestations. These modifications of the ecological niche, in principle always beneficial for traditional medicine, on the contrary for evolutionary medicine are potentially harmful and dangerous.

Delayed exposure to poliovirus is a likely cause of modern epidemics of poliomyelitis, a scourge till worldwide application of polio vaccines [209]. Poliovirus has been for thousands of years an endemic pathogen, which rarely caused poliomyelitis or infantile paralysis, until to the 1880s, when major epidemics of poliomyelitis began to occur in Europe and, soon after, in the United States [213].

Reduced exposure to allergens, especially in early life, caused by modern extreme hygiene, is a significant risk factor for allergy and is the most likely explanation, at present, for the extraordinary worldwide increase in atopic allergy [51].

"Hygiene hypothesis" maintains that exposure to bacteria, viruses and parasitic worms during childhood protects against the development of allergies [214] and atopic diseases [215]. Allergies may be caused by a delayed establishment of gut flora in infants [216].

For diabetes mellitus type 1, an autoimmune disorder, it is hypothesised that "... increased hygiene may contribute to an imbalance of the immune system, facilitating autoimmune reactions [against β-cells] when virus infections, or proteins like cow's milk or gluten, provoke." [217]

Some intestinal worms secrete chemicals that suppress the immune system to prevent the host from attacking the parasite [218] and without these substances the immune system becomes unbalanced and oversensitive [219]. Clinical trials have been initiated to test the effectiveness of certain worms in treating some allergies [220].

The deliberate infestation with a parasitic worm (helminthic therapy) is a promising treatment for several autoimmune diseases such as Crohn's disease [221,222,223], ulcerative colitis [223], multiple sclerosis [224], allergic asthma [220,225], etc., whose incidence is greatly increased in recent years and, moreover, is greater in industrialised countries in comparison with developing countries with less strict hygienic habits [225,226,227,228]. These autoimmune and allergic disorders, and others, are explained by the Hygiene hypothesis, which is in short a thesis of evolutionary medicine.

4) The abuse of soaps, deodorants, detergents, disinfectants, etc., modifies normal microbial flora of epidermis and external mucosae (especially of armpits, genitals and hands) and causes the spreading of pathogens, in particular fungi (personal observation).

D. Interactions between Diseases Caused by Alterations of the Ecological Niche (Category 2) and Ageing (Category 5.3.2)

Various alterations of the ecological niche and the diseases caused by them (cigarette smoking, diabetes mellitus, hypertension, hypercholesteremia, obesity, alcoholism, etc.; "risk factors") increase physiological cell turnover, likely provoking a greater apoptosis rate, and therefore accelerate the onset of manifestations that without them should be present only in older individuals [193]. The effects of risk factors are countered by drugs with organ protection qualities ("protective drugs") such as statins [193,229], ACE-inhibitors and sartans [230], probably by normalisation of apoptosis rate.

Risk factors increase the frequency of cardiovascular diseases and accelerate their onset [195]. Smoking, diabetes, and obesity are risk factors for AMD [231]. There is association between Alzheimer disease and risk factors [232].

Protective drugs reduce the risk of cardiovascular diseases [229,230] and of diabetes [233,234], are effective in the prevention of atrial fibrillation [235,236] and against Alzheimer disease [237].

Statins reduce decline in lung function [238] and lower the risk of nuclear cataract [239].

Some diseases caused by alterations of the genotype, such as Werner syndrome and dyskeratosis congenita have analogous effects of risk factors on cells with moderate and high turnover, respectively [182] (Figure 19).

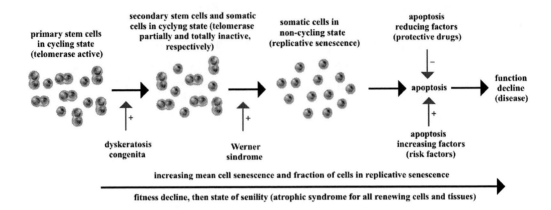

Figure 19. Risk factors (and some genetic diseases) increase apoptosis rate and cell turnover. Protective drugs counter the effect of risk factors but it is not documented the capacity of reducing physiological turnover rate.

Comparison between Evolutionary Disease Categories and the Breakdown Types of a Machine

It is possible a comparison between the various disease categories classified in evolutionary terms and the various types of breakdowns of a machine (e.g., a car) (Figure 20).

The industrialist is certainly very careful in its manufacture, but it is inevitable that some cars will be sold with one or more faults in construction. As for more frequent defects the manufacturer will adopt opportune measures, it is predictable that each particular defect will have a limited frequency. The breakdowns caused by these defects are analogous to the diseases caused by alterations of the genotype.

A car has a range of operative conditions, e.g., specific types of oil, lubricants and fuel to be used, particular maintenance operations to be observed, etc. The owners not observing manufacturer indications expose their cars to conditions for which the car is not designed and therefore they will risk failures. The breakdowns with these causes are analogous to the diseases caused by alterations of the ecological niche.

In their use, cars can collide with other motor-vehicles or be damaged by vandals. These harms are analogous to the diseases caused by interactions with other species.

If the owner uses the car on roads with gravely uneven surface or to cross a stream or for other conditions for which the car is by no means designed, it is probable a damage, which is analogous to the diseases caused by conditions beyond adaptation range.

As years go, the car wears out, breakdowns becomes more and more frequent, repairs more and more expensive and difficult, spare parts are of not easy finding, until to the car is unusable and must be scraped. In part, this is due to mechanical wear and to some components that cannot be substituted (or with replacements too expensive). In part, this is because cars have a built-in obsolescence, that is they are designed not for the greatest duration but to last for a certain period after which the machine must begin to break down with increasing frequency and with increasing costs for the owner until to he is induced to buy a new machine. Built-in obsolescence and its consequences are analogous to ageing manifestations.

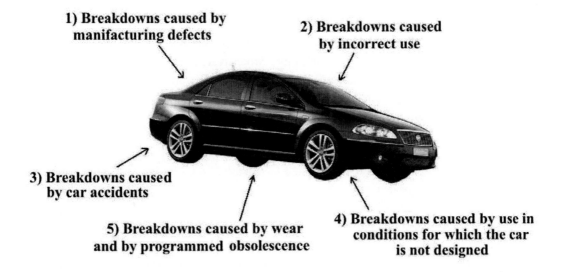

Figure 20. Categories of car breakdowns, in analogy with the evolutionary classification of diseases and the peculiar phenomenon of ageing.

The concept of planned or built-in obsolescence is less known and obvious than that of mechanical wear.

In 1983, I wrote:

"Built-in obsolescence is that characteristic of an industrial product, specifically planned and pursued, for which the product deteriorates and becomes more and more hardly repairable after a definite time, even though being reliable and fully usable before that time.

Built-in obsolescence causes a waste of materials and a considerable economic overload for the consumer, but has at least three important advantages.

The first is to avoid that the annual part of renewal of a product in a stable market be minimal. For example, a nation in which there are 10 millions of motor-vehicles, with a mean duration of ten years, demands for replacement an annual production of 1 million of motor-vehicles. If the mean duration of a car would increase to 20 years, the annual production should fall to 0.5 millions, with catastrophic consequences for proceeds and employment. The second advantage is the introduction of new technologies with speed inversely proportional to the mean duration of the product. A product with unlimited duration would delay or even make economically disadvantageous the use of new and more effective technologies. The third advantage is that a productive system organised for a quick and continuous renewal is easily adaptable to: a) an unexpected market growth; b) the opening of new markets; c) the conversion to the production of other items; d) the transformation in military industry, etc. On the contrary, the production of goods with very long duration, as there is a minimal annual production, is not much fit to the aforesaid events.

In this regard, I have the following beliefs.

Built-in obsolescence is a hidden pillar of the modern "consumer culture". Neither manufacturers nor trade unions, nor politicians have interest to publicise such pillar.

The consumer believes that it is not possible to make products with greater duration or that the necessary modifications would render the product too expensive. These opinions are wrong and on the contrary considerable efforts in the design of an industrial consumer product are directed to make the product both accurate and reliable until to a certain time and afterwards not much reliable and more and more expensively repairable.

Built-in obsolescence of an industrial product and the programmed senescence of a living being are two very different phenomena, yet the analogies are considerable and not superficial. With opportune modifications of the terms, the main common aim is that to allow to the industrial product or to the living being the greatest evolution, the greatest adaptability to new conditions, the greatest competitiveness in the struggle.

If the considerations stated regarding senescence are true:

It is tragic to observe that the man and his machines share a last fate similar in its essence.

It is ironic to consider that the modern technology even in this has been preceded and exceeded by the Nature.

It is incredible that in a civilisation in which built-in obsolescence is fundamental, it is not known that the living world obeys to a parallel logic" (translated from Italian [10]).

From Wikipedia (14/08/2008)
Article: Planned Obsolescence

"Planned obsolescence (also built-in obsolescence in the United Kingdom) is the process of a product becoming obsolete and/or non-functional after a certain period or amount of use in a way that is planned or designed by the manufacturer. Planned obsolescence has potential benefits for a producer because the product fails and the consumer is under pressure to purchase again, whether from the same manufacturer (a replacement part or a newer model), or from a competitor, which might also rely on planned obsolescence. For an industry, planned obsolescence stimulates demand by encouraging purchasers to buy again sooner if they still want a functioning product. Built-in obsolescence is in many different products, from vehicles to light bulbs, from buildings to software. There is, however, the potential backlash of consumers who learn that the manufacturer invested money to make the product obsolete faster; such consumers might turn to a producer, if any, which offers a more durable alternative.

Planned obsolescence was first developed in the 1920s and 1930s when mass production had opened every minute aspect of the production process to exacting analysis.

Estimates of planned obsolescence can influence a company's decisions regarding product engineering. Therefore, the company can use the least expensive components that satisfy product lifetime projections. Such decisions are part of a broader discipline known as value engineering.

The use of planned obsolescence is not always easy to pinpoint, and it is complicated by related problems, such as competing technologies or creeping featurism, which expands functionality in newer product versions.

- Rationale behind the strategy

A new product development strategy that seeks to make existing products obsolete may appear counter intuitive, particularly if coming from a leading marketer of the existing products. Why would a firm deliberately endeavour to reduce the value of its existing product portfolio?

The rationale behind the strategy is to generate long-term sales volume by reducing the time between repeat purchases (referred to as shortening the replacement cycle). Firms that pursue this strategy believe that the additional sales revenue it creates more than offsets the additional costs of research and development and opportunity costs of existing product line cannibalization. However, the rewards are by no means certain: in a competitive industry, this can be a risky strategy because consumers may decide to buy from competitors. Because of this, gaining by this strategy requires fooling the consumers on the actual cost per use of the item in comparison to the competition.

Shortening the replacement cycle has many critics as well as supporters. Critics such as Vance Packard claim the process wastes resources and exploits customers. Resources are used up making changes, often cosmetic changes, that are not of great value to the customer. Supporters claim it drives technological advances and contributes to material well-being. They claim that a market structure of planned obsolescence and rapid innovation may be preferred to long-lasting products and slow innovation. In a fast paced competitive industry, market success requires that products are made obsolete by actively developing replacements. Waiting for a competitor to make products obsolete is a sure guarantee of future demise ..."

An Example of Difference between the Current Classification of Diseases and the Evolutionary Classification

Some subjects suffer in juvenile age from myocardial infarction or cerebral ischemia as outcome of serious hereditary hypercholesteremia or other genetic diseases. Others, smokers and/or obese and/or diabetic and/or hypertensive middle-aged subjects, are hit by the same affections. Others, non-smokers non-obese non-diabetic old subjects, suffer from the same diseases.

In the traditional classification, the three groups of patients are classified together, while in the evolutionary classification their affections are divided in three distinct groups of diseases.

It being understood that the aforesaid diseases in their manifestations are treated in the same way, in the evolutionary classification there is a clear-cut distinction.

In the first case, we have diseases deriving from alterations of the genotype: practically they are not preventable (with the exception of therapeutic abortion that is not exactly a prevention), it is possible a precocious identification, pharmacological treatment reduces the risk, ideal therapy is genetic, ideal prevention is eugenics before conception.

In the second case, we have diseases deriving from alterations of the ecological niche. Effective prevention is possible and should be the best choice. Pharmacological treatment reduces the risk of new events but the correction of ecological niche alterations should be the main measure.

In the third case, we have diseases deriving from a physiological function as ageing appears to be. Prevention is not possible. Pharmacological treatment could reduce but not cancel the risk, which increases with the age. The only effective measure could be a genetic modification of ageing regulating and determining mechanisms.

Strategies to Reduce Morbidity Rates and to Increase Life Span and Longevity

1. Actions for the First Evolutionary Category of Diseases (Caused by Alterations of the Genotype)

Today: If possible, precocious identification of subjects with genetic diseases and their pharmacological treatment. Therapeutic abortion in some cases.

In the future:

- Option A - Overcoming the limits of current gene therapy [240], in particular the transitory success of the therapy, caused by cell turnover if the corrected gene is not inserted in stem cells, and the possibility that an insertion may inactivate a suppressor oncogene and arouse a cancer (insertional oncogenesis) [241] (Figure 21), development of methods with which it will possible to insert in a sure way in the genome of the patient the corrected gene in a position not causing possible dangerous interference with other genes. Treatment of genetic diseases with gene therapy, in a way that the therapeutic method is unvarying and only the genetic inserted sequence changes. Limitation of the reproduction of subjects with genetic alterations, subordinating the reproduction to controls, if possible, of the genetic condition of the foetus.

- Option B - Development of methods with which it will possible to substitute in a sure way the altered gene with the corrected gene in the genome of the patient and in all his cells, germinal cells included (Figures 22 and 23). Reproduction without restrictions as long as it is verified that the substitution has been made correctly.

- Effects: Limitation of morbidity and mortality deriving from genetic diseases. Limitations of the progressive increase in their incidence in the future generations. Limited increase in the mean duration of life. No increase in longevity.

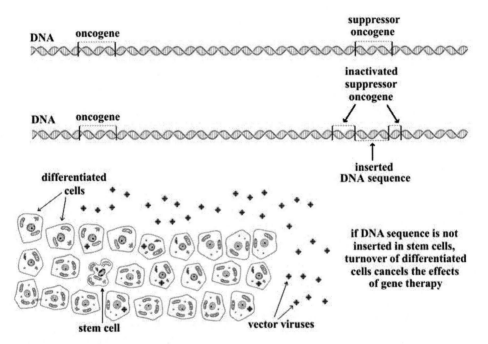

Figure 21. Current gene therapy. DNA sequence is inserted in a random position by a vector virus. If an insertion inactivates a suppressor oncogene, this may cause a cancer. The type of vector virus and/or limits in the dose of viruses inoculated may cause the transformation only of differentiated cells and not of the rare stem cells and, consequently, the transitory success of the therapy, because cell turnover gradually substitutes differentiated cells with new cells originated from non-transformed stem cells.

2. Actions for the Second Category of Diseases (Caused by Alterations of the Ecological Niche)

Today: Generally, after the manifestation of the disease, it is strongly advised to avoid risk factors. The people and many physicians have not a precise knowledge of the risk factors. The affection is defined disease and there is not a full awareness that the pathological condition is the alteration of the ecological niche.

In the future: Optimal knowledge of the ecological conditions to which our species is adapted. It is necessary to define the risk for each alteration of the ecological niche and to spread in the population and the medical categories the knowledge of the risks. Prevalent utilisation of the resources for prevention. Adoption of measures discouraging risk behaviours. The cures for subjects not observing preventive measures and advice must be the last bastion.

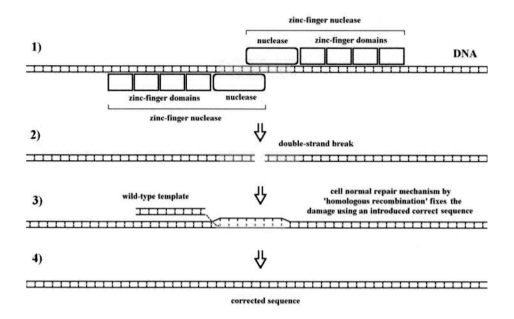

Figure 22. Option B. The corrected gene is inserted in substitution of the altered gene. With the use of two zinc-finger nucleases, composed of zinc-finger domains (each specific for a particular three-base DNA sequence) and a nuclease (a Type IIS restriction enzyme), it is possible to break DNA double-strand in a precise point with the successive correction by normal cell DNA-repair system by using an introduced DNA corrected sequence [242]. This method appears very promising [243].

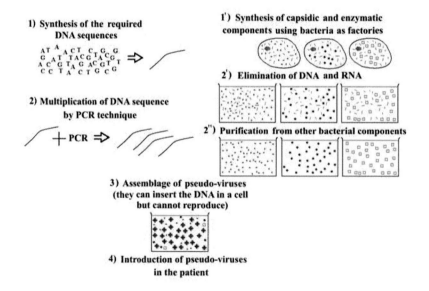

Figure 23. Creation of gene vectors (hypothetical scheme). The required DNA sequences (for the specific zinc-finger nucleases, for the gene to be modified, etc.) are created starting from defective viral sequences and from single nucleotides and multiplied by using PCR technique. Capsidic components and enzymes essential for the assemblage and activation of pseudo-virus are synthesised by using transformed bacteria and later eliminating DNA, RNA and other bacterial components. DNA sequence and capsidic and enzymatic components are assembled creating pseudo-viruses able to insert or substitute a DNA sequence in a cell but not to reproduce.

Effects: Drastic reduction of all the pathologies classifiable in this category with parallel reduction of morbidity and mortality. Reduction of the related sanitary costs. Increase in life span. No increase in longevity.

3. Actions for the Third Category of Diseases (Caused by Interactions with Other Species)

Today: Indiscriminate actions against any type of infection or parasitosis. Excessive or inappropriate use of antibiotics. Scarce attention to the ancestral ecological relationship between man and microbial species and parasites.

In the future: Widening of the study of the relations between man and his parasites. Reduction or elimination of the circumstances that increase the danger of parasitic infection and epidemics. Limits in the excessive or inappropriate use of antibiotics. A greater and prevalent use of preventive measures and vaccines.

Effects: Reduction of morbidity and mortality. Reduction of antibiotic-resistance cases. Increase in life span. No increase in longevity.

4. Actions for the Fourth Category of Diseases (Caused by Conditions beyond Adaptation Range)

Today: Actions that reduce risk conditions.

In the future: More careful actions to reduce risk conditions (e.g., safer cars and roads, greater severity and observance of safety measures at work, etc.)

Effects: Reduction of morbidity and mortality. Increase in life span. No increase in longevity.

5. Actions for Ageing

Today: Ageing is considered not a physiological event but a mixed set of diseases with age-related increasing frequency and severity. Ageing manifestations are empirically treated for their dysfunctions and in analogy with diseases showing the same dysfunctions. The cures allow often an increase in survival time in conditions of low quality of life.

In future: It is indispensable to acquire the awareness that ageing is something other than a disease phenomenon and that needs specific measures. It is possible to conceive an ambitious project for the solution of the problem in four steps:

Step 1
Parallel pursuit of various targets (duration: at least a decade)

a)   Widening of the studies on the telomere-telomerase system;
b)   The same for apoptosis phenomenon;

c) The same for cell turnover of all tissues and its effect on the functions of the organs;
d) The same for the morphogenesis of the organs, in particular for the dentition;
e) Development of genetic techniques for the effective and precise insertion of a genetic sequence in a point of the genome not causing dangerous alterations;
f) Development of genetic techniques for the effective and precise substitution of a genetic sequence with another sequence;
g) Research of possible safe drugs to modify the telomere-telomerase system and/or cell turnover (or other) so that longevity is increased.

Step 2

Parallel pursuit of various targets (duration: at least a decade)

a) Experiments on animals of insertion of genetic sequences to modify the modulation of the telomere-telomerase system for increasing longevity;
b) The same with techniques of genetic substitution;
c) First applications of the above-mentioned techniques for the treatment of severe genetic diseases;
d) First applications of the above-mentioned techniques for the treatment of age-related severe diseases such as age-related macular degeneration and Alzheimer's disease;
e) As with (a) and (b) to obtain multiple dentitions;
f) Experiments on animals of possible drugs with increasing longevity qualities.

Step 3

Duration: at least two decades

a) First experiments on man of gene therapy (but not on germinal cells) and of possible drugs with increasing longevity qualities;
b) Verification of the results and progressive widening of the experiments.

Step 4

Duration: indeterminate

a) Possible experimentation and application of gene therapy on human germinal cells;
b) Applications on a large scale of safe and tested techniques and drugs

Effects: Increase in the mean duration of life deriving from longevity increase.

For the extreme weight of the argument, the creation of an apposite international agency, adequately funded, could be useful, with the specific aim of controlling ageing and, as a very important corollary, genetic diseases, following the example and the wonderful outcomes of NASA (Figure 24).

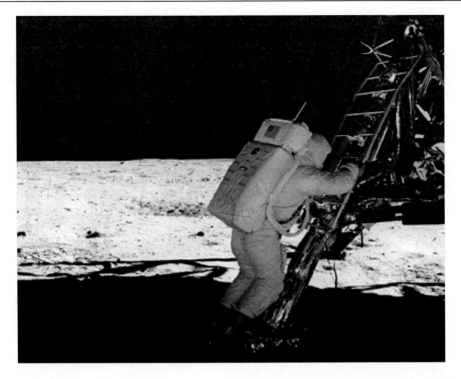

Figure 24. President John F. Kennedy focused NASA, founded in 1958 by Eisenhower, on sending astronauts to the moon by the end of the 1960s. This aim was achieved on July 20, 1969 (from NASA official site http://www.nasa.gov/).

Characteristics of a Future Age with Unlimited Longevity

When Moses, by then very old and just before his death, saw from the mountain of Nebo the Promised Land [Deuteronomy, 34], certainly the Hebrews wept for joy and imagined the ending of all their torments. However, the Promised Land, though ending the many pains they had suffered in Sinai, was the beginning of many other sufferings, struggles and disillusions.

A world with unlimited longevity would be as the Promised Land: many pains of today would end, but many others would begin. Our descendants would commiserate with us for our limited life span and longevity but would envy us for so many other things.

A society composed of individuals with very long longevity cannot be in a simple way the same society of today. All or most would have to change.

A very small risk to life considered today acceptable because the expectation of life is a few decades becomes unacceptable if there is a very long expectation of life. Rigorous measures to prevent incidents—with a severity currently unimaginable—would be the rule.

Today, procreation is free and one of the rights considered inviolable. The limitation of only one child per family imposed in China seems to most people an unacceptable limitation. In a society with a very long life span, births would be regulated and limited in proportion.

Children would be a rare exception, cuddled and protected by whole communities. Motherhood would become a rare privilege.

Today, marriage is a life-long oath and its break is a trauma strongly discouraged. Marriage would be transformed into a temporary engagement with specific rules and limitations.

Powerful and/or rich persons would be able to obtain peaks of power and/or wealth today inconceivable. Many rules would be arranged to limit the excesses and to assure turnover in power management.

Today, a man studies for a certain period of his life, then works for another period and then retires on a pension, enjoying the fruits of his work. This way of life would not be possible any longer. Perhaps there would be an alternation between periods of work and others of rest or study.

The mean level of education would increase enormously, and cases of persons with various degrees and specialisations would be frequent as well, because after a certain period there would be a psychological demand to change the object of study and work.

There would be extreme attention to beautiful, artistic and poetical things, and there would be supreme examples of lovers of artistic disciplines, but also monstrous examples of egoism and wickedness.

But there would be also the spread of what the Romans called *tedium vitae*, and perhaps suicide would become the main cause of death.

The wars—in memory—would become a symbol of extreme madness, but the world would be static and uniform. Our descendants would commiserate with us for our innumerable wars and yet in historical action representations would pursue those emotions that they would lack entirely in everyday life—a little like when we deplore the troubles of the past centuries but are fascinated by representations of warriors fighting with swords, bows and other ancient weapons.

And what are we to say of philosophy, religion, politics, poetry, sociology, psychology, etc.? All changes if the expectation of life is immensely great.

Cynics and unbelievers would state that God, religion and philosophy are reformulated and adapted to the new society, showing once again to be only creations of the human mind.

Mystics and believers would state instead that God, religion and philosophy are unchanged in their essence and that a life unlimited in its duration allows a better level of comprehension, because we would be less limited by physical ties.

Economics and politics would have radically different aims. Today, we plan for the contemporary generation and a little—if one is farsighted—for the next. In the future, men would think first to the future, as the contemporary generation would have to live in that time.

Conclusion

The development and the efficacious application on a large scale of safe techniques of gene therapy would reduce the consequences of diseases of category 1 (diseases caused by alterations of the genotype).

Respect for the ecological conditions to which the human species is adapted would largely reduce morbidity and mortality of diseases of category 2 (diseases caused by alterations of the ecological niche).

A better comprehension of the interactions between our species and its parasites and of the ecological conditions that minimise their damage, a greater use of vaccines and a more intelligent use of antibiotics would relieve the impact of diseases of category 3 (diseases caused by interactions with other species).

Strong precautionary measures would reduce the impact of diseases of category 4 (diseases caused by conditions beyond adaptation range).

Improvements in health cures and greater social assistance would improve the survival and the quality of life of elderly persons.

The entirety of the aforesaid measures would increase the mean duration of life, but longevity would be unvaried (Figure 25), except for a greater survival in very bad conditions of older persons.

A modification of our genetic program in the part that limits longevity would increase life span and longevity without a theoretical limit. It will be essential to make decisions regarding the ethical nature and advisability of this possibility, but here there is a boundary between science and politics, religion and human free will.

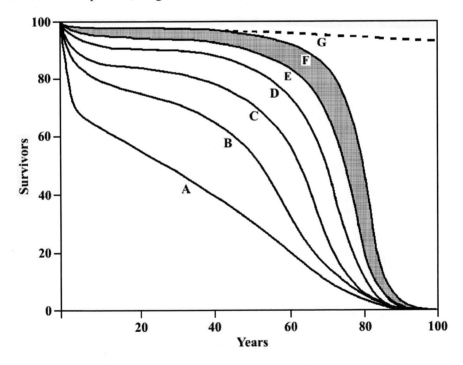

Figure 25. Life tables of human species (inspired by Figure 0.1 in [244]) illustrating a historical progressive increase in life span while longevity appears unchanged (curves A-E). Actual condition in developed countries is roughly indicated by curve E. With good preventive measures and better health treatment curve F is a likely outcome, with a little further increase in life span (dashed area) but not in longevity. Only with a modification of the progressive increase in mortality caused by intrinsic factors (ageing) will a drastic increase in life span and longevity be possible (curve G).

Appendix: Calculation of Equilibrium Frequencies

C is a gene having an advantage or disadvantage s in the homozygous condition and s' in the heterozygote condition. C' is its inactive allele. The notations C_n and C'_n indicate the frequency at the n-th generation of C and C', respectively. The frequency of mutation of C' in C is indicated with v and that of C in C' with u.

The frequencies of C_{n+1} and C'_{n+1} are given by:

$$C_{n+1} = \frac{C_n + C_n^2\, s + 2\, C_n\, C'_n\, s' + C'_n\, v - C_n\, u}{T} \tag{A1}$$

$$C'_{n+1} = \frac{C'_n + 2\, C_n\, C'_n\, s' - C'_n\, v + C_n\, u}{T} \tag{A2}$$

where T is the sum of numerators.

Formula (A1) can be written as:

$$C_{n+1} == \frac{C_n\, [1 + C_n\, s + 2\, (1 - C_n)\, s' - v - u] + v}{1 + 4\, C_n\, s' + C_n^2\, (s - 4\, s')} \tag{A3}$$

There is equilibrium condition when the frequency of C does not change passing from a generation to the next, that is, when:

$$C_{n+1} = C_n = C_e \tag{A4}$$

Substituting in (A3), we have:

$$C_e\, [1 + 4\, C_e\, s' + C_e^2\, (s - 4\, s')] = C_e\, [1 + C_e\, s + 2\, (1 - C_e)\, s' - v - u] + v \tag{A5}$$

The solutions of this third grade equation are long and complex.

With a recessive harmful gene (s' = 0), supposing the simplification: s < 0; u = 0, formula (A5) becomes:

$$C_e\, (1 + C_e^2\, s) = C_e\, (1 + C_e\, s - v) + v \tag{A6}$$

and the solutions are:

$$1, \; -\sqrt{-v/s}, \; \sqrt{-v/s} \tag{A7}$$

Discarding solutions 1 and 2 and recalling that s < 0, we can write:

$$C_e = \sqrt{v/[s]} \tag{A8}$$

where [s] means the absolute value of s.

For Hardy-Weinberg equilibrium (CC + 2 CC' + C'C' = 1), the equilibrium frequency of the phenotype expressing the disadvantageous condition will be:

$$P_e = C_e^2 = v/[s] \tag{A9}$$

In the case of a dominant harmful gene, with the simplification: s = s' < 0; u = 0, formula (A5) becomes:

$$C_e (1 - 3 C_e^2 s + 4 C_e s) = C_e (1 - C_e s + 2 s - v) + v \tag{A10}$$

and the solutions are:

$$1, \quad \frac{2 s - 2 \sqrt{s^2 + 3 s v}}{6 s}, \quad \frac{2 s + 2 \sqrt{s^2 + 3 s v}}{6 s} \tag{A11}$$

Discarding solutions 1 and 2:

$$C_e = \frac{2 s + 2 \sqrt{s^2 + 3 s v}}{6 s} \approx 0{,}5 \ v/[s] \tag{A12}$$

For Hardy-Weinberg equilibrium, the equilibrium frequency of the phenotype expressing the disadvantageous condition (P_e) will be:

$$P_e = C_e C_e + 2 C_e C'_e = 2 C_e - C_e^2 = \frac{(1 - \sqrt{1 + 3 v/s}) (5 + \sqrt{1 + 3 v/s})}{9} \approx v/[s] \tag{A13}$$

that is, for a dominant harmful gene the frequency of the phenotype is almost identical to that for a recessive gene.

In the case of a gene harmful in the recessive condition (s < 0) and advantageous in the heterozygote condition (s' > 0), with the simplifications u = 0; v = 0, formula (A5) becomes:

$$C_e [1 + 4 C_e s' + C_e^2 (s - 4 s')] = C_e [1 + C_e s + 2 (1 - C_e) s'] \tag{A14}$$

and the solutions are:

$$0, \quad 1, \quad - \frac{2 s'}{s - 4 s'} \tag{A15}$$

The first solution is valid if s < 0 and s' < 0. The second solution is valid if s > 0 and s' <= 0. The third solution is valid if s' > 0. Therefore, discarding solutions 1 and 2:

$$C_e = - \frac{2\,s'}{s - 4\,s'} = \frac{2\,s'}{[s] + 4\,s'} \tag{A16}$$

For Hardy-Weinberg equilibrium, equilibrium frequencies of phenotypes in homozygous and heterozygote conditions are given by C_e^2 and $2\,C_e\,(1 - C_e)$, respectively.

For chromosome alterations, it is useful to consider a chromosome alteration as an altered gene in a haploid organism, underlining that equilibrium frequency of a chromosome alteration (C_e) and equilibrium phenotypic frequency (P_e) coincide.

Therefore, supposing $s < 0$ and $u = 0$:

$$C_{n+1} = \frac{C_n - C_n\,s + (1 - C_n)\,v}{C_n - C_n\,s + (1 - C_n)\,v - (1 - C_n)\,v} = \frac{C_n\,(1 - s - v) + v}{1 - C_n\,s} \tag{A17}$$

$$C_e\,(1 - C_e\,s) = C_e\,(1 - s - v) + v \tag{A18}$$

The solutions are:

$$1, \quad -v/s \tag{A19}$$

that is: $C_e = P_e = v/[s]$ \hfill (A20)

as for P_e of recessive or dominant genes in a diploid organism.

Reviewed by

Theodore C. Goldsmith, former NASA project manager, recipient of NASA's Exceptional Service Medal, author of the book *The Evolution of Aging* and of articles regarding genetics, evolution theory, and aging theories.

References

[1] Dobzhansky, T (1973) Nothing in biology makes sense except in the light of evolution. *Am. Biol. Teach.* 35, 125-9.

[2] Williams, GC & Nesse, R.M. (1991) The dawn of Darwinian medicine. *Quart. Rev. Biol.* 66, 1-22.

[3] Nesse, RM & Williams, GC (1994) *Why we get sick.* New York (USA), Times Books.

[4] Trevathan, WR, Smith, EO & McKenna, JJ (eds) (1999) *Evolutionary Medicine.* New York (USA), Oxford University Press.

[5] Trevathan, WR, Smith, EO & McKenna, JJ (eds) (2008) *Evolutionary Medicine: new perspectives.* New York (USA), Oxford University Press.

[6] Stearns, SC (ed) (1999) *Evolution in health and disease* (1st ed.). Oxford (UK), Oxford University Press.

[7]   Stearns, SC & Koella, JC (eds) (2008) *Evolution in health and disease* (2nd ed.). Oxford (UK), Oxford University Press.

[8]   Trevathan, WR, Smith, EO & McKenna, JJ (2008) Introduction and overview of Evolutionary Medicine. In: Trevathan, WR, Smith, EO & McKenna, JJ (eds) *Evolutionary Medicine: new perspectives*. New York (USA), Oxford University Press.

[9]   Eaton, SB, Shostak, M & Konner, M (1988) *The paleolithic prescription: a program of diet & exercise and a design for living*. New York (USA), Harper & Row.

[10]   Libertini, G (1983) [*Evolutionary Arguments*] [Book in Italian]. Naples (Italy), Società Editrice Napoletana.

[11]   Kirkwood, TBL & Austad, SN (2000) Why do we age? *Nature* 408, 233-8.

[12]   Austad, SN & Finch, CE (2008) The evolutionary context of human aging and degenerative disease. In: Stearns, CS & Koella, JC (eds) *Evolution in health and disease* (2nd ed.). Oxford (UK), Oxford University Press.

[13]   Libertini, G (1988) An Adaptive Theory of the Increasing Mortality with Increasing Chronological Age in Populations in the Wild. *J. Theor. Biol.* 132, 145-62.

[14]   Weismann, A (1884) *Über Leben und Tod*, Jena. Reprinted in: *Essays upon Heredity and Kindred Biological Problems* (1889), Oxford (UK), Clarendon Press.

[15]   Skulachev, VP (1997) Aging is a specific biological function rather than the result of a disorder in complex living systems: biochemical evidence in support of Weissmann's hypothesis. *Biochemistry (Mosc)* 62, 1191-5.

[16]   Goldsmith, TC (2003) *The Evolution of Aging: How Darwin's Dilemma is Affecting Your Chance for a Longer and Healthier Life*. Lincoln, Nebraska (USA), iUniverse.

[17]   Goldsmith TC (2004) Aging as an evolved characteristic – Weismann's theory reconsidered. *Med. Hypotheses* 62, 304-8.

[18]   Goldsmith, TC (2006) *The Evolution of Aging*. Lincoln, Nebraska (USA), Azinet.

[19]   Goldsmith TC (2008) Aging, evolvability, and the individual benefit requirement; medical implications of aging theory controversies. *J. Theor. Biol.* 252, 764-8.

[20]   Longo, VD, Mitteldorf, J & Skulachev, VP (2005) Programmed and altruistic ageing. *Nat. Rev. Genet.* 6, 866-72.

[21]   Libertini, G (2006) Evolutionary explanations of the "actuarial senescence in the wild" and of the "state of senility". *The Scientific World JOURNAL* 6, 1086-108 DOI 10.1100/tsw.2006.209.

[22]   Libertini, G (2008) Empirical evidence for various evolutionary hypotheses on species demonstrating increasing mortality with increasing chronological age in the wild. *TheScientificWorldJOURNAL* 8, 182-93 DOI 10.1100/tsw.2008.36.

[23]   Nesse, RM (2008) The importance of evolution for medicine. In: Trevathan W.R., Smith E.O. & McKenna J.J.(eds) *Evolutionary Medicine: new perspectives*. New York (USA), Oxford University Press.

[24]   Stearns, SC, Nesse, RM & Haig, D (2008) Introducing evolutionary thinking for medicine. In: Stearns, SC & Koella, JC (eds) *Evolution in health and disease* (2nd ed.). Oxford (UK), Oxford University Press.

[25]   Price, WA (1939) *Nutrition and Physical Degeneration*. New York – London, Paul B. Hoeber.

[26] Eaton, SB, Konner, M, Shostak, M (1988) Stone agers in the fast lane: chronic degenerative diseases in evolutionary perspective. *Am. J. Med.* 84, 739-49.

[27] Blurton Jones, NG, Hawkes, K & O'Connell, JF (2002) Antiquity of postreproductive life: are there modern impacts on hunter-gatherer postreproductive life spans? *Am. J. Hum. Biol.* 14, 184-205.

[28] Bragulat, E & de la Sierra, A (2002) Salt intake, endothelial dysfunction, and salt-sensitive hypertension. *J. Clin. Hypertens. (Greenwich).* 4, 41-6.

[29] Rodriguez-Iturbe, B, Romero, F & Johnson, RJ (2007) Pathophysiological mechanisms of salt-dependent hypertension. *Am. J. Kidney Dis.* 50, 655-72.

[30] Morse, SA, Bravo, PE, Morse, MC & Reisin, E (2005) The heart in obesity-hypertension. *Expert. Rev. Cardiovasc. Ther.* 3, 647-58.

[31] Fredrick, DR (2002) Myopia. *BMJ.* 324, 1195-9.

[32] Chow, YC, Dhillon, B, Chew, PT & Chew, SJ (1990) Refractive errors in Singapore medical students. *Singapore Med J.* 31, 472–3.

[33] Wong, TY, Foster, PJ, Hee, J, Ng, TP, Tielsch, JM, Chew, SJ, Johnson GJ & Seah SK (2000) Prevalence and risk factors for refractive errors in an adult Chinese population in Singapore. *Invest. Ophthalmol. Vis. Sci.* 41, 2486-94.

[34] Kee, CS & Deng, L (2008) Astigmatism associated with experimentally induced myopia or hyperopia in chickens. *Invest. Ophthalmol. Vis. Sci.* 49, 858-67.

[35] Lipworth, L, Tarone, RE & McLaughlin, JK (2006) The epidemiology of renal cell carcinoma. *J. Urol.* 176, 2353-8.

[36] Fransen, E, Topsakal, V, Hendrickx, JJ, Van Laer, L, Huyghe, JR, Van Eyken, E, Lemkens, N, Hannula, S, Mäki-Torkko, E, Jensen, M, Demeester, K, Tropitzsch, A, Bonaconsa, A, Mazzoli, M, Espeso, A, Verbruggen, K, Huyghe, J, Huygen, PL, Kunst, S, Manninen, M, Diaz-Lacava, A, Steffens, M, Wienker, TF, Pyykkö, I, Cremers, CW, Kremer, H, Dhooge, I, Stephens, D, Orzan, E, Pfister, M, Bille, M, Parving, A, Sorri, M, Van de Heyning, P & Van Camp, G (2008) Occupational noise, smoking, and a high Body Mass Index are risk factors for age-related hearing impairment and moderate alcohol consumption is protective: a European population-based multicenter study. *J. Assoc. Res. Otolaryngol.* 9, 264-76.

[37] Daniel, E (2007) Noise and hearing loss: a review. *J. Sch. Health* 77, 225-31.

[38] Viegi, G, Maio, S, Pistelli, F, Baldacci, S & Carrozzi, L (2006) Epidemiology of chronic obstructive pulmonary disease: health effects of air pollution. *Respirology* 11, 523-32.

[39] Taraseviciene-Stewart, L & Voelkel, NF (2008) Molecular pathogenesis of emphysema. *J. Clin. Invest.* 118, 394-402.

[40] Giovino, GA (2007) The tobacco epidemic in the United States. *Am. J. Prev. Med.* 33, S318-26.

[41] Clavel, J (2007) Progress in the epidemiological understanding of gene-environment interactions in major diseases: cancer. *C. R. Biol.* 330, 306-17.

[42] La Vecchia, C, Zhang, ZF & Altieri, A (2008) Alcohol and laryngeal cancer: an update. *Eur. J. Cancer Prev.* 17, 116-24.

[43] Janković, S & Radosavljević, V (2007) Risk factors for bladder cancer. *Tumori* 93, 4-12.

[44] Hart, A.R., Kennedy, H. & Harvey, I. (2008) Pancreatic cancer: a review of the evidence on causation. *Clin. Gastroenterol. Hepatol.* 6, 275-82.

[45] Halter, F & Brignoli, R (1998) *Helicobacter pylori* and smoking: two additive risk factors for organic dyspepsia. *Yale J. Biol. Med.* 71, 91-9.

[46] Parasher, G, Eastwood, GL (2000) Smoking and peptic ulcer in the Helicobacter pylori era. *Eur. J. Gastroenterol. Hepatol.* 12, 843-53.

[47] Trepel, F (2004) [Dietary fibre: more than a matter of dietetics. II. Preventative and therapeutic uses][Article in German] *Wien. Klin. Wochenschr.* 116, 511-22.

[48] Arnbjörnsson, E (1983) Acute appendicitis and dietary fiber. *Arch. Surg.* 118, 868-70.

[49] Adamidis, D, Roma-Giannikou, E, Karamolegou, K, Tselalidou, E & Constantopoulos, A (2000) Fiber intake and childhood appendicitis. *Int. J. Food. Sci. Nutr.* 51, 153-7.

[50] National Institutes of Health, USA (2000) Osteoporosis prevention, diagnosis, and therapy. *NIH Consens. Statement.* 17, 1-45.

[51] Janeway, C, Travers, P, Walport, M & Shlomchik, M (2001). *Immunobiology* (5th Ed.). New York and London, Garland Science.

[52] Kirchner, DB (2002) The spectrum of allergic disease in the chemical industry. *Int. Arch. Occup. Environ. Health.* 75, S107-12.

[53] Greaves, MF (2000) *Cancer: The Evolutionary Legacy.* Oxford (UK), Oxford University Press.

[54] Adachi, M & Brenner, DA (2005) Clinical syndromes of alcoholic liver disease. *Dig. Dis.* 23, 255-63.

[55] Truswell, AS, Kennelly, BM, Hansen, JD & Lee, RB (1972) Blood pressure of !Kung bushmen in northern Botswana. *Am. Heart J.* 84, 5-12.

[56] Wild, S, Roglic, G, Green, A, Sicree, R & King, H (2004) Global prevalence of diabetes: estimates for the year 2000 and projections for 2030. *Diabetes Care* 27, 1047-53.

[57] Mullard, A (2008) Microbiology: the inside story. *Nature* 453, 578-80.

[58] Woolhouse, M & Antia, R (2008) Emergence of new infectious diseases. In: Stearns, CS & Koella, JC (eds) *Evolution in health and disease* (2nd ed.). Oxford (UK), Oxford University Press.

[59] Wilson, EO (1975) *Sociobiology, The New Synthesis.* Cambridge (UK), Harvard University Press.

[60] Denic, S & Agarwal, MM (2007) Nutritional iron deficiency: an evolutionary perspective. *Nutrition* 23, 603-14.

[61] Doherty, CP (2007) Host-pathogen interactions: the role of iron. *J. Nutr.* 137, 1341-4.

[62] Flaxman, SM & Sherman, PW (2000) Morning sickness: a mechanism for protecting mother and embryo. *Quart. Rev. Biol.* 75, 113-48.

[63] Flaxman, SM & Sherman, PW (2008) Morning sickness: adaptive cause or nonadaptive consequence of embryo viability? *Am. Nat.* 172, 54-62.

[64] Vanden Broeck, D, Horvath, C & De Wolf, MJ (2007) *Vibrio cholerae*: cholera toxin. *Int. J. Biochem. Cell Biol.* 39, 1771-5.

[65] Lechler, R & Warrens, A (2000) *HLA in Health and Disease.* San Diego, California (USA), Academic Press.

[66] Shiina, T, Inoko, H & Kulski, JK (2004) An update of the HLA genomic region, locus information and disease associations: 2004. *Tissue Antigens* 64, 631-49.

[67] Slev, PR, Nelson, AC & Potts, WK (2006) Sensory neurons with MHC-like peptide binding properties: disease consequences. *Curr. Opin. Immunol.* 18, 608-16.

[68] Wedekind, C, Seebeck, T, Bettens, F & Paepke, AJ (1995) MHC-dependent mate preferences in humans. *Proc. Biol. Sci.* 260, 245-9.

[69] Wedekind, C & Füri, S (1997) Body odour preferences in men and women: do they aim for specific MHC combinations or simply heterozygosity? *Proc. Biol. Sci.* 264, 1471-9.

[70] Ober, C, Weitkamp, LR, Cox, N, Dytch, H, Kostyu, D & Elias, S (1997) HLA and mate choice in humans. *Am. J. Hum. Genet.* 61, 497-504.

[71] Ober, C, Weitkamp, L & Cox, N (1999) HLA and mate choice. In: Johnston, RE, Muller-Schwarze, D & Sorenson, PW (eds) *Advances in Chemical Signals in Vertebrates*. New York (USA), Kluwer Academic Press.

[72] Loisel, DA, Alberts, SC & Ober, C (2008) Functional significance of MHC variation in mate choice, reproductive outcome, and disease risk. In: Stearns SC & Koella JC (eds) *Evolution in health and disease* (2nd ed.). Oxford (UK), Oxford University Press.

[73] Apanius, V, Penn, D, Slev, PR, Ruff, LR & Potts, WK (1997) The nature of selection on the major histocompatibility complex. *Crit. Rev. Immunol.* 17, 179-224.

[74] Tregenza, T & Wedell, N (2000) Genetic compatibility, mate choice and patterns of parentage: invited review. *Mol. Ecol.* 9, 1013-27.

[75] Dorak, MT, Lawson, T, Machulla, HK, Mills, KI & Burnett, AK (2002) Increased heterozygosity for MHC class II lineages in newborn males. *Genes Immun.* 3, 263-9.

[76] Ober, C & van der Ven, K (1997) Immunogenetics of reproduction: an overview. In: Olding, L.B. (ed) *Current Topics in Microbiology and Immunology*. Berlin (Germany), Springer-Verlag.

[77] Ober, C (1992) The maternal-fetal relationship in human pregnancy: an immunogenetic perspective. *Exp. Clin. Immunogenet.* 9, 1-14.

[78] Ober, C, Hyslop, T, Elias, S, Weitkamp, LR & Hauck, WW (1998) Human leukocyte antigen matching and fetal loss: results of a 10 year prospective study. *Hum. Reprod.* 13, 33-8.

[79] Scrimshaw, SCM (1984) Infanticide in human populations: societal and individual concerns. In: Hausfater, G & Hrdy, S.B. (Eds.) *Infanticide: comparative and evolutionary perspectives*. New York (USA), Aldine.

[80] Hamilton, WD (1964) The genetical evolution of social behaviour, I, II. *J. Theor. Biol.* 7, 1-52.

[81] Hamilton, WD (1970) Selfish and spiteful behaviour in an evolutionary model. *Nature* 228, 1218-20.

[82] Trivers, RL (1971) The evolution of reciprocal altruism. *Quart. Rev. Biol.* 46, 35-57.

[83] Trivers, RL & Hare, H (1976). Haploidiploidy and the evolution of the social insect. *Science,* 191, 249-63.

[84] Altman, SA & Altmann, J (1970) *Baboon ecology: African field research*. Chicago (USA), The University of Chicago Press.

[85] Hall, KR (1960) Social vigilance behaviour in of the chacma baboon, *Papio ursinus. Behaviour,* 16, 261-94.

[86] Kerr, JFR, Wyllie, AH & Currie, AR (1972) Apoptosis: a basic biological phenomenon with wide-ranging implications in tissue kinetics. *Br. J. Cancer,* 26, 239-57.

[87] Fröhlich, KU, Fussi, H & Ruckenstuhl, C (2007) Yeast apoptosis - from genes to pathways. *Semin. Cancer Biol.* 17, 112-21.

[88] Büttner, S, Eisenberg, T, Herker, E, Carmona-Gutierrez, D, Kroemer, G & Madeo, F (2006) Why yeast cells can undergo apoptosis: death in times of peace, love, and war. *J. Cell Biol.* 175, 521–5.

[89] Fröhlich, KU & Madeo, F (2000) Apoptosis in yeast - a monocellular organism exhibits altruistic behaviour. *FEBS Lett.* 473, 6-9.

[90] Silk, JB (1980) Adoption and kinship in Oceania. *Am. Anthropol.* 82, 799–820.

[91] Rachlin, H, Jones, BA (2008) Altruism among relatives and non-relatives. *Behav. Processes.* 79, 120-3.

[92] Deevey, ESJr. (1947) Life tables for natural populations of animals. *Quart. Rev. Biol.* 22, 283-314.

[93] Laws, RM (1966). Age criteria for the African elephant, *Loxodonta a. africana. E. Afr. Wildl. J.* 4, 1-37.

[94] Laws, RM (1968). Dentition and ageing of the hippopotamus. *E. Afr. Wildl. J.* 6, 19-52.

[95] Laws, RM & Parker, ISC (1968) Recent studies on elephant populations in East Africa. *Symp. Zool. Soc. Lond.* 21, 319-59.

[96] Spinage, CA (1970) Population dynamics of the Uganda Defassa Waterbuck (*Kobus defassa Ugandae* Neumann) in the Queen Elizabeth park, Uganda. *J. Anim. Ecol.* 39, 51-78.

[97] Spinage, CA (1972) African ungulate life tables. *Ecology,* 53, 645-52.

[98] Finch, CE (1990) *Longevity, Senescence, and the Genome.* Chicago (USA), The University of Chicago Press.

[99] Holmes, DJ & Austad, SN (1995) Birds as animal models for the comparative biology of aging: a prospectus. *J. Gerontol. A Biol. Sci. Med. Sci.* 50, B59-66.

[100] Ricklefs, RE (1998) Evolutionary theories of aging: confirmation of a fundamental prediction, with implications for the genetic basis and evolution of life span. *Am. Nat.* 152, 24-44.

[101] Williams, GC (1957) Pleiotropy, natural selection and the evolution of senescence. *Evolution,* 11, 398-411.

[102] Medawar, PB (1952) An Unsolved Problem in Biology. London (UK), H. K. Lewis. Reprinted in: Medawar, P.B. (1957) *The Uniqueness of the Individual.* London (UK), Methuen.

[103] Hamilton, WD (1966) The moulding of senescence by natural selection. *J. Theor. Biol.* 12, 12-45.

[104] Edney, EB & Gill, RW (1968) Evolution of senescence and specific longevity. *Nature,* 220, 281-2.

[105] Mueller, LD (1987) Evolution of accelerated senescence in laboratory populations of *Drosophila. Proc. Natl. Acad. Sci. USA* 84, 1974-7.

[106] Partridge, L & Barton, NH (1993) Optimality, mutation and the evolution of ageing. *Nature,* 362, 305-11.

[107] Rose, MR (1991) *Evolutionary biology of aging*. New York (USA), Oxford University Press.

[108] Kirkwood, TBL (1977) Evolution of ageing. *Nature* 270, 301-4.

[109] Kirkwood, TBL & Holliday, R (1979) The evolution of ageing and longevity. *Proc. R. Soc. Lond. B Biol. Sci.* 205, 531-46.

[110] Le Bourg, É (2001) A mini-review of the evolutionary theories of aging. Is it the time to accept them? *Demogr. Res.* 4, 1-28.

[111] Finch, CE & Austad, SN (2001) History and prospects: symposium on organisms with slow aging. *Exp. Gerontol.* 36, 593-7.

[112] Vaupel, JW, Baudisch, A, Dölling, M, Roach, DA & Gampe, J (2004) The case for negative senescence. *Theor. Popul. Biol.* 65, 339-51.

[113] Fossel, MB (2004) *Cells, Aging and Human Disease*. New York (USA), Oxford University Press.

[114] Campisi, J (1997) The biology of replicative senescence. *Eur. J. Cancer* 33, 703-9.

[115] Wright, WE & Shay, JW (2005) Telomere biology in aging and cancer. *J. Am. Geriatr. Soc.* 53, S292-4.

[116] Campisi, J (2000) Cancer, aging and cellular senescence. *In Vivo* 14, 183-8.

[117] Klapper, W, Heidorn, H, Kühne, K, Parwaresch, R & Krupp, G (1998) Telomerase activity in 'immortal' fish. *FEBS Letters* 434, 409-12.

[118] Klapper, W, Kühne, K, Singh, KK, Heidorn, K, Parwaresch, R & Krupp, G (1998). Longevity of lobsters is linked to ubiquitous telomerase expression. *FEBS Letters* 439, 143-6.

[119] Rosen, P (1985) Aging of the immune system. *Med. Hypotheses* 18, 157-61.

[120] DePinho, RA (2000) The age of cancer. *Nature* 408, 248-54.

[121] Artandi, SE (2002) Telomere shortening and cell fates in mouse models of neoplasia. *Trends Mol. Med.* 8, 44-7.

[122] Jazwinski, SM (1993) The genetics of aging in the yeast *Saccharomyces cerevisiae*. *Genetica* 91, 35-51.

[123] Laun, P, Bruschi, CV, Dickinson, JR, Rinnerthaler, M, Heeren, G, Schwimbersky, R, Rid, R & Breitenbach, M (2007) Yeast mother cell-specific ageing, genetic (in)stability, and the somatic mutation theory of ageing. *Nucleic Acids Res.* 35, 7514-26.

[124] Fabrizio, P & Longo, VD (2007) The chronological life span of *Saccharomyces cerevisiae*. *Methods Mol. Biol.* 371, 89-95.

[125] Laun, P, Pichova, A, Madeo, F, Fuchs, J, Ellinger, A, Kohlwein, S, Dawes, I, Fröhlich, KU & Breitenbach, M (2001) Aged mother cells of *Saccharomyces cerevisiae* show markers of oxidative stress and apoptosis. *Mol. Microbiol.* 39, 1166-73.

[126] Kaeberlein, M, Burtner, CR & Kennedy, BK (2007) Recent developments in yeast aging *PLoS Genet.* 3(5): e84.

[127] Mitteldorf, J (2006) How evolutionary thinking affects people's ideas about aging interventions. *Rejuvenation Res.* 9, 346-50.

[128] Skulachev, VP (2002) Programmed death in yeast as adaptation? *FEBS Lett.* 528, 23-6.

[129] Skulachev, VP (2003) Aging and the programmed death phenomena. In: *Topics in Current Genetics*, Vol. 3, Nyström, T & Osiewacz HD (eds) *Model Systems in Aging*. Berlin Heidelberg (Germany), Springer-Verlag.

[130] Herker, E, Jungwirth, H, Lehmann, KA, Maldener, C, Fröhlich, KU, Wissing, S, Büttner, S, Fehr, M, Sigrist, S and Madeo, F (2004) Chronological aging leads to apoptosis in yeast *J. Cell Biol.*, 164, 501-7.

[131] Skulachev, VP & Longo, VD (2005) Aging as a mitochondria-mediated atavistic program: can aging be switched off? *Ann. N. Y. Acad. Sci.* 1057, 145-64.

[132] Hayflick, L & Moorhead, PS (1961) The serial cultivation of human diploid cell strains. *Exp. Cell Res.* 25, 585-621.

[133] Hayflick, L (1965) The limited *in vitro* lifetime of human diploid cell strains. *Exp. Cell Res.* 37, 614-36.

[134] Schneider, EL & Mitsui, Y (1976) The relationship between in vitro cellular aging and in vivo human age. *Proc. Natl. Acad. Sci. USA* 73, 3584-8.

[135] Rheinwald, JG & Green, H (1975) Serial cultivation of strains of human epidermal keratinocytes: the formation of keratinizing colonies from single cells. *Cell*, 6, 331-44.

[136] Bierman, EL (1978) The effect of donor age on the in vitro life span of cultured human arterial smooth-muscle cells. *In Vitro*, 14, 951-5.

[137] Tassin, J, Malaise, E & Courtois, Y (1979) Human lens cells have an in vitro proliferative capacity inversely proportional to the donor age. *Exp. Cell Res.* 123, 388-92.

[138] Röhme, D (1981) Evidence for a relationship between longevity of mammalian species and life spans of normal fibroblasts *in vitro* and erythrocytes *in vivo*. *Proc. Natl. Acad. Sci. USA* 78, 5009-13.

[139] Martin, GM, Sprague, CA & Epstein, CJ (1970) Replicative life-span of cultivated human cells. Effects of donor's age, tissue, and genotype. *Lab. Invest.* 23, 86-92.

[140] Wright, WE & Hayflick, L (1975) Nuclear control of cellular ageing demonstrated by hybridization of anucleate and whole cultured normal human fibroblasts. *Exp. Cell. Res.* 96, 113-21.

[141] Olovnikov, AM (1973) A theory of marginotomy: The incomplete copying of template margin in enzyme synthesis of polynucleotides and biological significance of the problem. *J. Theor. Biol.* 41, 181-90.

[142] Watson, JD (1972) Origin of concatemeric T7 DNA. *Nature New Biol.* 239, 197-201.

[143] Blackburn, EH & Gall, J.G. (1978) A tandemly repeated sequence at the termini of the extrachromosomal ribosomal RNA genes in *Tetrahymena*. *J. Mol. Biol.* 120, 33-53.

[144] Moyzis, RK, Buckingham, JM, Cram, LS, Dani, M, Deaven, LL, Jones, MD, Meyne, J, Ratliff, RL & Wu, JR (1988) A highly conserved repetitive DNA sequence, (TTAGGG)n, present at the telomeres of human chromosomes. *Proc. Natl. Acad. Sci. USA*. 85, 6622-6.

[145] Blackburn, EH (1991) Structure and function of telomeres. *Nature*, 350, 569-73.

[146] Harley, CB, Futcher, AB & Greider, CW (1990) Telomeres shorten during ageing of human fibroblasts. *Nature*, 345, 458-60.

[147] Greider, CW & Blackburn EH (1985) Identification of a specific telomere terminal transferase activity in *Tetrahymena* extracts. *Cell*, 51, 405-13.

[148] Morin, GB (1989) The human telomere terminal transferase enzyme is a ribonucleoprotein that synthesizes TTAGGG repeats. *Cell,* 59, 521-9.

[149] van Steensel, B & de Lange, T (1997) Control of telomere length by the human telomeric protein TRF1. *Nature,* 385, 740-3.

[150] Yu, GL, Bradley, JD, Attardi, LD & Blackburn, EH (1990) *In vivo* alteration of telomere sequences and senescence caused by mutated *Tetrahymena* telomerase RNAs. *Nature,* 344, 126-32.

[151] Bodnar, AG, Ouellette, M, Frolkis, M, Holt, SE, Chiu, C, Morin, GB, Harley, CB, Shay, JW, Lichsteiner, S & Wright, WE (1998) Extension of life-span by introduction of telomerase into normal human cells. *Science,* 279, 349-52.

[152] Counter, CM, Hahn, WC, Wei, W, Caddle, SD, Beijersbergen, RL, Lansdorp, PM, Sedivy, JM & Weinberg, RA (1998) Dissociation among *in vitro* telomerase activity, telomere maintenance, and cellular immortalization. *Proc. Natl. Acad. Sci. USA* 95, 14723-8.

[153] Vaziri, H (1998) Extension of life span in normal human cells by telomerase activation: a revolution in cultural senescence. *J. Anti-Aging Med.* 1, 125-30.

[154] Vaziri, H & Benchimol, S (1998) Reconstitution of telomerase activity in normal cells leads to elongation of telomeres and extended replicative life span. *Cur. Biol.* 8, 279-82.

[155] de Lange, T & Jacks, T (1999) For better or worse? Telomerase inhibition and cancer. *Cell* 98, 273-5.

[156] Pontèn, J, Stein, WD & Shall, S (1983) A quantitative analysis of the aging of human glial cells in culture. *J. Cell Phys.* 117, 342-52.

[157] Jones, RB, Whitney, RG & Smith, JR (1985) Intramitotic variation in proliferative potential: stochastic events in cellular aging. *Mech. Ageing Dev.* 29, 143-9.

[158] Blackburn, EH (2000) Telomere states and cell fates. *Nature* 408, 53-6.

[159] Holt, SE, Shay, JW & Wright, WE (1996) Refining the telomere-telomerase hypothesis of aging and cancer. *Nat. Biotechnol.* 14, 836-9.

[160] Slijepcevic, P & Hande, MP (1999) Chinese hamster telomeres are comparable in size to mouse telomeres. *Cytogenet. Cell Genet.* 85, 196-9.

[161] Reed, JC (1999) Dysregulation of Apoptosis in Cancer. *J. Clin. Oncol.* 17, 2941-53.

[162] Anversa, P & Nadal-Ginard, B (2002) Myocyte renewal and ventricular remodelling. *Nature* 415, 240-3.

[163] Schultz, E & Lipton, BH (1982) Skeletal muscle satellite cells: changes in proliferation potential as a function of age. *Mech. Age. Dev.* 20, 377-83.

[164] Carlson, BM & Faulkner, JA (1989) Muscle transplantation between young and old rats: age of host determines recovery. *Am. J. Physiol.* 256, C1262-6.

[165] Adams, V, Gielen, S, Hambrecht, R & Schuler, G (2001) Apoptosis in skeletal muscle. *Front. Biosci.* 6, D1-D11.

[166] Wyllie, AH, Kerr, JFR & Currie, AR (1980) Cell death: the significance of apoptosis. *Int. Rev. Cytol.* 68, 251-306.

[167] Lynch, MP, Nawaz, S & Gerschenson, LE (1986) Evidence for soluble factors regulating cell death and cell proliferation in primary cultures of rabbit endometrial cells grown on collagen. *Proc. Natl. Acad. Sci. USA* 83, 4784-8.

[168] Medh, RD & Thompson, EB (2000) Hormonal regulation of physiological cell turnover and apoptosis. *Cell Tissue Res.* 301, 101-24.

[169] Harada, K, Iwata, M, Kono, N, Koda, W, Shimonishi, T & Nakanuma, Y (2000) Distribution of apoptotic cells and expression of apoptosis-related proteins along the intrahepatic biliary tree in normal and non-biliary diseased liver. *Histopathology,* 37, 347-54.

[170] Cardani, R & Zavanella T. (2000) Age-related cell proliferation and apoptosis in the kidney of male Fischer 344 rats with observations on a spontaneous tubular cell adenoma. *Toxicol. Pathol.* 28, 802-6.

[171] Finegood, DT, Scaglia, L & Bonner-Weir, S (1995) Dynamics of beta-cell mass in the growing rat pancreas. Estimation with a simple mathematical model. *Diabetes,* 44, 249-56.

[172] Benedetti, A, Jezequel, AM & Orlandi, F (1988) A quantitative evaluation of apoptotic bodies in rat liver. *Liver,* 8, 172-7.

[173] Dremier, S, Golstein, J, Mosselmans, R, Dumont, JE, Galand, P & Robaye, B (1994) Apoptosis in dog thyroid cells. *Biochem. Biophys. Res. Comm.* 200, 52-8.

[174] Sutherland, LM, Edwards, YS & Murray, AW (2001) Alveolar type II cell apoptosis. *Comp. Biochem. Physiol.* 129, 267-85.

[175] Héraud, F, Héraud, A & Harmand, MF (2000) Apoptosis in normal and osteoarthritic human articular cartilage. *Ann. Rheum. Dis.* 59, 959-65.

[176] Xia, SJ, Xu, CX, Tang, XD, Wang, WZ & Du, DL (2001) Apoptosis and hormonal milieu in ductal system of normal prostate and benign prostatic hyperplasia. *Asian J. Androl.* 3, 131-4.

[177] Prins, JB & O'Rahilly, S (1997) Regulation of adipose cell number in man. *Clin. Sci. (Lond.)* 92, 3-11.

[178] Spelsberg, TC, Subramaniam, M, Riggs, BL & Khosla, S (1999) The actions and interactions of sex steroids and growth factors/cytokines on the skeleton. *Mol. Endocrinol.* 13, 819-28.

[179] Migheli, A, Mongini, T, Doriguzzi, C, Chiadò-Piat, L, Piva, R, Ugo, I & Palmucci, L. (1997) Muscle apoptosis in humans occurs in normal and denervated muscle, but not in myotonic dystrophy, dystrophinopathies or inflammatory disease. *Neurogenetics,* 1, 81-7.

[180] Pollack, M. & Leeuwenburgh, C (2001) Apoptosis and aging: role of the mitochondria. *J. Gerontol. A Biol. Sci. Med. Sci.* 56, B475-82.

[181] Andreeff, M, Goodrich, DW & Pardee, AB (2000) Cell proliferation, differentiation, and apoptosis. In: Holland, J.F. et al. (eds) Holland-Frei. *Cancer Medicine* (5th Ed.), Hamilton, Ontario, USA, & London, B. C. Decker.

[182] Marciniak, R & Guarente, L (2001) Human genetics. Testing telomerase. *Nature,* 413, 370-2.

[183] Horner, PJ & Gage, FH (2000) Regenerating the damaged central nervous system. *Nature,* 407, 963-70.

[184] Tyner, SD, Venkatachalam, S, Choi, J, Jones, S, Ghebranious, N, Igelmann, H, Lu, X, Soron, G, Cooper, B, Brayton, C, Hee Park, S, Thompson, T, Karsenty, G, Bradley, A

& Donehower, LA (2002) p53 mutant mice that display early ageing-associated phenotypes. *Nature,* 415, 45-53.

[185] Dokal, I (2000) Dyskeratosis congenita in all its forms. *Br. J. Haematol.* 110, 768-79.

[186] Mitchell, JR, Wood, E & Collins, K (1999) A telomerase component is defective in the human disease dyskeratosis congenita. *Nature,* 402, 551-5.

[187] Artandi, SE, Chang, S, Lee, SL, Alson, S, Gottlieb, GJ, Chin, L & DePinho, RA (2000) Telomere dysfunction promotes non-reciprocal translocations and epithelial cancers in mice. *Nature,* 406, 641-5.

[188] Yu, CE, Oshima, J, Fu, YH, Wijsman, EM, Hisama, F, Alisch, R, Matthews, S, Nakura, J, Miki, T, Ouais, S, Martin, GM, Mulligan, J & Schellenberg, GD (1996) Positional cloning of the Werner's syndrome gene. *Science,* 272, 258-62.

[189] Fukuchi, K., Martin, G.M. & Monnat, R.J., Jr. (1989) Mutator phenotype of Werner syndrome is characterized by extensive deletions. *Proc. Natl. Acad. Sci. USA* 86, 5893-7. [Published erratum appears in *Proc. Natl. Acad. Sci. USA,* 86, 7994 (1989)].

[190] Martin, GM & Oshima, J (2000) Lessons from human progeroid syndromes. *Nature* 408, 263-6.

[191] Barker, N, van Es, JH, Kuipers, J, Kujala, P, van den Born, M, Cozijnsen, M, Haegebarth, A, Korving, J, Begthel, H, Peters, PJ & Clevers, H (2007) Identification of stem cells in small intestine and colon by marker gene Lgr5. *Nature,* 449, 1003-7.

[192] Webster, SGP (1978) The gastrointestinal system – c. The pancreas and the small bowel. In: Brocklehurst, JC (ed) *Textbook of Geriatric Medicine and Gerontology* (2nd Ed.). New York (USA), Churchill Livingstone.

[193] Hill, JM, Zalos, G, Halcox, JPJ, Schenke, WH, Waclawiw, MA, Quyyumi, AA & Finkel, T (2003) Circulating endothelial progenitor cells, vascular function, and cardiovascular risk. *N. Engl. J. Med..* 348, 593-600.

[194] Werner, N, Kosiol, S, Schiegl, T, Ahlers, P, Walenta, K, Link, A, Böhm, M & Nickenig, G (2005) Circulating endothelial progenitor cells and cardiovascular outcomes. *N. Engl. J. Med.* 353, 999-1007.

[195] Tallis, RC, Fillit, HM & Brocklehurst, JC (eds) (1998) *Brocklehurst's Textbook of Geriatric Medicine and Gerontology* (5th ed.). New York (USA), Churchill Livingstone.

[196] Griffiths, CEM (1998) Aging of the Skin. In: Tallis, RC et al. (eds), *Brocklehurst's Textbook of Geriatric Medicine and Gerontology* (5th Ed.). New York (USA), Churchill Livingstone.

[197] Fine, SL, Berger, JW, Maguire, MG & Ho, AC (2000) Age-related macular degeneration. *N. Engl. J. Med.* 342, 483-92.

[198] Berger JW, Fine SL & Maguire, MG (1999) *Age-related macular degeneration*, Mosby (USA).

[199] Fossel, MB (1996) *Reversing Human Aging.* New York (USA), William Morrow and Company.

[200] Qiu, WQ, Walsh, DM, Ye, Z, Vekrellis, K, Zhang, J, Podlisny, MB, Rosner, MR, Safavi, A, Hersh, LB & Selkoe, DJ (1998) Insulin-degrading enzyme regulates extracellular levels of amyloid beta-protein by degradation. *J Biol Chem.* 273, 32730-8.

[201] Vekrellis, K, Ye, Z, Qiu, WQ, Walsh, D, Hartley, D, Chesneau, V, Rosner, MR & Selkoe, DJ (2000) Neurons regulate extracellular levels of amyloid beta-protein via proteolysis by insulin-degrading enzyme. *J. Neurosci.* 20, 1657-65.

[202] Bertram, L, Blacker, D, Mullin, K, Keeney, D, Jones, J, Basu, S, Yhu, S, McInnis, MG, Go, RC, Vekrellis, K, Selkoe, DJ, Saunders, AJ & Tanzi, RE (2000) Evidence for genetic linkage of Alzheimer's disease to chromosome 10q. *Science,* 290, 2302-3.

[203] von Zglinicki, T, Serra, V, Lorenz, M, Saretzki, G, Lenzen-Grossimlighaus, R, Gessner, R, Risch, A & Steinhagen-Thiessen, E (2000) Short telomeres in patients with vascular dementia: an indicator of low antioxidative capacity and a possible risk factor? *Lab. Invest.* 80, 1739-47.

[204] Gorelick, PB (2004) Risk factors for vascular dementia and Alzheimer disease. *Stroke* 35, 2620-2.

[205] National vital statistics reports, Vol. 56, no. 10, April 24, 2008. (http://www.cdc.gov/nchs/data/nvsr/nvsr56/nvsr56_10.pdf).

[206] Cohn, SK Jr (2002) The Black Death: end of a paradigm. *Amer. Histor. Rev.* 107, 703-38.

[207] Patterson, KD & Pyle, GF (1991). The geography and mortality of the 1918 influenza pandemic. *Bull. Hist. Med.* 65, 4–21.

[208] Knobler, SL, Mack, A, Mahmoud, A & Lemon, SM (eds) (2005) *The Threat of Pandemic Influenza: Are We Ready? Workshop Summary.* Washington, D.C. (USA), The National Academies Press.

[209] McMichael, AJ (2004) Environmental and social influences on emerging infectious diseases: past, present and future. *Philos. Trans. R. Soc. Lond. B Biol. Sci.* 359, 1049-58.

[210] Armstrong, GL, Conn, LA & Pinner, RW (1999) Trends in infectious disease mortality in the United States during the 20th century. *JAMA* 281, 61-6.

[211] Bergstom, CT & Feldgarden, M (2008) The ecology and evolution of antibiotic-resistant bacteria. In: Stearns, SC & Koella, JC (eds) *Evolution in health and disease* (2st ed.). Oxford (UK), Oxford University Press.

[212] Read, AF & Mackinnon, MJ (2008) Pathogen evolution in a vaccinated world. In: Stearns, SC & Koella, JC (eds) *Evolution in health and disease* (2nd ed.). Oxford (UK), Oxford University Press.

[213] Trevelyan, B, Smallman-Raynor, M & Cliff, AD (2005) The Spatial Dynamics of Poliomyelitis in the United States: From Epidemic Emergence to Vaccine-Induced Retreat, 1910-1971. *Ann. Assoc. Am. Geogr.* 95, 269-293.

[214] Cooper, PJ (2004). Intestinal worms and human allergy. *Parasite Immunol.* 26, 455–67.

[215] von Mutius, E (2002). Environmental factors influencing the development and progression of pediatric asthma. *J. Allergy Clin. Immunol.* 109, S525–32.

[216] Emanuelsson, C. & Spangfort, M.D. (2007). Allergens as eukaryotic proteins lacking bacterial homologues. *Mol. Immunol.* 44, 3256–60.

[217] Ludvigsson, J. (2006) Why diabetes incidence increases - a unifying theory. *Ann. N. Y. Acad. Sci.* 1079, 374-82.

[218] Carvalho, EM, Bastos, LS & Araújo, MI (2006). Worms and allergy. *Parasite Immunol.* 28, 525–34.

[219] Yazdanbakhsh, M, Kremsner, PG & van Ree, R (2002). Allergy, parasites, and the hygiene hypothesis. *Science* 296, 490–4.

[220] Falcone, FH & Pritchard, DI (2005). Parasite role reversal: worms on trial. *Trends Parasitol.* 21, 157–60.

[221] Hunter, MM & McKay, DM (2004). Review article: helminths as therapeutic agents for inflammatory bowel disease. *Aliment. Pharmacol. Ther.* 19, 167–77.

[222] Croese, J, O'Neil, J, Masson, J, Cooke, S, Melrose, W, Pritchard, D & Speare, R (2006). A proof of concept study establishing *Necator americanus* in Crohn's patients and reservoir donors. *Gut* 55: 136–137.

[223] Summers, RW, Elliott, DE, Urban, JF Jr, Thompson, R, & Weinstock, JV (2005). *Trichuris suis* therapy in Crohn's disease. *Gut* 54, 87–90.

[224] Correale, J & Farez, M (2007). Association between parasite infection and immune responses in multiple sclerosis. *Annals Neurol.* 61, 97–108.

[225] Leonardi-Bee, J, Pritchard, D & Britton, J (2006). Asthma and current intestinal parasite infection: systematic review and meta-analysis. *Amer. J. Resp. Crit. Care Med.* 174, 512–523.

[226] Zaccone, P, Fehervari, Z, Phillips, JM, Dunne, DW & Cooke, A (2006). Parasitic worms and inflammatory diseases. *Parasite Immunol.* 28, 515–23.

[227] Pugliatti, M, Sotgiu, S & Rosati, G (2002). The worldwide prevalence of multiple sclerosis. *Clin. Neurol. Neurosurg.* 104, 182–91.

[228] Weinstock, JV, Summers, R & Elliott, DE (2004). Helminths and harmony. *Gut* 53, 7–9.

[229] Davidson, MH (2007) Overview of prevention and treatment of atherosclerosis with lipid-altering therapy for pharmacy directors. *Am. J. Manag. Care* 13, S260-9.

[230] Weir, MR (2007) Effects of renin-angiotensin system inhibition on end-organ protection: can we do better? *Clin. Ther.* 29, 1803-24.

[231] Klein, R, Deng, Y, Klein, BE, Hyman, L, Seddon, J, Frank, RN, Wallace, RB, Hendrix, SL, Kuppermann, BD, Langer, RD, Kuller, L, Brunner, R, Johnson, KC, Thomas, AM & Haan, M (2007) Cardiovascular disease, its risk factors and treatment, and age-related macular degeneration: Women's Health Initiative Sight Exam ancillary study. *Am. J. Ophthalmol.* 143, 473-83.

[232] Vogel, T, Benetos, A, Verreault, R, Kaltenbach, G, Kiesmann, M & Berthel, M (2006) [Risk factors for Alzheimer: towards prevention?] [Article in French] *Presse Med.* 35, 1309-16.

[233] McCall, KL, Craddock, D & Edwards, K (2006) Effect of angiotensin-converting enzyme inhibitors and angiotensin II type 1 receptor blockers on the rate of new-onset diabetes mellitus: a review and pooled analysis. *Pharmacotherapy* 26, 1297-306.

[234] Ostergren, J (2007) Renin-angiotensin-system blockade in the prevention of diabetes. *Diabetes Res. Clin. Pract.* 78, S13-21.

[235] Jibrini, MB, Molnar, J & Arora, RR (2008) Prevention of atrial fibrillation by way of abrogation of the renin-angiotensin system: a systematic review and meta-analysis. *Am. J. Ther.* 15, 36-43.

[236] Fauchier, L, Pierre, B, de Labriolle, A, Grimard, C, Zannad, N & Babuty, D (2008) Antiarrhythmic effect of statin therapy and atrial fibrillation a meta-analysis of randomized controlled trials. *J. Am. Coll. Cardiol.* 51, 828-35.

[237] Ellul, J, Archer, N, Foy, CM, Poppe, M, Boothby, H, Nicholas, H, Brown, RG & Lovestone, S (2007) The effects of commonly prescribed drugs in patients with Alzheimer's disease on the rate of deterioration. *J. Neurol. Neurosurg. Psychiatry* 78, 233-9.

[238] Alexeeff, SE, Litonjua, AA, Sparrow, D, Vokonas, PS & Schwartz, J (2007) Statin use reduces decline in lung function: VA Normative Aging Study. *Amer. J. Respir. Crit. Care Medic.* 176, 742-7.

[239] Klein, BE, Klein, R, Lee, KE & Grady, LM (2006) Statin use and incident nuclear cataract. *JAMA* 295, 2752-8.

[240] Dropulic, B & Carter, B (Eds.) (2008) *Concepts in Genetic Medicine.* Hoboken, New Jersey (USA), John Wiley & Sons.

[241] Porteus, MH, Connelly, JP & Pruett, SM (2006) A look to future directions in gene therapy research for monogenic diseases. *PLoS Genet.* 2(9):e133.

[242] Urnov, FD, Miller, JC, Lee, YL, Beausejour, CM, Rock, JM, Augustus, S, Jamieson, AC, Porteus, M.H., Gregory, PD & Holmes, MC (2005) Highly efficient endogenous human gene correction using designed zinc-finger nucleases. *Nature* 435, 646-51.

[243] High, KA (2005) Gene therapy: the moving finger. *Nature* 435, 577-9.

[244] Comfort, A. (1979). *The Biology of Senescence.* London (UK), Livingstone.

In: Handbook on Longevity: Genetics, Diet and Disease   ISBN 978-1-60741-075-1
Editors: Jennifer V. Bentely and Mary Ann Keller   © 2009 Nova Science Publishers, Inc.

Chapter V

Stress Resistance and Aging in Long-Lived Rodent Models

James M. Harper[1]* and Adam B. Salmon[2]

[1]Department of Pathology and Geriatrics Center, University of Michigan School of Medicine, Ann Arbor, MI, USA

[2]The Sam and Ann Barshop Institute for Longevity and Aging Studies, University of Texas Health Science Center at San Antonio, San Antonio, TX, USA

Abstract

The aging process affects nearly every biochemical and physical system measured to date. Nevertheless, the mechanism(s) responsible for modulating the rate of aging have yet to be identified. A number of mechanistic theories have predicted that the accumulation of damage to cellular macromolecules could be key determinants of the rate of aging and the progression of age-related disease. These theories also predict that aging may be slowed by the attenuation of damage accumulation, a process that may be accomplished by enhanced resistance to stress.

Treatments that extend lifespan, for example the restriction of caloric intake, are known to reduce the accumulation of cellular damage, including oxidation and DNA mutation, as well as increase the resistance to numerous stressors such as oxidative stress, DNA damage and heat. In addition, genetic mutations that extend murine lifespan have consistently shown a corresponding increase in resistance to multiple types of stress. For instance, dwarf mutations, like the Snell and Ames dwarf, have been shown to extend lifespan by 40-60% while delaying multiple age-related pathologies. Dwarf mice also

---

* Address correspondence to:
James M. Harper, Ph.D.
109 Zina Pitcher Pl, Room 3005 BSRB
Ann Arbor, MI 48109-2200
Email: jmharper@umich.edu
Phone: 734-615-0494
FAX: 734-936-9220

show an increased resistance to oxidative stress *in vivo*, as well as cellular resistance to multiple cytotoxic and metabolic insults.

In addition to these well-characterized mutant mouse models, wild-derived and free-living rodent populations are a virtually untapped resource in the context of stress resistance, aging and disease. Recent studies have shown that wild-derived mouse stocks are very different physiologically from laboratory mouse stocks and that they exhibit significant differences in life span. Work in these underutilized strains and other long-lived rodent models, has suggested that they also exhibit enhanced stress resistance, and especially an enhanced resistance to oxidative stress. Hence, it may be that among models of extended longevity, resistance to stress plays an important role in the maintenance of cellular homeostasis, thereby preserving cell and tissue function and delaying the progression of age-related phenotypes.

Introduction

In this chapter, we explore the hypothesis that the aging rate of mammalian species is a reflection of alterations to multiple pathways that also play a role in regulating resistance to many different forms of cellular stress. The relationship between these seemingly disparate mechanisms has previously been rooted in theory, but recent evidence has shown that extension of lifespan through dietary treatments or through genetic mutation also commonly has a positive affect on cellular stress resistance. We will show that this relationship is present even in relatively simple eukaryotes, and thus the particulars of the stress resistance and longevity link may have evolved relatively early. Further, this relationship exists even in more recently derived animals like mammals, suggesting this may be a fundamental phenotype found in the regulation of aging across all eukaryotic species. We will also argue that development of experimental approaches to study the regulation of stress resistance, and in particular, cellular stress resistance, can likely contribute much to our understanding of the processes that regulate aging and the common pathologies that accompany advancing age.

Background

Aging is a universal phenomenon, yet despite years of investigation little is known of the mechanisms that regulate this process. In mammals, the aging process is a gradual, progressive decline in function that turns healthy, young adult organisms into frail, old organisms with a greater susceptibility to illness, injury and death (Miller 1999). The aging process affects multiple organs, tissues and cell types and has been shown to have distinct effects on nearly every biochemical and physical function of the body that has been measured (Finch 1990). Under this definition, the aging process is generally thought to begin at attainment of maturity though many of the phenotypes of aging are not visible until late in life. In part because of the relative ease of observing the physical attributes of the aged, much is known about what defines an old individual but little is known about the processes that regulate the aging process in early adult life. The general knowledge of phenotypes of aging often complicates our understanding of the aging process; it is quite easy to see the effects of aging in these phenotypes, but it is generally much more difficult to determine the causes of the aging process. As such, it has been proposed that the goal of aging research should be the discrimination of cause and effect in an effort to narrow down the physiological regulatory mechanisms of the aging process (Medawar 1955).

Through the years, a number of different mechanistic theories have proposed that the accumulation of macromolecular damage could be an important regulator of the aging process. The earliest formal theories of why an organism ages proposed that aging was programmed and regulated by biological clocks, some of which may be controlled by the accumulation of damage or by general wear and tear. One of the first theories to actually propose a molecular mechanism for aging, and probably the most popular and well-studied theory since its proposal, has been the oxidative stress theory of aging. First proposed in 1956 by Denham Harman, the general tenets of this theory are that normal cell physiological processes generate reactive oxygen species as by-products and these free radicals react with many cellular macromolecules, damaging them and producing toxic products, the accumulation of which ultimately regulates the rate of aging (Harman 1956). Under this theory, the aging process is regulated by a balance reflecting the deleterious reactions that produce free radicals, the capabilities of the cell or tissue to protect from these radicals, and the ability of the cell or tissue to repair damaged macromolecules.

A second mechanistic theory (though it is not necessarily completely independent from the oxidative stress theory) has suggested that DNA damage and mutation accumulation can drive the aging process. Cellular DNA is under constant challenge by exogenous and endogenous sources of genotoxic stress that can cause both transient and accumulated damage and genome instability. Damaged DNA may be particularly deleterious because it may lead to cellular death or may become a permanent mutation passed among dividing cells that can lead to aberrant cell function. The maintenance of the genome thus seems to be quite important in the prevention of organismal pathologies associated with the accumulation of DNA damage and mutations. It may well be then that processes that improve DNA repair, diminish DNA damage and mutations, or protect from oxidative damage can extend mammalian longevity.

There is a generally consistent trend among animals that increasing age results in an accumulation of oxidative damage to multiple cellular macromolecules as well as accumulated DNA damage. For instance, past reports using primarily rodent models tend to agree that levels of oxidized lipids and proteins accumulate in numerous tissues with advancing age (reviewed in Bokov et al. 2004). There is also a consistent trend for oxidative DNA damage to increase as rodents age (Hamilton et al. 2001). Other forms of DNA damage, such as double-stranded breaks, and mutations have been less well-studied, but again there tends to be a general association for increased accumulation of these types of DNA alterations with age in rodents (Sedelnikova et al. 2004; Crowley and Curtis 1963; Tucker et al. 1999; Jones et al. 1995; Dempsey et al. 1993a; Dolle et al. 1997). The data supporting these trends were mostly generated by examining how old animals differed from young animals, and thus it is unclear whether the accumulation of these forms of damage are general causes of aging or if they are merely effects of the aging process itself. Importantly, calorie restriction (CR) has often been found to diminish the accumulation of many of these forms of damage. For nearly 70 years, it has been known that CR, or limiting caloric intake by approximately 1/3 that consumed by control animals without malnutrition, can significantly extend the lifespan of rodents and delay age-related changes in numerous physiological, biochemical and pathological processes (reviewed in Weindruch and Walford 1988). In general, most reports have suggested that CR in rodents can reduce the age-related accumulation of oxidized lipids (Ward et al. 2005; Davis et al. 1993; Laganiere and Yu 1987; Rao et al. 1990), the accumulation of several forms of protein oxidative damage in different tissues (Lass et al. 1998; Dubey et al. 1996; Sohal et al. 1994; Youngman et al. 1992), and the accumulation of oxidized DNA (Hamilton et al. 2001). CR has also been shown to reduce the age-associated accumulation of DNA mutations at particular chromosomal locations both for spontaneous mutations and for chemically-induced mutations (Aidoo et al. 1999; Dempsey et al. 1993b). And while the effect of CR on the accumulation of other forms of DNA damage has not been directly measured, CR has been shown to increase the rate of repair of multiple forms of DNA lesions (Lipman et al. 1989; Licastro et al. 1988; Tilley et al. 1992; Weraarchakul et al. 1989; Shaddock et al. 1993; Shaddock et al. 1995). It remains speculative, but the reduction of cellular damage by CR could be the root mechanism by which by which CR can both extend lifespan and reduce age-related pathology.

As the accumulated damage in cells reaches a critical point, ultimately they may succumb to apoptotic or non-apoptotic cell death pathways, or differentiate to alternate states such as neoplasia or other changes that put tissue or organismal function at risk. By reducing the accumulation of these forms of damage, CR, or other means by which lifespan is extended, may then delay the onset of of these physiological processes. Thus, it appears that the diminishment of stress-induced damage may be important in the determination of healthy slow aging and reducing age-related pathologies. As a whole, the processes that diminish the accumulation of damage may be described by the general term stress resistance. Further, alterations that protect from damage, or enhance repair of damage, or otherwise maintain cellular homeostasis might be described as a process that increases stress resistance.

At this point, it would be a good idea to define our usage of the term stress in this chapter. Organisms in general can be stressed by a variety of means, from cytotoxic stresses that cause molecular damage to cellular components, to more physiological and psychological stresses such as extremes of temperature or pressure, mechanical trauma, or even lack of sleep or loud noises. In this chapter, stress will primarily refer to cellular stresses that are thought to damage cellular molecules and cause cell death or dysfunction. Commonly, these stresses may fall into particular, though not necessarily discreet, categories, generally based on their modes of action such as oxidative stress, genotoxic stress, or translational stress.

These different types of stress also highlight the differences between cellular stress and stress to whole organisms. It is relatively easy to follow damage to cells or to smaller, lower-order organisms when they are exposed to the types of cellular stressors discussed above. However, higher order animals, mammals in particular, have evolved multiple different pathways to maintain homeostasis that often time can make interpretation of stress resistance difficult, and it may be somewhat naïve to attribute these results solely to stress resistance mechanisms acting at the cellular level. Some cellular stressors may generate a specific form of tissue injury in whole animals that leads to death and thus may be only a distant and indirect surrogate for cellular injury induced by the agent itself. For instance, paraquat is often described as a systemic oxidative stress and has been shown to increase superoxide anion production *in vivo,* but animal death due to paraquat is most often attributed to lung damage that leads to respiratory arrest (Bus et al. 1976). In this case, the specific form of tissue injury that leads to the animal's death may be only a distant and indirect surrogate for cellular injury induced by the agent itself. In addition, mammals have many complex regulatory mechanisms which they use to buffer the effects of harmful agents, such as evaporative heat loss and blood flow to regulate overheating, or the distribution and activation of inflammatory cells in response to oxidative damage. Further, the effects of stress in mammals are complicated because these animals are made of many vastly different cell types that may be differentially protected from the toxic agent due to tissue-specific protective factors, variation in exposure to and accumulation of the test agent, etc. Thus, experimental procedures that expose mice to agents like paraquat provide only limited information about cellular resistance to that agent.

Another approach to address whether relatively long-lived mammals are resistant to stress is by using cells derived from these animals to assay their cellular resistance to cytotoxic agents. Approaches using cell culture may eliminate many of the complicating factors of assaying organismal stress resistance addressed above. In particular, cell-based assays can provide information about the response to the specific action of a stressing agent rather than the multitude of secondary responses that may contribute to an organism's death. Another important benefit of assays that utilize short- or long-term cell cultures is that multiple experiments could be run in parallel testing the effects of different agents. Such experiments might rapidly determine if long-lived animals are resistant to multiple different agents and in particular to agents whose mechanisms of action are different. The rather limited use of cell-based assays of stress resistance in long-lived mammals renders this a fertile area for future study. There is obviously much to be learned about whether long-lived animals are resistant to cellular stresses, particularly if they are resistant to multiple forms of cellular stress.

However, using cellular approaches to study stress resistance in mammals poses both technical and strategic problems. Evaluation of several cell types, from different tissues, will be needed to clarify the relevance of stress resistance on aging in mammals. In part, the difficulty of cell culture for most cell types from adult animals may limit these choices, as may the growth and survival characteristics of each cell type that can be cultured. Such problems can complicate the evaluation of results from these experiments and complicate interpretation of the role of cell stress resistance in the modulation of the aging process in the animal from which cells were derived. Because of these inherent complexities of interpreting stress resistance using either *in vitro* or *in vivo* studies, we will discuss both experimental procedures that expose whole animals to cellular stressors as well as those that specifically examine cellular stress resistance.

Stress Resistance and Life Span in Laboratory Models of Aging

Invertebrate Models: The First to Show a Correlation between Long Lifespan and Stress Resistance

While the focus of this chapter will be on mammalian models of extended lifespan, the origins of much of the research we will discuss is rooted in work utilizing invertebrate models for aging research. One of the most important and widely used models for studying the mechanisms of aging has been the nematode *Caenorhabditis elegans*. Prior to the development of *C. elegans* as a biogerontological model, aging research was largely performed using comparative studies; that is, measuring how a particular phenotype differs between young and old organisms. The first reports that mutations to single genes could extend longevity in *C. elegans* represented a major paradigm shift in the manner that biogerontological research could be performed. After this finding, it was possible to use genetic tools to dissect the potential of specific mechanisms, such as the role of particular signaling pathways, and their role in regulating the aging process by utilizing these gerontogenes.

Subsequent exploration into the mechanisms by which lifespan was extended in these models hinted at the importance of the mechanisms of stress resistance in the regulation of longevity. Two of the earliest published gerontogenes in *C. elegans* were *age-1*, which encodes a homologue of the mammalian phosphatidyl inositol 3-kinase (PI3K), and *daf-2*, which encodes an insulin receptor (IR) tyrosine kinase that is the worm homologue of the mammalian insulin receptor (Friedman and Johnson 1988a; Kenyon et al. 1993). Both mutations were found to extend worm lifespan nearly two-fold and were also subsequently shown to induce, at non-permissive temperatures, an alternate developmental pathway in which larvae enter a diapause state called the dauer (Riddle 1988). In wild-type worms, unfavorable or stressful conditions such as limited food supply and high population density favor dauer formation. During this time, dauer larvae are developmentally arrested and express sets of genes that protect them from harsh conditions such as elevated temperature, desiccation, oxidation and intense γ-radiation (Riddle 1988; Anderson 1978; Yeargers 1981). Worms with mutations in *age-1* and *daf-2* undergo dauer formation at high temperatures (>35° C), but at permissive temperatures these mutations have little effect on fertility or the rate of development and reproduction (Friedman and Johnson 1988a; Kenyon et al. 1993; Friedman and Johnson 1988b; Johnson et al. 2000). It has then been suggested that the regulation of dauer-related transcripts may be responsible for the effect of longevity of these mutations.

Further, there is evidence that the dauer-specific regulation of these gene mutations that can extend *C. elegans* lifespan also often renders those worms relatively resistant to a variety of different lethal agents, even though the worms themselves were adults and not dauer larvae. When *age-1* mutants were cultured in the presence of the oxidizing agent hydrogen peroxide, they were found to live significantly longer than control worms (Larsen 1993). Subsequently, *age-1* mutant worms were found to be resistant to other oxidative stressors including paraquat, an herbicide that stimulates intrinsic reactive oxygen species production

(Vanfleteren 1993), and juglone, which causes intracellular redox cycling and superoxide production (Johnson et al. 2001), and also to be resistant to culture at high oxygen concentrations (Adachi et al. 1998). In addition, *age-1* mutants have been found to be resistant to agents that are thought to act, at least in part, independently of oxidative stress; *age-1* mutants are resistant to the lethal effects caused by UV light (Murakami and Johnson 1996), to incubation at high temperature (Lithgow G.J. et al. 1994) and to incubation with the heavy metals cadmium or copper (Barsyte et al. 2001). Mutations in *daf-2* exhibit a similar pattern of stress resistance to all agents tested including an increased resistance to oxidative stress induced by paraquat or menadione (Honda and Honda 1999), increased resistance to UV (Murakami and Johnson 1996), increased resistance to heat (Lithgow et al. 1995), and increased resistance to cadmium and copper (Barsyte et al. 2001). Additional reports utilizing other long-lived mutant *C. elegans* have shown a general, though not universal, correlation between stress resistance and longevity; thus, these early findings have generally supported the idea that pathways that extend nematode lifespan may do so, in part, by increasing resistance to stress.

The finding in *C. elegans* that genetic mutations could extend lifespan and enhance stress resistance has stimulated many new studies using genetic approaches to explore ideas about aging in flies as well. While *Drosophila* are particularly adept for random mutation approaches due to the availability of well-developed molecular genetic tools and their relatively short lifespan, only a few long-lived mutant strains have been developed in this manner. For example, flies with a mutation of the gene *methuselah (mth)*, which encodes a G protein-coupled transmembrane, receptor-like molecule, emerged from a screen for long-lived mutants among randomly mutated flies. *Mth* mutations can extend lifespan of both male and female flies by about 35% without reduction of fecundity; mutation of *mth* also renders flies resistant to lethality induced by heat and by paraquat (Lin et al. 1998). The function of *mth* is still not clear, but mutations of the endogenous ligands of the gene product of *mth* also extend lifespan about 50% compared to a control, and render flies relatively resistant to paraquat (Cvejic et al. 2004). A second long-lived fly strain generated by random mutagenesis has a mutation in the gene *I'm not dead yet (Indy); Indy* flies have an average lifespan nearly two-fold that of control flies (Rogina et al. 2000). Similar to *mth* mutant flies, *Indy* flies are resistant to paraquat toxicity (Oliver 2005). The *Indy* gene encodes a dicarboxylate transporter which is thought to be involved in the transport of metabolites from the gut into nutrient storage sites and metabolic tissues such as the fat body, but mutations of *Indy* do not decrease basal metabolic rate, do not affect physiological measures such as flight or activity and do not reduce fecundity under normal laboratory rearing conditions (Rogina et al. 2000; Helfand and Rogina 2003; Marden et al. 2003). Thus, even though the genes products of *mth* and *Indy* have not been reported to modulate stress resistance directly, mutation of these genes can render flies resistant to stress and extend longevity.

Extended longevity and stress resistance have been found using directed mutagenesis in flies in addition to the random screens described above. For instance, diminishment of insulin-like signaling through ablation of the neuroendocrine cells that produce *Drosophila* insulin-like peptides (DILPs) can extend lifespan 10-35% depending on sex and reproductive status and render these flies resistant to heat and paraquat (Broughton et al. 2005). The *Drosophila* homologue of the forkhead transcription factor (*dFOXO*) has recently been shown to extend lifespan 20-50% when overexpressed and also to confer resistance to paraquat when overexpressed in the fat body of adult flies (Giannakou et al. 2004; Hwangbo et al. 2004). In addition, flies overexpressing *d4E-BP*, a regulatory element of the *dFOXO* downstream effector eIF4E, are long-lived and peroxide resistant (Tettweiler et al. 2005). In a related line of investigation, enhancement of Jun N-terminal kinase (JNK) signaling, and subsequent antagonism of insulin-like signaling, by overexpression of a JNK-specific phosphatase, was shown to extend fly longevity up to about 30% and to increase resistance to paraquat (Wang et al. 2003; Wang et al. 2005). However, other mutations that extend *Drosophila* lifespan have been shown to have little affect on stress resistance; mutation of the insulin receptor gene (*InR*) yields dwarf flies that live about 85% longer than the control for females and 50% longer for males (Tatar et al. 2001) and some mutations of an insulin receptor substrate *(chico)* also yield long-lived dwarf flies live up to 48% longer than control (Clancy et al. 2001). For *chico* and *InR* mutants, age-related changes to the heart, including stress-induced failure, are reduced suggesting that these mutations can delay the progression of age-related pathologies (Wessells et al. 2004). But the *chico* mutation does not seem to render flies stress resistant; female *chico* heterozygotes and homozygotes are not resistant to heat or paraquat relative to control flies, and male *chico* homozygotes are more sensitive than controls to these stresses (Clancy et al. 2001). Further, larvae with loss of function *chico* mutations are sensitive to γ-irradiation as measured by eclosion of larvae to adult, though this may represent the adverse effects of reduced insulin signaling on eclosion more than stress resistance (Jaklevic et al. 2006). Many of the mutations discussed above are within the same general signaling pathway, so it is unclear why there has been a discrepancy in the stress resistance of these long-lived flies. It may be particulars in the means of assay or that particular mediators of signals through this pathway are more important for stress resistance than others. In general though, these mutations suggest that, like in *C. elegans*, mutations that extend lifespan in *Drosophila* tend to enhance resistance to multiple forms of stress.

Thus, these findings in invertebrates suggest that longevity in lower organisms may be regulated by many of the same pathways that regulate resistance to stress. A larger question is whether higher order organisms like mammals show a similar relationship.

Is There a Correlation between Lifespan and Stress Resistance in Mammals?

Traditionally, studies of the mechanisms of aging in mammals (mostly in mice and rats) have generally been designed to address how young animals differ from old animals. However, this type of design suffers because while it is relatively simple test a hypothesis on how "young" differ from "old", it is much more difficult to test hypotheses on the mechanisms that determine those final phenotypes. Another approach is to utilize two groups of animals that age at different rates to test hypotheses on how the aging rate can be modulated. This approach, described above for several invertebrate models, can then be used to address the role of specific treatments, genes, or gene pathways on aging in general or on the progression of age-related phenotypes. Thus, this approach may be used to focus on specific mechanisms that regulate aging.

In mammals, aging rate can be modified by two primary means: 1. modification of dietary intake (restriction of either calories or specific dietary components) or by 2. genetic mutation, either by single gene mutation, through selection for particular niches, or by the evolution of separate species. There is now accumulating evidence that lifespan extension by both means is associated with an increase in the resistance to multiple types of stress and/or an increase in the processes associated with stress resistance.

Calorie Restriction and Resistance to Stress

For more than seventy years now, it has been known that lifespan in rodents can be extended by restricting caloric intake without causing malnutrition (McCay et al. 1935). Since McCay's first report in 1935, calorie restriction (CR) has been the most commonly utilized model of extended longevity, and for most of that time the only model of extended longevity, and has been utilized to explore many of the potential mechanisms that regulate aging in mammals (Weindruch and Walford 1988). The CR-mediated extension of lifespan of rodents is also accompanied by CR-mediated delay of age-related changes in numerous physiological, biochemical and pathological processes and a delayed onset of most age-related diseases relative to ad libitum (AL) fed controls (reviewed in Weindruch and Walford 1988). Studies of CR in other laboratory models, including invertebrate models, have shown that many species respond to low calorie diets by increased lifespan, with only a few exceptions (reviewed in Weindruch and Walford 1988). Many reports have suggested that one of the many phenotypes of CR in rodent models is an upregulation of pathways that may regulate resistance to stress. It is still relatively unclear whether the stress-resistant phenotype of CR contributes directly to lifespan extension (i.e. protects from the accumulation of deleterious end-products such as oxidative or genotoxic damage or the accumulation of dead cells) or if this correlation results from concurrent upregulation of pathways common both to stress resistance and longevity. Regardless, these two phenotypes, stress resistance and longevity, are often correlated in CR studies and thus an understanding of how CR affects stress resistance can lead to a greater understanding of its effects on the aging process.

Studies of stress resistance of rodents under CR have utilized a great range of stresses, toxins and carcinogens to measure the resistance to injury of both the animals and of their tissues *in vivo*. For instance, C57BL/6 mice that have undergone CR are resistant to death due to injection of paraquat (Richardson et al. 2004; Sun et al. 2001). In studies using Fisher 344 rats, CR protected these animals from death when they were exposed to high temperature (>33° C for several hours) relative to AL control (Heydari et al. 1993; Hall et al. 2000), although this result is somewhat complicated by the fact that rats under CR are smaller than those under AL and thus the heat resistance of CR rats may be due to a greater evaporative heat loss potential rather than heat resistance directly. CR has also been shown to reduce the effects of chronic cadmium toxicity in rats as measured by urinary excretion of proteins and glucose and by loss of bone density over time (Shaikh et al. 1999). CR is effective in protecting rats against methylmercury-induced pathological changes in skeletal muscle (Usuki et al. 2004) and can protect rats from excitatory neurodegeneration in hippocampus caused by kainic acid treatment or from striatal neurodegeneration caused by 3-nitropropionic acid (3-NPA) and malonate (Bruce-Keller et al. 1999). CR also protects rodents from mortality caused by several toxins with differing actions including ganciclovir (a hematopoetic toxin), cyclosporin A, phenobarbitol, clofibrate, L-647,318 (an inhibitor of 3-hydroxy-3-methyl-glutaryl coenzyme A (HMG-CoA) reductase), and MK-458 (a dopamine agonist) (Berg et al. 1994; Keenan et al. 1997). Finally, rats undergoing CR are resistant to liver damage caused by the hepatotoxin thiacetoamide, with an increased rate of liver regeneration following thiacetoamide treatment (Apte et al. 2003) as well as to the the hepatotoxin acetaminophen (Harper et al. 2006c).

Rodents undergoing CR have long been known to show diminished spontaneous cancer rates (Weindruch and Walford 1988) and also appear to be resistant to many types of DNA damaging insults. For instance, the mutation frequency in splenic T-cells is reduced in CR-fed mice subjected to bleomycin, a radiomimetic drug that causes DNA damage through a free radical-dependent mechanism (Aidoo et al. 1999). CR has been shown to inhibit the formation of skin tumors in mice and rats following treatment with benzo(a)pyrene (Tannenbaum 1942) or with methylcholanthrene (Lavick and Baumann 1943) as well as reduce the incidence of mammary tumors caused by DMBA injection (Kritchevsky et al. 1984; Klurfeld et al. 1989), intestinal tumors caused by methylazoxymethanol acetate injection (Pollard and Luckert 1985), and myeloid leukemia caused by X-ray irradiation (Yoshida et al. 1997). From these data, it is clear that the effects of CR are far-reaching, and that CR provides protection from different sources of insult to many tissues and organs.

For reasons discussed above, the interpretation of stress resistance in whole animals is often complicated by the complex mechanisms utilized by mammals to maintain homeostasis. Thus, often a reductionist approach utilizing tissues or cells derived from animals can help directly delineate phenotypes of interest, such as stress resistance. As discussed above, much has been published on the stress and toxin response of CR-treated rodents as whole animal studies, but there has been relatively little published on the characteristics of cells derived from CR animals. Probably the most well-studied stress resistance-associated mechanism that has been studied in cellular studies of the effects of CR has been the ability of cells from CR- and AL-fed animals to repair different types of DNA lesions. For instance, hepatocytes from CR rats repair UV irradiation-induced cyclobutane pyrimidine dimers (CPD) more rapidly than in cells from AL animals (Guo et al. 1998). These assays, which specifically measured nucleotide excision repair (NER), showed that cells in culture could retain the effects of CR even after being removed from the animal. Similarly, a mixture of cell types freshly isolated from the skin of CR-fed rats were protected from UV light and methyl methanesulfonate (MMS) as measured by unscheduled DNA synthesis, a measure of general DNA repair (Lipman et al. 1989). This same measure of DNA repair has shown that CR in rats can increase the rate of DNA repair of UV damage in primary cultures of splenic lymphocytes (Licastro et al. 1988), in secondary fibroblast cultures derived from lung (Tilley et al. 1992) and in cultured liver and kidney cells (Weraarchakul et al. 1989). CR also enhanced the rate of repair of genotoxic lesions caused by the carcinogens 2-acetylaminofluorane, aflatoxin B_1, DMBA, dimethylnitrosamine and tacrine in primary hepatocytes derived from rats (Shaddock et al. 1993; Shaddock et al. 1995) and of the lesions caused by tacrine in primary hepatocytes from mice (Shaddock et al. 1995).

Others have attempted to show that CR of rodents can enhance oxidative stress resistance of cells from those animals. These sparse data on cellular oxidative stress resistance have often shown a less consistent correlation between stress resistance and CR than have results for DNA repair. For instance, lens epithelial cells isolated from mice that have undergone CR have been shown to resist the induction of cell death in response to high doses of hydrogen peroxide (Li et al. 1997). However, later work utilizing the same model suggested that with extended culturing of cells utilizing standard cell culture techniques, the resistance of CR-derived cells is lost (Li et al. 1997). This particular result might suggest that the effects of CR on cells may be transient in nature. Further supporting this idea are data showing that fibroblasts derived from the skin of CR- and AL-fed mice showed no difference in resistance to cell death caused by hydrogen peroxide (Harper et al. 2006c). In this study, primary fibroblasts were sub-cultured for a period greater than two weeks utilizing standard culture techniques; i.e. both CR- and AL-derived fibroblasts were cultured using the same media containing the serum derived from fetal bovine sources. This study showed that cells from CR-fed mice not only showed no difference from AL-derived cells in their resistance to hydrogen peroxide, but also no difference from AL-derived cells to the cytotoxic effects of UV light or the heavy metal cadmium, both of which may act in part through the generation of free radicals (Harper et al. 2006c). However, some data have been presented that suggest using cell culture techniques that utilize serum from CR-fed animals can extend "CR-like" phenotypes to cell culture lines, including resistance to cell death induced by peroxide or heat (de Cabo et al. 2003; Cohen et al. 2004). Deciding how such experiments relate to the *in vivo* environment of CR rodents can be difficult because the particular components of "CR-serum" are still unknown. However, it is clear that CR affects multiple circulating factors *in vivo* (Weindruch and Walford 1988), and these cell culture models might still be used to determine the direct effects to cells of these alterations. Additional studies on how CR influences cellular resistance to stress are clearly needed.

Very little is known about the mechanisms that regulate stress resistance among the rodents on longevity extending CR diets. It may be that these animals have increased activity of the proteins that protect from stress-induced tissue damage or animal death. This hypothesis has been primarily addressed by surveying multiple tissues of long-lived and control animals for the expression of proteins that protect from particular forms of damage, such as the antioxidants that protect from oxidative stress. However, there seems to be no clear consensus among these studies suggesting that CR consistently upregulates these proteins.

For instance, catalase is an antioxidant that protects cells by its enzymatic conversion of peroxide to water and oxygen. Mice fed a CR diet seem to express lower levels of catalase mRNA and protein and have lower catalase activity in the liver, eye lens, kidney and skeletal muscle (Usuki et al. 2004; Mura et al. 1996; Gong et al. 1997). However, some of these results did suggest that the loss of catalase activity in these tissues with age is attenuated in CR mice (Mura et al. 1996; Gong et al. 1997). Others have suggested that mice undergoing CR have higher levels of catalase activity in the liver, brain, heart and kidney (Wu et al. 2003; Sohal et al. 1994) or that CR attenuates an age-related increase in catalase (Luhtala et al. 1994). There is also inconsistency in the association of the antioxidant enzymes CuZn-superoxide dismutase (Sod1) and Mn-superoxide dismutase (Sod2) with differences in longevity. These enzymes convert oxygen free radicals to oxygen and peroxide with Sod1 acting primarily in the cytosol and Sod2 primarily in the mitochondria. CR also has been shown to have no effect on the expression or activity of Sod1 or Sod2 in liver, kidney, skeletal muscle or eye lens (Usuki et al. 2004; Mura et al. 1996; Gong et al. 1997). In contrast, however, there are reports of increases in activity of the Sod proteins in CR models (Wu et al. 2003; Sohal et al. 1994). Lastly, there is also inconsistency in reports on modulation of the activity of glutathione peroxidase (GpX), which protects mitochondria from oxygen free radicals, with CR. In CR models, GpX has been suggested to be higher, lower and unchanged depending on the tissue, age of the animal, and length of time on CR (Usuki et al. 2004; Mura et al. 1996; Gong et al. 1997; Wu et al. 2003; Sohal et al. 1994). Thus, in the published literature there is no clear cut support for the idea that the mechanisms that increase longevity do so by increasing the expression of GpX, or any other antioxidants examined. These data thus make it difficult to support a relationship between oxidative stress defense and lifespan.

There are more consistent data for protein expression patterns that may protect from sources of damage that might be, in part, oxidation-independent, though much less has been published on this topic. The activity of glutathione-s-transferase, which detoxifies many compounds by conjugation with reduced glutathione, decreases with age and CR prevents the loss of its activity with age in kidney (Cho et al. 2003). CR also seems to prevent the loss of the heat shock proteins HSP-27, HSP-72, and HSP-90 with age in the skeletal muscle in rats (Selsby et al. 2005). These limited data thus suggest that agents that prevent multiple types of damage, rather than merely oxidative damage, may be more closely tied to the mechanisms that regulate longevity.

Recently, it has been shown that mammalian lifespan can be extended through another form of dietary restriction. A diet restricted in the level of the essential amino acid methionine, provided ad libitum and thus without restriction of caloric intake, has been shown to extend lifespan in rats about 30-40% (Orentreich et al. 1993; Zimmerman et al. 2003) and the lifespan of mice by about 10% (Miller et al. 2005). The limited information on the effects of methionine restriction (MR) suggests that, like CR, MR is able to lengthen lifespan by delaying the rate of aging and progression of age-related pathologies. In mice, MR retards the development of cataracts and can delay the senescence of the immune system (Miller et al. 2005) while in rats, MR inhibits chronic progressive nephropathy, the major cause of aging-related mortality of F344 rats, and testicular cancer, a common neoplasia in aged rats (Komninou et al. 2002). Little is known about the stress resistance of these animals, but like CR-treated rodents, mice undergoing MR show less liver damage following acetaminophen treatment (Miller et al. 2005). MR also seems to increase glutathione levels in the blood of rats, suggesting an increase in the protection from oxidative damage (Richie, Jr. et al. 1994). In addition, MR in rats seems to diminish mitochondrial production of reactive oxygen species and reduce the amount of oxidative damage found in DNA and in proteins (Sanz et al. 2006). MR-fed rodents also may be resistant to chemically-induced cancer; treatment of rats with an MR diet inhibits the formation of colon tumors following azoxymethane treatment (Komninou et al. 2002; Komninou et al. 2006).

To date, only one report has attempted to define the effects of MR on cellular stress resistance in rodents. In this study, primary fibroblasts derived from the skin of mice on a MR diet or fed AL with all amino acids provided at normal levels were tested for their resistance to hydrogen peroxide, UV light and the heavy metal cadmium (Harper et al. 2006c). MR-derived fibroblasts were found to be no different from AL-derived in their resistance to any of these stresses, similarly to what was discussed above for CR-derived fibroblasts. It may be that for MR, like proposed for CR, the effects of stress resistance are transient and through several generations of subculturing using standard cell culture techniques, MR-associated stress resistance may be lost. It will require reexamination of this question utilizing different techniques, or cell types, to determine if restriction of methionine has a positive effect on cellular resistance to stress.

Overall, the data discussed above suggest that dietary treatments like CR and MR positively affect the mechanisms regulating stress resistance in addition to modulating mechanisms that extend lifespan. It remains to be determined whether this relationship results from shared pathways between these mechanisms, such as by signaling through insulin/IGF-I signaling or through reduction of mTOR activity, or whether these two phenotypes result from simultaneous stimulation of independent pathways through some CR or MR-mediated signal.

Genetic Mutations and Resistance to Stress

For over 70 years, CR was the only consistent means of extending rodent lifespan. Within the last dozen years however, a number of single-gene mutants have been shown to also extend lifespan in mice. The discovery of these mutants has represented a major paradigm shift in the way one can study aging in mammals; CR is a complex phenotype that has been shown to have multiple effectors and downstream phenotypes, as discussed above. With the utilization of single gene mutations that extend lifespan, for the first time researchers could investigate the role that a particular protein, or signaling pathway, has on the regulation of aging and address specific scientific questions about what may be necessary for long lifespan. In addition, these mutant strains can used to examine how long-lived animals differ from controls to provide information on the mechanisms that may delay the aging process. The utilization of these long-lived genetic models has contributed, and will continue to contribute, much to our understanding of the mechanisms that regulate the aging process in mammals. Subsequent exploration into these mechanisms has hinted at the importance of stress resistance in the regulation of longevity in mammals.

Dwarf Mice

In many cases, the lifespan-extending mutations in mice are orthologous to known longevity mutants found in invertebrate models. For instance, past studies have shown the importance of the insulin/insulin-like growth factor I (IGF-I) signaling pathway in the regulation of lifespan in both *C. elegans* (e.g. *age-1* and *daf-2* mutants discussed above) and in *Drosophila* (e.g. *InR* and *chico* mutants discussed above) and thus hint at the importance of this pathway for regulating aging across multiple phylogenetic groups (Braeckman et al.

2001; Tatar et al. 2003). In mammals, the first report of a single-gene mutation that extended life span was that of the Ames dwarf mouse, which has a homozygous recessive mutation in *Prop-1* (Prophet of Pit1) (Brown-Borg et al. 1996a). A similar mutant, originally described in 1929, is the Snell dwarf mouse, which has a mutation of the gene *Pit1* (pituitary-specific transcription factor 1) which is downstream of *Prop-1* signaling (Snell 1929; Camper et al. 1990; Andersen et al. 1995). Both mutations interfere with the cellular processes necessary for the differentiation of pituitary somatotrophs, thyrotrophs and lactotrophs in the anterior pituitary, the cells responsible for secretion of growth hormone (GH), thyroid stimulating hormone and prolactin, respectively (Camper et al. 1990; Li et al. 1990). Therefore, Snell and Ames dwarf mice are deficient for these hormones, as well as their secondary effectors, like IGF-I, shortly after birth, which highlights the presumed importance of the IGF-I signaling pathway in regulating aging across species. Further supporting this idea, mutations to the IGF-I receptor ($IGF-IR^{+/-}$), to $p66^{Shc}$ (a downstream effector of IGF-IR) and to *Klotho* (thought to inhibit signaling through the insulin/IGF-I signaling pathway) have also been reported to also extend mouse lifespan and affect stress resistance (discussed below).

The hormonal alterations that accompany the Snell and Ames dwarf mutations make these mice small, approximately 1/3 the size of control mice (Flurkey et al. 2001; Cheng et al. 1983)) and also make these mice long-lived compared to their littermate controls. Initial reports of the lifespan of the Snell dwarf mouse were contrary to this and showed that this mutant strain was rather short-lived (3 – 5.5 months) and suggested that the dwarf mice represented a potential model of accelerated aging, particularly of the immune system (Silberberg 1972). However, even control mice were relatively short lived in this study (maximum lifespan ~2 years or roughly 1/3 shorter than generally recognized as the maximum lifespan of most mouse strains reared under standard laboratory conditions) suggesting that poor housing conditions probably contributed to the diminished lifespan of the dwarf animals. Further, many of the parameters of aging other than lifespan that were used in this study, such as hair graying and loss, atrophy, and *in vivo* cellular turnover are more indicative of illness rather than aging. Others reported that a coallelic dwarf strain, the Jackson dwarf mice ($Pit1^{dw-J}$) had no lifespan reduction compared to control and hinted that these mice may actually outlive their littermate controls (Eicher and Beamer 1980). This strain has a separate mutation in the *Pit1* locus than the Snell dwarf, but the two mutations have similar effects on the differentiation of the pituitary cells and an indistinguishable phenotype. This study suffered due to small sample sizes and a lack of statistical analysis of lifespan data. Therefore, an independent lifespan study was performed, which found that coallelic hybrid Snell dwarf mice carrying ($Pit1^{dw}/Pit1^{dw-J}$) have a mean lifespan >40% greater than that of their littermate controls (Snell dwarf mean $1,178 \pm 235$ days vs. control mean 832 ± 158 days) when housed in specific-pathogen free conditions and with a control littermate to provide warmth to the hypothermic dwarf mice (Flurkey et al. 2001). It was also found that maximum longevity was approximately 37% greater in Snell dwarf mice (Snell dwarf 1,451 days vs. control 1060 days). Further, analysis of mortality curves suggested that the effects of aging on lethal illness in dwarf animals are delayed by about 12 months, but that once initiated these effects increase at approximately the same rate in each genotype. These results were replicated by a study of the Snell dwarf mutation on a second mouse strain (Flurkey et al. 2002), suggesting that the mutation and its effects can extend lifespan regardless of genetic background. Because the both the *Prop-1* and *Pit1* mutations share the same pituitary development pathway, the Ames dwarf and Snell dwarf mice share most of the same endocrinological phenotypes. In addition, Ames dwarf mice were found to have a mean lifespan of 49-68% greater than their littermate controls, and a maximum lifespan of 20-50% greater than control, depending on sex (Brown-Borg et al. 1996).

Not only are both of these hypopituitary dwarf models long-lived, but evidence also suggests that the extension of longevity is accompanied by delay or diminution of many late-life pathologies. Because of their similar genetic mutations and the resulting similar patterns of alterations in the endocrine system, the delayed and diminished pathologies of Ames and Snell dwarf mice will be discussed in parallel. Snell dwarf mice show a decline in the rate at which collagen cross-links occur during aging (Flurkey et al. 2001). The proportion of CD4 and CD8 T-cells that express markers of memory and P-glycoprotein activity is significantly lower in old Snell dwarf mice, indicative of a lower degree of immunosenescence than that of control mice (Flurkey et al. 2001). Age-dependent pathology of the knee joints and vertebral column is greatly retarded in Snell dwarf mice and age-related osteoarthritis is completely prevented (Silberberg 1972). The incidence of cataract formation with age is greatly reduced in Snell dwarf mice, as is the severity of glomerular basement membrane damage in the kidneys (Vergara et al. 2004). Tests of mental acuity and measures of locomotion show that Ames dwarf mice have a delay in the rate of age-related cognitive decline (Kinney et al. 2001; Mattison et al. 2000), perhaps because of a higher level of neurogenesis in the brain (Sun et al. 2005). Both Snell and Ames dwarf mice have been shown to have lower incidence and presumably slower progression of multiple forms of spontaneous neoplasia (Ikeno et al. 2003; Vergara et al. 2004). Further, Snell dwarf mice are resistant to the development of neoplasia in multiple tissues when induced by at least three different chemical mutagens (Bielschowsky and Bielschowsky 1960; Bielschowsky and Bielschowsky 1961; Bickis et al. 1956), perhaps due to DNA damage protection; the frequency of X-ray- or mitomycin C-induced mutagenic lesions are significantly lower in Snell dwarf bone marrow cells and spermatagonia relative to controls (van Buul and van Buul-Offers 1982; van Buul and van Buul-Offers 1988).

The pathways that have led to an extension of lifespan in dwarf mice also appear to have positively affected mechanisms responsible for regulating stress resistance. In particular, most previous reports suggest that proteins that protect from many types of damage are more active in tissues from long-lived dwarf mice. For instance, the activity of Sod1 has been shown to be higher in the hypothalamus (the only tissue tested) of young and middle-aged Ames dwarf, but not in old animals (Hauck and Bartke 2000). However, GpX activity was found to be lower in the liver and heart of Ames dwarf mice and no different from control in the kidney (Al-Regaiey et al. 2005). Methionine sulfoxide reductase, which repairs oxidized methionine residues in proteins, has been shown to be expressed at higher levels in the liver and kidney of Ames dwarf mice (Brown-Borg 2006). The mRNA encoding metallothionein, an antioxidant and chelator of heavy metals, was shown to be expressed at higher levels in the liver, heart, kidney and brain of Ames dwarf mice (Brown-Borg 2006). Glutathione-s-transferase, which detoxifies many compounds by conjugation with reduced glutathione, is found at higher levels in the kidney of Ames dwarf mice (Brown-Borg and Rakoczy 2005). The heat shock protein HSP-70 is found at higher levels in the Ames dwarf kidney (Brown-

Borg 2006). These limited data thus suggest that agents that prevent multiple types of damage, rather than merely oxidative damage, may be more closely tied to the mechanisms that regulate longevity in dwarf mice.

The data above show that cellular defenses to stress, primarily oxidative stress, are upregulated in many tissues from the Ames and Snell dwarf mice. Recently, it has also been shown that these long-lived mice display cellular resistance to not only to oxidative stress, but also to several other forms of cytotoxic stress. Primary fibroblasts derived from Snell dwarf mice were shown to be resistant to cell death induced by agents that cause oxidative stress, such as hydrogen peroxide and the superoxide generator paraquat, as well as to the heavy metal cadmium, UV light, and methyl methanesulfonate (MMS) that cause cell death mainly through non-oxidative pathways (Murakami et al. 2003; Salmon et al. 2005). Thus it seems that this phenotype is a result of alterations of multiple pathways which act together to concordantly increase resistance to multiple forms of cytotoxic stress, both oxidative and non-oxidative related (Leiser et al. 2006). Primary fibroblasts from Ames dwarf mice have been subsequently shown to be resistant to the same panel of stressors (Salmon et al. 2005; Salmon et al. 2008a). It appears that the stress resistant phenotype is regulated by the hormone alterations in the dwarf animal; even though fibroblasts derived from adult dwarf mice are stress resistant, cells derived from newborn, and thus mice that have not yet been exposed to the low GH and IGF-I are not more resistant to most stressors (Salmon et al. 2005). Serially passaged cells from Snell dwarf mice are also delayed in their entry into "growth crisis," characterized by a failure of logarithmic expansion and the emergence of transformed aneuploid variants (Maynard and Miller 2006), suggesting that they are resistant to the oxygen-dependent accumulation of mutations and chromosomal rearrangements characteristic of mouse cells grown under 20% O_2 concentrations. In addition, the UV resistance of cells from Snell dwarf mice appears to be due to a greater ability to repair the DNA lesions caused by UV light (Salmon et al. 2008b). These results are consistent with the idea that that fibroblasts from these mice, like many long-lived nematode mutants, exhibit resistance to multiple forms of stress.

Surprisingly, recent evidence suggests that in contrast to their resistance to multiple other forms of stress, Snell dwarf cells are sensitive to agents that cause ER stress such as thapsigargin and tunicamycin (Salmon et al. 2008a). These agents cause accumulation of unfolded or misfolded proteins in the endoplasmic reticulum which causes ER stress, and instigates a concerted adaptive program known as the unfolded protein response (UPR) that alleviates ER stress through reduction of protein load, increase in folding capacity, and eliminating irreparably misfolded proteins. It is possible that the sensitivity of Snell dwarf cells, if it occurred in appropriate cells *in vivo*, might help to rid the organism of defective cells and thus postpone pathological outcomes. It is also possible that heightened sensitivity to ER stress might induce compensatory increases in pathways that protect against the lethal effects of some of the other agents tested in these *in vitro* analyses. It is of interest to note, that cells from the longest-living rodent, the naked mole-rat, are also sensitive to the induction of ER stress by thapsigargin and tunicamycin (Salmon et al. 2008a).

There is also limited experimental evidence supporting the prediction of multiple stress resistance in dwarf animals when testing the stress resistance of animals *in vivo*. Dwarf mice are relatively resistant to death caused by paraquat; they live about 40% longer than their controls following paraquat injection than do paraquat-treated control mice (Bartke et al. 2001). Further, responses in the MAPK/ERK kinase signaling cascade and in the phosphorylation of c-Jun are reduced in the liver of Snell dwarf mice after treatment with 3-NPA, which induces mitochondrial free radical generation (Madsen et al. 2004). In addition, tissues from the Ames dwarf mice tend to exhibit lower levels of oxidative damage with increasing age as measured by inorganic peroxides in the liver and kidney (Bartke et al. 1998; Carlson et al. 1999), protein carbonyls in the liver and brain (Brown-Borg et al. 2001), and oxidative damage to the mitochondrial DNA in the heart and brain (Sanz et al. 2002). This suggests that the changes that lengthen life in Snell dwarf mice can also confer oxidative stress resistance to particular tissues *in vivo*. It remains to be seen if other pathways that regulate resistance to non-oxidative stresses are similarly upregulated in dwarf mice; however, the diminished cancer rates in these dwarf mice and resistance of Snell dwarf mice to the development of carcinogen-induced tumors suggests there may be fundamental differences in DNA repair (Ikeno et al. 2003; Vergara et al. 2004; Bielschowsky and Bielschowsky 1960; Bielschowsky and Bielschowsky 1961; Bickis et al. 1956).

In many ways, mice lacking the growth hormone receptor (GHR-KO) are phenotypically similar to dwarf mice. These mice lack functional GH receptors due to targeted gene disruption resulting in GH resistance and dwarfism (Zhou et al. 1997). GHR-KO mice differ in their hormonal profile from Ames and Snell dwarf mice in that GHR-KO mice have high levels of GH, modest declines in thyroid hormones, yet are similar to dwarf mice in that they have very low IGF-I levels (Coschigano et al. 2000; Coschigano et al. 2003). Like dwarf mice, GHR-KO mice are long-lived; GHR-KO mice live up to 55% longer than their controls, depending on sex and genetic background (Coschigano et al. 2000; Coschigano et al. 2003). There is some discrepancy in whether these animals resemble dwarf mice in their resistance to stress. For instance, the activity of GPX in kidney was 25% higher in GHR-KO compared with wild-type mice, but catalase and GPX activities were decreased in the liver (Hauck et al. 2002). Sod2 mRNA levels were also found to be higher in GHR-KO mice (Al-Regaiey et al. 2005) and GHR-KO mice also show high levels of metallothionein in kidney, liver, and heart (Brown-Borg 2006). Cells derived from GHR-KO mice do seem to be resistant to a variety of different cytotoxic stressors, including hydrogen peroxide, paraquat, UV light, and MMS, but surprisingly were found to be no different from control in their resistance to cadmium (Salmon et al. 2005; Salmon et al. 2008a). GHR-KO mice differed from dwarf mice in their *in vivo* response to paraquat; female GHR-KO mice died at the same rate as controls and male GHR-KO actually died more rapidly than control (Hauck et al. 2002). Further, GHR-KO mice are sensitive to liver damage caused by acetaminophen, the toxicity of which is thought to be in part due to induced oxidative stress (Harper et al. 2006c). Snell dwarf mice were also found to be sensitive to acetaminophen, in contrast to their resistance to paraquat and 3-NPA (Harper et al. 2006c). In part, the sensitivity of GHR-KO and Snell dwarf mice to acetaminophen might represent differences in conversion to a toxic metabolite rather than resistance to oxidative stress. The lack of consistent stress response between the pituitary dwarf models and GHR-KO mice might be merely an effect of background strain, housing conditions, or experimental protocol. Alternatively, the absence of evidence for cadmium resistance in GHR-KO cell lines and paraquat sensitivity of GHR-KO mice might suggest these phenotypes may depend on hormonal, or perhaps other, factors that differ between the pituitary mutants and the GHR-KO model. However, these stress sensitive phenotypes also suggest that we cannot rule out that stress resistance and longevity may not always be common factors.

Other Long-Lived IGF-I Signaling Mutants

As discussed above, mutations within the insulin/IGF-I signaling pathway have been shown to regulate lifespan across multiple species and thus IGF-I signaling has been predicted to be an important regulator of lifespan. However, the dwarf mutant mice discussed above have alterations to a number of other hormones, thus the direct role of IGF-I in regulating lifespan and stress resistance can be difficult to interpret. To test whether IGF-I signaling could directly regulate lifespan, another long-lived model was developed, mice carrying a heterozygous deletion of the IGF-I receptor ($IGF\text{-}IR^{+/-}$). Female $IGF\text{-}IR^{+/-}$ were shown to live up to 33% longer than their controls, but there was no significant extension of lifespan in male mice with the same genotype (Holzenberger et al. 2003). In addition, female $IGF\text{-}IR^{+/-}$ mice, but not males, live significantly longer following paraquat injection, suggesting an concomitant increases in oxidative stress resistance in addition to the lifespan extending effects (Holzenberger et al. 2003). This was further supported by the finding that murine embryonic fibroblast (MEF) cultures derived from $IGF\text{-}IR^{+/-}$ mice are significantly more resistant to cell death induced by hydrogen peroxide relative to those from control mice (Holzenberger et al. 2003). A similar IGF-I receptor deficiency has also been shown to render mice relatively resistant to death caused by hyperoxia-induced lung damage (Ahamed et al. 2005). Interpretation of the lifespan and stress resistance data of $IGF\text{-}IR^{+/-}$ mice requires some caution because the mice were reared in a colony that was not specific pathogen free, and the mean longevity of both control (568 days) and mutant mice (756 days) is lower than the mean survival of many other laboratory stocks. Thus, the differences in lifespan, and perhaps resistance to paraquat, may in part reflect differences in response to infectious agents.

Mice lacking the gene product of $p66^{shc}$, a downstream effector of IGF-IR, were also shown to live 30% longer than their controls (Migliaccio et al. 1999). In addition, these mice were shown to survive significantly longer than control following administration of paraquat (Migliaccio et al. 1999). Further, $p66^{shc}$ knock-out mice show reduced necrosis and apoptosis of muscle and endothelial cells following induction of localized oxidative stress by ischemia and ischemia with reperfusion (Zaccagnini et al. 2004). MEF cultures derived from $p66^{shc}$ knock-out mice are resistant to apoptosis induced by peroxide, UV light, and staurosporine, which non-selectively inhibits protein kinase activity, relative to MEF cultures from control mice (Migliaccio et al. 1999; Orsini et al. 2004). Thymic and splenic T-cells from $p66^{shc}$ knock-out mice are resistant to dexamethasone-induced cell death, although this finding is somewhat confounded in that death in untreated cells was lower in $p66^{shc}$ knockout mice than in controls (Pacini et al. 2004). Mesangial cells derived from the kidneys of these mice are resistant, relative to control-derived cells, to death caused by incubation in culture media containing high glucose, a rather ill-defined cellular stress (Menini et al. 2006). These reports on $p66^{shc}$ knock-out mice show that this particular mutation confers resistance to many types of stress upon multiple cell types within the mouse. However, similar to the *IGF-IR*[+/-] mice, some reservation on the lifespan-extending effects of this mutation must be warranted due to the small sample size and relatively short lifespan in the original report, in addition to the lack of replication of this survival study.

The gene product of *Klotho* is thought to inhibit signaling through the insulin/IGF-I signaling pathway. While deficiency of this gene leads to multiple phenotypes associated with "accelerated aging" (Kuro-o et al. 1997), overexpression of *Klotho* has been shown to extend lifespan by up to 30% (Kurosu et al. 2005). Administration of the *Klotho* gene product was shown to protect immortalized HeLa cell lines from paraquat and mice overexpressing this gene are resistant to paraquat-induced death (Yamamoto et al. 2005). In addition, these transgenic *Klotho* mice showed reduced DNA damage and increased MnSOD levels, suggesting that *Klotho* has the ability to upregulate multiple stress protective mechanisms, such as DNA repair and antioxidant defenses.

Other Transgenic Mice

While the regulation of IGF-I signaling has been shown to play an integral role in aging of both invertebrates and mammals, lifespan has also been shown to be extended in invertebrates by alterations in pathways that do not directly affect IGF-I signaling pathways. Of particular interest to this chapter, overexpression of several different cellular stress protective proteins have been shown to not only increase stress resistance of *C. elegans* and *Drosophila*, but have also commonly, though not uniformly, been shown to extend lifespan. The protective proteins shown to have a positive effect on invertebrates have included heat shock proteins and factors, antioxidants, and DNA repair proteins (Yokoyama et al. 2002; Morrow et al. 2004; Morley and Morimoto 2004; Hsu et al. 2003; Orr and Sohal 2003; Sun and Tower 1999; Sun et al. 2002; Sun et al. 2004; Hertweck et al. 2004; Symphorien and Woodruff 2003).

Mammalian lifespan might also be extended by transgenic overexpression of genes whose products act to protect cells from oxidative stress. For instance, overexpression of human catalase specifically in mitochondria (MCAT) can extend both maximal and median longevity by about 20% in mice relative to controls (Schriner et al. 2005). MCAT mice were not tested for resistance to stress, but they did exhibit diminished age-related accumulation of oxidative damage to the nucleic acids in skeletal muscle compared to wild-type. The heart-specific overexpression of metallothionein, an antioxidant and metal chelator, can extend the mean lifespan of mice by about 15%, although it does not extend maximum lifespan (Yang et al. 2006). Because maximum longevity was unchanged, it may be that aging was not altered in these animals, per se. Instead, overexpression of metallothionein in the heart may protect from some common pathology that contributes to death, thereby increasing the average age at which mice die, but not changing the overall aging rate. Again, resistance to stress was not directly tested, but cardiomyocytes from these animals displayed lower levels of apoptosis due to free radical production. Finally, overexpressing human thioredoxin, which acts as an antioxidant by reducing oxidized proteins, extends mouse mean (35%) and maximum (22%) longevity relative to control (Mitsui et al. 2002). However, the mean longevity of both transgenic (~22 months) and control mice (~15 months) was relatively short compared to that which is typically found for laboratory stocks of the same genetic background (C57BL/6). These mice were bred in a specific-pathogen free environment and no data were provided on causes of death, so it is difficult to explain why control mice in this experiment are so much shorter lived than in other laboratories. These mice seemed to be resistant to ischemia-induced oxidative stress in the brain as measured by infarct area following treatment (Takagi et al. 1999) and bone marrow cells from these mice were more resistant to UV radiation than those from normal mice (Mitsui et al. 2002).

The three transgenic stress protein models above provide modest support for the idea that lifespan can be extended by upregulation of oxidative stress defenses. However, each report must be evaluated with some caution for reasons described above. In addition, the relative lifespan extension of these transgenic mutant strains tends to be rather modest compared to that insulin/IGF-I mutant mouse strains. This suggests that the aging process is unlikely to be regulated by oxidative stress alone. In support of this idea, long-lived male GHR-KO mice are sensitive to paraquat and female GHR-KO are no different from control (Hauck et al. 2002). Lifespan is extended by about 20% in transgenic mice generated to overexpress α-MUPA (urokinase-type plasminogen activator), a protease whose overexpression is thought to inhibit feeding (Miskin and Masos 1997). Like GHR-KO male mice, female α-MUPA mice were found to be sensitive to the effects of paraquat injection; male α-MUPA mice were not tested (Tirosh et al. 2005). Also, Snell dwarf and GHR-KO mice are sensitive to the hepatotoxicity of acetaminophen, the toxicity of which may be partly due to oxidative stress (Harper et al. 2006c). These results cast doubt on the hypothesis that longevity is regulated principally by the level of response to oxidative stress. The oxidative stress theory of aging would predict that long-lived mice would be more resistant to agents that induce oxidative stress and conversely, that animals sensitive to oxidative stress should be shorter lived. Mice generated to express a 50% reduction in levels of Mn-superoxide dismutase ($Sod2^{+/-}$) show high levels of oxidative damage to nucleic acids in many tissues and are sensitive to organismal death by injection of paraquat. However, the lifespan of these mice is no different that that of mice expressing normal levels of $Sod2$ (Van Remmen et al. 2003).

It may well be that the regulation of longevity does not solely affect, or require, resistance to oxidative stress, but that the mechanisms that affect resistance to other types of damaging insults may also be important. For instance, both Snell and Ames dwarf mice exhibit lower incidences of spontaneous cancer (Vergara et al. 2004; Ikeno et al. 2003), suggesting that hypopituitary dwarf mice may be protected from the effects of endogenous DNA damage. However, the development of spontaneous neoplasia may be, in part, caused by the development of oxidative lesions in DNA (Halliwell 2007). Further, the progression of cancer in these models may be hindered by the low levels of IGF-I, which has been shown to be an important factor in neoplastic growth. While resistance to oxidative stress is most commonly addressed, some of these long-lived mutants have been assayed for their resistance to other forms of insult. Snell dwarf mice have been shown to be resistant to multiple types of DNA damaging agents that do not cause oxidative damage. In particular, development of skin neoplasia caused by topical application of the chemical carcinogens dimethylbenzanthracene (DMBA) or methylcholanthrene is reduced in Snell dwarf mice compared to controls (Bielschowsky and Bielschowsky 1961; Bickis et al. 1956). Development of tumors in multiple tissue types following injection with 2-aminofluorene is also reduced in Snell dwarf mice relative to control (Bielschowsky and Bielschowsky 1960). Following X-ray irradiation of mice, the frequency of mutagenic lesions is significantly lower in the bone marrow cells and spermatogonia of Snell dwarf mice than in control mice (van Buul and van Buul-Offers 1988). In addition, the frequency of mutagenic lesions formed by mitomycin C treatment is significant lower in erythropoietic bone marrow cells from Snell dwarf mice compared to controls (van Buul and van Buul-Offers 1982). In long-lived α-MUPA mice, the incidence of spontaneous tumors, particularly in the lung, is lower than in control mice (Tirosh et al. 2003), as is the formation of precancerous lesions and tumors in the colon, stomach and skin following injection with the carcinogens diethylhydrazine or DMBA (Tirosh et al. 2005). The brains of at least two long-lived models show resistance to neurodegeneration induced by kainic acid, an excitotoxic agent that acts independently of oxidative stress. Hippocampal neurodegeneration in regions CA1 and CA3 is lower in thioredoxin overexpressing mice following kainic acid treatment (Takagi et al. 2000). A similar result was found in transgenic mice lacking the gene *Surf1*, which encodes a subunit of the mitochondrial respiratory chain. These mice have a mean lifespan about 20% greater than that of their controls; maximum lifespan has not been reported (Dell'Agnello et al. 2007). Following kainic acid injection, *Surf1-/-* mice had diminished neuronal loss in both the hippocampus and the thalamus. These reports suggest that the mutations that lead to long life also render many of the tissues of these mice resistant to multiple forms of injury.

Taken together, the results presented above suggest that long-lived mutant mice tend to be resistant, *in vivo*, to the effects of organismal stress. Some models have shown have been shown to be sensitive to oxidative stress, suggesting oxidation resistance alone may not be required for long life. However, the results suggest that resistance to multiple types of stress, including both oxidative and non-oxidative stresses, may be a better indicator of longevity than resistance to a single form of organismal stress alone.

Laboratory versus Wild-Derived Mouse Stocks

Typical laboratory stocks of the house mouse (*Mus musculus*), for example C57BL/6, DBA/2, and Swiss Webster, have been in use for decades; hence they are familiar to the biomedical research community and there is an extensive body of knowledge regarding the development, reproduction, physiology, behavior and genetics of these strains. Indeed, C57BL/6 mice have been the subject of hundreds of aging studies and our understanding of the genetics of this, as well as other, laboratory strains has provided significant insight into the molecular mechanisms of stress resistance, age-related disease and the regulation of life span, as outlined in the preceding sections. However, a genetic resource that is often overlooked by the biogerontological community, but has much to offer, is wild-derived and free-living populations of *Mus musculus*, as well as other species of rodent (Harper 2008).

For the purpose of this discussion wild-derived stocks will be defined as wild-caught individuals or the recent progeny of wild-caught individuals (e.g., offspring or grandoffspring), in addition to commercially available stocks such as MOLF/Ei and CAST/Ei (Klebanov et al. 2001; Bektas et al. 2004; Roberts et al. 2007). Although these commercially available stocks are very different from populations of live-trapped individuals and their recently captive-born progeny (Harper, 2008), they were still somewhat recently derived from wild-caught individuals and are often not of the European *domesticus* subspecies group (Yoshiki and Moriwaki 2006). Moreover, despite their being the product of multiple generations of brother-sister matings, inbreeding in commercially available wild-derived stocks generally occurred prior to being domesticated. This is significant because the domestication process itself has dramatic behavioral and physiological consequences (Blottner et al. 2000; Stuermer et al. 2006; Blottner and Stuermer 2006; Kunzl and Sachser 1999; Künzl et al. 2003); hence it has been argued that "wild alleles" have been maintained within these strains (Klebanov et al. 2001). As the name implies, free-living populations refer to individuals in their natural environment.

Aside from commercially available stocks, wild-derived and free-living populations are composed of genetically heterogeneous individuals whose genetic repertoire is the product of selection under "real world" conditions. Obviously, this is in stark contrast to a standard laboratory stock and the consequences of this difference are many. For example, laboratory mouse stocks are often genetically identical and homozygous at essentially all loci, an abnormal condition not likely to be found in free-living populations, animal, or human, In addition, laboratory stocks represent the endpoint of tremendous selection pressures for docility, rapid growth, and successful propagation under laboratory conditions   (Miller et al. 1999); and of particular relevance to this discussion, the creation of laboratory stocks can result in the loss of naturally occurring alleles that may act to slow the aging process through their effects on stress resistance and disease processes (Miller et al. 2000; Harper et al. 2006a). This is well illustrated by a study of viral resistance conducted in populations of feral house mice where a heretofore unknown allele that conferred resistance to murine leukemia virus (MuLV) was found (Gardner 1993). Likewise, genome polymorphism studies have identified numerous alleles in both inbred wild-derived and wild caught mouse stocks that were not present in typical laboratory mice (Campino et al. 2002; Salcedo et al. 2007), while the gene for granzyme B, a pro-apoptotic protease, is essentially invariant in laboratory mice but is highly polymorphic in feral and wild-derived mouse populations (Thia and Trapani 2007). Hence, by studying wild-derived populations biogerontologists may also (re)discover key alleles involved in the regulation of aging.

Relative to their laboratory counterparts, wild-derived mouse stocks are typically long-lived, even after multiple generations in captivity under both specific pathogen free (SPF) (Miller et al. 2002; Harper et al. 2006a) and conventional colony conditions (Harper et al. 2006b). And, as is the case for most laboratory mouse stocks, end-of-life pathology of wild-derived mice has indicated that neoplastic disease is the leading cause of death (Harper et al. 2006b). The degree of "lifespan extension" seen in these wild-derived mouse stocks is rather substantial, and provides a point of comparison to nutritional (e.g., caloric restriction, low methionine diets) and laboratory genetic models of life span extension; in particular, wild-derived mouse stocks typically live about 15 – 20% longer than laboratory control stocks. Although this is only half of what can be achieved by life-long calorie restriction (Weindruch and Walford 1988a) or by mutation in dwarf and growth hormone receptor knockout (GHRKO) mice (Brown-Borg et al. 1996b; Coschigano et al. 2000), this degree of increase it is similar to the that seen with mutations in the genes for the growth hormone releasing hormone receptor (Ghrhr), the insulin receptor (IR), the insulin-like growth factor I receptor (IGF-1R), insulin receptor substrate-2 (IRS-2), pregnancy associated plasma protein A (PAPP-A), and Surfeit locus protein 1 (Surf1) (Flurkey et al. 2001b; Bluher et al. 2003; Holzenberger et al. 2003; Conover and Bale 2007; Dell'Agnello et al. 2007; Taguchi et al. 2007). Notably, however, wild-derived stocks are not exposed to any experimental treatment with a presumptive effect on lifespan, and the longest-lived wild-derived mouse to date reached the impressive age of 4.1 years (Harper et al. 2006a), much greater than that seen in a typical laboratory mouse. In fact, the maximum life span of wild-derived stocks rivals that of the longest-lived mutant stocks.

Genetics of Wild-Derived Mouse Stocks

Although the data are not unequivocal, there is evidence to suggest that the superior longevity of wild-derived stocks is the result of delayed reproductive maturation, a reduction in circulating IGF-I levels, and/or altered growth trajectories relative to laboratory mice (Harper et al. 2006a). Importantly, these features are also common to long-lived mutant strains, most notably Ames and Snell dwarf mice, and at least some of the difference is likely the result of underlying genetic variation. Unfortunately, inter-strain comparisons still tell us very little about which genes are responsible.

The construction of hybrid stocks, which can then be compared to each of its parental strains, provides a useful tool to inquire whether genetically based differences exist amongst strains, as well as whether or not they are the result of additive allelic effects, or are simply the result of directional dominance or epistatic interactions. The construction of reciprocal crosses also allows us to take go one step further and assess whether maternal effects are involved. Nonetheless, these approaches still have limitations, the most important being that they do not address whether the observed phenotypic differences simply represent coincidence, or instead are the outcome of a set of causal relationships based upon pleiotropic effects of polymorphic alleles. To answer this question, the construction of F2 intercross stocks is needed (i.e., by crossing F1 hybrids). This results in a significant degree of genome reshuffling, thereby producing offspring with variable combinations of alleles (Jansen 2003) with three possible genotypes for each: (a) homozygous for parent A; (b) heterozygous; or (c) homozygous for parent B. Here, the co-occurrence of traits in the segregating population is indicative that they are regulated to some degree by common, and potentially genetic, factors. See Guénet and Bonhomme (2003) for a more detailed discussion.

Segregating populations of (wild x laboratory) F2 hybrid stocks have been generated and have clearly implicated a genetic component to the observed differences in growth, maturation, hormone levels and aging in wild-derived versus laboratory mice. In particular, in F2 hybrid stocks crossing [X] with [Y] the level of each of these measures was intermediate to those seen in the parental stocks, suggesting that they are modulated by co-dominant loci that distinguish wild-derived from laboratory mice (Harper et al. 2006a). Interestingly, in an unrelated study Klebanov et al. (2001) used a different approach, the construction of 4-way crosses of mice involving 3 laboratory and 1 wild-derived stock, to identify quantitative trait loci (QTL) that were associated with increased life span. In each case the QTL involved an allele from one of two undomesticated wild-derived stocks (MOLD/Rk and CAST/Ei). Finally, the increased life span of one wild-derived stock (SPRET/Ei) has been suggested to be secondary to increased *klotho* expression, a putative anti-aging gene, and its beneficial effects on cardiovascular health (Bektas et al. 2004). The next challenge is to identify other candidate genes that may be involved in modulating life span via a conventional gene mapping approach.

Stress Resistance and Aging in Wild-Derived Mice

In terms of stress resistance, there is evidence to suggest that, similar to long-lived mutant laboratory strains, wild-derived mouse stocks may also better resist toxic and metabolic insults both *in vivo* and *in vitro*. For example, in a study using primary dermal fibroblast cell lines, those cells derived from a wild-derived stock were better able to resist changes associated with cellular senescence and oxidative stress-induced apoptosis than cell lines from laboratory C57BL/6J mice (Yuan et al. 2006). In a second study also using primary dermal fibroblast cell lines, enhanced resistance to a variety of cytotoxic agents and metabolic insults was also found in cell lines generated from wild-caught house mice relative to those derived from a laboratory stock (Harper et al. 2007).

Significant changes in the expression of xenobiotic metabolism genes with advancing age has been documented in laboratory rodents (Lee et al. 2008b), and more recently it was shown that in long-lived Little mice harboring a mutation in the *ghrhr* gene there is a significant alteration in xenobiotic metabolism in intact animals (Amador-Noguez et al. 2007). Unfortunately, there is essentially nothing known about *in vivo* stress resistance in wild-derived mouse stocks except that the tissue-specific expression of glutathione S-transferases, important for detoxification of xenobiotic compounds, tends to be higher in wild-derived versus laboratory mice; however the functional consequence of these differences has not been evaluated (Ruiz-Laguna et al. 2005). And although it is not a measure of stress resistance *per se*, it is interesting that inbreeding significantly impairs resistance to pathogenic infection in mice (Ilmonen et al. 2008). It is not difficult to imagine that stress resistance pathways are similarly affected; in fact captive populations of wild-caught *Drosophila melanogaster* (Hoffman et al. 2001) maintained under laboratory conditions exhibit a rapid decline in whole animal stress resistance with time.

At present the mechanistic bases for the improved stress resistance of wild-derived cell lines is unknown, but two candidate pathways have emerged. First, in addition to maintaining genomic stability (Siderakis and Tarsounas 2007) and cell cycle control (Matulic et al. 2007), telomere biology may be an important mediator of cellular stress resistance, either due to differences in telomere length (Rubio et al. 2004) and/or in the expression of telomerase reverse transcriptase (TERT), the telomerase catalytic subunit (Lee et al. 2008a). It is now well-known that inbreeding in laboratory stocks significantly alters telomere length in both *Mus musculus* and *Peromyscus* sp. (Bickle et al. 2001; Manning et al. 2002; Hemann and Greider 2000) such that the telomeres of wild-derived stocks are significantly shorter than those in laboratory mice; however a direct relationship between telomere length/TERT activity in wild-derived cell lines and their degree of stress resistance has not been established.

Second, the ratio of specific lipids in cellular membranes is thought to be an important mediator of membrane susceptibility to peroxidation, and perhaps life span, in a broad range of animal species (Hulbert et al. 2007). Indeed, caloric restriction in mice significantly alters membrane composition such that the peroxidation index (PI), a composite score of peroxidation susceptibility, was reduced in a number of tissues (Hulbert et al. 2007), while the PI of membranes prepared from whole tissue lysates generated from two distinct wild-derived stocks was significantly lower than the PI of a laboratory control stock (Hulbert et al. 2006); however, the PI of primary cell lines has not been assessed in these mice. Recently, the cysteine content of proteins has also been postulated to play an important role in oxidative stress sensitivity (Moosmann and Behl 2008). These data are intriguing, but there is currently nothing known about cysteine levels in wild-derived versus laboratory stocks; although basal levels of endogenous free radical production by isolated mitochondria does not differ (Lambert et al. 2007).

Looking Beyond Wild-Derived House Mice

In general, biogerontological research makes use of only handful of inbred laboratory mouse stocks, and while significant gains have been made in identifying putative aging genes using these models, it is still rather short-sighted. To date, single-gene mutations and selective breeding regimens have failed to increase life span by much more than 40% within rodents, while natural selection has produced differences of much greater magnitude within this same order, upwards of 25-fold. The differences are even more dramatic if all mammalian orders are included, on the order of 100-fold or more. It remains to be seen how evolutionary processes can produce this dramatic degree of variation in life span, and more importantly, if long-lived animals from different taxa share common genetic pathways for slowed aging (Austad 2005).

Taking a cue from studies done in long-lived strains harboring mutations in the GH axis (Murakami et al. 2003; Salmon et al. 2005), Harper et al. (2007) demonstrated that the maximum life span of the test species was associated with the degree of resistance to some, but not all, cytotoxic and metabolic insults using fibroblast cell lines derived from seven species of wild-trapped rodents, in addition to a single species of bat. Likewise, primary fibroblast cell lines grown from the skin of naked mole rats, the longest-lived rodent, were more resistant to a number of stressors relative to mouse cell lines grown and tested in parallel (Salmon et al. 2008a), while some bats exhibit a high degree of endogenous antioxidant protection (Wilhelm Filho et al. 2007). Similarly, Kapahi et al. (1999) showed that dermal-derived fibroblasts from mammalian species across orders showed a correlation between cellular oxidative stress resistance and species maximal lifespan. Further, Ogburn et al. (1998, 2001) have shown that fibroblasts from birds, which are in general much longer-lived than similarly sized mammals, are resistant to a number of oxidative stressors. There is also mounting evidence that vascular aging, which is at least in part a consequence of cumulative oxidative damage, is significantly delayed in long-lived mammalian species

(Ungvari et al. 2008). Interestingly, differences in vascular aging, and perhaps enhanced longevity itself, may be a byproduct of reduced mitochondrial free radical production (Lambert et al. 2007; Brunet-Rossinni 2004). Taken together, these data are consistent with the notion that enhanced stress resistance is a prerequisite for the evolution of enhanced longevity in mammalian species, yet virtually nothing is known about how this might come about in species other than mice and rats; although recent studies using heterologous microarray hybridization will surely begin to fill in the blanks (Eddy and Storey 2008; Storey 2006). In addition, the study of wild-derived mouse stocks, as well as other species of rodent, may soon provide important insight into age-related disease processes; for example, the evolution of telomere biology as a function of body size in mammals due to its association with cancer risk (reviewed in Gorbunova and Seluanov 2008) and patterns of adult neurogenesis (Amrein et al. 2004b; Amrein et al. 2004a).

In summary, laboratory mouse stocks have experienced tens-to-hundreds of generations of selective pressure for alleles that lead to high fecundity, rapid growth, excessive food intake, and abnormal behavior, thereby creating experimental animals that differ dramatically from the natural condition (Ellegren and Sheldon 2008). Although these stocks of mice clearly have their uses, and have unquestionably made significant contributions to our understanding of aging and age-related disease, the process of creating laboratory stocks has likely resulted in less-than-ideal experimental subjects for aging research. This is because the selective pressures that mold fitness traits early in life are likely to impact aging as a consequence of their secondary or pleiotropic effects on gerontologically important factors. These selection pressures are also likely to have resulted in the loss of naturally-occurring alleles that significantly impact the aging process. The study of wild-derived mouse stocks, whether they are commercially available strains or are the progenitors of live-trapped animals can overcome these limitations. Finally, by looking beyond the mouse the plausibility of specific hypotheses of aging generated in mice can be tested, as well as raising the possibility that heretofore underappreciated, or unknown, genetic pathways important in the regulation of mammalian aging will be discovered.

Conclusion

Although the exact mechanisms responsible for controlling the aging rate have yet to be identified there is mounting evidence from a number of animal models that stress resistance is an important player in this process. In general, slow aging may be may be a consequence of attenuated damage accumulation secondary to enhanced stress resistance. In mice and rats, this is evident from dietary treatments that extend lifespan, such as caloric restriction and a reduction in dietary methionine, as well as genetic mutations the extend life span. In each case, increased longevity is often accompanied by a reduction in the accumulation of various forms of damage, including oxidative damage and DNA mutation, and increases in resistance to different forms of cytotoxic stress. Finally, in addition to these well-characterized laboratory mouse models of aging, studies done in wild-derived and free-living rodent populations has suggested that they too exhibit enhanced stress resistance, especially enhanced resistance to oxidative stress, in conjunction with the evolution of long-life.

Overall, studies done in these rodent models of extended longevity clearly suggest that an increased resistance to stress may play an important role in the maintenance of cellular homeostasis, thereby preserving cell and tissue function and delaying the progression of age-related disease.

References

Adachi H, Fujiwara Y, Ishii N (1998). Effects of oxygen on protein carbonyl and aging in *Caenorhabditis elegans* mutants with long (age-1) and short (mev-1) life spans. *Journals of Gerontology A Biological Sciences and Medical Sciences 53*, B240-B244.

Ahamed K, Epaud R, Holzenberger M, Bonora M, Flejou JF, Puard J, Clement A, Henrion-Caude A (2005). Deficiency in type 1 insulin-like growth factor receptor in mice protects against oxygen-induced lung injury. *Respiratory Research 6*, 31.

Aidoo A, Desai VG, Lyn-Cook LE, Chen JJ, Feuers RJ, Casciano DA (1999). Attenuation of bleomycin-induced *Hprt* mutant frequency in female and male rats by calorie restriction. *Mutation Research 430*, 155-163.

Al-Regaiey KA, Masternak MM, Bonkowski M, Sun L, Bartke A (2005). Long-lived growth hormone receptor knockout mice: interaction of reduced insulin-like growth factor I/insulin signaling and caloric restriction. *Endocrinology 146*, 851-860.

Amador-Noguez D, Dean A, Huang W, Setchell K, Moore D, Darlington G (2007). Alterations in xenobiotic metabolism in the long-lived Little mice. *Aging Cell 6*, 453-470.

Amrein I, Slomianka L, Lipp H (2004a). Granule cell number, cell death and cell proliferation in the dentate gyrus of wild-living rodents. *European Journal of Neuroscience 20*, 3342-3350.

Amrein I, Slomianka L, Poletaeva I, Bologova N, Lipp H (2004b). Marked species and age-dependent differences in cell proliferation and neurogenesis in the hippocampus of wild-living rodents. *Hippocampus 14*, 1000-1010.

Andersen B, Pearse II RV, Jenne K, Sornson M, Lin SC, Bartke A, Rosenfeld MG (1995). The Ames dwarf gene is required for Pit-1 gene activation. *Developmental Biology 172*, 495-503.

Anderson GL (1978). Responses of dauer larvae of *Caenorhabditis elegans* (Nematoda: Rhabditidae) to thermal stress and oxygen deprivation. *Canadian Journal of Zoology 56*, 1786-1791.

Apte UM, Limaye PB, Desaiah D, Bucci TJ, Warbritton A, Mehendale HM (2003). Mechanisms of increased liver tissue repair and survival in diet-restricted rats treated with equitoxic doses of thioacetamide. *Toxicological Science 72*, 272-282.

Austad SN (2005). Diverse aging rates in metazoans: targets for functional genomics. *Mechanisms of Ageing and Development 126*, 43-49.

Barsyte D, Lovejoy DA, Lithgow GJ (2001). Longevity and heavy metal resistance in daf-2 and age-1 long-lived mutants of *Caenorhabditis elegans*. *FASEB Journal 15*, 627-634.

Bartke A, Brown-Borg H, Mattison J, Kinney B, Hauck S, Wright C (2001). Prolonged longevity of hypopituitary dwarf mice. *Experimental Gerontology 36*, 21-28.

Bartke A, Brown-Borg HM, Bode AM, Carlson J, Hunter WS, Bronson RT (1998). Does growth hormone prevent or accelerate aging? *Experimental Gerontology 33*, 675-687.

Bektas A, Schurman SH, Sharov AA, Carter MG, Dietz HC, Francomano CA (2004). Klotho gene variation and expression in 20 inbred mouse strains. *Mammalian Genome 15*, 759-767.

Berg TF, Breen PJ, Feuers RJ, Oriakus ET, Chen FX, Hart RW (1994). Acute toxicity of ganciclovir: Effect of dietary restriction and chronobiology. *Food Chemistry and Toxicology 32*, 45-50.

Bickis I, Estwick RR, Campbell JS (1956). Observations on initiation of skin carcinoma in pituitary dwarf mice. I. *Cancer 9*, 763-767.

Bickle C, Cantrell M, Austad S, Wichman H (2001). Effects of domestication on telomere length in Mus musculus and Peromyscus maniculatus. *FASEB Journal 12*, A317.

Bielschowsky F, Bielschowsky M (1960). Carcinogenesis in the pituitary dwarf mouse. The response to 2-aminofluorene. *British Journal of Cancer 14*, 195-199.

Bielschowsky F, Bielschowsky M (1961). Carcinogenesis in the pituitary of dwarf mouse. The response to dimethylbenzanthracene applied to the skin. *British Journal of Cancer 15*, 257-262.

Blottner S, Franz C, Rohleder M, Zinke O, Stuermer IW (2000). Higher testicular activity in laboratory gerbils compared to wild Mongolian gerbils (Meriones unguiculatus). *Journal of Zoology 250*, 461-466.

Blottner S, Stuermer IW (2006). Reproduction of wild Mongolian gerbils bred in the laboratory with respect to generation and season 2. Spermatogenic activity and testicular testosterone concentration. *Animal Science 82*, 389-395.

Bluher M, Kahn BB, Kahn CR (2003). Extended longevity in mice lacking the insulin receptor in adipose tissue. *Science 299*, 572-574.

Bokov A, Chaudhuri A, Richardson A (2004). The role of oxidative damage and stress in aging. *Mechanisms of Ageing and Development 125*, 811-826.

Braeckman BP, Houthoofd K, Vanfleteren JR (2001). Insulin-like signaling, metabolism, stress resistance and aging in *Caenorhabditis elegans*. *Mechanisms of Ageing and Development 122*, 673-693.

Broughton SJ, Piper MDW, Ikeya T, Bass TM, Jacobson J, Driege Y, Martinez P, Hafen E, Withers DJ, Leevers SJ, Partridge L (2005). Longer lifespan, altered metabolism, and stress resistance in Drosophila from ablation of cells making insulin-like ligands. *Proceedings of the National Academy of Sciences USA 102*, 3105-3110.

Brown-Borg H (2006). Longevity in mice: is stress resistance a common factor? *AGE 28*, 145-162.

Brown-Borg HM, Borg KE, Meliska CJ, Bartke A (1996a). Dwarf mice and the ageing process. *Nature 384*, 33.

Brown-Borg HM, Rakoczy SG (2005). Glutathione metabolism in long-living Ames dwarf mice. *Experimental Gerontology 40*, 115-120.

Brown-Borg H, Johnson W, Rakoczy S, Romanick M (2001). Mitochondrial oxidant generation and oxidative damage in Ames dwarf and GH transgenic mice. *AGE 24*, 85-96.

Bruce-Keller AJ, Umberger G, McFall R, Mattson MP (1999). Food restriction reduces brain damage and improves behavioral outcome following excitotoxic and metabolic insults. *Annals of Neurology 45*, 8-15.

Brunet-Rossinni AK (2004). Reduced free-radical production and extreme longevity in the little brown bat (Myotis lucifugus) versus two non-flying mammals. *Mechanisms of Ageing and Developmentelop 125*, 11-20.

Bus JS, Cagen SZ, Olgaard M, Gibson JE (1976). A mechanism of paraquat toxicity in mice and rats. *Toxicology and Applied Pharmacology 35*, 501-513.

Camper SA, Saunders TL, Katz RW, Reeves RH (1990). The Pit-1 transcription factor gene is a candidate for the murine Snell dwarf mutation. *Genomics 8*, 586-590.

Campino S, Behrschmidt C, Bagot S, Guénet JL, Cazenave PA, Holmberg D, Penha-Gonτalves C (2002). Unique genetic variation revealed by a microsatellite polymorphism survey in ten wild-derived inbred strains. *Genomics 79*, 618-620.

Carlson J, Bharadwaj R, Bartke A (1999). Oxidative stress in hypopituitary dwarf mice and in transgenic mice overexpressing human and bovine GH. *AGE 22*, 181-186.

Cheng TC, Beamer WG, Phillips JA, Bartke A, Mallonee RL, Dowling C. (1983). Etiology of growth hormone deficiency in little, Ames, and Snell dwarf mice. *Endocrinology 113*, 1669-1678.

Cho CG, Kim HJ, Chung SW, Jung KJ, Shim KH, Yu BP, Yodoi J, Chung HY (2003). Modulation of glutathione and thioredoxin systems by calorie restriction during the aging process. *Experimental Gerontology 38*, 539-548.

Clancy DJ, Gems D, Harshman LG, Oldham S, Stocker H, Hafen E, Leevers SJ, Partridge L (2001). Extension of life-span by loss of CHICO, a Drosophila insulin receptor substrate protein. *Science 292*, 104-106.

Cohen HY, Miller C, Bitterman KJ, Wall NR, Hekking B, Kessler B, Howitz KT, Gorospe M, de Cabo R, Sinclair DA (2004). Calorie restriction promotes mammalian cell survival by inducing the SIRT1 deacetylase. *Science 305*, 390-392.

Conover CA, Bale LK (2007). Loss of pregnancy-associated plasma protein A extends lifespan in mice. *Aging Cell 6*, 727-729.

Coschigano KT, Clemmons D, Bellush LL, Kopchick JJ (2000). Assessment of growth parameters and life span of GHR/BP gene-disrupted mice. *Endocrinology 141*, 2608-2613.

Coschigano K, Holland AN, Riders ME, List EO, Flyvbjerg A, Kopchick JJ (2003). Deletion, but not antagonism, of the mouse growth hormone receptor results in severely decreased body weights, insulin, and insulin-like growth factor I levels and increased life span. *Endocrinology 144*, 3799-3810.

Crowley C, Curtis HJ (1963). The development of somatic mutations in mice with age. *Proceedings of the National Academy of Sciences USA 49*, 626-628.

Cvejic S, Zhu Z, Felice SJ, Berman Y, Huang XY (2004). The endogenous ligand Stunted of the GPCR Methuselah extends lifespan in Drosophila. *Nature Cell Biology 6*, 540-546.

Davis LJ, Tadolini B, Luigi Biagi a, Walford R, Licastro F (1993). Effect of age and extent of dietary restriction on hepatic microsomal lipid peroxidation potential in mice. *Mechanisms of Ageing and Development 72*, 155-163.

de Cabo R, Furer-Galban S, Anson RM, Gilman C, Gorospe M, Lane MA (2003). An *in vitro* model of caloric restriction. *Experimental Gerontology 38*, 631-639.

Dell'Agnello C, Leo S, Agostino A, Szabadkai G, Tiveron C, Zulian A, Prelle A, Roubertoux P, Rizzuto R, Zeviani M (2007). Increased longevity and refractoriness to Ca2+-dependent neurodegeneration in Surf1 knockout mice. *Human Molecular Genetics 16*, 431-444.

Dempsey JL, Odagiri Y, Morley AA (1993a). *In vivo* mutations at the H-2 locus in mouse lymphocytes. *Mutation Research 285*, 45-51.

Dempsey JL, Pfeiffer M, Morley AA (1993b). Effect of dietary restriction on *in vivo* somatic mutation in mice. *Mutation Research 291*, 141-145.

Dolle MET, Giese H, Hopkins CL, Martus HJ, Hausdorff JM, Vijg J (1997). Rapid accumulation of genome rearrangements in liver but not in brain of old mice. *Nature Genetics 17*, 431-434.

Dubey A, Forster MJ, Lal H, Sohal RS (1996). Effect of age and caloric intake on protein oxidation in different brain regions and on behavioral functions of the mouse. *Archives of Biochemistry and Biophysics 333*, 189-197.

Eddy S, Storey K (2008). Comparative molecular physiological genomics. Heterologous probing of cDNA arrays. *Methods in Molecular Biology 410*, 81-110.

Eicher EM, Beamer WG (1980). New mouse dw allele: Genetic location and effects on lifespan and growth hormone levels. *Journal of Heredity 71*, 187-190.

Ellegren H, Sheldon BC (2008). Genetic basis of fitness differences in natural populations. *Nature 452*, 169-175.

Finch CE (1990). *Longevity, Senescence and the Genome*. University of Chicago Press.

Flurkey K, Papaconstantinou J, Miller RA, Harrison DE (2001). Lifespan extension and delayed immune and collagen aging in mutant mice with defects in growth hormone production. *Proceedings of the National Academy of Sciences USA 98*, 6736-6741.

Flurkey K, Papaconstantinou J, Harrison DE (2002). The Snell dwarf mutation Pit1dw can increase life span in mice. *Mechanisms of Ageing and Development 123*, 121-130.

Friedman DB, Johnson TE (1988a). A mutation in the age-1 gene in *Caenorhabditis elegans* lengthens life and reduces hermaphrodite fertility. *Genetics 118*, 75-86.

Friedman DB, Johnson TE (1988b). Three mutants that extend both mean and maximum life span of the nematode, *Caenorhabditis elegans*, define the age-1 gene. *Journals of Gerontology 43*, B102-B109.

Gardner M (1993). Genetic control of retroviral disease in aging wild mice. *Genetica 91*, 199-209.

Giannakou ME, Goss M, Junger MA, Hafen E, Leevers SJ, Partridge L (2004). Long-lived drosophila with overexpressed dFOXO in adult fat body. *Science 305*, 361.

Gong X, Shang F, Obin M, Palmer H, Scrofano MM, Jahngen-Hodge J, Smith DE, Taylor A (1997). Antioxidant enzyme activities in lens, liver and kidney of calorie restricted Emory mice. *Mechanisms of Ageing and Development 99*, 181-192.

Gorbunova V, Seluanov A (2008) Coevolution of telomerase activity and body mass in mammals: From mice to beavers. *Mechanisms of Ageing and Development 130*, 3-9.

Guo Z, Heydari A, Richardson A (1998). Nucleotide excision repair of actively transcribed versus nontranscribed DNA in rat hepatocytes: effect of age and dietary restriction. *Experimental Cell Research 245*, 228-238.

Guénet JL, Bonhomme F (2003). Wild mice: an ever-increasing contribution to a popular mammalian model. *Trends in Genetics 19*, 24-31.

Hall DM, Oberely TD, Mosely PM, Buettner G, Oberely LW, Weindruch R, Kregel KC (2000). Caloric restriction improves thermotolerance and reduces hyperthermia-induced cellular damage in old rats. *FASEB Journal 14*, 78-86.

Halliwell B (2007). Oxidative stress and cancer: have we moved forward? *Biochemical Journal 401*, 1-11.

Hamilton ML, Van Remmen H, Drake JA, Yang H, Guo ZM, Kewitt K, Walter CA, Richardson A (2001). Does oxidative damage to DNA increase with age? *Proceedings of the National Academy of Sciences USA 98*, 10469-10474.

Harman D (1956). Aging: a theory based on free radical and radiation chemistry. *Journals of Gerontology 11*, 298-300.

Harper JM, Durkee SJ, Dysko R, Austad SN, Miller RA (2006a). Genetic modulation of hormone levels and life span in hybrids between laboratory and wild-derived mice. *Journals of Gerontology A Biological Sciences and Medical Sciences 61*, 1019-1029.

Harper JM, Leathers CW, Austad SN (2006b). Does caloric restriction extend life in wild mice? *Aging Cell 5*, 441-449.

Harper JM, Salmon AB, Chang Y, Bonkowski M, Bartke A, Miller RA (2006c). Stress resistance and aging: Influence of genes and nutrition. *Mechanisms of Ageing and Development 127*, 687-694.

Harper JM, Salmon AB, Leiser SF, Galecki AT, Miller RA (2007). Skin-derived fibroblasts from long-lived species are resistant to some, but not all, lethal stresses and to the mitochondrial inhibitor rotenone. *Aging Cell 6*, 1-13.

Harper J (2008). Wild-derived mouse stocks: an underappreciated tool for aging research. *AGE 30, 135-145.*

Hauck SJ, Aaron JM, Wright C, Kopchick JJ, Bartke A (2002). Antioxidant enzymes, free-radical damage, and response to paraquat in liver and kidney of long-living growth hormone receptor/binding protein gene-disrupted mice. *Hormone and Metabolism Research 34*, 481-486.

Hauck SJ, Bartke A (2000). Effects of growth hormone on hypothalamic catalase and Cu/Zn superoxide dismutase. *Free Radicals in Biology and Medicine 28*, 970-978.

Helfand SL, Rogina B (2003). Genetics of aging in the fruit fly, *Drosophila melanogaster*. *Annual Review of Genetics 37*, 329-348.

Hemann MT, Greider CW (2000). Wild-derived inbred mouse strains have short telomeres. *Nucleic Acids Research 28*, 4474-4478.

Hertweck M, Gobel C, Baumeister R (2004). C. elegans SGK-1 Is the critical component in the Akt/PKB kinase complex to control stress response and life span. *Developmental Cell 6*, 577-588.

Heydari AR, Wu B, Takahashi R, Strong R, Richardson A (1993). Expression of heat shock protein 70 is altered by age and diet at the level of transcription. *Molecular Cell Biology 13*, 2909-2918.

Hoffman A, Hallas R, Sinclair C, Partridge L (2001). Rapid loss of stress resistance in *Drosophila melanogaster* under adaptation to laboratory culture. *Evolution 55*, 436-438.

Holzenberger M, Dupont J, Ducos B, Leneuve P, Geloen A, Even PC, Cervera P, Le Bouc Y (2003b). IGF-1 receptor regulates lifespan and resistance to oxidative stress in mice. *Nature 421*, 182-187.

Honda Y, Honda S (1999). The daf-2 gene network for longevity regulates oxidative stress resistance and Mn-superoxide dismutase gene expression in *Caenorhabditis elegans*. *FASEB Journal13*, 1385-1391.

Hsu AL, Murphy CT, Kenyon C (2003). Regulation of aging and age-related disease by DAF-16 and Heat-Shock Factor. *Science 300*, 1142-1145.

Hulbert AJ, Faulks SC, Harper JM, Miller RA, Buffenstein R (2006). Extended longevity of wild-derived mice is associated with peroxidation-resistant membranes. *Mechanisms of Ageing and Development 127*, 653-657.

Hulbert AJ, Pamplona R, Buffenstein R, Buttemer WA (2007). Life and death: Metabolic rate, membrane composition, and life span of animals. *Physiological Reviews 87*, 1175-1213.

Hwangbo DS, Gersham B, Tu MP, Palmer M, Tatar M (2004). Drosophila dFOXO controls lifespan and regulates insulin signalling in brain and fat body. *Nature 429*, 562-566.

Ikeno Y, Bronson RT, Hubbard GB, Lee S, Bartke A (2003). Delayed occurrence of fatal neoplastic diseases in Ames dwarf mice: correlation to extended longevity. *Journals of Gerontology A Biological Sciences and Medical Sciences 58*, 291-296.

Ilmonen P, Penn D, Damjanovich K, Clarke J, Lamborn D, Morrison L, Ghotbi L, Potts W (2008). Experimental infection magnifies inbreeding depression in house mice. *Journal of Evolutionary Biology 21*, 834-841.

Jaklevic B, Uyetake L, Lemstra W, Chang J, Leary W, Edwards A, Vidwans S, Sibon O, Tin Su T (2006). Contribution of growth and cell cycle checkpoints to radiation survival in Drosophila. *Genetics 174*, 1963-1972.

Jansen RC (2003). Studying complex biological systems using multifactorial perturbation. *Nature Reviews Genetics 4*, 145-151.

Johnson TE, Cypser J, de Castro E, de Castro S, Henderson S, Murakami S, Rikke B, Tedesco P, Link C (2000). Gerontogenes mediate health and longevity in nematodes through increasing resistance to environmental toxins and stressors. *Experimental Gerontology 35*, 687-694.

Johnson TE, de Castro E, Hegi de Castro S, Cypser J, Henderson S, Tedesco P (2001). Relationship between increased longevity and stress resistance as assessed through gerontogene mutations in *Caenorhabditis elegans*. *Experimental Gerontology 36*, 1609-1617.

Jones IM, Thomas CB, Tucker B, Thompson CL, Plesnaova P, Vorobtsova I, Moore DH (1995). Impact of age and environment on somatic mutation at the hprt gene of T lymphocytes in humans. *Mutation Research 338*, 129-139.

Kapahi P, Boulton ME, Kirkwood TB (1999). Positive correlation between mammalian life span and cellular resistance to stress. *Free Radicals in Biology and Medicine 26*, 495-500.

Keenan KP, Ballam GC, Dixit R, Soper KA, Laroque P, Mattson BA, Adams SP, Coleman JB (1997). The effects of diet, overfeeding and moderate dietary restriction on Sprague-Dawley rat survival, disease and toxicology. *Journal of Nutrition 127*, 851S.

Kenyon C, Chang J, Gensch E, Rudner A, Tabtiang R (1993). A C. elegans mutant that lives twice as long as wild type. *Nature 366*, 461-464.

Kinney BA, Meliska CJ, Steger RW, Bartke A (2001). Evidence that Ames dwarf mice age differently from their normal siblings in behavioral and learning and memory parameters. *Hormones and Behavior 39*, 277-284.

Klebanov S, Astle CM, Roderick TH, Flurkey K, Archer JR, Chen J, Harrison DE (2001). Maximum life spans in mice are extended by wild strain alleles. *Experimental Biology and Medicine 226*, 854-859.

Klurfeld DM, Welch CB, Davis MJ, Kritchevsky D (1989). Determination of degree of energy restriction necessary to reduce DMBA-induced mammary tumorigenesis in rats during the promotion phase. *Journal of Nutrition 119*, 286-291.

Komninou D, Leutzinger Y, Reddy BS, Richie J (2006). Methionine restriction inhibits colon carcinogenesis. *Nutrition and Cancer 54*, 202-208.

Komninou D, Malloy V, Krajcik R, Rivenson D, Orentreich N, Richie JP (2002). Methionine restriction inhibits age-related spontaneous tumorigenesis in F344 rats. *Proceedings of the American Association of Cancer Research 45*, 3919.

Kritchevsky D, Weber MM, Klurfeld DM (1984). Dietary fat versus caloric content in initiation and promotion of 7,12-dimethylbenz(a)anthracene-induced mammary tumorigenesis in rats. *Cancer Research 44*, 3174-3177.

Künzl C, Kaiser S, Meier E, Sachser N (2003). Is a wild mammal kept and reared in captivity still a wild animal? *Hormones and Behavior 43*, 187-196.

Kunzl C, Sachser N (1999). The behavioral endocrinology of domestication: A comparison between the domestic guinea pig (*Cavia aperea porcellus*) and its wild ancestor, the cavy (*Cavia aperea*). *Hormones and Behavior 35*, 28-37.

Kuro-o M, Matsumura Y, Aizawa H, Kawaguchi H, Suga T, Utsugi T, Ohyama Y, Kurabayashi M, Kaname T, Kume E, Iwasaki H, Iida A, Shiraki-Iida T, Nishikawa S, Nagai R, Nabeshima Yi (1997). Mutation of the mouse klotho gene leads to a syndrome resembling ageing. *Nature 390*, 45-51.

Kurosu H, Yamamoto M, Clark JD, Pastor JV, Nandi A, Gurnani P, McGuinness OP, Chikuda H, Yamaguchi M, Kawaguchi H, Shimomura I, Takayama Y, Herz J, Kahn CR, Rosenblatt KP, Kuro-o M (2005). Suppression of aging in mice by the hormone Klotho. *Science 309*, 1829-1833.

Laganiere S, Yu BP (1987). Anti-lipoperoxidation action of food restriction. *Biochemical and Biophysical Research Communications 145*, 1185-1191.

Lambert AJ, Boysen HM, Buckingham JA, Yang T, Podlutsky A, Austad SN, Kunz TH, Buffenstein R, Brand MD (2007). Low rates of hydrogen peroxide production by isolated heart mitochondria associate with long maximum lifespan in vertebrate homeotherms. *Aging Cell 6*, 607-618.

Larsen PL (1993). Aging and resistance to oxidative damage in *Caenorhabditis elegans*. *Proceedings of the National Academy of Sciences USA 90*, 8905-8909.

Lass A, Sohal BH, Weindruch R, Forster MJ, Sohal RS (1998). Caloric restriction prevents age-associated accrual of oxidative damage to mouse skeletal muscle mitochondria. *Free Radicals in Biology and Medicine 25*, 1089-1097.

Lavick PS, Baumann CA (1943). Further studies on the tumor promoting action of fat. *Cancer Research 3*, 749-756.

Lee J, Sung YH, Cheong C, Choi YS, Jeon HK, Sun W, Hahn WC, Ishikawa F, Lee HW (2008a). TERT promotes cellular and organismal survival independently of telomerase activity. *Oncogene 27*, 3754-3760.

Lee JS, Ward WO, Wolf DC, Allen JW, Mills C, DeVito MJ, Corton JC (2008b). Coordinated changes in xenobiotic metabolizing enzyme gene expression in aging male rats. *Toxicological Sciences 106*, 263-283.

Leiser SF, Salmon AB, Miller RA (2006). Correlated resistance to glucose deprivation and cytotoxic agents in fibroblast cell lines from long-lived pituitary dwarf mice. *Mechanisms of Ageing and Development 127*, 821-829.

Li S, Crenshaw EB, Rawson EJ, Simmons DM, Swanson LW, Rosenfeld MG (1990). Dwarf locus mutants lacking three pituitary cell types result from mutations in the POU-domain gene Pit-1. *Nature 347*, 528-533.

Li Y, Yan Q, Wolf NS (1997). Long-term caloric restriction delays age-related decline in proliferation capacity of murine lens epithelial cells *in vitro* and *in vivo*. *Investigations in Ophthalmologic and Vision Science 38*, 100-107.

Licastro F, Weindruch R, Davis L, Walford R (1988). Effect of dietary restriction upon the age-associated decline of lymphocyte DNA repair activity in mice. *AGE 11*, 48-52.

Lin YJ, Seroude L, Benzer S (1998). Extended life-span and stress resistance in the Drosophila mutant methuselah. *Science 282*, 943-946.

Lipman JM, Turturro A, Hart RW (1989). The influence of dietary restriction on DNA repair in rodents: A preliminary study. *Mechanisms of Ageing and Development 48*, 135-143.

Lithgow G.J., White TM, Hinerfeld DA, Johnson TE (1994). Thermotolerance of a long-lived mutant of *Caenorhabditis elegans*. *Journals of Gerontology 49*, B270-B276.

Lithgow GJ, White TM, Melov S, Johnson TE (1995). Thermotolerance and extended life-span conferred by single-gene mutations and induced by thermal stress. *Proceedings of the National Academy of Sciences USA 92*, 7540-7544.

Luhtala TA, Roecker EB, Pugh T, Feuers RJ, Weindruch R (1994). Dietary restriction attenuates age-related increases in rat skeletal muscle antioxidant enzyme activities. *Journals of Gerontology A Biological Sciences and Medical Sciences 49*, B231-B238.

Madsen MA, Hsieh CC, Boylston WH, Flurkey K, Harrison D, Papaconstantinou J (2004). Altered oxidative stress response of the long-lived Snell dwarf mouse. *Biochemical and Biophysical Research Communications 318*, 998-1005.

Manning EL, Crossland J, Dewey MJ, Van Zant G (2002). Influences of inbreeding and genetics on telomere length in mice. *Mammalian Genome 13*, 234-238.

Marden JH, Rogina B, Montooth KL, Helfand SL (2003). Conditional tradeoffs between aging and organismal performance of Indy long-lived mutant flies. *Proceedings of the National Academy of Sciences USA 100*, 3369-3373.

Mattison J, Wright C, Bronson R, Roth G, Ingram D, Bartke A (2000). Studies of aging in ames dwarf mice: Effects of caloric restriction. *AGE 23*, 9-16.

Matulic M, Sopta M, Rubelj I (2007). Telomere dynamics: the means to an end. *Cell Proliferation 40*, 462-474.

Maynard SP, Miller RA (2006). Fibroblasts from long-lived Snell dwarf mice are resistant to oxygen-induced *in vitro* growth arrest. *Aging Cell 5*, 89-96.

McCay CM, Crowell MF, Maynard LA (1935). The effect of retarded growth upon the length of life span and upon the ultimate body size. *Journal of Nutrition 10*, 63-79.

Medawar, P. 1955. The definition and measurement of senescence. Pages 4-15 In: G. E. W. Wolstenhilme, ed. *Ciba Foundation colloquia on ageing, Volume 1*. J & A Churchill, London.

Menini S, Amadio L, Oddi G, Ricci C, Pesce C, Pugliese F, Giorgio M, Migliaccio E, Pelicci P, Iacobini C, Pugliese G (2006). Deletion of p66Shc longevity gene protects against experimental diabetic glomerulopathy by preventing diabetes-induced oxidative stress. *Diabetes 55*, 1642-1650.

Migliaccio E, Giorgi M, Mele S, Pelicci G, Reboldi P, Pandolfi PP, Lanfrancone L, Pelicci PG (1999). The p66shc adaptor protein controls oxidative stress response and life span in mammals. *Nature 402*, 309-313.

Miller RA (1999). Kleemeier Award Lecture: Are there genes for aging? *Journals of Gerontology A Biological Sciences and Medical Sciences 54A*, B297-B307.

Miller RA, Austad SN, Burke D, Chrisp C, Dysko R, Galecki A, Jackson A, Monnier VM (1999). Exotic mice as models for aging research: polemic and prospectus. *Neurobiology of Aging 20*, 217-231.

Miller RA, Dysko R, Chrisp C, Seguin R, Linsalata L, Buehner G, Harper JM, Austad S (2000). Mouse (*Mus musculus*) stocks derived from tropical islands: New models for genetic analysis of life history traits. *Journal of Zoology 250*, 95-104.

Miller RA, Harper JM, Dysko R, Durkee SJ, Austad SN (2002). Longer life spans and delayed maturation in wild-derived mice. *Experimental Biology and Medicine 227*, 500-508.

Miller RA, Buehner G, Chang Y, Harper JM, Sigler R, Smith-Wheelock M (2005). Methionine-deficient diet extends mouse lifespan, slows immune and lens aging, alters glucose, T4, IGF-I and insulin levels, and increases hepatocyte MIF levels and stress resistance. *Aging Cell 4*, 119-125.

Miskin R, Masos T (1997). Transgenic mice overexpressing urokinase-type plasminogen activator in the brain exhibit reduced food consumption, body weight and size, and increased longevity. *Journals of Gerontology A Biological Sciences and Medical Sciences. 52A*, B118-B124.

Mitsui A, Hamuro J, Nakamura H, Kondo N, Hirabayashi Y, Ishizaki-Koizumi S, Hirakawa T, Inoue T, Yodoi J (2002). Overexpression of human thioredoxin in transgenic mice controls oxidative stress and life span. *Antioxidants and Redox Signaling 4*, 693-696.

Moosmann B, Behl C (2008). Mitochondrially encoded cysteine predicts animal lifespan. *Aging Cell 7*, 32-46.

Morley JF, Morimoto RI (2004). Regulation of longevity in *Caenorhabditis elegans* by heat shock factor and molecular chaperones. *Molecular Biology of the Cell 15*, 657-664.

Morrow G, Samson M, Michaud S, Tanguay RM (2004). Overexpression of the small mitochondrial Hsp22 extends Drosophila life span and increases resistance to oxidative stress. *FASEB Journal 18*, 598-599.

Mura CV, Gong X, Taylor A, Villalobos-Molina R, Scrofano MM (1996). Effects of calorie restriction and aging on the expression of antioxidant enzymes and ubiquitin in the liver of Emory mice. *Mechanisms of Ageing and Development 91*, 115-129.

Murakami S, Johnson TE (1996). A genetic pathway conferring life extension and resistance to UV stress in *Caenorhabditis elegans. Genetics 143*, 1207-1218.

Murakami S, Salmon AB, Miller RA (2003). Multiplex stress resistance in cells from long-lived dwarf mice. *FASEB Journal 17*, 1565-1566.

Ogburn CE, Austad SN, Holmes DJ, Kiklevich JV, Gollahon K, Rabinovitch PS, Martin GM (1998). Cultured renal epithelial cells from birds and mice: enhanced resistance of avian cells to oxidative stress and DNA damage. *Journals of Gerontology A Biological Sciences and Medical Sciences 53*, B287-B292.

Ogburn CE, Carlberg K, Ottinger MA, Holmes DJ, Martin GM, Austad SN (2001). Exceptional cellular resistance to oxidative damage in long-lived birds requires active gene expression. *Journals of Gerontology A Biological Sciences and Medical Sciences 56*, B468-474.

Oliver,SN. Caloric restriction, stress resistance and longevity in *Drosophila melanogaster*. 2005. University of Connecticut.

Orentreich N, Matias JR, DeFelice A, Zimmerman JA (1993). Low methionine ingestion by rats extends life span. *Journal of Nutrition 123*, 269-274.

Orr WC, Sohal RS (2003). Does overexpression of Cu,Zn-SOD extend life span in *Drosophila melanogaster? Experimental Gerontology 38*, 227-230.

Orsini F, Migliaccio E, Moroni M, Contursi C, Raker VA, Piccini D, Martin-Padura I, Pelliccia G, Trinei M, Bono M, Puri C, Tacchetti C, Ferrini M, Mannucci R, Nicoletti I, Lanfrancone L, Giorgio M, Pelicci PG (2004). The life span determinant p66Shc localizes to mitochondria where it associates with mitochondrial heat shock protein 70 and regulates trans-membrane potential. *Journal of Biological Chemistry 279*, 25689-25695.

Pacini S, Pellegrini M, Migliaccio E, Patrussi L, Ulivieri C, Ventura A, Carraro F, Naldini A, Lanfrancone L, Pelicci P, Baldari CT (2004). p66SHC promotes apoptosis and antagonizes mitogenic signaling in T cells. *Molecular and Cellular Biology 24*, 1747-1757.

Pollard M, Luckert PH (1985). Tumorigenic effects of direct- and indirect-acting chemical carcinogens in rats on a restricted diet. *Journal of the National Cancer Institute 74*, 1347-1349.

Rao G, Xia E, Nadakavukaren MJ, Richardson A (1990). Effect of dietary restriction on the age-dependent changes in the expression of antioxidant enzymes in rat liver. *Journal of Nutrition 120*, 602-609.

Richardson A, Liu F, Adamo ML, Remmen HV, Nelson JF (2004). The role of insulin and insulin-like growth factor-I in mammalian ageing. *Best practice & research. Clinical endocrinology & metabolism, 18*, 393-406.

Richie JP, Jr., Leutzinger Y, Parthasarathy S, Malloy V, Orentreich N, Zimmerman JA (1994). Methionine restriction increases blood glutathione and longevity in F344 rats. *FASEB Journal 8*, 1302-1307.

Riddle, D. L. 1988. The dauer larva. Pages 393-412 In: W. B. Wood, ed. *The nematode Caenorhabditis elegans*. Cold Spring Harbor Laboratory Press, Cold Spring Harbor, NY.

Roberts A, Pardo-Manuel de Villena F, Wang W, McMillan L, Threadgill D (2007). The polymorphism architecture of mouse genetic resources elucidated using genome-wide resequencing data: implications for QTL discovery and systems genetics. *Mammalian Genome 18*, 473-481.

Rogina B, Reenan RA, Nilsen SP, Helfand SL (2000). Extended life-span conferred by cotransporter gene mutations in Drosophila. *Science 290*, 2137-2140.

Rubio MA, Davalos AR, Campisi J (2004). Telomere length mediates the effects of telomerase on the cellular response to genotoxic stress. *Experimental Cell Research 298*, 17-27.

Ruiz-Laguna J, Abril N, Prieto-Alamo M, López-Barea J, Pueyo C (2005). Tissue, species, and environmental differences in absolute quantities of murine mRNAs coding for alpha, mu, omega, pi, and theta glutathione S-transferases. *Gene Expression 12*, 165-176.

Salcedo T, Geraldes A, Nachman MW (2007). Nucleotide variation in wild and inbred mice. *Genetics 177*, 2277-2291.

Salmon AB, Murakami S, Bartke A, Kopchick J, Yasumura K, Miller RA (2005). Fibroblast cell lines from young adult mice of long-lived mutant strains are resistant to multiple forms of stress. *American Journal of Physiology Endocrinology and Metabolism 289*, E23-E29.

Salmon AB, Sadighi Akha AA, Buffenstein R, Miller RA (2008a). Fibroblasts from naked mole-rats are resistant to multiple forms of cell injury, but sensitive to peroxide, ultraviolet light, and endoplasmic reticulum stress. *Journals of Gerontology Series A: Biological Sciences and Medical Sciences 63*, 232-241.

Salmon AB, Ljungman M, Miller RA (2008b). Cells from long-lived mutant mice exhibit enhanced repair of ultraviolet lesions. *Journals of Gerontology A Biological Sciences and Medical Sciences 63*, 219-231.

Sanz A, Bartke A, Barja G (2002). Long-lived Ames dwarf mice: oxidative damage to mitochondrial DNA in heart and brain. *AGE 25*, 119-122.

Sanz A, Caro P, Ayala V, Portero-Otin M, Pamplona R, Barja G (2006). Methionine restriction decreases mitochondrial oxygen radical generation and leak as well as oxidative damage to mitochondrial DNA and proteins. *FASEB Journal 20*, 1064-1073.

Schriner SE, Linford NJ, Martin GM, Treuting P, Ogburn CE, Emond M, Coskun PE, Ladiges W, Wolf N, Van Remmen H, Wallace DC, Rabinovitch PS (2005). Extension of murine life span by overexpression of catalase targeted to mitochondria. *Science 308*, 1909-1911.

Sedelnikova OA, Horikawa I, Zimonjic DB, Popescu NC, Bonner WM, Barrett JC (2004). Senescing human cells and ageing mice accumulate DNA lesions with unrepairable double-strand breaks. *Nature Cell Biology 6*, 168-170.

Selsby JT, Judge AR, Yimlamai T, Leeuwenburgh C, Dodd SL (2005). Life long calorie restriction increases heat shock proteins and proteasome activity in soleus muscles of Fisher 344 rats. *Experimental Gerontology 40*, 37-42.

Shaddock JG, Feuers RJ, Chou MW, Pegram RA, Casciano DA (1993). Effects of aging and caloric restriction on the genotoxicity of four carcinogens in the *in vitro* rat hepatocyte/DNA repair assay. *Mutation Research 295*, 19-30.

Shaddock JG, Feuers RJ, Chou MW, Swenson GH, Casciano DA (1995). Genotoxicity of tacrine in primary hepatocytes isolated from B6C3F1 mice and aged ad libitum and calorie restricted Fischer 344 rats. *Mutation Research 344*, 79-88.

Shaikh ZA, Jordan SA, Tang W (1999). Protection against chronic cadmium toxicity by caloric restriction. *Toxicology 133*, 93-103.

Siderakis M, Tarsounas M (2007). Telomere regulation and function during meiosis. *Chromosome Research 15*, 667-679.

Silberberg R (1972). Articular aging and osteoarthrosis in dwarf mice. *Pathologia et Microbiologia (Basel). 38*, 417-430.

Snell GD (1929). Dwarf, a new mendelian recessive character of the house mouse. *Proceedings of the National Academy of Sciences USA 15*, 733-734.

Sohal RS, Ku HH, Agarwal S, Forster MJ, Lal H (1994). Oxidative damage, mitochondrial oxidant generation and antioxidant defenses during aging and in response to food restriction in the mouse. *Mechanisms of Ageing and Development 74*, 121-133.

Storey K (2006). Gene hunting in hypoxia and exercise. *Advances in Experimental Medicine and Biology 588*, 293-309.

Stuermer IW, Tittman C, Schilling C, Blottner S (2006). Reproduction of wild Mongolian gerbils bred in the laboratory with respect to generation and season 1. Morphological changes and fertility lifespan. *Animal Science 82*, 377-387.

Sun D, Muthukumar AR, Lawrence RA, Hernandes G (2001). Effects of calorie restriction on polymicrobial peritonitis induced by cecum ligation and puncture in young C57BL/6 mice. *Clinical Diagnostic Laboratory Immunology 8*, 1003-1011.

Sun J, Tower J (1999). FLP recombinase-mediated induction of Cu/Zn-superoxide dismutase transgene expression can extend the life span of adult *Drosophila melanogaster* flies. *Molecular and Cellular Biology 19*, 216-218.

Sun J, Folk D, Bradley TJ, Tower J (2002). Induced overexpression of mitochondrial Mn-superoxide dismutase extends the life span of adult *Drosophila melanogaster*. *Genetics 161*, 661-672.

Sun J, Molitor J, Tower J (2004). Effects of simultaneous over-expression of Cu/ZnSOD and MnSOD on *Drosophila melanogaster* life span. *Mechanisms of Ageing and Development 125*, 341-349.

Sun LY, Evans MS, Hsieh J, Panici J, Bartke A (2005). Increased neurogenesis in dentate gyrus of long-lived Ames dwarf mice. *Endocrinology 146*, 1138-1144.

Symphorien S, Woodruff RC (2003). Effect of DNA repair on aging of transgenic *Drosophila melanogaster*: I. mei-41 locus. *Journals of Gerontology A Biological Sciences and Medical Sciences 8*, B782-B787.

Syntichaki P, Troulinaki K, Tavernarakis N (2007). eIF4E function in somatic cells modulates ageing in *Caenorhabditis elegans*. *Nature 445*, 922-926.

Taguchi A, Wartschow LM, White MF (2007). Brain IRS2 signaling coordinates life span and nutrient homeostasis. *Science 317*, 369-372.

Takagi Y, Hattori I, Nozaki K, Mitsui A, Ishikawa M, Hashimoto N, Yodoi J (2000). Excitotoxic hippocampal injury is attenuated in thioredoxin transgenic mice. *Journal of Cerebral Blood Flow and Metabolism 20*, 829-833.

Takagi Y, Mitsui A, Nishiyama A, Nozaki K, Sono H, Gon Y, Hashimoto N, Yodoi J (1999). Overexpression of thioredoxin in transgenic mice attenuates focal ischemic brain damage. *Proceedings of the National Academy of Sciences USA 96*, 4131-4136.

Tannenbaum A (1942). The genesis and growth of tumors. II. Effects of calorie restriction per se. *Cancer Research 2*, 460-467.

Tatar M, Bartke A, Antebi A (2003). The endocrine regulation of aging by insulin-like signals. *Science 299*, 1346-1351.

Tatar M, Kopelman A, Epstein D, Tu MP, Yin CM, Garofalo RS (2001). A mutant Drosophila insulin receptor homolog that extends life-span and impairs neuroendocrine function. *Science 292*, 107-110.

Tettweiler G, Miron M, Jenkins M, Sonenberg N, Lasko PF (2005). Starvation and oxidative stress resistance in Drosophila are mediated through the eIF4E-binding protein, d4E-BP. *Genes and Development 19*, 1840-1843.

Thia K, Trapani J (2007). The granzyme B gene is highly polymorphic in wild mice but essentially invariant in common inbred laboratory strains. *Tissue Antigens 70*, 198-204.

Tilley R, Miller S, Srivastava V, Busbee D (1992). Enhanced unscheduled DNA synthesis by secondary cultures of lung cells established from calorically restricted aged rats. *Mechanisms of Ageing and Development 63*, 165-176.

Tirosh O, Aronis A, Zusman I, Kossoy G, Yahav S, Shinder D, Abramovitz R, Miskin R (2003). Mitochondrion-mediated apoptosis is enhanced in long-lived α-MUPA transgenic mice and calorically restricted wild-type mice. *Experimental Gerontology 38*, 955-963.

Tirosh O, Pardo M, Schwartz B, Miskin R (2005). Long-lived α-MUPA transgenic mice show reduced SOD2 expression, enhanced apoptosis and reduced susceptibility to the carcinogen dimethylhydrazine. *Mechanisms of Ageing and Development 126*, 1262-1273.

Tucker JD, Spruill MD, Ramsey MJ, Director AD, Nath J (1999). Frequency of spontaneous chromosome aberrations in mice: effects of age. *Mutation Research 425*, 135-141.

Ungvari Z, Buffenstein R, Austad S, Podlutsky A, Kaley G, Csiszar A (2008). Oxidative stress in vascular senescence: lessons from successfully aging species. *Frontiers in Bioscience 13*, 5056-5070.

Usuki F, Yasutake A, Umehara F, Higuchi I (2004). Beneficial effects of mild lifelong dietary restriction on skeletal muscle: prevention of age-related mitochondrial damage, morphological changes, and vulnerability to a chemical toxin. *Acta Neuropathologica 108*, 1-9.

van Buul PPW, van Buul-Offers S (1982). Effect of hormone treatment on spontaneous and radiation-induced chromosomal breakage in normal and dwarf mice. *Mutation Research 106*, 237-246.

van Buul PPW, van Buul-Offers SC (1988). Effects of hormone treatment on chromosomal radiosensitivity of somatic and germ cells of Snell's dwarf mice. *Mutation Research 198*, 263-268.

Van Remmen H, Ikeno Y, Hamilton M, Pahlavani M, Wolf N, Thorpe SR, Alderson NL, Baynes JW, Epstein CJ, Huang TT, Nelson J, Strong R, Richardson A (2003). Life-long reduction in MnSOD activity results in increased DNA damage and higher incidence of cancer but does not accelerate aging. *Physiological Genomics 16*, 29-37.

Vanfleteren JR (1993). Oxidative stress and ageing in *Caenorhabditis elegans. Biochem Journal 292*, 605-608.

Vellai T, Takacs-Vellai K, Zhang Y, Kovacs AL, Orosz L, Muller F (2003). Genetics: influence of TOR kinase on lifespan in C. elegans. *Nature 426*, 620.

Vergara M, Smith-Wheelock M, Harper JM, Sigler R, Miller RA (2004). Hormone-treated Snell dwarf mice regain fertility but remain long-lived and disease resistant. *Journals of Gerontology A Biological Sciences and Medical Sciences 59*, 1244-1250.

Wang MC, Bohmann D, Jasper H (2003). JNK signaling confers tolerance to oxidative stress and extends lifespan in Drosophila. *Developmental Cell 5*, 811-816.

Wang MC, Bohmann D, Jasper H (2005). JNK extends life span and limits growth by antagonizing cellular and organism-wide responses to insulin signaling. *Cell 121*, 115-125.

Ward WF, Qi W, Remmen HV, Zackert WE, Roberts LJ, II, Richardson A (2005). Effects of age and caloric restriction on lipid peroxidation: measurement of oxidative stress by F2-isoprostane levels. *Journals of Gerontology A Biological Sciences and Medical Sciences 60*, 847-851.

Weindruch R, Walford RL (1988) *The Retardation of Aging and Disease by Dietary Restriction*. Springfield, IL: Charles C. Thomas.

Weraarchakul N, Strong R, Wood WG, Richardson A (1989). The effect of aging and dietary restriction on DNA repair. *Experimental Cell Research 181*, 197-204.

Wessells RJ, Fitzgerald E, Cypser JR, Tatar M, Bodmer R (2004). Insulin regulation of heart function in aging fruit flies. *Nature Genetics 36*, 1275-1281.

Wilhelm Filho D, Althoff SL, Dafré AL, Boveris A (2007). Antioxidant defenses, longevity and ecophysiology of South American bats. *Comparative Biochemistry and Physiology Part C: Toxicology & Pharmacology 146*, 214-220.

Wu A, Sun X, Wan F, Liu Y (2003). Modulations by dietary restriction on antioxidant enzymes and lipid peroxidation in developing mice. *Journal of Anatomy 94*, 947-952.

Yamamoto M, Clark JD, Pastor JV, Gurnani P, Nandi A, Kurosu H, Miyoshi M, Ogawa Y, Castrillon DH, Rosenblatt KP, Kuro-o M (2005). Regulation of oxidative stress by the anti-aging hormone Klotho. *Journal of Biological Chemistry 280*, 38029-38034.

Yang X, Doser TA, Fang CX, Nunn JM, Janardhanan R, Zhu M, Sreejayan N, Quinn MT, Ren J (2006). Metallothionein prolongs survival and antagonizes senescence-associated cardiomyocyte diastolic dysfunction: role of oxidative stress. *FASEB Journal 20*, 1024-1026.

Yeargers E (1981). Effect of gamma-radiation on dauer larvae of *Caenorhabditis elegans. Journal of Nematology 13*, 235-237.

Yokoyama K, Fukumoto K, Murakami T, Harada Si, Hosono R, Wadhwa R, Mitsui Y, Ohkuma S (2002). Extended longevity of *Caenorhabditis elegans* by knocking in extra copies of hsp70F, a homolog of mot-2 (mortalin)/mthsp70/Grp75. *FEBS Letters 516*, 53-57.

Yoshida K, Inoue T, Nojima K, Hirabayashi Y, Sado T (1997). Calorie restriction reduces the incidence of myeloid leukemia induced by a single whole-body radiation in C3H/He mice. *Proceedings of the National Academy of Sciences USA 94*, 2615-2619.

Yoshiki A, Moriwaki K (2006). Mouse phenome research: implications of genetic background. *ILAR Journal 47*, 94-102.

Youngman LD, Park JK, Ames BN (1992). Protein oxidation associated with aging is reduced by dietary restriction of protein or calories. *Proceedings of the National Academy of Sciences USA 89*, 9112-9116.

Yuan R, Flurkey K, Van Aelst-Bouma R, Zhang W, King B, Austad S, Miller R, Harrison D (2006). Altered growth characteristics of skin fibroblasts from wild-derived mice, and genetic loci regulating fibroblast clone size. *Aging Cell 5*, 203-212.

Zaccagnini G, Martelli F, Fasanaro P, Magenta A, Gaetano C, Di Carlo A, Biglioli P, Giorgio M, Martin-Padura I, Pelicci PG, Capogrossi MC (2004). p66[ShcA] modulates tissue response to hindlimb ischemia. *Circulation 109*, 2917-2923.

Zhou Y, Xu BC, Maheshwari HG, He L, Reed M, Lozykowski M, Okada S, Cataldo L, Coschigano K, Wagner TE, Baumann G, Kopchick JJ (1997). A mammalian model for Laron syndrome produced by targeted disruption of the mouse growth hormone receptor/binding protein gene (the Laron mouse). *Proceedings of the National Academy of Sciences USA 94*, 13215-13220.

Zimmerman JA, Malloy V, Krajcik R, Orentreich N (2003). Nutritional control of aging. *Experimental Gerontology 38*, 47-52.

In: Handbook on Longevity: Genetics, Diet and Disease   ISBN 978-1-60741-075-1

Editors: Jennifer V. Bentely and Mary Ann Keller   © 2009 Nova Science Publishers, Inc.

Chapter VI

Longevity-Associated Mitochondrial DNA 5178 C/A Polymorphism Modifies the Effect of Coffee Consumption on Glucose Tolerance in Middle-Aged Japanese Men

Akatsuki Kokaze,[a,b]* Mamoru Ishikawa,[b,c] Naomi Matsunaga,[b] Kanae Karita,[b] Masao Yoshida,[b] Tadahiro Ohtsu,[a] Takako Shirasawa,[a] Yahiro Haseba,[a] Masao Satoh,[d] Koji Teruya,[e] Hiromi Hoshino[a] and Yutaka Takashima[b]

[a]Department of Public Health, Showa University School of Medicine,
Shinagawa-ku, Tokyo, Japan
[b]Department of Public Health, Kyorin University School of Medicine,
Mitaka-shi, Tokyo, Japan
[c]Mito Red Cross Hospital, Mito-shi, Ibaraki, Japan
[d]School of Medical Technology and Health, Faculty of Health and Medical Care, Saitama
Medical University, Hidaka-shi, Saitama, Japan
[e]Department of Public Health, Kyorin University School of Health Sciences,
Hachioji-shi, Tokyo, Japan

* Correspondence to: Akatsuki Kokaze,
Department of Public Health, Showa University School of Medicine,
1-5-8 Hatanodai, Shinagawa-ku, Tokyo 142-8555, Japan
Tel: +81(3)3784-8133; Fax: +81(3)3784-7733; E-mail: akokaze@med.showa-u.ac.jp

Abstract

Mitochondrial DNA 5178 C/A (Mt5178 C/A), NADH dehydrogenase subunit-2 237 leucine/methionine (ND2-237 Leu/Met), polymorphism is reported to be associated with longevity, blood pressure, serum lipid levels, fasting plasma glucose levels, glucose tolerance, serum uric acid levels, pulmonary function, hematological parameters, intraocular pressure, serum electrolyte levels, and serum protein fraction levels in the Japanese population. Mt5178A (ND2-237lMet) genotype reportedly provides resistance to diabetes and atherosclerotic diseases, such as myocardial infarction and cerebrovascular diseases. Several epidemiological studies have shown that habitual coffee consumption exerts a protective effect against abnormal glucose tolerance in a Japanese population. This study investigated whether longevity-associated Mt5178 C/A (ND2-237 Leu/Met) polymorphism modifies the effects of coffee consumption on the risk of abnormal glucose tolerance in middle-aged Japanese men. A total of 332 male subjects (age, 52.8 ± 7.8 years; mean $\pm$ SD) were selected from individuals visiting the hospital for regular medical check-ups. After adjustment, the odds ratio (OR) for abnormal glucose tolerance was significantly lower in subjects with Mt5178C (ND2-237Leu) who consume more than four cups of coffee daily compared with those who consume less than one cup of coffee daily (OR = 0.245; 95% CI: 0.066 - 0.914). On the other hand, the association between Mt5178A genotype and risk for abnormal glucose tolerance did not depend on coffee consumption. These results suggest that longevity-associated Mt5178 C/A (ND2-237 Leu/Met) polymorphism modifies the effects of coffee consumption on reduced abnormal glucose tolerance risk in middle-aged Japanese men. This novel diet-gene interaction may contribute to the individualized prevention of lifestyle-related adult-onset diseases and allow for healthy aging and longevity.

Introduction

Mitochondrial DNA 5178 C/A Polymorphism

Longevity is a consequence of a complicated interaction between genetic, behavioral, and environmental factors. One of the genetic variations influencing life expectancy is mitochondrial DNA polymorphism [1, 2]. Mitochondrial DNA 5178 cytosine/adenine (Mt5178 C/A) polymorphism, which results in NADH dehydrogenase subunit-2 237 leucine/methionine (ND2-237 Leu/Met) polymorphism, is one of the longevity-associated mitochondrial DNA polymorphisms [3-9].

Tanaka et al. suggested that Mt5178 C/A polymorphism was associated with longevity in Japanese people [3, 4]. They reported that the frequency of Mt5178A, one of two genetic markers of mitochondrial DNA haplogroup D, was significantly higher in centenarians than in the general population [3]. Their reports on Mt5178 C/A polymorphism inspired researchers to perform genetic epidemiological studies on the association of Mt5178 C/A polymorphism and various diseases [10-17].

The clinical, biochemical, and biophysical properties of Mt5178 C/A polymorphism and its interaction with lifestyle factors are discussed below.

Mitochondrial DNA 5178 C/A Polymorphism and Atherogenic Diseases

Several clinical studies show that the Mt5178C genotype is more susceptible to atherogenic diseases than the Mt5178A genotype [10-12].

Mukae et al. reported that the frequency of the Mt5178C genotype was significantly higher in patients with acute myocardial infarction than in control subjects, and that this difference was more apparent in younger patients [10]. They concluded that Mt5178C may promote the occurrence of acute myocardial infarction, and that the Mt5178C genotype was a possible genetic risk factor for coronary disease in Japanese individuals. Takagi et al. also reported that the frequency of Mt5178C genotype was significantly higher in subjects with myocardial infarction than in controls after adjustment for age, gender, body mass index (BMI), smoking habits, hypertension, hypercholesterolemia, diabetes, and hyperuricemia [11].

Ohkubo et al. investigated Mt5178 C/A polymorphism and angiotensin I-converting enzyme gene polymorphism in patients with cerebrovascular disorders and age-matched normal controls [12]. Although there was no significant difference in the frequencies of angiotensin I-converting enzyme genotypes between patients with cerebrovascular disorders and age-matched normal controls, the frequency of Mt5178C was significantly higher in cerebrovascular disorder patients than in normal controls. They thus suggested that the Mt5178C genotype is a genetic risk factor for cerebrovascular disease in Japanese subjects.

Mitochondrial DNA 5178 C/A Polymorphism, Blood Pressure and Hypertension

Blood pressure is a crucial factor in the pathology of age-related circulatory diseases. We previously reported that Mt5178 C/A polymorphism may influence both diastolic blood pressure (DBP) in Japanese women and the blood-pressure-increasing effect of habitual drinking in Japanese men [18]. In healthy Japanese women, DBP was significantly higher in those with Mt5178A than in those with Mt5178C. After adjusting for age, BMI, habitual drinking, and habitual smoking, this difference remained. In healthy Japanese men, Mt5178 C/A polymorphism was not found to be associated with blood pressure. However, the results of a thorough data analysis suggested that Mt5178 C/A polymorphism may be indirectly associated with systolic blood pressure (SBP) and DBP via drinking frequency. After adjusting for age, BMI, and habitual smoking, SBP was shown to be significantly higher in daily drinkers with Mt5178C than in occasional drinkers and non-drinkers with Mt5178C. Moreover, DBP was observed to be significantly higher in daily drinkers with Mt5178C than in occasional drinkers and non-drinkers with Mt5178C. However, in men with Mt5178A, no significant differences in blood pressure among daily drinkers, occasional drinkers, and non-drinkers were observed.

To investigate whether Mt5178 C/A polymorphism is associated with a risk of hypertension, we conducted a cross-sectional study [19]. The frequency of hypertension was significantly higher in Mt5178C genotypic men than in Mt5178A genotypic men. Multiple logistic regression analysis revealed that the Mt5178A genotype, particularly in younger subjects (<60 years), had a lower odds ratio (OR) for hypertension than the Mt5178C genotype. Moreover, the association of Mt5178 C/A polymorphism with hypertension may depend on the frequency of alcohol consumption. The OR for hypertension was significantly higher in daily drinkers with Mt5178C compared with non- or ex-drinkers with Mt5178C. However, the association between the Mt5178A genotype and hypertension may not depend on the frequency of alcohol consumption. Mt5178C genotypic men may have a higher risk of hypertension than Mt5178A genotypic men. However, even with the Mt5178C genotype, positive changes in habitual drinking behavior may reduce the risk of hypertension and subsequent atherosclerotic diseases.

Mitochondrial DNA 5178 C/A Polymorphism and Serum Lipid Levels

We previously reported that Mt5178 C/A polymorphism may be associated with serum lipid levels in Japanese subjects [20]. In healthy Japanese men, after adjusting for age and BMI, serum high-density lipoprotein cholesterol (HDLC) levels were significantly higher in those with the Mt5178A genotype than in those with the Mt5178C genotype. However, this significant difference disappeared after adjusting for drinking frequency. We then investigated the interaction between Mt5178 C/A polymorphism and habitual alcohol drinking on serum lipid levels [21]. An interaction between Mt5178 C/A polymorphism and daily drinking on serum triglyceride (TG) levels was observed. Moreover, an interaction between Mt5178 C/A polymorphism and cigarette consumption on serum TG levels was also observed. Multiple regression analysis showed that in men with Mt5178A, daily drinking decreased serum TG levels and cigarette consumption increased serum TG levels, whereas in men with Mt5178C, the effects of daily drinking and cigarette consumption on serum TG levels were unclear. Considering that cigarette smoking influences serum cholesterol levels [22, 23], we performed a cross-sectional study to investigate the interaction between Mt5178 C/A polymorphism and habitual smoking on serum lipid levels. In that study, healthy Japanese male subjects were classified into two groups based on BMI: BMI ≤ 22 and BMI > 22 [24]. An interaction between Mt5178 C/A polymorphism and cigarette smoking was observed with regard to serum TG levels in subjects with a BMI ≤ 22, and with regard to serum total cholesterol (TC) levels and serum low-density lipoprotein cholesterol (LDLC) levels in subjects with a BMI > 22. In subjects with a BMI > 22, serum TC levels were significantly lower in non-smokers with Mt5178A than in smokers with Mt5178A, whereas serum LDLC levels were lower in non-smokers with Mt5178A than in those with Mt5178C or in smokers with Mt5178A. Although an interaction between Mt5178 C/A polymorphism and habitual smoking was not observed with regard to serum TG levels in subjects with a BMI > 22, serum TG levels were significantly higher in smokers with Mt5178A than in non-smokers with Mt5178A as well as in non-smokers with Mt5178C. Taken together, these results suggest that habitual smoking may deprive Japanese Mt5178A genotypic men with a BMI > 22 of their antiatherogenic advantage.

In healthy Japanese women, serum TG levels were significantly lower in those with the Mt5178A genotype than in those with the Mt5178C genotype [20]. This difference in serum

TG levels between the Mt5178 C/A genotypes was more evident in postmenopausal women than in premenopausal women.

In Asian populations outside Japan, there was reportedly no significant difference either in serum TG levels or in serum HDLC levels between Mt5178 C/A genotypes [25]. However, plasma apolipoprotein B levels were significantly higher in Chinese men with Mt5178A than in those with Mt5178C.

Mitochondrial DNA 5178 C/A Polymorphism and Serum Uric Acid Levels

Hyperuricemia is a risk factor for cardiovascular disease [26, 27]. We investigated whether Mt5178 C/A polymorphism is associated with serum uric acid (UA) levels [28]. In non-obese (BMI < 25) male subjects, an interaction between Mt5178 C/A genotypes and drinking frequency on serum UA levels was observed. Serum UA levels were significantly higher in daily drinkers with Mt5178C than in non-daily drinkers with Mt5178C. In non-obese men, after adjusting for covariates, daily drinkers with Mt5178C had a significantly higher OR for hyperuricemia (serum UA level $\geq$ 6.5 mg/dl). However, in obese (BMI $\geq$ 25) men, no significant interaction between Mt5178 C/A polymorphism and habitual drinking on serum UA levels or on risk for hyperuricemia was observed. These results suggest that Mt5178 C/A polymorphism modulates the effects of daily alcohol consumption on serum UA levels in non-obese Japanese men. Even among non-obese men, those with the Mt5178C genotype should avoid daily alcohol consumption to lower the risk of hyperuricemia.

Mitochondrial DNA 5178 C/A Polymorphism and Pulmonary Function

Respiratory function is also associated with longevity [29, 30]. Among younger subjects (<55 years), forced vital capacity (FVC) and forced expiratory volume in 1 s (FEV$_1$) were significantly higher in men with Mt5178A than in men with Mt5178C [31]. These findings may help elucidate the biological significance of the relationship between mitochondrial function, respiratory function, and longevity. Moreover, smoking-related decreases in the FEV$_1$/FVC ratio were more evident for men with Mt5178C than for those with Mt5178C. Cigarette consumption (pack-years of smoking) was significantly and negatively associated with FEV$_1$/FVC ratio for men with Mt5178C. Among older subjects ($\geq$55 years), the FEV$_1$/FVC ratio was significantly lower for current smokers with Mt5178C than for never smokers with Mt5178C or for never smokers with Mt5178A. In addition to antiatherogenic advantages, higher FVC and higher FEV$_1$ are probably biophysical factors associated with longevity in individuals with the Mt5178A genotype. Moreover, these findings may assist in establishing personalized prevention strategies for pulmonary dysfunction and individualized guidance for smoking cessation on the basis of genetic information on Mt5178 C/A polymorphism.

Mitochondrial DNA 5178 C/A Polymorphism and Hematological Parameters

Hematological parameters, such as erythrocytosis and increased hematocrit levels, are thrombogenic risk factors for myocardial infarction [32] and stroke [33]. Therefore, we investigated the association between Mt5178 C/A genotypes and hematological parameters in healthy Japanese male subjects [34]. In subjects with a BMI $\leq$ 23, Mt5178 C/A polymorphism influenced the effects of habitual smoking on hematological parameters. Red blood cell (RBC) counts were significantly lower and mean corpuscular hemoglobin (MCH) levels were significantly higher in smokers with Mt5178A than non-smokers with Mt5178A. Platelet counts were significantly higher in smokers with Mt5178C than in non-smokers with Mt5178C. Cigarette consumption was strongly associated with RBC counts, mean corpuscular volume levels, and MCH levels for men with Mt5178A, and was associated with platelet counts for those with Mt5178C. However, these results do not let us state that thrombogenic risk is lower in men with Mt5178A than those with Mt5178C.

Mitochondrial DNA 5178 C/A Polymorphism and Intraocular Pressure

Age-related changes in intraocular pressure (IOP) are known to vary with ethnicity [35-41]. In analyses of the relationship between aging and IOP, it may be essential to account for genetic factors. Therefore, we investigated whether Mt5178 C/A polymorphism was associated with IOP [42]. Mean IOP was significantly lower in men with Mt5178A than in those with Mt5178C. This difference in mean IOP between Mt5178 C/A genotypes remained evident after adjusting for age, BMI, blood pressure, habitual smoking, and habitual drinking. Moreover, interactions between Mt5178 C/A polymorphism and habitual smoking or habitual drinking with regard to IOP were observed. Habitual smoking was significantly associated with IOP in men with Mt5178A, whereas daily alcohol consumption was significantly associated with IOP in those with Mt5178C. These results suggest that Mt5178 C/A polymorphism is associated with IOP in middle-aged Japanese men.

Mitochondrial DNA 5178 C/A Polymorphism and Serum Electrolyte Levels

Physiological factors are involved in age-associated changes in water and electrolyte balance [43]. We investigated the relationship between Mt5178 C/A polymorphism and serum sodium, potassium, chloride, and calcium levels [44]. Serum sodium and serum chloride levels were significantly lower in subjects with Mt5178A than in those with Mt5178C. Cigarette consumption and BMI were significantly and positively associated with serum chloride levels, and hemoglobin levels were significantly and negatively associated with serum chloride levels in subjects with Mt5178C. In men with Mt5178A, hemoglobin levels were significantly and negatively associated with serum chloride levels. After adjusting for covariates, serum sodium and chloride levels remained significantly lower only in obese (BMI $\geq$ 25) subjects, and serum calcium levels appeared to be significantly higher in

Mt5178A genotypic men than in Mt5178C genotypic men. It is uncertain whether or how these differences in serum electrolyte levels influence the aging process, onset of age-related diseases, or longevity. However, mitochondrial function may be involved in age-related changes in water and electrolyte balance.

Mitochondrial DNA 5178 C/A Polymorphism and Serum Protein Fraction Levels

Some researchers have reported a change in serum protein, albumin, and globulin levels during the aging process [45-48]. Therefore, we investigated whether Mt5178 C/A polymorphism was associated with serum protein fraction levels [49]. Alpha-1, alpha-2, and beta globulin proportions were significantly higher in women with Mt5178A than in those with Mt5178C. Moreover, alpha-1, alpha-2, and beta globulin levels were significantly higher in Mt5178A genotypic women than in Mt5178C genotypic women. These differences in serum globulin levels between the Mt5178 C/A genotypes were more apparent in premenopausal women than in postmenopausal women. On the other hand, no such biochemical differences in serum protein fraction levels were observed in men. Considering that tobacco smoke influences serum protein fraction levels [50-53], we assessed whether Mt5178 C/A polymorphism influenced the effects of habitual smoking on serum protein fraction levels in Japanese men [54]. In men with Mt5178C, alpha-1 and alpha-2 globulin levels were significantly lower in non-smokers than in smokers, and the influence of smoking on these globulin levels depended on daily cigarette consumption. However, in men with Mt5178A, no significant differences were observed in alpha-1 or alpha-2 globulin levels between smokers and non-smokers.

Mitochondrial DNA 5178 C/A Polymorphism and Diabetes

Diabetes and its subsequent complications threaten healthy aging and longevity. Several mitochondrial DNA mutations are associated with type 2 diabetes [13, 55-59]. Wang et al. reported the association of longevity-associated Mt5178 C/A polymorphism with the occurrence and clinical features of type 2 diabetes [13]. The frequency of the Mt5178A genotype was lower in patients with type 2 diabetes than in controls. Moreover, patients with a maternal history of diabetes tended to carry the Mt5178C genotype more frequently compared with those without a maternal history of diabetes and controls. Mean age at onset of diabetes was significantly lower in patients with Mt5178C than in those with Mt5178A, whereas insulin treatment tended to be more frequent in Mt5178C genotypic patients.

Diabetes is one of the risk factors for atherosclerotic diseases (Janka et al., 1996) [60]. Using ultrasonography, Matsunaga et al. assessed the association between the Mt5178 C/A genotypes and early atherosclerotic changes of the bilateral carotid arteries in patients with type 2 diabetes [14]. Mean intima-media thickness in the bilateral arteries was significantly greater in patients with Mt5178C than in those with Mt5178A. The Mt5178 C/A polymorphism was significantly correlated with mean intima-media thickness and the presence of plaque. They concluded that the Mt5178A genotype exerted an antiatherogenic effect even in patients with type 2 diabetes.

To investigate whether Mt5178 C/A polymorphism is associated with glucose tolerance, we conducted a cross-sectional study using the 75-g oral glucose tolerance test (OGTT). Non-diabetic Japanese male subjects were classified into three subgroups by BMI: BMI < 22; 22 ≤ BMI < 25; and BMI ≥ 25 [61]. The frequency of Mt5178A was significantly lower among subjects with BMI < 22 exhibiting impaired fasting glucose and impaired glucose tolerance than among those with normal glucose tolerance. In the BMI < 22 group, fasting plasma glucose (FPG) levels and plasma glucose levels at 60 and 120 min after glucose load (OGTT-1h and OGTT-2h, respectively) were significantly lower in subjects with Mt5178A than in those with Mt5178C. After adjusting for age, BMI, habitual smoking, habitual drinking, and family history of diabetes, FPG levels and OGTT-2h levels were still significantly lower in subjects with Mt5178A than in those with Mt5178C. However, after adjusting for covariates, in both the 22 ≤ BMI < 25 and BMI ≥ 25 groups, FPG levels were significantly higher in subjects with the Mt5178A genotype than in those with the Mt5178C genotype. In the BMI < 22 group, FPG levels were significantly higher in drinkers with Mt5178C than in non-drinkers with Mt5178A. OGTT-1h and OGTT-2h levels were significantly higher in drinkers with Mt5178C than in drinkers with Mt5178A. Thus, Mt5178 C/A polymorphism may be associated with FPG levels and glucose tolerance in middle-aged Japanese men.

Aim of this Study

Several large-scale epidemiological studies have shown that coffee consumption is a potential lifestyle habit to reduce the risk of type 2 diabetes [62-69]. These preventive medical reports encouraged us to perform a nutrigenetic study on glucose tolerance. The objective of this study was to investigate whether Mt5178 C/A polymorphism modifies the effects of coffee consumption on the risk of abnormal glucose tolerance in middle-aged Japanese male subjects.

Methods

Subjects

Participants were recruited from among individuals visiting the Mito Red Cross Hospital for regular medical check-ups between August 1999 and August 2000. This study was conducted in accordance with the Declaration of Helsinki and was approved by the Ethics Committee of the Kyorin University School of Medicine. Written informed consent was obtained from 602 volunteers before participation. Among these, 449 men were enrolled in the study. One hundred and seventeen individuals with unclear data or lack of data were excluded. Therefore, subjects comprised 332 Japanese men (age, 52.8 ± 7.8 years; mean ± SD).

Clinical Characteristics of Subjects

Determination of blood, chemical, and physical data was conducted as described previously [20, 61]. All subjects except those with diabetes underwent OGTT. Normal glucose tolerance was defined as FPG < 110 mg/dl and OGTT-2h < 140 mg/dl. Abnormal glucose tolerance was defined as FPG $\geq$ 110 mg/dl and/or OGTT-2h $\geq$ 140 mg/dl or diagnosed with diabetes. BMI was defined as the ratio of subject weight (kg) to the square of subject height (m). A survey of coffee intake, alcohol consumption, and habitual smoking was performed by means of a questionnaire. Coffee consumption was classified based on number of cups of coffee per day (fewer than one cup per day, one to three cups per day, and more than four cups per day). Alcohol consumption was classified based on drinking frequency (daily drinkers; occasional drinkers, which include those who drink several times per week or per month; and non- or ex-drinkers). Habitual smoking was classified as non- or ex-smokers and current smokers.

Genotyping

DNA was extracted from whole blood using the DNA Extractor WB kit (Wako Pure Chemical Industries, Osaka, Japan). The forward and reverse oligonucleotide primers used to determine the Mt5178 C/A genotype were: 5'-CTTAGCATACTCCTCAATTACCC-3' and 5'-CTGAATTCTTCGATAATGGCCCA-3'. Polymerase chain reaction (PCR) was performed with 50 ng genomic DNA in buffer containing 1.5 mM MgCl$_2$, 1.25 mM dNTPs and 0.5 µl Amplitaq DNA polymerase (GeneAmp, Perkin Elmer, Waltham, MA, USA). After initial denaturation at 94°C for 5 min, PCR was conducted through 40 cycles as follows: denaturation at 94°C for 30 s, annealing at 60°C for 60 s, and polymerase extension at 72°C for 10 min. The PCR product was then digested with restriction enzyme *Alu*I (Nippon Gene, Tokyo, Japan) and electrophoresed on 1.5% agarose gels. Gels were stained with ethidium bromide, visualized under UV light, and photographed. The absence of an *Alu*I site was designated as Mt5178A, and the presence of this restriction site was designated as Mt5178C.

Statistical Analyses

Statistical analyses were performed using SAS statistical software, version 9.1 for Windows (SAS Institute, Inc., Cary, NC, USA). Multiple logistic regression analysis was used to calculate ORs for abnormal glucose tolerance. For multiple logistic regression analysis, habitual alcohol consumption (non- or ex-drinkers = 0, occasional drinkers = 1, daily drinkers = 2) and habitual smoking (non- or ex-smokers = 0, current smokers = 1) were numerically coded. Differences with *P* values of less than 0.05 were considered statistically significant.

Results

No significant differences in biophysical or biochemical characteristics were observed between the Mt5178C and Mt5178A genotypes (Table 1). No significant difference in the frequency of abnormal glucose tolerance was observed between the Mt5178 C/A genotypes.

On multiple logistic regression analysis (Table 2), associations between Mt5178 C/A polymorphism and abnormal glucose tolerance depended on coffee consumption. The OR for abnormal glucose tolerance was lower in subjects with Mt5178C who consume more than four cups of coffee per day compared with those who consume fewer than one cup of coffee per day (several cups of coffee per week or month) (OR = 0.344, 95% CI: 0.106 - 1.113, P = 0.075). After adjustment for age, BMI, habitual alcohol consumption, habitual smoking, and serum TG levels, a significant OR was observed (OR = 0.245, 95% CI: 0.066 - 0.914, P = 0.036). On the other hand, the association between Mt5178A genotype and abnormal glucose tolerance did not appear to depend on coffee consumption.

Table 1. Clinical characteristics of study subjects by Mt5178 C/A genotype

	Mt5178C	**Mt5178A**	*P* value
	n = 197	n =135	
Age (y)	53.0 ± 7.9	52.6 ± 7.8	0.602
Body mass index (kg/m^2)	23.3 ± 2.6	23.6 ± 2.5	0.165
Systolic blood pressure (mmHg)	125.0 ± 15.6	125.2 ± 13.8	0.872
Diastolic blood pressure (mmHg)	72.8 ± 10.1	72.5 ± 8.5	0.788
Total cholesterol (mg/dl)	204.9 ± 35.8	204.8 ± 32.0	0.982
HDL cholesterol (mg/dl)	54.6 ± 13.6	56.2 ± 16.1	0.344
Triglyceride (mg/dl)	143.1 ± 97.5	139.9 ± 90.2	0.764
Fasting plasma glucose (mg/dl)	96.4 ± 8.7	97.0 ± 9.1	0.517
Uric acid (mg/dl)	5.99 ± 1.24	5.96 ± 1.22	0.798
Coffee consumption (<1 cup per day/1 - 3 cups per day/≥4 cups per day) (%)	40.1/48.7/11.2	39.3/48.9/11.8	0.977
Alcohol consumption (daily/occasionally/non- or ex-) (%)	19.3/36.5/44.2	12.6/38.5/48.9	0.267
Current smokers (%)	43.2	41.5	0.763
Abnormal glucose tolerance (%)	33.5	31.1	0.648

Values are means ± S.D. unless otherwise noted.
All *P* values depict significance of differences between Mt5178C and Mt5178A. For coffee consumption, alcohol consumption, current smokers, and abnormal glucose tolerance, *P* values were calculated by chi-squared test.

Discussion

In the present study, we found that Mt5178 C/A polymorphism modulates the effects of coffee consumption on reducing the risk of abnormal glucose tolerance in middle-aged Japanese men. For Mt5178C genotypic men, habitual coffee drinking may reduce the risk of abnormal glucose tolerance.

There have been a number of reports regarding the association between mitochondrial DNA polymorphism and lifestyle-related adult-onset diseases in Japanese subjects [10-14, 70-72]. Judging from the case-control studies on Mt5178 C/A polymorphism [10-14], individuals with Mt5178A appear to be resistant to lifestyle-related atherosclerotic diseases. Though the frequency of Mt5178A genotype is rare worldwide [25, 73, 74], it is assumed to be as high as 40 - 45% in the Japanese population [3, 10-14, 75]. Because the Mt5178A genotype, namely mitochondrial haplotype D, occurs in a relatively high number of Japanese subjects, this genetic property may help explain why life expectancy in Japan is one of the longest in the world.

Table 2. Odds ratios and 95% confidence intervals for abnormal glucose tolerance by Mt5178 C/A genotype and coffee consumption

Genotype and coffee consumption	Frequency		OR (95% CI)	Adjusted OR† (95% CI)
	NGT	AGT		
Mt5178C				
<1 cup per day (%)	48 (60.8)	31 (39.2)	1	1
1 - 3 cups per day (%)	65 (67.7)	31 (32.3)	0.738 (0.369 - 1.376)	0.790 (0.405 - 1.539)
≥4 cups per day (%)	18 (81.8)	4 (18.2)	0.344 (0.106 - 1.113)	0.245 (0.066 - 0.914)*
Mt5178A				
<1 cup per day (%)	35 (66.0)	18 (34.0)	1	1
1 - 3 cups per day (%)	48 (72.7)	18 (27.3)	0.729 (0.333 - 1.599)	0.880 (0.344 - 2.247)
≥4 cups per day (%)	10 (62.5)	6 (37.5)	1.167 (0.365 - 3.725)	2.467 (0.560 - 10.87)

NGT; normal glucose tolerance, AGT; abnormal glucose tolerance, OR; odds ratio; 95% CI; 95% confidence interval. †OR adjusted for age, body mass index, habitual alcohol consumption, habitual smoking, and serum triglyceride levels. *$P < 0.05$.

Individuals with Mt5178A (ND2-237Met) genotype may be more resistant to atherosclerosis than those with Mt5178C (ND2-237Leu) genotype [10-14]. The antiatherogenic advantages of ND2-237Met genotype may be brought about by the biophysical and biochemical properties of ND2-237Met. Methionine residues have an antioxidant potential for scavenging reactive oxygen species (ROS) [76]. NADH dehydrogenase is involved in the production of ROS [77] and is a target of attack by ROS. Our previous reports have suggested that longevity-associated Mt5178 C/A polymorphism modifies the effects of habitual alcohol consumption on blood pressure [18], increased risk of hypertension [19], serum lipid levels [21], serum UA levels [28], and IOP [42], and the effects of habitual smoking on serum lipid levels [21, 24], respiratory function [31], hematological parameters [34], IOP [42], and serum protein fraction levels [54]. Habitual alcohol drinking influences the production of ROS by NADH dehydrogenase [78], and modifies the susceptibility of mitochondrial proteins, including NADH dehydrogenase, to ROS [79]. Habitual smoking attenuates the activity of NADH dehydrogenase [80]. We hypothesize that differences in ethanol-related or smoking-related ROS production and/or sensitivity between ND2-237 Leu/Met bring about the differences in biophysical or biochemical status described above. The rate of mitochondrial ROS production is probably one of the determinant factors for the lifespan of animal species [81-83]. Moreover, considering that ROS are pathophysiologically involved with diabetes [84], atherosclerosis, and aging [85], the protective potential of ND2-237Met against ROS may play a crucial role in resistance to diabetes and atherosclerotic diseases and in realizing longevity.

Chlorogenic acid, a major component of coffee, affects glucose tolerance [86-90]. One of the proposed mechanisms for the beneficial effects of chlorogenic acid on glucose metabolism is its antioxidant effects [91]. Using an *in vitro* model, Pavlica and Gebhatdt reported the protective effects of chlorogenic acids against ROS [92]. Chlorogenic acids also inhibit excessive ROS production in rats [93]. Therefore, chlorogenic acid is assumed to be involved in the mechanism by which Mt5178 C/A (ND2-237 Leu/Met) polymorphism modulates the effects of coffee intake on risk reduction of abnormal glucose tolerance. Further biophysical and biochemical investigations are required to validate the mechanisms responsible for the differences in the effects of chlorogenic acids on glucose tolerance between the Mt5178 C/A (ND2-237 Leu/Met) genotypes. Moreover, considering other genetic factors potentially associated with glucose tolerance through oxidative stress [94], investigations into gene-gene or gene-gene-environment interactions of ROS with glucose tolerance or risks of diabetes are needed.

In addition to the preventive effects on diabetes [66, 67], coffee consumption has preventive effects on metabolic syndrome [95] and hyperuricemia [96] in Japanese subjects. Moreover, habitual coffee drinking reduces the risks of hepatocellular carcinoma [97-99], colorectal cancer [100, 101], and endometrial cancer [102, 103] in Japanese subjects. For Mt5178C (ND2-237Leu) genotypic men, habitual daily drinking increases the risk of hypertension [19] or hyperuricemia [28]. Therefore, considering the results in this study, in addition to avoiding daily alcohol consumption, intake of four or more cups of coffee is recommended for men with Mt5178C (ND2-237Leu) to reduce the risk of atherosclerotic disease. However, considering that excessive coffee intake reportedly increases the risk for pancreatic cancer [104] or hip fracture [105] in Japanese subjects, total risk management for lifestyle-related adult-onset diseases is needed to ensure successful aging and longevity.

From a nutrigenetic point of view, Aoyama et al. conducted a cross-sectional analysis of Trp64Arg polymorphism in the beta 3-adrenergic receptor gene (BAR-3) and Mt5178 C/A polymorphism to determine whether these polymorphisms are correlated with lifestyle-related phenotypes and nutrient intake [106]. Body fat content was significantly higher in subjects with the BAR-3 variant genotype (Arg/Arg or Arg/Trp) and Mt5178A compared with those with the BAR-3 normal genotype (Trp/Trp) and Mt5178A, and those with the BAR-3 normal genotype and Mt5178C. Carbohydrate energy ratio was significantly higher and animal protein intake was significantly lower in subjects with the BAR-3 normal genotype and Mt5178A than in those with the other three genotypic combinations. This gene-gene interaction, that is, combinations of BAR-3 polymorphism and Mt5178 C/A polymorphism, therefore appear to influence eating behavior and diet-related health conditions in Japanese subjects. The consideration of a diet-gene interaction on health conditions, such as an interaction between perilipin gene polymorphism and a high-saturated fat, low-carbohydrate diet on insulin resistance [107], may help establish individualized prevention strategies for lifestyle-related diseases. Health education or health guidance based on genetic susceptibility is a potential tool of prevention for lifestyle-related diseases. However, even in the case of cancer prevention, an interventional study showed that it is difficult for participants to stop their negative and/or risk-inducing behaviors [108]. Whether individualized prevention is efficient for lifestyle-related diseases may depend on improvement of health education and health guidance supported by progress in behavioral science, psychology, and genetic literacy.

In addition to the small sample size, a limitation of this study was the evaluation of habitual coffee consumption based on the number of cups consumed per day. Whether there is any interaction between Mt5178 C/A polymorphism and volume of chlorogenic acids, caffeine, or other compounds in coffee on glucose tolerance or risk of diabetes warrants further investigation.

In conclusion, longevity-associated Mt5178 C/A (ND2-237 Leu/Met) polymorphism may modify the effects of habitual coffee consumption on glucose tolerance in middle-aged Japanese men. For men with the Mt5178C (ND2-237Leu) genotype, habitual drinking of four or more cups of coffee may reduce the risk of abnormal glucose tolerance. Therefore, although individuals with Mt5178C (ND2-237Leu) may have a higher risk of diabetes than those with Mt5178A (ND2-237Met), preferable lifestyle habits may reduce the risk of diabetes and subsequent atherosclerotic diseases. These findings may inspire further investigations of gene-diet or gene-gene-diet interactions involving habitual coffee intake on diabetes, and may contribute to the establishment of individualized nutritional strategies for diabetes, thereby lowering the incidence of atherosclerotic diseases and leading to healthy aging and longevity.

Acknowledgements

This study was supported in part by Grants-in-Aid from the Ministry of Education, Culture, Sports, Science and Technology of Japan (No. 14570355 and No. 18590572) and the Chiyoda Mutual Life Foundation.

References

[1]   Santoro, A., Salvioli, S., Raule, N., Capri, M., Sevini, F., Valensin, S., Monti, D., Bellizzi, D., Passarino, G., Rose, G., De Benedictis, G. & Franceschi, C. (2006). Mitochondrial DNA involvement in human longevity. *Biochim. Biophys. Acta 1757*: 1388-1399.

[2]   Salvioli, S., Capri, M., Santoro, A., Raule, N., Sevini, F., Lukas, S., Lanzarini, C., Monti, D., Passarino, G., Rose, G., De Benedictis, G. & Franceschi, C. (2008). The impact of mitochondrial DNA on human lifespan: A view from studies on centenarians. *Biotechnol. J. 3*: 740-749.

[3]   Tanaka, M., Gong, J. S., Zhang, J., Yoneda, M. & Yagi, K. (1998). Mitochondrial genotype associated with longevity. *Lancet 351*: 185-186.

[4]   Tanaka, M., Gong, J. S., Zhang, J., Yamada, Y., Borgeld, H. J. & Yagi, K. (2000). Mitochondrial genotype associated with longevity and its inhibitory effect on mutagenesis. *Mech. Ageing Dev. 116*: 65-76.

[5]   Ivanova, R., Lepage, V., Charron, D. & Schächter, F. (1998). Mitochondrial genotype associated with French Caucasian centenarians. *Gerontology 44*: 349.

[6]   De Benedictis, G., Rose, G., Carrieri, G., De Luca, M., Falcone, E., Passarino, G., Bonafé, M., Monti, D., Baggio, G., Bertolini, S., Mari, D., Mattace, R. & Franceschi, C. (1999). Mitochondrial DNA inherited variants are associated with successful aging and longevity in humans. *FASEB J. 13*: 1532-1536.

[7]   Ross, O. A., McCormack, R., Curran, M. D., Duguid, R. A., Barnett, Y. A., Rea, I. M. & Middleton, D. (2001). Mitochondrial DNA polymorphism: its role in longevity of the Irish population. *Exp. Gerontol. 36*: 1161-1178.

[8]   Niemi, A. -K., Moilanen, J. S., Tanaka, M., Hervonen, A., Hurme, M., Lehtimaki, T., Arai, Y., Hirose, N. & Majamaa, K. (2005). A combination of three common inherited mitochondrial DNA polymorphisms promotes longevity in Finnish and Japanese subjects. *Eur. J. Hum. Genet. 13*: 166-170.

[9]   Alexe, G., Fuku, N., Bilal, E., Ueno, H., Nishigaki, Y., Fujita, Y., Ito, M., Arai, Y., Hirose, N., Bhanot, G. & Tanaka, M. (2007). Enrichment of longevity phenotype in mtDNA haplogroups D4b2b, D4a, and D5 in the Japanese population. *Hum. Genet. 121*: 347-356.

[10]   Mukae, S., Aoki, S., Itoh, S., Satoh, R., Nishio, K., Iwata, T. & Katagiri, T. (2003). Mitochondrial 5178A/C genotype is associated with acute myocardial infarction. *Circ. J. 67*: 16-20.

[11]   Takagi, K., Yamada, Y., Gong, J. S., Sone, T., Yokota, M. & Tanaka, M. (2004). Association of a 5178C→A (Leu237Met) polymorphism in the mitochondrial DNA with a low prevalence of myocardial infarction in Japanese individuals. *Atherosclerosis 175*: 281-286.

[12]   Ohkubo, R., Nakagawa, M., Ikeda, K., Kodama, T., Arimura, K., Akiba, S., Saito, M., Ookatsu, Y., Atsuchi, Y., Yamano, Y. & Osame, M. (2002). Cerebrovascular disorders and genetic polymorphisms: mitochondrial DNA5178C is predominant in cerebrovascular disorders. *J. Neurol. Sci. 198*: 31-35.

[13] Wang, D., Taniyama, M., Suzuki, Y., Katagiri, T. & Ban, Y. (2001). Association of the mitochondrial DNA 5178 A/C polymorphism with maternal inheritance and onset of type 2 diabetes in Japanese patients. *Exp. Clin. Endocrinol. Diabetes 109*: 361-364.

[14] Matsunaga, H., Tanaka, Y., Tanaka, M., Gong, J. S., Zhang, J., Nomiyama, T., Ogawa, O., Ogihara, T., Yamada, Y., Yagi, K. & Kawamori, R. (2001). Antiatherogenic mitochondrial genotype in patients with type 2 diabetes. *Diabetes Care 24*: 500-503.

[15] Kato, T., Kunugi, H., Nanko, S. & Kato, N. (2000). Association of bipolar disorder with the 5178 polymorphism in mitochondrial DNA. *Am. J. Med. Genet. 96*: 182-186.

[16] Iwao, N., Iwao, S., Kobayashi, F., Tajima, K., Tanaka, M., Atsuta, Y., Tamakoshi, A. & Hamajima, N. (2003). No association of the mitochondrial genotype (Mt5178A/C) with six cancers in a Japanese population. *Asian Pacific J. Cancer Prev. 4*: 331-336.

[17] Yamaguchi, J., Hasegawa, Y., Kawasaki, T. Masui, T, Kanoh, T., Ishiguro, N. & Hamajima, N. (2006). ALDH2 polymorphisms and bone mineral density in an elderly Japanese population. *Osteoporos. Int. 17*: 908-913.

[18] Kokaze, A., Ishikawa, M., Matsunaga, N., Yoshida, M., Sekine, Y., Sekiguchi, K., Harada, M., Satoh, M., Teruya, K., Takeda, N., Fukazawa, S., Uchida, Y. & Takashima, Y. (2004). Longevity-associated mitochondrial DNA 5178 A/C polymorphism and blood pressure in the Japanese population. *J. Hum. Hypertens. 18*: 41-45.

[19] Kokaze, A., Ishikawa, M., Matsunaga, N., Yoshida, M., Satoh, M., Teruya, K., Honmyo, R., Masuda, Y., Uchida, Y. & Takashima, Y. (2007). NADH dehydrogenase subunit-2 237 Leu/Met polymorphism modifies the effects of alcohol consumption on risk for hypertension in middle-aged Japanese men. *Hypertens. Res. 30*: 213-218.

[20] Kokaze, A., Ishikawa, M., Matsunaga, N., Yoshida, M., Sekine, Y., Teruya, K., Takeda, N., Sumiya, Y., Uchida, Y. & Takashima, Y. (2001). Association of the mitochondrial DNA 5178 A/C polymorphism with serum lipid levels in the Japanese population. *Hum. Genet. 109*: 521-525.

[21] Kokaze, A., Ishikawa, M., Matsunaga, N., Yoshida, M., Sekine, Y., Sekiguchi, K., Satoh, M., Harada, M., Teruya, K., Takeda, N., Uchida, Y., Tsunoda, T. & Takashima, Y. (2003). Longevity-associated mitochondrial DNA 5178 A/C polymorphism modulates effects of daily drinking and cigarette consumption on serum triglyceride levels in middle-aged Japanese men. *Exp. Gerontol. 38*: 1071-1076.

[22] Freeman, D. J., Griffin, B. A., Murray, E., Lindsay, G. M., Gaffney, D., Packard, C. J. & Shepherd, J. (1993). Smoking and plasma lipoproteins in man: effects on low density lipoprotein cholesterol levels and high density lipoprotein subfraction distribution. *Eur. J. Clin. Invest. 23*: 630-640.

[23] Freeman, D. J., Caslake, M. J., Griffin, B. A., Hinnie, J., Tan, C. E., Watson, T. D. G., Packard, C. J. & Shepherd, J. (1998). The effect of smoking on post-heparin lipoprotein and hepatic lipase, cholesteryl ester transfer protein and lecithin: cholesterol acyl transferase activities in human plasma. *Eur. J. Clin. Invest. 28*: 584-591.

[24] Kokaze, A., Ishikawa, M., Matsunaga, N., Yoshida, M., Makita, R., Satoh, M., Teruya, K., Sekiguchi, K., Masuda, Y., Harada, M., Uchida, Y. & Takashima, Y. (2006). Overview of longevity-associated mitochondrial DNA 5178 C/A polymorphism and a discussion of its modulation of the effects of habitual smoking on serum total and LDL

cholesterol levels in middle-aged Japanese men. In C. R. Woods (Eds.) *Trends in DNA research* (pp. 33-51). New York, U. S. A.: Nova Science Publishers.

[25] Lal, S., Madhavan, M. & Heng, K. (2005). The association of mitochondrial DNA 5178 C > A polymorphism with plasma lipid levels among three ethnic groups. *Ann. Hum. Genet. 69*: 639-644.

[26] Johnson, R. J., Kang, D. H., Feig, D., Kivilighn, S., Kanellis, J., Watanabe, S., Tuttle, K. R., Rodrigues-Itube, B., Herrera-Acosta, J. & Mazzali, M. (2003). Is there a pathogenetic role for uric acid in hypertension and cardiovascular and renal disease? *Hypertension 41*: 1183-1190.

[27] Tomita, M., Mizuno, S., Yamanaka, H., Hosoda, Y., Kakuma, K., Matsuoka, Y., Okada, M., Yakaguchi, M., Yoshida, H., Morisawa, H. & Murayama, T. (2000). Does hyperuricemia affect mortality? A prospective cohort study of Japanese male workers. *J. Epidemiol. 10*: 403-409.

[28] Kokaze, A., Ishikawa, M., Matsunaga, N., Yoshida, M., Satoh, M., Teruya, K., Honmyo, R., Yorimitsu, M., Masuda, Y., Uchida, Y. & Takashima, Y. (2006). Longevity-associated NADH dehydrogenase subunit-2 237 Leu/Met polymorphism influences the effects of alcohol consumption on serum uric acid levels in nonobese Japanese men. *J. Hum. Genet. 51*: 765-771.

[29] Jedrychowski, W. (1990). Effects of smoking and longevity of parents on lung function in apparently healthy elderly. *Arch. Gerontol. Geriatr. 10*: 19-26.

[30] Goldberg, R. J., Larson, M. & Levy, D. (1996). Factors associated with survival to 75 years of age in middle-aged men and women. The Framingham Study. *Arch. Intern. Med. 156*: 505-509.

[31] Kokaze, A., Ishikawa, M., Matsunaga, N., Yoshida, M., Satoh, M., Teruya, K., Honmyo, R., Shirasawa, T., Hoshino, H. & Takashima, Y. (2007). Longevity-associated mitochondrial DNA 5178 C/A polymorphism and its interaction with cigarette consumption are associated with pulmonary function in middele-aged Japanese men. *J. Hum. Genet. 52*: 680-685.

[32] Puddu, P. E., Lanti, M., Menotti, A., Mancini, M., Zanchetti, A., Cirillo, M., Angeletti, M. & Gubbio Study Research Group. (2002). Red blood cell count in short-term prediction of cardiovascular disease incidence in Gubbio population study. *Acta Cardiol. 57*: 177-185.

[33] Tegos, T. J., Kalodiki, E., Daskalopoulou, S. S. & Nicolaides, A. N. (2000). Stroke: epidemiological, clinical picture, and risk factors Part I of III. *Angiology 51*: 793-808.

[34] Kokaze, A., Ishikawa, M., Matsunaga, N., Yoshida, M., Makita, R., Satoh, M., Teruya, K., Sekiguchi, K., Masuda, Y., Harada, M., Uchida, Y. & Takashima, Y. (2005). Interaction between longevity-associated mitochondrial DNA 5178 C/A polymorphism and cigarette smoking on hematological parameters in Japanese men. *Arch. Gerontol. Geriatr. 40*: 113-122.

[35] Shiose, Y. & Kawase, Y. (1986). A new approach to stratified normal intraocular pressure in a general population. *Am. J. Ophthalmol. 101*: 714-721.

[36] David, R., Zangwill, L., Stone, D. & Yassur, Y. (1987). Epidemiology of intraocular pressure in population screened for glaucoma. *Br. J. Ophthalmol. 71*: 766-771.

[37] Klein, B. E. K., Klein, R. & Linton, K. L. P. (1992). Intraocular pressure in an American community. The Beaver Dam Eye Study. *Invest. Ophthalmol. Vis. Sci. 33*: 2224-2228.

[38] Lesk, M. C., Connell, A. M. S., Wu, S. Y., Hyman, L. & Schachat, A. P. (1997). Distribution of intraocular pressure. The Barbados Eye Study. *Arch. Ophthalmol. 115*: 1051-1057.

[39] Bonomi, L., Marchini, G., Marraffa, M., Bernardi, P., De Franco, I., Perfetti, S., Varotto, A. & Tenna, V. (1998). Prevalence of glaucoma and intraocular pressur distribution in a defined population. The Egna-Neumarkt Study. *Ophthalmology 105*: 209-215.

[40] Nomura, H., Shimokata, H., Ando, F., Miyake, Y. & Kuzuya, F. (1999). Age-related changes in intraocular pressure in a large Japanese population. *Ophthalmology 106*: 2016-2022.

[41] Lee, J. S., Lee, S. H., Oum, B. S., Chung, J. S., Cho, B. M. & Hong, J. W. (2002). Relationship between intraocular pressure and systemic health parameters in a Korean population. *Clin. Experiment. Ophthalmol. 30*: 237-241.

[42] Kokaze, A., Yoshida, M., Ishikawa, M., Matsunaga, N., Makita, R., Satoh, M., Sekiguchi, K., Masuda, Y., Uchida, Y. & Takashima, Y. (2004). Longevity-associated mitochondrial DNA 5178 A/C polymorphism is associated with intraocular pressure in Japanese men. *Clin. Experiment. Ophthalmol. 32*: 131-136.

[43] Miller, M. (2003). Disorders of fluid balance. In W. R. Hazzard, J. P. Blass, J. B. Halter, J. G. Ouslander, & M. E. Tinetti (Eds.) *Principles of geriatric medicine and gerontology* (pp. 581-592). New York, U. S. A.: McGraw-Hill.

[44] Kokaze, A., Ishikawa, M., Matsunaga, N., Yoshida, M., Makita, R., Satoh, M., Teruya, K., Sekiguchi, K., Masuda, Y., Harada, M., Uchida, Y. & Takashima, Y. (2005). Longevity-associated NADH dehydrogenase subunit-2 polymorphism and serum electrolyte levels in middle-aged obese Japanese men. *Mech. Ageing Dev. 126*: 705-709.

[45] Herrmann, F. R., Safran, C., Levkoff, S. E. & Minaker, K. L. (1992). Serum albumin level on admission as a predictor of death, length of stay, and readmission. *Arch. Int. Med. 152*: 125-130.

[46] Sahyoun, N. R., Jacques, P. F., Dallal, G. & Russell, R. M. (1996). Use of albumin as a predictor of mortality in community-dwelling and institutionalized elderly populations. *J. Clin. Epidemiol. 49*: 981-988.

[47] Nozaki, H., Nohara, Y., Ashitomi, I., Zukeran, R., Inafuku, T., Akisaka, M. & Suzuki, M. (1998). Serum globulin levels and activities of daily living in centenarians. *Jpn. J. Geriatr. 35*: 680-685.

[48] Sullivan, D. H. (2001). What do the serum proteins tell us about our elderly patients? *J. Gerontol. A Biol. Sci. Med. Sci. 56*: M71-M74.

[49] Kokaze, A., Ishikawa, M., Matsunaga, N., Yoshida, M., Sekine, Y., Teruya, K., Takeda, N., Satoh, M., Sumiya, Y., Uchida, Y. & Takashima, Y. (2002). Association of the longevity-associated mitochondrial DNA 5178 A/C polymorphism with serum protein fraction levels in healthy Japanese women. *Exp. Gerontol. 37*: 931-936.

[50] Wolf, G. T., Chretien, P. B., Weiss, J. F., Edwards, B. K. & Spiegel, H. E. (1982). Effects of smoking and age on serum levels of immune reactive proteins. *Otolaryngol. Head Neck Surg. 90*: 319-326.

[51] Banedek, I. H., Blouin, R. A. & McNamara, P. J. (1984). Influence of smoking on serum protein composition and the protein binding of drugs. *J. Pharm. Pharmacol. 36*: 214-216.

[52] Lindberg, G., Råstam, L., Gullberg, B., Lundbald, A., Nilsson-Ehle, P. & Hanson, B. S. (1993). Serum concentrations of total sialic acid and sialoglycoproteins in relation to coronary heart disease risk markers. *Atherosclerosis 103*: 123-129.

[53] Shima, M. & Adachi, M. (1996). Effects of environmental tobacco smoke on serum levels of acute phase proteins in schoolchildren. *Prev. Med. 25*: 617-624.

[54] Kokaze, A., Ishikawa, M., Matsunaga, N., Yoshida, M., Sekine, Y., Sekiguchi, K., Satoh, M., Harada, M., Teruya, K., Takeda, N., Uchida, Y. & Takashima, Y. (2003). Longevity-associated mitochondrial DNA 5178 A/C polymorphism influences effects of cigarette smoking on serum protein fraction levels in Japanese men. *Mech. Ageing Dev. 124*: 765-770.

[55] Nakagawa, Y., Ikegami, H., Yamato, E., Takekawa, K., Fujisawa, T., Hamada, Y., Ueda, H., Uchigata, Y., Miki, T., Kumahara, Y. & Ogihara, T. (1995). A new mitochondrial DNA mutation associated with non-insulin-dependent diabetes mellitus. *Biochem. Biophys. Res. Commun. 212*: 664-668.

[56] Hirai, M., Suzuki, S., Onoda, M., Hinokio, Y., Ai, L., Hirai, A., Ohtomo, M., Komatsu, K., Kasuga, S., Satoh, Y., Akai, H. & Toyota, T. (1996). Mitochondrial DNA 3394 mutation in the NADH dehydrogenase subunit 1 associated with non-insulin-dependent diabetes mellitus. *Biochem. Biophys. Res. Commun. 219*: 951-955.

[57] Hattori, Y., Nakajima, K., Eizawa, T., Ehara, T., Koyama, M., Hirai, T., Fukuda, Y. & Kinoshita, M. (2003). Heteroplasmic mitochondrial DNA 3310 mutation in NADH dehydrogenase subunit 1 associated with type 2 diabetes, hypertrophic cardiomyopathy, and mental retardation in single patient. *Diabetes Care 26*: 952-953.

[58] Kahn, S. E. & Porte Jr., D. (2003). The pathophysiology and genetics of type 2 diabetes mellitus. In D. Porte Jr., R. S. Sherwin, & A. B. Baron (Eds.) *Diabetes Mellitus* (6th ed. pp. 331-365). New York, U. S. A.: McGraw-Hill.

[59] Guo, L. J., Oshida, Y., Fuku, N., Takeyasu, T., Fujita, Y., Kurata, M., Ito, M & Tanaka, M. (2005). Mitochondrial genome polymorphisms associated with type-2 diabetes or obesity. *Mitochondrion 5*: 15-33.

[60] Janka, H. U. (1996). Increased cardiovascular morbidity and mortality in diabetes mellitus: identification of high risk patients. *Daibetes Res. Clin. Pract. 30 Suppl.*: 85-88.

[61] Kokaze, A., Ishikawa, M., Matsunaga, N., Yoshida, M., Makita, R., Satoh, M., Teruya, K., Sekiguchi, K., Masuda, Y., Harada, M., Uchida, Y. & Takashima, Y. (2005). Longevity-associated mitochondrial DNA 5178 C/A polymorphism is associated with fasting plasma glucose levels and glucose tolerance in Japanese men. *Mitochondrion 5*: 418-425.

[62] van Dam, R. M. & Feskens, E. J. (2002). Coffee consumption and risk of type 2 diabetes mellitus. *Lancet 360*: 1477-1478.

[63] Agardh, E. E., Carlsson, S., Ahlbom, A., Efendic, S., Grill, V., Hammar, N, Hilding, A. & Östenson, C. -G. (2004). Coffee consumption, type 2 diabetes and impaired glucose tolerance in Swedish men and women. *J. Intern. Med. 255*: 645-652.

[64] Salazar-Martinez, E., Willett, W. C., Ascherio, A., Manson, J. E., Leitzmann, M. F., Stampfer, M. J. & Hu, F. B. (2004). Coffee consumption and risk for type 2 diabetes mellitus. *Ann. Intern. Med. 140*: 1-8.

[65] Tuomilehto, J., Hu, G., Bidel, S., Lindstrom, J. & Jousilahti, P. (2004). Coffee consumption and risk of type 2 diabetes mellitus among middle-aged Finnish men and women. *JAMA 291*: 1213-1219.

[66] Yamaji, T., Mizoue, T., Tabara, S., Ogawa, S., Yamaguchi, K., Shimizu, E., Mineshita, M. & Kono, S. (2004). Coffee consumption and glucose tolerance status in middle-aged Japanese men. *Daibetologia 47*: 2145-2151.

[67] Iso, H., Date, C., Wakai, K., Fukui, M., Tamakoshi, A. & JACC Study Group. (2006). The relationship between green tea and total caffeine intake and risk for self-reported type 2 diabetes among Japanese adults. *Ann. Intern. Med. 144*: 554-562.

[68] van Dam, R. M., Willett, W. C., Manson, J. E. & Hu, F. B. (2006). Coffee, caffeine, and risk of type 2 diabets: a prospective cohort study in younger and middle-aged U. S. women. *Diabetes Care 29*: 398-403.

[69] Pereira, M. A., Parker, E. D. & Folsom, A. R. (2006). Coffee consumption and risk of type 2 diabetes mellitus: an 11-year prospective study of 28,812 postmenopausal women. *Arch. Intern. Med. 166*: 1311-1316.

[70] Fuku, N., Park, K. S., Yamada, Y., Nishigaki, Y., Cho, Y. M., Matsuo, H., Segawa, T., Watanabe, S., Kato, K., Yokoi, K., Nozawa, Y., Lee, H. K. & Tanaka, M. (2007). Mitochondrial haplogroup N9a confers resistance against type 2 diabetes in Asians. *Am. J. Hum. Genet. 80*: 407-415.

[71] Nishigaki, Y., Yamada, Y., Fuku, N., Matsuo, H., Segawa, T., Watanabe, S., Kato, K., Yokoi, K., Yamaguchi, S., Nozawa, Y. & Tanaka, M. (2007). Mitochondrial haplogroup N9b is protective against myocardial infarction in Japanese males. *Hum. Genet. 120*: 827-836.

[72] Nishigaki, Y., Yamada, Y., Fuku, N., Matsuo, H., Segawa, T., Watanabe, S., Kato, K., Yokoi, K., Yamaguchi, S., Nozawa, Y. & Tanaka, M. (2007). Mitochondrial haplogroup A is a genetic risk factor for atherothrombotic cerebral infarction in Japanese females. *Mitochondrion 7*: 72-79.

[73] Cann, R. L., Stoneking, M. & Wilson, A. C. (1987). Mitochondrial DNA and human evolution. *Nature 325*: 31-36.

[74] Yao, Y. G., Kong, Q. G. & Zhang, Y., P. (2002). Mitochondrial DNA 5178A polymorphism and longevity. *Hum. Genet. 111*: 462-463.

[75] Shimokata, H., Yamada, Y., Nakagawa, M., Okubo, R., Saido, T., Funakoshi, A., Miyasaka, K., Ohta, S., Tsujimoto, G., Tanaka, M., Ando, F. & Niino, N. (2000). Distribution of geriatric disease-related genotypes in the National Institute for Longevity Science, Longevity Study of Aging (NILS-LSA). *J. Epidemiol. 10*: S46-S55.

[76] Stadtman, E. R., Moskovitz, J. & Levine, R. L. (2003). Oxidation of methionine residues of proteins: biological consequences. *Antioxid. Redox Signal. 5*: 577-582.

[77] Lenaz, G., Bovina, C., D'Aurelio, M., Fato, R., Formiggini, G., Genova, M. L., Giuliano, G., Merlo Pich, M., Paolucci, U., Parenti Castelli, G. & Ventura, B. (2002). Role of Mitochondria in oxidative stress and aging. *Ann. N. Y. Acad. Sci. 959*: 199-213.

[78] Bailey, S. M. & Cunningham, C. C. (2002). Contribution of mitochondria to oxidative stress associated with alcoholic liver disease. *Free Radic. Biol. Med. 32*: 11-16.

[79] Bailey, S. M., Pietsch, E. C & Cunningham, C. C. (1999). Ethanol stimulates the production of reactive oxygen species at mitochondrial complex I and III. *Free Radic. Biol. Med. 27*: 891-900.

[80] Smith, P. R., Cooper, J. M., Govan, G. G., Harding, A. E. & Scapira, A. H. (1993). Smoking and mitochondrial function: a model for environmental toxins. *Q. J. Med. 86*: 657-660.

[81] Barja, G. (2004). Free radicals and aging. *Trends Neurosci. 27*: 595-600.

[82] Lambert, A. J., Boysen, H. M., Buckingham, J. A., Yang, T., Podlutsky, A., Austad, S. N., Kurz, T. H., Buffenstein, R. & Brand, M. D. (2007). Low rates of hydrogen peroxide production by isolated heart mitochondria associate with long maximum lifespan in vertebrate homeotherms. *Aging Cell 6*: 607-618.

[83] Robert, K. A., Brunet-Rossinni, A. & Bronikowski, A. M. (2007). Testing the "free radical theory of aging" hypothesis: physiological differences in long-lived and short-lived colubrid snakes. *Aging cell 6*: 395-404.

[84] Van Houten, B., Woshner, V. & Santos, J. H. (2006). Role of mitochondrial DNA in toxic responses to oxidative stress. *DNA Repair (Amst) 5*: 145-152.

[85] Valko, M., Leibfritz, D., Moncol, J., Cronin, M. T. D., Mazur, M. & Telser, J. (2007). Free radicals and antioxidants in normal physiological functions and human disease. *Int. J. Biochem. Cell Biol. 39*: 44-84

[86] Andrade-Cetto, A. & Wiedenfeld, H. (2001). Hypoglycemic effect of Cecrooia obtusifolia on streptozotocin diabetic rats. *J. Ethnopharmacol. 78*: 145-149.

[87] Rodriguez de Sotillo, D. V. & Hadley, M. (2002). Chlorogenic acid modifies plasma and liver concentrations of: cholesterol, triacylglycerol, and minerals in (fa/fa) Zucker rats. *J. Nutr. Biochem. 13*: 717-726.

[88] Shearer, J., Farah, A., de Paulis, T., Bracy, D. P., Pencek, R. R., Graham, T. E. & Wasserman, D. H. (2003). Quinides of roasted coffee enhance insulin action in conscious rats. *J. Nutr. 133*: 3529-3532.

[89] Herrera-Arellano, A., Aguilar-Santamaria, L., Garcia-Hernandez, B., Nicasio-Torres, P. & Tortoriello, J. (2004). Clinical trial of *Cecropia obtusifolia* and *Marrubium vulgare* leaf extracts on blood glucose and serum lipids in type 2 diabetics. *Phytomedicine 11*: 561-566.

[90] Bassoli, B. K., Cassolla, P., Borba-Murad, G. R., Constantin, J., Salgueiro-Pagadigorria, C. L., Bazotte, R. B., da Silva, R., S. & de Souza, H. M. (2008). Chlorogenic acid reduces the plasma glucose peak in the oral glucose tolerance test: effects on hepatic glucose release and glycaemia. *Cell Biochem. Funct. 26*: 320-328.

[91] van Dam, R. M. (2006). Coffee and type 2 diabetes: from beans to beta-cells. *Nutr. Metab. Cardiovasc. Dis. 16*: 69-77.

[92] Pavlica, S. & Gebhardt, R. (2005). Protective effects of ellagic and chlorogenic acids against oxidative stress in PC12 cells. *Free Radic. Res. 39*: 1377-1390.

[93] Suzuki, A., Yamamoto, N., Jokura, H., Yamamoto, M., Fujii, A., Tokumitsu, I. & Saito, I. (2006). Chlorogenic acid attenuates hypertension and improves endothelial function in spontaneously hypertensive rats. *J. Hypertens. 24*: 1065-1073.

[94] Nakanishi, S., Yamane, K., Ohishi, W., Nakashima, R., Yoneda, M., Nojima, H., Watanabe, H. & Kohno, N. (2008) Manganese superoxide dismutase Ala16Val polymorphism is associated with the development of type 2 diabetes in Japanese-Americans. *Diabetes Res. Clin. Pract.81*: 381-385.

[95] Hino, A., Adachi, H., Enomoto, M., Furuki, K., Shigetoh, Y., Otsuka, M., Kumagae, S., Hirai, Y., Jalaldin, A., Satoh, A. & Imaizumi, T. (2007). Habitual coffee but not green tea consumption in inversely associated with metabolic syndrome. An epidemiology study in a general Japanese population. *Diabetes Res. Clin. Pract. 76*: 383-389.

[96] Kiyohara, C., Kono, S., Honjo, T., Todoroki, I., Sakurai, Y., Nishiwaki, M., Hamada, H., Nishikawa, H., Koga, H., Ogawa, S. & Nakagawa, K. (1999). Inverse association between coffee drinking and serum uric acid concentrations in middle-aged Japanese males. *Br. J. Nutr. 82*: 125-130.

[97] Inoue, M., Yoshimi, I., Sobue, T., Tugane, S. & JPHC Study Group. (2005). Influence of coffee drinking on subsequent risk of hepatocellular carcinoma: a prospective study in Japan. *J. Natl. Cancer Inst. 97*: 293-300.

[98] Kurozawa, Y., Ogimoto, I., Shibata, A., Nose, T., Yoshimura, T., Suzuki, H., Sakata, R., Fujita, Y., Ichikawa, S., Iwai, N., Tamakoshi, A. & JACC Study Group (2005). Coffee and risk of death from hepatocellular carcinoma in a large cohort study in Japan. *Br. J. Cancer 93*: 607-610.

[99] Ohishi, W., Fujiwara, S., Cologne, J. B., Suzuki, G., Akahoshi, M., Nishi, N., Takahashi, I. & Chayama, K. (2008). Risk factors for hepatocellular carcinoma in a Japanese population: a nested case-control study. *Cancer Epidemiol. Biomarkers Prev. 17*: 846-854.

[100] Oba, S., Shimizu, N., Nagata, C., Shimizu, H., Kametani, M., Takeyama, N., Ohnuma, T. & Matsushita, S. (2006) The relationship between the consumption of meat, fat, and coffee and the risk of colon cancer: a prospective study in Japan. *Cancer Lett. 244*: 260-267.

[101] Lee, K. J., Inoue, M., Otani, T., Iwasaki, M., Sasazuki, S., Tsugane, S. & JPHC Study Group. (2007). Coffee consumption and risk of colorectal cancer in a population-based prospective cohort of Japanese men and women. *Int. J. Cancer 121*: 1312-1318.

[102] Hirose, K., Niwa, Y., Wakai, K., Matsuo, K., Nakanishi, T. & Tajima, K. (2007). Coffee consumption and the risk of endometrial cancer: evidence from a case-control study of female hormone-related cancers in Japan. *Cancer Sci. 98*: 411-415.

[103] Koizumi, T., Nakaya, N., Okamura, C., Sato, Y., Shimazu, T., Nagase, S., Niikura, H., Kuriyama, S., Tase, T., Ito, K., Tsubono, Y., Okamura, K., Yaegashi, N. & Tsuji, I. (2008). Case-control study of coffee consumption and risk of endometrial endometrioid adenocarcinoma. *Eur. J. Cancer Prev. 17*: 358-363.

[104] Lin, Y., Tamakoshi, A., Kawamura, T., Inaba, Y., Kikuchi, S., Motohashi, Y., Kurosawa, M., Ohno, Y. & JACC Study Group. (2002). Risk of pancreatic cancer in relation to alcohol drinking, coffee consumption and medical history: findings from the

Japan collaborative cohort study for evaluation of cancer risk. *Int. J. Cancer 99*: 742-746.

[105] Yoshimura, N., Suzuki, T., Hosoi, T. & Orimo, H. (2005). Epidemiology of hip fracture in Japan: incidence and risk factors. *J. Bone Miner. Metab. 23 Suppl*: 78-80.

[106] Aoyama, M., Shidoji, Y., Saimei, M., Tsunawake, N. & Ichinose, M. (2003). Phenotypic linkage between single-nucleotide polymorphisms of β_3-adrenergic receptor gene and NADH dehydrogenase subunit-2 gene, with special reference to eating behavior. *Biochem. Biophys. Res. Commun. 309*: 261-265.

[107] Corella, D., Qi, L., Tai, E. S., Deurenberg-Yap, M., Tan, C. E., Chew, S. K. & Ordovas, J. M. (2006). Perilipin gene variation determines higher susceptibility to insulin resistance in Asian women when consuming a high-saturated fat, low-carbohydrate diet. *Diabetes Care 29*: 1313-1319.

[108] Ito, H., Matsuo, K., Wakai, K., Saito, T., Kumimoto, H., Okuma, K., Tajima, K. & Hamajima, N. (2006). An intervention study of smoking cessation with feedback on genetic cancer susceptibility in Japan. *Prev. Med. 42*: 102-108.

In: Handbook on Longevity: Genetics, Diet and Disease   ISBN 978-1-60741-075-1
Editors: Jennifer V. Bentely and Mary Ann Keller   © 2009 Nova Science Publishers, Inc.

Chapter VII

Pesticides and Longevity

Sáenz de Cabezón Irigaray, Francisco Javier; Carvajal Montoya,
Luz Dary and Moreno Grijalba, Fernando

Unidad de Protección de Cultivos. Departamento de Agricultura y Alimentación
Universidad de La Rioja. C/ Madre de Dios, 51. 26006-Logroño (La Rioja), Spain

Abstract

Most common and effective way of a pesticide to take effect is through direct ingestion via food, water or air. Once the active ingredient is inside the body of the target (pest) or non-target organism (humans, environment, wild and domesticated fauna), it can either affect vital processes killing the organism, or display single or multiple side effects that can have serious effects on other life processes affecting the longevity of the organism. After more than 7 decades depending on heavy use of chemical in agriculture, the rise of concern about how these active ingredients affect the physiology of different organisms, have developed ways to analyze and to describe the deleterious effects of pesticides on human and environmental health. In this chapter, we will discuss the interaction of pesticides, with target and non target physiological systems, giving emphasis on secondary effects (hormonal, developmental, genetic, general homeostatic changes) that can impair not only the life (longevity) of the affected organism but can have effects on successive generations. In this way, we will obtain an idea of how pesticide exposure can have various effects on human health, those effects can interact, synergize and lead to chronic damage at various physiological systems and organizational levels, as a result, if damages are important enough to impair or interfere with metabolic, homeostatic or/and functional responses, the target can view its lifespan, including reproductive outcomes, reduced.

1. Introduction

Aging is a consequence of accumulation of damage that affects one or several physiological functions endangering the survival of an organism (Murphy and Patridge, 2008). Therefore, agents that can cause aging-related damage would affect longevity by exerting function failures to the different physiological systems that sustain life (nervous system, respiratory system, circulatory system, immune system, etc.). Organisms are constantly exposed to threats that can cause a decline in their longevity; those can be generated by the environment or by metabolic pathways inherent to the individual. In addition, exposures to different man-made sources (i.e. environmental pollution, xenobiotics) pose a risk on human health and therefore to life. To cope with these molecules, organisms have different detoxifying mechanisms than pose a challenge in terms of energy and metabolic byproducts which can also result in a decline of the organism lifespan.

Synthetic pesticides were introduced in the 30ties to give solution to insect vector diseases and afterwards applied to agriculture as an easy and cheap way to ensure the farmer investment against noxious organisms and provide safe food production for the community. Thus, modern agriculture is based on the use of a great amount of chemicals that ensure growers with the net profit of the crop. The overall cost of these prophylactic measures is not well understood by conventional farmers and people in general (see Pimentel, 2005 for review). Those costs have an environmental, health or social nature that can have deleterious effects not only at food security or ecological level but also at economic level (soil, water quality, crop productivity, fauna, etc.). Once pesticides were introduced, their active ingredients became part of the different trophic webs reaching unwanted locations endangering not only human health but the environment. Fungicides, herbicides, insecticides, acaricides, rodenticides, nematicides (hence pesticides for simplicity), are the most commonly man-made xenobiotics used to ensure yields. Exposure to these chemicals can result in direct acute poisoning or long term/chronic effects that finally reduce the organisms probability of surviving as a consequence of physiological system failures. For example, pesticides that interfere with the immune system can expose the individual to a greater susceptibility in contracting a disease, allergy or even cause death by promoting carcinogenic cells.

In this chapter we will give a general overview on the effects and known interferences with the physiological systems of different families of pesticides used in agriculture, that results on deleterious effects not only to humans beings eventually driving to the death of the individual, but their progeny, endangering the continuity of an specific/local population. To fulfill this purpose we will separate the chapter into the different known effects on physiological systems that affect human health based on literature review. We do not intend to write an extensive review of all pesticide effects on human health literature, but give a broad view on how pesticides can generate a risk on human health. We will focus on chemicals used to combat arthropod pests, although references to other important pesticides, like fungicides, will be given.

2. Exposure to Pesticides

People throughout the world are exposed to pesticides from different sources; the final effects of such exposures are determined by how much contact they have within each pathway of exposure. Individual's lifestyle choices, like where they live or their daily diet, are determinant in the overall pesticide exposure profile. Sectors that routinely use pesticides like agriculture or pest control are more exposed to pesticides. Farmer families are then more exposed to pesticide contamination than people living in urban areas. An study in various German winegrowing communities, shown that people who live close to heavy pesticide users like winegrowers, had more risk to certain types of cancer than people who live further away, due to pesticide exposure related to lifestyle habits (see bellow, section 3.5.). Pesticide residues can be taken into homes on shoes, clothes or pets, being a major source of exposition within the home. Exposures via food and water are both chronic exposure routes affecting the entire population. Surface and ground water has detectable but low level residues of known endocrine disruptor pesticides with unknown chronic effects after long term exposure. Also rainfall can contain pesticide residues that can reach unwanted locations. Contamination by food is an obvious pathway, strongly influenced by lifestyle habits, moreover, food residues are currently thought to be the most important exposure pathway. The use of pesticides in the home, aircraft traveling, pet ownership, and gardening are not well known exposure routes that should claim our attention. Persistence of some pesticides like DDT and HCH, which have low water solubility, and high lipophilicity allow them to bioaccumulate in the fatty tissues of living organisms. Residues of these compounds and their metabolites resulted from detoxification processes or degradation, can be found in blood or breast milk, at low levels than in the past (Aballe et al. 2008).

Continuous or even short term exposure to low level chronic doses has been studied by different authors, concluding that pesticides can have deleterious effects depending on the kind of chemical exposed to, the degree of exposure and showing different effects on the target depending in this two factors. Of course other factors to have in account are the physiology and genetics of the individual affected, and protective measures of the applicator, manufacturer, harvester in other words the person exposed. As we will show, Pyrethroids and Pyrethrins; Carbamates and Organophosphates (OP) are acetylcholinesterase inhibitors, and both of them target the nervous system. Exposition to high doses of either chemical will result in death by overall nervous system failure due to interaction at the synaptic level, although other physiological systems would be affected as a result of interactions with the nervous system. At high doses we can not identify each cause of death, but chronic exposure to lower doses could lead to different and accumulative physiological system failures that can impair our live expectancy and thus have effects in our longevity. It is, therefore essential to find out the exact mechanisms of action and its meaning at different physiological systems and survey the effects at chronic exposure levels.

3. Effects of Pesticides on Longevity

As we stated above, a dramatic or chronic damage on an important physiological system will reduce the probability of surviving of a giving being. Thus, accumulated damage at molecular, gene, cell and therefore tissue level will lead to, for example, cell dysfunction and disorganization, fails on detoxifying systems, and eventually death by cancer or system malfunction (see Murphy and Patridge, 2008 for a comprehensive review). How a pesticide leads to death is hard to explain. For example, cytochrome P450 (CYP) enzymes involved in first step detoxification processes, metabolizing lipophilic exogenous substrates, can be induced by several pesticides, and thus may lead to the production of carcinogenic and mutagenic molecules; how this can be translated to a physiological level is not a simple task, because many biological processes are involved and have to be explored to reach a clear explanation of the cause of death.

Since the discovery of DDT and other synthetically generated chemicals before and after Second World War, chemical companies had put lot of efforts in the discovering, synthesis and marketing of new active molecules than can kill injurious organisms without harming or risking nontarget organisms. Several classes of pesticides with varied modes of action are now available in the market. For some of these pesticides if not for all of them, the exact mode of action is unknown. The problem of indexing the effects of pesticides on health and therefore on longevity as the probability of survival of an organism, is that in the majority of studies there is no evidence that a single pesticide cause certain effect. In some cases the pesticide is not identified while others a mixture of pesticides was used by the tested individual or individuals. In other cases lack of significative results can lead to conclude that the observed effect was provoked by the pesticide, individual health condition or medical history, or a combination of all. Here in we describe the studies reported in the literature that link exposure to pesticides (mainly by ingestion) with the risk of a deleterious outcome on important physiological systems. Other effects such as dermatitis or ocular toxicity are no reviewed here as we believe that those outcomes have much less deleterious effects than in other physiological systems studied.

3.1. Digestive System

The gastro intestinal tract digest and absorbs nutrients and water from drink and food, being highly exposed to exogenous substances and functioning as a detoxification barrier equipped with metabolic enzymes similar to those from liver. Few studies have attempted to understand the influence of intestinal metabolism on the bioavailability of food contaminants, giving more relevance to the hepatic metabolism, ignoring intestinal metabolism (Poet et al. 2003). Intestinal tract is exposed to higher levels of contaminants than other organs besides skin or respiratory system; also most of the cytochrome P450 (CYP) enzymes expressed in the liver (the main detoxifying organ) are present in the intestine, at different levels and may be with a different regulation.

Pesticides can be substrates of biotransformation and also influence enzymes involved in detoxifying processes inside the intestinal tract and the liver (See Sergent et al. 2008, for a review). A detoxification process consists in three steps that involve three main systems: at CYP level (phase I), phase II conjugation enzymes and phase III involving efflux pumps. Induction of CYP enzymes by pesticides is well documented in hepatic targets but information related to the interaction between pesticides and intestinal CYPs is scarce. CYP enzymes that mediate detoxification reactions can, under certain circumstances, process their substrates into carcinogenic or mutagenic products. Endosulfan, for example, increases the CYP3A7 and CYP3A1 transcript levels leading to high genotoxic metabolites. Treatment with OCs caused an increase of toxic Benzo[a]Pyrene CYP1A-dependent metabolites in rat and human hepatic cells (Haake et al. 1987). Exposure to captan in mouse induced CYP3A1/2 and CYP1A2, which could have adverse effects with typical substrates of CYP3A (aflatoxins, 1-nitrpyrene, PAHs) or CYP1A2 (aromatic amines, PCBs, dioxins and PAHs) (Paolini et al, 1999). Some OCs can activate the nuclear hormone receptor PXR, which leads to the activation of CYP3A4 gene transcription (Coumoul et al. 2002). Oxidation reactors resulting from metabolization of OPs can result in a desulfuration reaction generating the more neurotoxic oxon form or in a dearylation reaction, which degrades the parent toxic compound to a non-toxic compound (Chamber, 1992). It has been shown that parathion, chlorpyrifos and diazinon are bioactivated by CYPs involving desulfuration and dearylation reactions (Poet et al. 2003). Also, OCs are reported as potent inhibitors of CYP, influencing the metabolic reactions of the parent drug, giving rise to high plasma levels of the parent drug, rising the possibility of the on set of adverse drug reactions (Hodgson and Rose, 2006; Di Consigilio et al. (2005). Metabolization of fungicides like benzimidazole, lead to the formation of thiabendazole metabolites, able to covalently bind with hepatic cells in the human liver (Coulet et al. 2000). Thiabendazoles, can also induce CYPs activities as well as gluthatione-S-tranferase mRNA levels (Prize et al, 2004). Metabolism of Imidacloprid, has been shown to involve CYPs. Vinclozolin enhanced B[a]P-induced micronucleus formation by increasing CYP1A1 expression, suggesting that the fungicide could be a potential comutagenic compound in human beings (Wu et al. 2005). Therefore, all these interactions at CYP level can activate many carcinogen substances to highly reactive electrophiles, which then react with targets such as DNA.

Products from phase I detoxification system are conjugated by phase II enzymes , such as UDP-glucuronosyltransferases (UGTs) sulfotransferases or glutathione S-transferases (GSTs). Those enzymes produce more lipophilic substances that can be excreted into urine or faeces. UGTs are a major clase of phase II enzymes. Inhibition of UGTs has been reviewed by Grancharov et al (2001). Recent studies shown that inhibition of SULTs by different compounds can lead to a greater bioavailability and in turn to the toxic effects of these compounds. Endocrine disruptors can inhibit the inactivation of estrogens by sulfonation, causing a rise on the levels of the free active endogenous estrogens (Waring and Harris 2005). Interaction of toxic compounds and SULTs has been reviewed by Wang and James (2006). Pesticides are also substrates of GSTs; anticarcinogens such as β-carotene or coumarin, enhance the activity of GSTs, which could lead to an increase in enzyme activity and to a more efficient detoxification of carcinogens (Van Lieshout et al. 1998). Pesticides like Methoxychlor and DDT were reported to enhance hepatic GST and CYP content. Captan and captafol inhibit GSTP1-1 isoform by acting as oxidizing agents (Di Ilio et al. 1996).

Excretion and disposition of diverse substances, including pesticides, is carried out by efflux pumps. This process is carrier-mediated as well as energy, species, substrate and site dependent. Known transporters belong to ATP-binding cassette (ABC) transporter superfamily that includes the multidrug resistance protein-1 (MDR1), multidrug resistance-associated proteins (MRPs) and breast cancer resistance protein (BCRP) (reviewed by Takano et al. 2006). Those transporters can determine the bioavailability of different compounds (substrates from phase I and II). Interactions between the three levels can lead to dramatic drug interactions. MDR1 shows extremely broad substrate specificity, with a predisposition towards lipophilic and cationic compounds. Many pesticides including OCs and OPs can inhibit its function. Chlorpyrifos-oxon metabolite is known to inhibit MDR1 transport in rat stomach. Chlorpyrifos induced expression of MDR1 gene, increasing efflux function. Inhibition of transport can have important clinical consequences, as shown by Cavret et al (2005). There is no evidence that the other transporters are implicated in pesticide transport. However studies with methoxychlor, shown a two-fold faster efflux than non treated cells, suggesting a role of MRP1 in modulating toxicity of this pesticide (Tribulli et al 2003).

3.2. Immune System

Immune system defends the body against infectious/foreign agents. Immune reactions to foreign substances can result in allergic reactions that produce an array of pathologies. Immunotoxic substances can be of any nature, and there is evidence that some pesticides can cause immune suppression and/or exacerbate allergic disease (Selgrade, 2005). Gene activation, induction of enzymes, altered T-lymphocyte/B-lymphocyte macrophage cooperation through impaired lymphokine function, altered homeostasis, altered signaling mechanism, have been suggested for induction of immunosupresion by the pesticide chemicals (Banerjee, 1999). OP, for example, induced immunotoxicity may be direct via inhibition of serine hydrolases or esterases in components of the immune system, through oxidative damage to immune organs, or by modulation of signal transduction pathways controlling immune functions. Indirect effects include modulation by nervous system, or chronic effects of altered metabolism on immune organs. Also decreased host resistance, hypersensitivity, pathology of immune organs are effects related to immunotoxicity (Galloway & Handy, 2003).

Studies on OP shown that immune response was related to diet, suppression of immune response by metabolites and the oxidative stress that can potentiate pesticide immune toxicity (Banerjee, 1999). The studies that clearly evidence immunotoxicity are scarce, sometimes contradictory results can be obtained, and from many of them health effects are not noticeable. In the other hand, the immunosuppressive response to pentachlorophenol and the increased immune response after hexachlorobenzene exposure was clearly evidenced. Also, there is consistent concordance with mancozeb enhanced immune response in the field and the use of other carbamates as immunostimulants in clinical therapy (Colosio et al. 2005).

Some pesticides interfere with the balance of the endocrine system, causing adverse effects on organisms and its progeny. Pesticides belonging to the endocrine disrupters group (those that interfere with the endocrine system) may modulate cytokine synthesis. Others have been shown to affect immunoglobulin synthesis. They also may have impact on immune cells survival, and laboratory studies demonstrated that endocrine disrupters can modulate allergic reactions (Chalubinski and Kowalski, 2006). Although, is suggested that endocrine disruptors have been involved in human pathologies, there is no clear relationship between adverse general health effects and this class of compounds. Recent studies (Hurs & Waxman, 2005) have demonstrated that toxicity is mediated, in part, by members of the nuclear receptor superfamily and also serve as activators of pregnane X receptor.

Current studies have shown poor relationship between *in utero* exposure to pesticides and immunotoxicity related systems due to interferences on immune system development. Although data is scarce, fungicides were associated with allergies and hayfever. Studies on DDT and other organochlorines have shown association between these pesticides and middle ear infections in Inuit children parentally exposed. Other studies have shown increased prevalence on middle ear or pulmonary diseases when Taiwan women were exposed to other environmental contaminants. But the small sample size, children age at diagnosis, and other limitations, make these studies inconclusive (Weselak et al. 2007).

3.3. Nervous System

Neurotoxicity is the production of an adverse change in the structure or function of the central or peripheral nervous system due to exposure to a chemical. The nervous system differs from most other organ systems in its limited capacity for repair and regeneration, which reduces its potential for recovery when cell death or damage has occurred. As we mentioned before, several pesticides like OP, carbamates and Organochlorines (OC), directly target nervous system as their mechanisms of toxicity. Several modes of action has been discovered and hypothesized. Among them, pesticides can disrupt the intracellular signalling, necessary for activation or inhibition of specific enzymes and/or opening ion channels changing the intracellular homeostasis, like ligand-gated chloride channels (GABA). Intracellular signalling is also important for nevous system development (Girard and Kuo, 1990). Disruption of Ca^{2+} homeostasis may have effects in several signal transduction pathways (see Kodavanti, 2005, for a review). Changes in neurotransmitters like dopamine, has been observed in mices with elevated motor levels. Exposure to OPs and their effects is well documented in the literature (Kodavanti, 2005). OPs inhibits the enzyme acetylcholinesterase, inactivating the neurotransmitter acetylcholine and leading to symptoms related to the autonomic and the central nervous systems. OP poisonings have shown decreased performance on visual attention and mood-scale tests, intellectual functioning, academic skills, flexibility of thinking, abstraction, motor speed, and coordination. Also hormonal imbalance has been documented as other mode of action on the nervous system. Many environmental pesticides alter thyroid function, inhibiting the thyroidal system or mimicking it, resulting in changes of thyroid hormone homeostasis, thus resulting in disorganization of the brain (Nunez, 1984), and effects on the formation and development of neural processes (Kimura-Koroda et al. 2005). Developmental neurotoxicity involves alterations in behaviour, neurophysiology, neurochemistry, and dysmorphology of the nervous system, occurring in the offspring as a consequence of pesticide exposure.

Parkinson's disease (PD) is a common neurodegenerative disorder, characterized by relatively selective degeneration of dopaminergic neurons in the *substantia nigra*. After more than 50% of dopamine neuronal loss in the substantia nigra and 75% depletion in striatal dopamine content, patients start to exhibit the cardinal symptoms of PD, which include resting tremor, bradykinesia, rigidity, and postural instability (Steece-Collier et al. 2002). Epidemiological studies indicate that pesticides are the leading candidates of environmental toxins that may contribute to the pathogenesis of PD. Rotenone, a common pesticide and an inhibitor of mitochondrial complex I, has been used to develop a PD model, with pathological features of degeneration of dopaminergic neurons and formation of cytoplasmic inclusions (Betarbet et al. 2000). Other pesticides, such as paraquat, dieldrin, and maneb, have been reported to cause degeneration of dopaminergic neurons (Wang et al. 2006). The mechanisms, however, remain largely unknown. Oxidative stress, mitochondrial dysfunction, protein aggregation, and apoptosis are key mediators of nigral dopaminergic neuronal cell death in PD. Many forms of familiar PD cases have been found to be caused by mutations in components related to the ubiquitin–proteasome system (UPS), highlighting the potential importance of UPS in PD (Greenamyre and Hastings, 2004; McNaught and Olanow, 2003). Pesticide-induced proteasome inhibition may be a significant contributor to the pathogenesis of PD. Further studies are necessary to determine the actual risk to human health including in vivo animal experiments. Ocular toxicity from direct entry of chemicals into the eye, results in the absorption of the chemical through the eye tissue and then into the circulation. Ocular toxiciy derived from exposure to pesticides is reviewed by Jaga & Dharmani (2006).

3.4. Genotoxicity

Genotoxic potential is a primary risk factor for long-term effects such as carcinogenic and reproductive toxicology. Most pesticides are tested in different mutagenicity assays covering gene mutation, chromosomal alteration and DNA damage (Bolognesi, 2003). Although genotoxic potential for agrochemical compounds is generally low, exposure to pesticides mixtures enhances the risk potential of a single pesticide by acting at different levels. Biomonitoring studies on human populations have focused on cytogenetic end-points: chromosomal aberration (CA), micronuclei (MN) frequency and sister-chromatid exchanges (SCE). As most exposures are to pesticide mixtures evaluation of single compounds are scarce.

Although millions of cases of pesticide poisonings were documented every year around the world, only few data on cytogenetic analysis are available (see Bolognesi 2003; Sailaja et al. 2006 and Remor et al. 2008 for reviews). Acute intoxication by OP resulted in a temporary by significant increase in the frequency of chromatid breaks and CAs. Intoxication with malathion and trichlorfon showed chromosomal damage and aneuploidy, although limited number of cases did not allow a clear conclusion (Czeizel, 1994). Genotoxic effects can vary depending on exposure degree, time of exposure, protective measures used and as we stated before exposure to a single or pesticide mixtures. Pesticide manufacturers are exposed not only to the active ingredient contained in the formulation but to the inert ingredients added to the formulation that can be more toxic than the active ingredient *per se*. Some studies have shown relationship between plant workers and genotoxicity but the heterogeneity of exposure in pesticide production plants does not allow to ascertain the casual agents (Bolognesi, 2003).

A number of studies have reported a significant incidence of cytogenetic damage among agricultural and forestry workers, floriculturist, vineyard cultivators, cotton field workers and others. However the lack of homogeneity in the exposure description prevents the use of this data in the comparision of different studies. Pesticide sprayers represent the most exposed group of agricultural workers. 18 out of 27 studies showed positive findings, 3 out of 10 concerning exposure to single compounds and 15 out of 17 studies for exposure to pesticide mixture (Bolognesi 2003). A positive dose-effects relationship was observed for cytogenetic damage in pesticide-exposed populations. Studies on agricultural workers with different degrees of exposure, different protective measures, and intensity of pesticide use showed differences on chromosomal damage as CA or MN (Bolognesi 2003). Also time-dependence of cytogenic damage was shown in workers with a long period of exposure (mainly floriculturist).

3.5. Cancer

Many of the several hundreds of pesticides that have been marketed for agriculture or domestic use, and specially those belonging to the organochlorates, carbamates, and carbinols are rated as probable or possible carcinogens, according to the US EPA and the IARC classification (Irigaray et al. 2007). They may act as endocrine disruptors, promoters, mutagenics, and of course immunosupressors. Pesticides that act like persistent organic pollutants, can, by definition, persist over long periods in the environment and contaminate water and food; moreover, they can contaminate the body through inhalation and skin contact, accumulate in adipose tissue, fatty breast tissue, pass through the placenta and accumulate in the milk of nursing mothers. All this can lead to the conclusion that children are at risk during pregnancy, breast feeding and childhood by inhalation, skin contact or contaminated food. A rise on the concern of childhood exposure to pesticides and cancer has lead to numerous reviews and studies summarized by Zahm and Ward (1998) and updated by Infante-Rivard and Weichenthal (2007). Those reviews showed some association between pesticide exposure and childhood cancer, however a case by case relationship does not exist between any single type of pesticide and a specific cancer.

Paternal exposure to pesticides, during pregnancy or post-natally is associated with an increase relative risk of children cancer. An excessive risk of leukemia, central nervous system tumors, Wilm's tumors, has been associated with parent exposure. Moreover, testing exposure of children to pesticides, a positive correlation was found with an overall increase in the risk ok leukemia, NHL, brain tumors, Wilm's tumors, Ewing sarcoma and germ cell tumors. Reproductive disorders on males has been associated with PCBs and testicular tumors, mothers of young man with testicular cancer that have been exposed to pesticides during pregnancy had higher levels of PCB than mother of the controls.

OC can combine with organic matter in drinking water originating chlorination disinfection byproducts like trihalomethanes and halocetic acids which have been demonstrated to be mutagenic *in vitro* and *in vivo*. Arsenic mixtures or derivates can cause lung cancer by inhalation but if ingested can cause bladder, kidney, liver or lung cancer. Thus arsenic exposure can deviate into a large spectrum of common cancer types. Arsenic and other kind of metals (cadmium, nickel) can damage zinc finger DNA repair proteins being mutagenic. Carbamates are rated as probable or possible carcinogens by the US EPA and the IARC classification. Novel C17 steroidal carbamates have shown to have effects on androgen receptor binding and prostate cancer cell growth (Moreira et al. 2008).

Increases of risk in certain types of cancer among farmers versus urban citizens have been reviewed elsewhere (McCauley et al. 2006), their review emphasized on the need of more studies needed to link exposure to pesticides in certain work environments like farms. Seidler at al. (2008) compared cancer incidence among residents of winegrowing communities with small areas under wine cultivation, they shown a potentially elevated skin, bladder and endocrine related cancer risks of the population in communities with a large area devoted to wine cultivation, although due to the methodology results are not conclusive for a causal relationship.

3.6. Reproduction

Epidemiologic studies have linked pre and postnatal exposures to pesticides with childhood cancers, birth defects, fetal death, etc, effects that basically impairs our reproduction and in consequence pose a risk of our future progeny. Reproduction can be affected on several ways, including seminal alterations, intrauterine problems and offspring malformation at different tissue levels. Reproductive effects of pesticides have been studied extensively but still conclusive information is scarce.

Carbaryl, a widely used broad-spectrum insecticide, was the first carbamate to be registered for use in cotton. Few epidemiological studies had identified carbamates exposure with effects on human health. Farm workers have shown to have more probability to have a miscarriage if the father was exposed to carbaryl in 3 month prior to conception or first trimester pregnancy (Savitz et al. 1997). Other studies shown that women over 35 yr old exposed to in the preconception period to carbaryl had a fourfold increase in risk of spontaneous abortion (Arbuckle et al. 2001); also Heeren et al. (2003) found a a significant increase of birth defects on women that use a mixture of carbaryl, carbufuran and camphechlor. Birth defects were detected in a woman who sprayed a combination of different insecticides including methomyl (Romero et al, 1989). However other studies showed no correlation between congenital anomalies, birth defects or neural-tube defects.

Banerjee et al. (1991) demonstrated the ability of commercial OP to alter significantly acetylcholine activity. Experimental studies with chlorpyrifos suggested that it can extend its action across pre and postnatal periods (Qiao et al. 2002; Richardson & Chambers, 2003). Chlorpyrifos acts by impairing neural development and affecting glia cells that are critical for brain development (Garcia et al. 2002, 2003). There are several reports in which OP have shown to be harmful to the developing fetus, however these reports lack a comparision group, and other factors may be related to the exposure and the outcome. Other studies have show that parental exposure to trichlorofon, malathion or temephos prior to pregnancy derived in congenital anormalities (Czeizel et al. 1993; Salazar-Garcia et al. 2004). Studies on animals have shown that OP may affect neurodevelopment and growth in developing animals, to date only one study on humans showed a relationship between OP exposure and infant reflexes (Young et al. 2005).

A study by Salazar-Garcia et al. (2004) found increased odds of any birth defect with parental exposure to DDT and lindane. Rita et al. (1987), found that Indian workers exposed to OC in grape gardens, experienced a six-fold increase on the risk of spontaneous abortion. Similarly, studies on cotton field, vineyard and malaria control workers exposed to OC and other pesticides showed significant increases in risk. Other studies found that high levels on serum levels of DDT, DDE, lindane, aldrin and hexachlorobenzene were related to spontaneous abortion or fetal death. However other studies reported no increase in serum levels of this compounds and the risk of a spontaneous abortion.

Pyrethroids are derivated from naturally occurring pyrethrins, extracted from chrysanthemum flowers. Pyrethrins are sodium channel modulators paralyzing the nervous system. There are potent lipophilic esters and synthetic pyretroids have an increased stability in the environment. Spontaneous abortion has been correlated from studies where the father has been exposed to pyrethroids (Rupa et al. 1991). Bell et al. (2001) fund an increased risk of fetal death due to congenital anomalies when synthetic pyrethroids where used in the same township, range or section during week 3 to 8 of pregnancy. Another study found a significant reduction on birth weight when mothers where exposed to pyrethroids (Hanke et al. 2003).

4. Conclusion

In this chapter we tried to give a general but detailed overview about the deleterious effects that exposure to pesticides, mainly by ingestion, can have on human health, and possibly the risk of a shortened lifespan due to development of various types of cancer; the raising cause of death in this century, on economically developed countries since World War II. First we distinguished between acute and chronic exposures and the ways that a pesticide can go into our organisms altering processes described before. We also consider of great importance to establish differences to the general public that should see pesticides as harmful molecules depending on the dose ingested or the dose that the individual is exposed to. It seems that is not well understood what a pesticide is: a biocide, a molecule intended to kill a noxious organism. Just by the fact that in most economically developed and developing countries one can buy pesticides from the storehouse without the need of an obtained license, we can have an idea about the situation. Although law is changing, it should change in a way that to buy a pesticide, one should show her/his ability to use it in a rational and not risky way, for example, in India, the first cause of suicide is self poisoning by pesticide ingestion (Gunnell et al. 2007). Free acquisition of pesticides enhanced the *per se* risk of exposition and poisoning by a pesticide. Pesticide use of $10 billion saves $40 billion in United States crops, based on direct costs and benefits (Pimentel, 2005). Indirect cost of pesticide use to the environment and public health rises to $12 billion, however if the full environmental, public health and social costs could be measured, total cost could be nearly double. Moreover, if we measure the number of pesticide induced cancers a year and net benefit of pesticide use, each case of cancer is equivalent to a benefit of $3.2 million, adding moral and ethical issues to this "cost benefit/approach".

As we have seen, pesticide exposure can have various effects on human health. Those effects can interact, synergize and lead to chronic damage at various physiological systems and organizational levels, as a result, if damages are important enough to impair or interfere with metabolic, homeostatic or/and functional responses, the target can view its lifespan reduced. As concluded by Murphy and Patridge (2008) in their review: "The accumulation of damage resulting in death, occurs at multiple levels, from physiological systems, through organs, to cells, and individual biomolecules". Another candidate mechanism in the generation of age related damage is the free radical theory. As we have seen pesticides can metabolize into reactive oxygen species and producing oxidative damage. Oxidative damage is a universal accompaniment of aging (Pletcher et al. 2008). Detoxifying systems like CYP and glutathione transferases have been implicated as components of a fundamental longevity assurance strategy (Zimniak, 2008).

Exposure to pesticide can generate a multitude of interactions at different levels, depending on the exposure profile. Sometimes the interaction is so strong that can have a profound effects on our survival, while other times, chronic exposure can have sublethal, non evidenced effects, that not only can impair our life but future generations. Currently, efforts are being invested in discovering persistent contaminants, that pose a higher risk due that they can bioaccumulate inside organism's tissues, and therefore become part of the food chain, travel further away from the spraying area and reach higher doses that those sprayed inside higher trophic levels. A simple increase of pesticide knowledge and prevention by applicators, farmworkers and pesticide users, should help in lowering the risk of pesticide use. Agricultural practices that enhance ecosystem functions without the use or limiting the use of pesticides, integrating them into the system, like Integrated Pest Management or Biological Control have demonstrated that reducing the dependence and therefore the use of pesticides is possible. Entomologist around the world are placing efforts in giving alternatives to the use of pesticides, and indirectly, maybe unconsciously, fighting against cancer and other deleterious diseases.

References

Aballe, A; Ballard, TJ; Dellatte, E; di Domenico, A; Ferri, F; Fulgenzi, AR; Grisanti, G; Iacovella, N; Ingelido, AM; Malisch, R; Miniero, R; Porpora, MG; Risica, S; Ziemacki, G; and De Felip, E. Persistent environmental contaminants in human milk: concentrations and time trends in Italy. *Chemosphere*, 2008. Doi: 10.1016/j.chemosphere.2007.12.036.

Arbuckle, TE; Lin, Z; and Mery, LS. An exploratory análisis of the effect of pesticida exposure on the risk of spontaneous abortion in an Notario faro population. *Environmental Health Perspectives*, 2001 109, 851-857.

Banerjee, BD. The influence of various factors on immune toxicity assessment of pesticide chemicals. *Toxicology Letters*, 1999 107, 21-31.

Banerjee, J; Ghosh, P; Mitra, S; Ghosh, N; and Bhattacharya, S. Inhibition of human fetal brain acetylcholinesterase: marker effect of neurotoxicity. *Journal of Toxicology and Environmental Health*, 1991 33, 283-290.

Bell, EM; Hertz-Picciotto, I; and Beaumont, JJ. Case-cohort analysis of agricultural pesticide applications near maternal residence and selected causes of fetal death. *American Journal of Epidemiology*, 2001 154, 702-710.

Betarbet, R; Sherer, TB; MacKenzie, G; Garcia-Osuna, M; Panov, AV; and Greenamyre, JT. Chronic systemic pesticide exposure reproduces features of Parkinson's disease. *Nature Neuroscience*, 2000 3, 1301-1306.

Bolognesi, C. Genotoxicity of pesticides: a review of human biomonitoring studies. *Mutation Research*, 2003 543, 251-272.

Cavret, S; Videmann, B; Mazallon, M; and Lecoeur, S. Diazinon cytotoxicity and transfer in Caco-2 cells: effect of long term exposure to the pesticide. *Environmental Toxicology and Pharmacology*, 2005 20, 375-380.

Chalubinski, M; and Kowalski, ML. Endocrine disrupters – potential modulators of the immune system and allergic response. *Alergy*, 2006 61, 1326-1335.

Chambers, H. Organophosphorous compounds: an overview. In: Chambers J, Levi P editors. Organophosphates: Chemistry, Fate, and Effects. San Diego: Academic Press; 1992; pp. 3-17.

Colosio, C; Birindelli, S; Corsini, E; Galli, CL; and Maroni, M. Low level exposure to chemicals and immune system. *Toxicology and Applied Pharmacology*, 2005 207, S320-S328.

Coulet, M; Eeckhoutte, C; Larrieu, G; Sutra, JF; Alvinerie, M; Mace, K; Pfeifer, A; Zucco, F; Stammati, AL; De Angelis, I; Vignoli, AL; and Galtier, P. Evidence of cytochrome P4501A2-mediated protein covalent binding of thiabendazole and for its passive intestinal transport: use of human and rabbit derived cells. *Chemico-Biological Interactions*, 2000 127, 109-124.

Coumoul, X; Diry, M; and Barouki, R. PXR-dependent induction of human CYP3A4 gene expression by organochlorine pesticides. *BiochemicalPharmacology*, 2002 64, 1513-1519.

Czeizel, AE. Phenotypic and cytogenetic studies in self-poisoned patients. *Mutation Research*, 1994 313, 175-181.

Czeizel, AE; Elek, C; Gundy, S; Metneki, J; Nemes, E; Reis, A; Sperling, K; Timar, L; Tusnady, G; and Viragh, Z. Environmental trichlorfon and cluster of congenital abnormalities. *Lancet*, 1993 341, 539-542.

Di Consiglio, E; Meneguz, A; Testai, E. Organophosphorothionate pesticides inhibit the activation of impramine by human hepatic cytochrome P450s. *Toxicology and Applied Pharmacology*, 2005 205, 237-246.

Di Ilio, C; Sacchetta, P; Angelucci, S; Buciarelli, T; Pennelli, A; Mazzetti, AP; LoBello, M; and Aceto, A. Interaction of glutathione transferase. *Toxicology Letters*, 1996 52, 43-48.

Galloway, T; and Handy, R. Immunotoxicity of organophosphorous pesticides. *Ecotoxicology*, 2003 12, 345-363.

García, SJ; Seidler, FJ, Qiao, D; and Slotkin, TA. Chlorpyrifos targets developing glia: effects on glial fibrillary acidic protein. *Brain Res. Dev. Brain Res*, 2002 133, 151-161.

García, SJ; Seidler, FJ; and Slotkin, TA. Developmental neurotoxicity elicited by prenatal or postnatal chlorpyrifos exposure: effects on neurospecific proteins indicate changing vulnerabilities. *Environmental Health Perspectives*, 2003 111, 297-304.

Girard, PR; and Kuo, JF. Protein kinase C and its 80-kilodalton substrate protein in neuroblastosoma cell neurite outgrowth. *Journal of Neurochemistry*, 1990 54, 300-306.

Grancharov, K; Naydenova, Z; Lozeva, S; and Golovinsky, E. Natural and synthetic inhibitors of UDP glucuronosyltransferase. Pharmacol. Therapeut, 2001 89,171-186.

Greenamyre, JT; and Hastings, TG. Biomedicine. Parkinson's-Divergent causes, convergent mechanisms. *Science*, 2004 304, 1120-1122.

Gunnel, D; Eddleston, M; Phillips, MR; and Konradsen, F. The global distribution of fatal pesticide self-poisoning: systematic review. *BMC Public Heatlh*, 2007 7, 357-371.

Haake, J; Kelley, M; Keys, B; and Safe, S. The effects of organochlorine pesticides as inducers of testosterone and benzo[*a*]pyrene hydroxilases. *General Pharmacology*, 1987 18, 165-169.

Hanke, W; Romitti, P; Fuortes, L; Sobala, W; and Mikulski, M. The use of pesticides in a Polish rural population and its effect on birth weight. *International Archives on Occupational and Environmental Health*, 2003 76, 614-620.

Heeren, GA; Tyler, J; and Mandeya, A. Agricultural chemical exposures and birth defects in the Eastern Cape Province, South Africa: a case control study. *Environmental Health*, 2003 2, 11.

Hurs, CH; and Waxman, DJ. Interactions of endocrine-active environmental chemicals with the nuclear receptor PXR. *Toxicological and Environmental Chemistry*, 2005 87, 299-311.

Infante-Rivard, C; and Weichenthal, S. Pesticides and childhood cancer: an update of Zahm and Ward's 1998 review. *Journal of Toxicology and Environmental Health Part B*, 2007 10, 81-99.

Irigaray, P; Newby, JA; Clapp, R; Hardell, L; Howard, V; Montagnier, L; and Epstein, S; Belpomme. Lifestyle-related factors and environmental agents causing cancer: an overview. *Biomedicine and Pharmacotherapy*, 2007 61, 640-658.

Jaga, K; and Dharmani, C. Ocular toxicity from pesticide exposure: a recient review. *Environmental Health and Preventive Medicine*, 2006 11, 102-107.

Kimura-Koroda, J; Nagata, I; and Kuroda, Y. Hydroxilated metabolites of polychlorinated biphenyls inhibit tyroid-hormone-dependent extensión of cerebellar Purkinje cell dendrites. *Developmental Brain Research*, 2005 154, 259-263.

Kodavanti, PRS. Neurotoxicity of persistent organic pollutants: possible mode(s) of action and further considerations. *Dose-Response*, 2005 3, 273-305.

McCauley, LA; Anger, K; Keifer, M; Langley, R; Robson, MG; and Rohlman, D. Studying health outcomes in farmworker populations exposed to pesticides. *Environmental Health Perspectives*, 2006 114, 953-960.

McNaught, KS; and Olanow, CW. Proteolytic stress: a unifying concept for the etiopathogenesis of Parkinson's disease. *Annals of Neurology*, 2003 53, S73-S84.

Moreira, VMA; Vasaitis, TS; Guo, Z; Njar VCO; and Salvador JAR. Síntesis of novel C17 steroidal carbamates, studies on CYP17 action, androgen receptor binding and function, and prostate cancer cell growth. *Steroids*, 2008 73, 1217-1227.

Murphy, MP; and Partridge, L. Toward a control theory of aging. *Annual Review of Biochemistry*, 2008 77, 777-798.

Nunez, J. Effects of thyroid hormones during brain differenciation. *Molecular and Cellular Endocrinology*, 1984 37, 125-132.

Paolini, M; Barillari, J; Trespidi, S; Valgimigli, L; Pedulli, GF; and Cantelli-Forti, G. Captan impairs CYP-catalyzed drug metabolism in the mouse. *Chemico-Biological Interactions*, 1999 123, 149-170.

Pimentel, D. Environmental and economic cost of the application of pesticides primarily in the United States. *Environment, Development and* Sustainability, 2005 7, 229-252.

Pletcher, SD; Kabil, H; and Partridge, L. Chemical complexity and the genetic of aging. *Annual Review of Ecology, Evolution, and Systematics*, 2007 38, 299-326.

Poet, T; Wu, H; and Kousba, A; Timchalk, C. In vitro rat hepatic and intestinal metabolism of the organophosphate pesticides chlorpyrifos and diazenon. *Toxicological Sciences*, 2003 72, 193-200.

Price, RJ; Scott, MP; Walters, D; Stierum, R; Groten, J; Meredith, C; and Lake, B. Effects of thiabendazole on some rat hepatic xenobiotic metabolising enzymes. *Food and Chemical Toxicology*, 2004 42, 899-908.

Qiao, D; Seidler, FJ; Padilla, S; and Slotkin, TA. Developmental neurotoxicity of chlorpyriphos: What is the vulnerable period?. *Environmental Health Perspectives*, 2002 110, 1097-1103.

Remor, AP; Totti, CC; Moreira, DA; Dutra, GP; Heuser, VD; and Boeira, JM. Occupational exposure of farm workers to pesticides: biochemical parameters and evaluation of genotoxicity. *Environmen Internatonal*, 2008 (in press). Doi:10.1016/j.envint.2008.06.011

Richardson, J; and Chambers, J. Effects of gestational exposure to chlorpyrifos on postnatal central and peripheral cholinergic neurochemistry. *Journal of Toxicology and Environmental Health A*, 2003 66, 275-289.

Rita, P; Reddy, PP; and Reddy, SV. Monitoring of workers occupationally exposed to pesticides in grape gardens of Andhra Pradesh. *Environmental Research*, 1987 44, 1-5.

Romero, P; Barnett, PG; and Midtling, JE. Congenital anomalies associated with maternal exposure to oxydemeton-methyl. *Environmental Research*, 1989 50, 256-261.

Rupa, DS; Reddy, PP; and Redd, O. Reproductive performance in population exposed to pesticides in cotton fields in India. *Environmental Research*, 1991 55, 123-128.

Sailaja, N; Chandrasekhar, M; Reckadevi, PV; Mahboob, M; Rahman, MF; Vuyyuri, SB; Danadevi, K; Hussain, SA; and Grover, P. Genotoxic evaluation of workers employed in pesticide production. *Mutation Research*, 2006 609, 74-80.

Salazar-Garcia, F; Gallardo-Diaz, E; Ceron-Mireles, P; Loomis, D; and Borja-Aburto, VH. Reproductive effects of occupational DDT exposure among male malaria control workers. *Environmental Health Perspectives*, 2004 112, 542-547.

Savitz, DA; Arbuckle, TE; Kaczor, D; and Curtis, KM. Male pesticida exposure and pregnancy outcome. *American Journal of Epidemiology*, 1997 146, 1025-1036.

Seidler, A; Hammer, GP; Husmann, G; Konig, J; Krtschil, A; Schmidtmann, I; and Blettner, M. Cancer risk among residents of Rhineland-Palatine winegrowing communities: a cancer-registry based ecological study. *Journal of Occupational Medicine and Toxicology*, 2008 3, 12-22.

Selgrade, MK. Biomarkers of effects: the immune system. *Journal of Biochemistry and Molecular Toxicology*, 2005 19, 177-179.

Sergent, T; Ribonnet, L; Kolosova, A; Garsou, S; Schaut, A; De Saeger, S; Van Peteghem, C; Larondelle, I; Pussemier, L; and Schneider, YJ. Molecular and cellular effects of food contaminants and secondary plant components and their plausible interactions at the intestinal level. *Food and Chemical Toxicology*, 2008 46, 813-841.

Steece-Collier, K; Maries, E; and Kordower, JH. Etiology of Parkinson's disease: genetics and environment revisited. *Proceedings of the Natural Academy of Science USA*, 2002 99, 13972-13974.

Takano, M; Yumoto, R; and Murakami, T. Expression and function of efflux drug transporters in the intestine. *Pharmacology and Therapeutics*, 2006 109, 137-161.

Tribull, T; Bruner, R; and Bain, L. The multidrug resistance-associated protein 1 transports methoxychlor and protects the seminiferous epithelium from injury. *Toxicology Letters*, 2003 142, 61-70.

Van Lieshout, E; Bedaf, M; Pieter, M; Ekkel, C; Nijhoff, W; and Peters, W. 1998. Effects of dietary anticarcinogens on rat gastrointestinal glutathione S-tranferase theta 1-1 levels. *Carcinogenesis*, 1998 19, 2055-2057.

Wang, LQ; and James, M. Inhibition of sulfonotranferases by xenobiotics. *Current Drug Metabolism*, 2006 7, 83-104.

Wang, XF; Li, S; Chou, AP; and Bronsteina, JM. Inhibitory effects of pesticides on proteasome activity: Implication in Parkinson's disease. *Neurobiology of Disease*, 2006 23, 198-205.

Waring, RH; and Harris, RM. Endocrine disrupters: a human risk?. *Molecular and Cellular Endocrinology*, 2005 244, 2-9.

Weselak, M; Arbuckle, TE; and Foster, W. Pesticide exposures and developmental outcomes: The epidemiological evidence. *Journal of Toxicology and Environmental Health, Part B*, 2007 10, 41-80.

Weselak, M; Arbuckle, TE; Wigle, DT; and Krewski, D. *In utero* pesticide exposure and childhood morbidity. *Environmental Research*, 2007 103, 79-86.

Wu, X; Lu, W; Roos, P; and Mersh-Sundermann, V. Vinclozolin, a widely used fungizide, ehanced BaP-induced micronucleous formation in human derived hepatoma cells by increasing CYP1A1 expression. *Toxicology Letters*, 2005 159, 83-88.

Young, JG; Eskenazi, B; Gladstone, EA; Bradman, A; Pedersen, L; Johnson, C; Barr, DB; Furlong, CE; and Holland, NT. Association between in utero organophosphate pesticide exposure and abnormal reflexes in neonates. *Neurotoxicology*, 2005 26, 199-209.

Zahm, SH; and Ward, MH. Pesticides and childhood cancer. Environmental and Heatlh Perspectives, 1998 106, 893-908.

Zimniak, P. Detoxification reactions: relevance to aging. *Ageing Research Reviews*, 2008. (in press) Doi: 10.1016/j.arr.2008.04.001

In: Handbook on Longevity: Genetics, Diet and Disease ISBN 978-1-60741-075-1
Editors: Jennifer V. Bentely and Mary Ann Keller © 2009 Nova Science Publishers, Inc.

Chapter VIII

The Optimal Human Diet: Theoretical Foundations of the Amen Protocol

Nūn Sava-Siva Amen-Ra
Amenta Press, Inc., Damascas, MD, USA*

Abstract

The purpose of this treatise is to explicate the central elements of a theoretically optimal human diet. Such a diet is herein defined as one that is plausibly capable of increasing human longevity, decreasing disease susceptibility, augmenting mental acuity and generally facilitating the attainment and maintenance of an aesthetic ideal encompassing muscularity, leanness and juvenescence. The main parameters pertinent to the conceptualization of this theoretical diet are temporal, quantitative and qualitative. That is, consideration is given to the frequency with which food is to be ingested and the time at which it should be ingested, the amount of calories that should be consumed and the composition of the food so consumed. This treatise will review and analyze scientific studies and fundamental physiological principles that form the theoretical and empirical bases of the diet. Caloric restriction and cyclic fasting—experimental interventions known to increase maximum mammalian lifespan—are the empirical cornerstones of the theoretically formulated regimen. As to the qualitative component of the diet, consideration is given to foods whose chemical constituents are known to influence the same physiological processes modulated by caloric restriction and cyclic fasting. Such processes include facilitation of detoxification, augmentation of antioxidant defense, attenuation of inflammation and oxidative damage, inhibition of glycation and maintenance of membrane, protein and genomic integrity. Thus, a major tenet of my theoretical complex is what I herein term *selective synergism*. In the context of this treatise, selective synergism entails ascertainment of the mechanisms involved in lifespan prolongation and disease diminution secondary to caloric restriction and attempting to

---

* AmentaPr@AmentaPress.com

augment these effects dietetically. Finally, consideration shall be given to psychological factors influencing compliance with such a restrictive protocol, including experiential insights gleaned from the author's own self-imposed adoption of the protocol in question spanning a period of four years.

Introduction

For nearly a century, it has been known that the lifespan of experimental animals can be lengthened by restricting the quantity of calories they are allowed to ingest and by reducing the rapidity with which they grow (Osborne TB et al. 1917). In the intervening years, scientists have sought to elucidate the molecular mechanisms mediating this phenomenon and ascertain its phylogenetic generality. In both respects, their efforts have been exemplar. Extraordinary innovations such as gene microarray analysis have enabled investigators to determine with impressive accuracy the physiological alterations induced by caloric curtailment. Moreover, myriad animal models have been employed in these analyses, leaving little doubt that diverse organisms respond in strikingly similar ways to dietary diminution. This latter point is important for our purposes inasmuch as direct confirmation of the efficacy of caloric restriction (CR) is empirically impractical in people, the population with which we are primarily concerned. We must therefore extrapolate from experiments involving animals if we are to formulate a theoretically optimal human diet. Indeed, evolutionary conservation enables such extrapolation. As we shall see, the phylogenetic generality of CR is evident in the evolutionary legacy of the human species and I shall argue that the optimality of a dietary regimen is partly determined by its similitude to the cardinal dietary habits of its evolutionary predecessors.

Discussion

It is repeatedly stressed in the literature that caloric restriction entails *energy* deprivation, not *nutrient* deprivation. Customarily, researchers ensure that CR subjects receive a quantity of micronutrients commensurate with their freely fed counterparts. Thus, while vitamins and minerals are maintained at acceptedly adequate levels, macronutrients—protein, carbohydrate, and fat—are restricted to specified levels. Generally, it is assumed that *caloric* restriction as such, and not restriction of any particular macronutrient, is efficacious in lifespan prolongation. As to the degree of restriction deemed adequate to augment longevity, Duffy and colleagues found that restricting the caloric intake of animals by as little as 10% relative to controls resulted in a significant increase in longevity on the order of 20% (Duffy PH et al. 2001). It is clear, however, that the more restrictive the regimen, the greater the gain in longevity. Indeed, a classic study by Weindruch and colleagues found that restricting the caloric intake of mice by 65% resulted in a proportionate 65% increase in maximum longevity (Weindruch R et al. 1986). As to the manner in which CR protocols are implemented, methodologies vary considerably. One type simply affords a control group unlimited access to food. The average daily caloric consumption of the control group is then calculated and the experimental group is given a fractional portion of this computed quantity on a daily basis. Alternatively, the control group may be given a predetermined portion of food while the experimental group is given a fractional allotment thereof. Another protocol provides experimental animals unfettered access to food for specific intervals, say 1 to 3 hours per day. Such "meal feeding" regimens have been found to result in substantial reductions in caloric intake and resultant increases maximum lifespan relative to controls (Nelson and Halberg 1986). A variant of the meal-feeding regimen combines quantitative and temporal caloric restriction, affording animals access to a restricted ration of food for a limited span of time. Yet another type of protocol involves intermittent feeding, wherein experimental animals are only allowed access to food on alternating days. The degree of restriction resulting from such regimens varies greatly however, with some investigators reporting substantial caloric deficits and others reporting equivalent intakes of food among experimental and control groups (Anson RM et al. 2003). From a human perspective, the latter protocol is of particular interest. Intermittent feeding permits unlimited access to food for limited periods, while significantly increasing mean and maximum lifespan (Goodrick CL et al. 1990). Because feeding is not limited quantitatively but only temporally, animals are ostensibly able to eat to the point of satiety. Psychologically (and perhaps physiologically), protracted bouts of food deprivation punctuated with intervals of unlimited access to food may be more satisfying and sustainable. I shall have more to say about this in a subsequent section but for now it is important to highlight a critical point. Because intermittent feeding protocols promote longevity even in the absence of appreciable caloric restriction, lifespan prolongation must be partly attributable to fasting as such. As shall be discussed more fully, fasting replicates many of the physiological effects of CR proper and it is the induction of these common physiological alterations that is responsible for the associated augmentation of longevity secondary to intermittent feeding. Therefore, the concept of caloric restriction should be understood to encompass both dimensions—quantitative and temporal.

Another methodological consideration is the juncture at which calorie restriction is imposed during the life of the organism. Many investigators initiate restriction in rodents immediately after weaning, though several sound studies suggest that anti-aging effects are incurred when initiated in adolescent and adult animals as well. Weindruch and Walford, for example, found that caloric restriction initiated in middle-aged mice (~1 year old) increased mean and maximum longevity by 10-20% (Weindruch and Walford 1982). Restriction at this advanced juncture also effected a significant suppression of spontaneous tumor formation and attenuated indices of immunologic aging (Weindruch R et al. 1982). An important study by Yu and colleagues found that CR was almost equally effective in rats when initiated after completion of skeletal development (~6 months) as when started shortly after weaning (~6 weeks) (Yu BP et al. 1985). Ostensibly, there is a point in the lifecycle at which CR is inefficacious and a point in advanced age at which CR may be deemed deleterious. Because humans exhibit different patterns of maturation and senescence, it is difficult to extrapolate an ideal initiation interval from rodents to humans. In light of the available evidence, however, it would seem that forestalling CR until the post-adolescent/early adult phase in humans might replicate the benefits of early initiation while ensuring that development is not unduly compromised. Considering the protracted developmental period of humans (particularly respecting the brain), the aforementioned admonition is especially important.

Mechanisms

There is no consensus as to how CR effectuates lifespan extension. Several theories have been forwarded, some more parsimonious than others. Though a consensus among scientists would be satisfying, it is ultimately unnecessary inasmuch as each of the interpretive theories explain aspects of aging and elucidate how particular aspects of aging are attenuated by caloric restriction. What is more, the various theories are nonexclusive and it is likely that each theoretical mechanism is operative to some degree in the mitigation of aging.

The oldest interpretation is probably the Metabolic Theory. This theory is based on the apparent inverse relationship between metabolic rate and maximum lifespan among species. Conceptually, this inter-specific relationship can be extended to longevity differences within a species. Perhaps, so the theory goes, metabolic reactions inevitably generate products that are deleterious to the organism, so that animals that produce these products profusely age more rapidly. Despite the intuitive appeal of this theory, empirical support for CR-mediated metabolic suppression has been inconsistent and equivocal (Speakman JR et al. 2002). In a paper published in the journal *Medical Hypotheses*, I invoke a variant of this theory. It posits that caloric restriction results in an alteration of energy expenditure such that resources are diverted from less essential processes (especially growth and reproductive receptivity) and instead allocated to preservative processes that ultimately elicit lifespan prolongation and, in humans, selective preservation of our most precious organ—the brain (Amen-Ra N 2006). However, as opined by some investigators, confirmation of the veracity of such theories as mine can only come from meticulous analyses of metabolic outputs of individual organs under conditions of caloric restriction.

The Free Radical Theory arguably has the most adherents and is buttressed by an impressive corpus of research. It is widely accepted that damage to macromolecules from oxygen-derived radicals underlies much of the aging process. Numerous studies have established the triumvirate efficacy of CR in inhibiting the generation of free radicals, attenuating the damaging effects of free radicals via endogenous antioxidants, and repairing oxidative damage incurred by membranes, proteins and DNA molecules. Nonetheless, questions remain. For example, while some studies show that CR increases the expression or activity of antioxidant enzymes, other investigators have reported either no effect or converse effects (Hart RW et al. 1992; Feuers RJ et al. 1993). In addition, it would seem that altering the genotypes of organisms such that they express elevated amounts of antioxidant enzymes would accordingly augment longevity. This has been demonstrated in some studies but not others (Schriner SE et al 2005). Thus, some doubt remains as to the centrality of oxidative damage in aging and the imperativeness of its attenuation in CR-mediated lifespan prolongation.

Glucose is central to the Glycation Theory. Despite the essentiality of glucose in animal metabolism, it is known to interact aberrantly with constitutive proteins, rendering them dysfunctional and resistant to degradation by proteolytic processes. This effect is termed *glycation* and the presence of such compromised proteins has been shown to increase with age. Because CR routinely results in significant suppression of circulating glucose, it is not surprising that it appreciably attenuates glycation (Masoro EJ et al. 1989). Thus, inhibition of glycation is thought to underlie the efficacy of CR in promoting longevity.

Caloric restriction has been shown to have a more marked effect on insulin than on its elicitor, glucose. An important study by Edward J. Masoro and colleagues found that CR reduced circulating glucose by 15% and insulin by 50% (Masoro EJ et al. 1992). An alteration of this magnitude, effectuated by an anti-aging intervention, automatically suggests a role for insulin in the aging process. Moreover, targeted genetic disruptions of insulin signaling have been shown to significantly extend the lifespan of animals (Barbieri M et al. 2003). Longevity-conferring genetic alterations have also been effected by suppressing the signaling of insulin-like growth factor I (IGF-I). What is more, CR similarly suppresses circulating levels of IGF-I. Simplistic reasoning therefore suggests a role for this anabolic peptide in the etiology of aging. Considering the role of insulin and IGF-I in mediating growth, development, and cell proliferation, combined with the observation that early-onset caloric restriction reduces the rapidity of growth, delays development, and generally inhibits cell proliferation, one is naturally lead to entertain the hypothesis that growth retardation (or protraction) is an operative phenomenon in CR-mediated life prolongation. This we might cumbersomely call the Insulin Signaling Theory.

Finally, there is the Hormesis Theory. This theory, based on compelling empirical evidence, holds that otherwise deleterious agents and conditions can exert beneficial physiological effects if sufficiently moderate in intensity. The mechanistic bases for these adaptive physiological responses involve enhancement of endogenous protective agents and processes that ultimately augment health and longevity. Caloric restriction is a physiological (and psychological) stressor that induces myriad adaptive responses such as heightened antioxidant defense, heightened protein replacement, heightened DNA repair, and heightened detoxification and elimination of toxic agents. CR is therefore considered a prime example of hormesis. The Hormesis Theory is particularly persuasive insofar as the modulation of maximum lifespan must necessitate a fundamental alteration of genetic expression. Hormesis hints at a mechanism whereby a single stressor can produce multifarious physiological alterations by modulating the expression of genes that protect organisms from numerous noxious agents. Wedded to the concept of differential gene expression, Hormesis harmonizes each of the aforementioned theoretical explanations for the anti-aging effect of CR. The ultimate source of the hormetic stress is the limitation of available energy. Because glucose is the central molecule of animal metabolism, limited intake of food necessarily lessens glycation—the pathological process of protein derangement implicated in aging. Insulin action is accordingly inhibited by depreciation of its chief elicitor, glucose. The combined curtailment of glucose and insulin interact with the genome in such ways as to alter the expression of myriad genes whose collective hormetic effects augment longevity and reduce susceptibility to diverse diseases. Though each of the aforementioned hypotheses has merit, the accumulated evidence leans in favor of Hormesis in the opinion of this theoretician.

Evolutionary Analyses Indicate the Applicability of CR to Humans

In an illuminative review article published in the journal *Biogerontology*, Edward J. Masoro enumerated a plethora of phylogenetically diverse organisms whose lifespan has been experimentally extended by CR. The efficacy of CR, he wrote, has been documented in species from three of the five Kingdoms of life—Protista, Fungi and Animalia:

> ...and within Animalia, it has been observed in species of four phyla: Rotifera, Nematoda, Arthopoda and Chordata. In the Phylum Chordata, dietary restriction-induced life extension has been reported for species in the Classes Pisces and Mammalia. In the Class Mammalia, dietary restriction has been shown to extend the life of rats, mice, hamsters and dogs, and there is suggestive evidence that it does so in the nonhuman primate species as well. (Masoro EJ 2006: 1)

Despite such phylogenetic generality, there are those who question whether caloric restriction can extend human longevity to an extent commensurate with experimental animals. While such scientific conservatism can be appreciated (especially in the absence of confirmatory empirical evidence) there are theoretically sound reasons for believing that caloric restriction will not only augment maximum human lifespan but that the human species is particularly amenable to the ameliorative effects thereof. In a pair of papers published in the journal *Medical Hypotheses*, I argue that humans bear physical and physiological attributes indicative of adaptations to ecologically imposed caloric restriction (Amen-Ra N 2007; Amen-Ra N 2006). As this topic is relevant to our present discussion, I shall summarize some of the major elements of my theoretical exposition.

In comparison to our closest extant relative, the chimpanzee (*Pan troglodytes*), humans are distinguished by four cardinal characteristics—a longer lifespan, lower reproductive receptivity relative to lifespan, a larger brain, and a longer period of maturation. These attributes—what I term the *quadripartite complex*—generally distinguish the simian superfamily from the larger Primate Order but are especially accentuated in the human lineage and likely conferred a decisive selective advantage upon our species. I surmise that the quadripartite complex was an adaptive response to changing climatic conditions. This supposition is based on evidence of substantial climatic change centered around 2-1.7 million years ago—a change characterized by increased aridity, cooler temperatures and general climatic flux (Ravelo AC et al. 2004; Reed KE 1997). These environmental alterations likely led to the extinction of *Paranthropus*, leaving *Homo* as the sole surviving representative of the hominin clade. Environmental alterations ostensibly led to ecological alterations, limiting the availability of exploitable food. Interestingly, the assemblage of adaptive attributes accentuated in man—long lifespan, lengthened development, high brain/bodyweight ratio and low reproductive receptivity—are consistently induced in organisms subjected to caloric restriction. What is more, the components of the quadripartite complex are controlled by a system of central importance in the mediation of CR—the neuro-endocrine system and its chief regulator, the hypothalamus. Let us consider how the hypothalamus could have mediated the metabolic changes evidenced by the quadripartite complex.

The rate and the extent to which mammalian organisms develop are dictated, principally, by two endocrine hormones: thyroid hormone (TH) and somatotropin (growth hormone, GH). Released by the thyroid and pituitary glands respectively, these hormones not only induce tissue growth but also elevate metabolism by increasing the influx of nutrients into the cells of proliferating or growing tissue. Under conditions of chronic caloric restriction, levels of these anabolic hormones are substantially reduced and, as a result, animals subjected to this restrictive regimen develop at a slower rate than control animals fed *ad libitum* (Weindruch and Walford 1988). The adaptive consequence of this effect is clear: Reducing the rate with which an organism grows reduces the quantity (and, indeed, quality) of food needed thereby. Developmental depression would have enabled hominins to support their young (and themselves) with less food. Further support for this line of reasoning is to be found in consideration of lactation. Lactation—a task that places high energetic demands on nursing females—is governed by the hypothalamus. Two hormones mediate hypothalamic control over lactation: thyrotropin releasing hormone (TRH) and prolactin inhibiting hormone (PIH). These hormones respectively prompt and inhibit pituitary release of prolactin, the proximal mediator of breast milk elaboration. In addition to eliciting exudation of breast milk, prolactin causes the breast to augment production of casein and lactalbumin, the principal protein constituents of milk. Interestingly, human breast milk has the lowest protein concentration of any primate—a value of 7% in comparison to the primate norm of ~20% (Oftedal OT 1991). This would seem to buttress the notion that humans are exquisitely adapted to dietary deprivation. Moreover, it underscores the role of the hypothalamus as the agent 'recruited' by natural selection to buffer the effects of ecologically induced dietary restriction. This adaptation—de-enrichment of human milk—is ostensibly tied to developmental depression: Slowly growing infants can be sustained on milk of a lower nutritional content. Conceivably, reduction of milk protein enrichment could have been effectuated by decreasing TRH or, alternatively, by increasing PIH. The phenomenon of milk de-enrichment also calls into question the prevailing notion that human evolution was contingent upon provisionment of meat. Clearly, the nutritional quality of milk—the sole source of sustenance for the growing human infant—should come to reflect a nutritional profile of dietary enrichment rather than dietary depreciation if, indeed, meat consumption was a formative factor in the evolution of the human species. Such is not the case. Rather, the nutritional profile of human breast milk suggests a perennial diet centered on low-calorie plant food. Interestingly, caloric restriction has been shown to result in decreased concentration of circulating levels of prolactin (Koizumi A et al. 1989). This further supports the adaptive role played by the hypothalamus in mitigating ecologically imposed nutritional stress during human evolution.

The maintenance of reproductive receptivity and procreative potential are energy intensive imperatives. These imperatives are, however, superfluous under conditions of caloric curtailment. It is therefore not surprising that animals subjected to CR are less fertile than freely fed controls. Female animals release fewer eggs during ovulation and have smaller litters while males exhibit suppressed spermatogenesis under conditions of chronic CR (Diskin MG et al. 2003; Wu A et al. 2002). These effects are mediated collectively by reductions in gonadotropins (i.e. luteinizing hormone, and follicle stimulating hormone) and by reductions in sex hormones (principally testosterone and estrogen). Interestingly, both testosterone and estrogen are known to increase whole body metabolic rate markedly (Guyton and Hall 2000). Thus, suppression of circulating sex hormones in hominins would have been doubly adaptive in that the likelihood of reproduction would have been reduced and the rate with which limited energy resources were utilized would have been curtailed considerably, augmenting the calorie conserving effects of low TH and GH noted previously.

When viewed in terms of the 'reproductive quotient'—that is, the ratio of reproductive lifespan to total lifespan—human females are far less fecund than chimpanzees. Viewed differently, the duration over which human females are reproductively receptive (relative to total lifespan) is reduced. If the reproductive range—the period from menarche to menopause or cessation of ovulation—of both chimpanzees and humans is approximated to be ~30 years and the maximum lifespan of chimpanzees and humans is approximated to be ~60 and ~120 years respectively, then humans have experienced a 2-fold relative reduction in their 'reproductive quotient'. It is conceivable that natural selection served to suppress human fertility (or more precisely, reduce reproductive range relative to lifespan) in the face of food scarcity, thereby preserving essential energy reserves. Indeed, it is estimated that energy expenditure is 7% lower in women when the endometrium is in a regressed (non-receptive) state (Strassman BI 1996). Clearly, the assumption of amenorreah (temporary cessation of menstruation) in the face of protracted caloric curtailment can ensure the conservation of copious amounts of energy and avert potential parental investment in offspring likely to suffer malnutrition and premature death due to food scarcity.

The human brain is three times more massive than the typical ape brain (~1/2 kilogram) and twice as massive as the first supposed member of the genus *Homo* (*H. habilis*). Encephalization—the pronounced disproportionate increase in the size of the brain— warrants particular attention due to the considerable metabolic expense of neural tissue, especially in light of the evidence that the formative period of human evolution was marked by food scarcity. The key to understanding the evolutionary accommodation of human encephalization may lie in the very nature of the nervous system. Not only is the brain a privileged organ, receiving a disproportionate allotment of nutrients, it is also exceptionally sensitive to metabolic deficits. Due to their high metabolic rate and limited capacity for anaerobic metabolism, neurons depend on an almost invariant supply of nutrients from the systemic circulation—an abrupt cessation of sustenance to the brain results in unconsciousness within seconds. Another indication of the brain's special status is the fact that it does not require insulin in order to effectuate influx of glucose, as do non-neural tissues. Consequently, the brain is perpetually provisioned with its full complement of glucose while the rest of the body must "make do" with the remainder. Moreover, when the level of circulating glucose is too sparse to meet the brain's needs, the body mobilizes its fat deposits, converting fatty acids into ketone bodies that are, in turn, preponderantly metabolized by the brain, kidneys and skeletal muscle. Thus, in the absence of abundant nutrient availability, the body is able to exploit its embedded energy reserves (fat) and convert this vital resource into a form (ketone bodies) utilizable by the nervous system to the exclusion of other organ systems. Though the liver plays a central role in the conversion of fatty acids into brain-bound ketone bodies, these volatile molecules are also produced locally in the brain by astrocytes (Guzman and Blazquez 2004). This mechanism would seem to ensure adequate appropriation of ketone body intermediates by the brain and, additionally, ensure exclusive sequestration of ketone bodies within the nervous system. There is, moreover, evidence which suggests that ketone bodies, in addition to serving as energy substrates for the brain, confer protection to the brain from toxic insults (Massieu L et al. 2003). Indeed, a study by Leite and colleagues found that brain-derived beta-hydroxy- butyrate (the most abundant circulating ketone body) induces increased secretion of a brain growth factor, which promotes nerve cell proliferation (Leite M et al. 2004). Two hormones in particular are crucial catalysts of ketogenesis: cortisol and epinephrine. Cortisol is released from the adrenal glands principally in response to food deprivation (more specifically, hypoglycemia). Ultimate control over cortisol secretion is exerted by the hypothalamus, however, through release of corticotropin releasing hormone. Cortisol thereupon accelerates gluconeogenesis and facilitates conversion of fatty acids into ketone bodies. The ketogenic compound epinephrine is also secreted by the adrenal gland, though the proximate cause of its release is direct discharge of sympathetic nerves from the hypothalamus in response to physical exertion (intensive foraging for example). Theoretically, by prompting increased secretion of the ketogenic compounds cortisol and epinephrine, the hypothalamus could augment availability of ketone body intermediates, thereby providing the brain with a plentiful supply of nutrients (ketone bodies) during bouts of malnourishment and by so doing provide protection to the brain as well as molecular stimuli for increased neural proliferation. This latter phenomenon is particularly intriguing in light of the teleological necessity of explaining human encephalization amidst apparent nutritional marginalization. Ketone-catalyzed neurogenesis is a clarifying component of a more comprehensive theoretical complex. Central to this complex is the corpus of research establishing the capacity of caloric restriction to increase expression of the neurotrophic factors BDNF, GDNF and NT-3 and its capacity to augment expression of neural chaperone proteins which play a role in ensuring proper protein conformation (Maswood N et al. 2004; Lee J et al 2002; Duan W et al. 2001; Aly KB et al. 1994). Tellingly, while there is no experimental evidence that caloric *enrichment* induces brain hyperplasia, there is compelling evidence that caloric *deprivation* does so. This calls into question theories of human brain evolution that invoke dietary enrichment, hunting and meat procurement to explain the augmentation of encephalization in hominins ancestral to humans (Aiello LC et al. 2002). Moreover, the importance of meat acquisition in human evolution is questionable considering the circumstantial nature of the evidence of early hominin hunting (Amen-Ra N 2003). Whereas dietary enrichment, meat eating and the hunting hypothesis have long been invoked to explain the evolution of the human brain, the available evidence indicates that dietary deprivation can appreciably augment neural accretion via enhanced expression of endogenous neurotrophic agents and this body of research may provide the most parsimonious explanatory framework for the evolutionary encephalization of the human brain. Altogether, the elements of this theoretical edifice are intriguing: Chronic caloric curtailment imposed during the formative stages of human evolution caused a substantial shift in energy allocation resulting in preferential provisionment of nutrients to the brain, an alteration which ultimately accelerated encephalization.

Maximum human lifespan is perhaps twice that of our nearest relative, the chimpanzee, with maximal human longevity exceeding 120 years and chimpanzees exceeding 60 years. As to which physiological phenomenon facilitated this accretion in lifespan, it should be reiterated that there exists a correlative relationship between the lifespan of animals and the rapidity with which they metabolize food—the longer the lifespan the lower the metabolism of the animal (Speakman JR et al. 2002). Though the underlying mechanism by which metabolic rate modulates aging and longevity is not altogether clear, a free radical-mediated mechanism may be operative. Presumably, because the generation of damaging free radicals is elicited upon ingestion of food, the more calories an animal intakes and the more precipitous the combustion of consumed calories, the more damage done to tissues and the more rapidly aging ensues. As previously discussed, one of the means by which caloric restriction is thought to augment longevity is via suppression of metabolic rate (Bevilacqua L et al. 2005; Greenberg and Boozer 2000). Moreover, CR seems to increase the efficiency of energy extraction and, accordingly, lower the levels of radicals released per calorie consumed. Considering the centrality of energy equilibration in determining the physiological disposition of organisms—rate of growth, rate of senescence, extent of encephalization and reproductive potential—it is plausible that the modulation of metabolism supervenes each component of the quadripartite complex. Evolutionary economization may have been effectuated by merely modulating the metabolic disposition of the hypothalamus, the body's chief homeostatic/regulatory organ. This economization may have afforded early *Homo* a selective advantage over sympatric hominins as members of this genus could subsist on foods of lower nutritional quality and consume less thereof. If indeed humans are evolutionarily adapted to caloric restriction, this may suggest that dietary indulgence is particularly deleterious for our species and, conversely, that caloric restriction is particularly beneficial. In light of this theoretical argument, the supposition that humans are unlikely to benefit significantly from CR is untenable.

Elements of the Amen Protocol

The lifestyle protocol that I have conceived and adopted—herein termed the *Amen Protocol*—is an intellectual amalgam comprised of theoretical extrapolations from scientific studies and experiential insights derived from self-experimentation. Primarily, the objective of the regimen is to integrate all that is known about experimental augmentation of lifespan and diminution of disease susceptibility. Secondary considerations include optimization of mental acuity and the attainment of an aesthetic ideal encompassing leanness, muscularity and juvenescence. That each of these stated ideals are promoted by caloric restriction is a testament to the centrality of metabolic modulation in controlling the physiological state and fate of organisms. It must be acknowledged at the outset that the protocol in question is not scientific *sensu stricto* but idealistic and synergistic. That is, our intent is to maximize human longevity and vitality by combining data from diverse biomedical domains operating, as it were, on the implicit 'Gestaltic' assumption that a synthesis of scientific knowledge will yield results more momentous than the myriad supporting studies may individually suggest. The cornerstone of the Amen Diet is caloric restriction—temporal and quantitative caloric restriction. To the degree that the operative mechanisms by which CR lengthens lifespan and lessens disease are known, I have sought to isolate these mechanisms and modulate them further so as to magnify or synergize the overall effects of a dietetically restrictive regimen. These effects are enhanced by another integral component of the protocol—exercise. As shall be discussed further, exercise influences important molecular mechanisms implicated in CR-mediated lifespan prolongation and disease diminution. I shall briefly delineate these mechanisms and expound upon them in subsequent sections on the elements of the Amen Fast, the Amen Diet, and the Amen Exercise Regimen. Most importantly, molecular defense is thought to be a crucial component of CR-mediated suppression of aging and disease. Molecular defense encompasses the main biochemical components of the body—proteins, lipids, and nucleic acids. Such defensive measures include suppression of circulating glucose, the effect of which is to lessen glycative damage to constitutive and catalytic proteins (Masoro EJ et al. 1989). CR also increases the expression of enzymes whose function involves recognition and replacement of damaged proteins (Radak Z et al. 2002). Additionally, CR augments production of chaperone proteins in various tissues, the effect of which is to protect proteins from diverse damage (Soti and Csermely 2002). CR suppresses free radical generation, thereby lessening oxidative damage to proteins, lipids, and DNA (Sohal and Weindruch 1996). Moreover, CR (equivocally) increases the expression of antioxidant enzymes that suppress and redress oxidative damage to cellular structures (Sohal RS 2002). Further, CR increases the expression of enzymes—polymerases—whose function involves recognition, repair and/or replacement of damaged DNA bases (Cabelof DC et al. 2003). CR-mediated DNA defense also involves a process known as gene silencing, whereby histone proteins bind to DNA more tightly, averting damage thereto and, ostensibly, inhibiting unnecessary transcription of inaccessible genes (Lamming DW et al. 2004). This latter mechanism conceivably forestalls the squandering of energy issuing from profuse production of nonnecessitous gene products. Such energy, it is supposed, can then be channeled into processes that promote organismic integrity and lengthen life. CR-mediated metabolic conservation/reallocation may play a key part in lifespan prolongation and this concept factors heavily in the theoretical framework of the Amen Protocol. In addition to promoting defense, CR promotes detoxification. Organisms are routinely exposed to environmental and dietary toxins and such exposure undoubtedly compromises longevity and promotes diseases, especially neoplasias. This problem is especially pertinent to humans given our exposure to numerous novel, synthetic chemicals whose physiological effects are yet unknown or incompletely understood. Organisms express enzymes that chemically convert toxins in such ways that generally render them less toxic and more easily excreted from the body. CR significantly increases the expression of enzymes dedicated to detoxification—so called xenobiotic enzymes—and this enhanced capacity to expunge toxins is thought to be a critical component of CR-mediated lifespan extension and cancer prevention (Leakey JA et al 1989). A related phenomenon is CR-mediated attenuation of adiposity. Expectedly, CR routinely results in appreciable weight loss. However, such weight loss is disproportionate, with fat being energetically exploited to a greater extent than skeletal muscle and other non-adipose tissue (Blanc S et al. 2003). Importantly, the most deleterious toxins are lipid soluble and consequently accumulate in adipose tissue (Hodgson E 2004). It would seem that elimination of superfluous stores of fat removes a reservoir for the sequestration of lipid-soluble toxins. Thus, leanness is not an entirely aesthetic ideal. What is more, the preferential preservation of muscle that CR promotes is not merely passive or incidental. An intriguing study by Hagopian and colleagues found that while the activities of most enzymes that catalyze the conversion of constitutive proteins into energy substrates were increased by caloric restriction, the activities of those enzymes that catabolize the amino acids predominant in skeletal muscles—the so-called branched chain amino acids—were unchanged (Hagopian K et al. 2003). Consequently, CR selectively spares skeletal muscle. Moreover, as with adipose extirpation, this effect is not entirely aesthetic. Muscle is replete with receptors for insulin. The relative abundance of muscle-borne insulin receptors in CR subjects undoubtedly augments their insulin sensitivity, contributing to a beneficial physiological profile characterized by sustainable, moderate hypoglycemia and hypoinsulinemia. Finally, CR evidently increases mental acuity and neurophysiological functioning and averts age-related cognitive decline (Arumugam TV et al. 2006). The means by which it does so include increasing the expression of neurotrophins that promote the generation and preservation of progenitor cells in the brain, especially those structures (i.e. the hippocampus) involved in learning and memory (Lee J et al. 2002). Another mechanism reportedly involves elevated elaboration of a hormone (specifically *ghrelin*) involved in synapse formation and spatial learning (Diano S et al. 2006).

Before I endeavor to explain the experimental, experiential, and theoretical bases of the Amen Protocol, I shall give a brief description of its design. The most distinctive feature of the protocol is its cyclicity: *23 hours of fasting, 1 hour of feeding.* Fasting commences at ~19:00 hours and ends on the following day with the evening meal (~18:00)[1]. Naturally, no calorific commodities are consumed during the fasting phase. Calorie-free beverages are consumed however and this is considered an important part of the regimen. Specifically, tea and botanical infusions are imbibed throughout the fast, with green tea and ginseng factoring prominently. Briefly, tea is prepared by steeping ~10 grams of whole, dried *Camellia senensis* leaves (of the green, white, black, or oolong variety) in 1 liter of water (~80° C). The tea is steeped for ~10 minutes and thereafter dispensed into an insulative steel vessel. Ginseng (specifically North American ginseng, *Panax quinquefolius* L.) is prepared by steeping ~15 grams of the dried roots in 1 liter of boiling water for ~2 hours. [The preferred method of preparation entails placing the ginseng in an insulative steel vessel and pouring boiling water over the dried roots. The strength (and palatability) of the infusion increases throughout the day and is culinarily optimal at ~6 hours.] Typically, 1-2 liters of tea and aqueous ginseng extract are imbibed daily. Within the last hour of the fast, the resistance exercise session commences, the details of which shall be discussed in the section on the Amen Exercise Regimen. Immediately following the evening exercise session, the feeding period commences. The composition of the diet is triumvirate, consisting of three components—supplemental, medicinal and saporal. The supplemental component contains protein (~15-25 grams), peptides, amino acids, fatty acids, minerals and vitamins, supplying at least the minimum recommended daily provision of nearly all essential nutrients in a liquid solution. The liquidity of the solution is considered important inasmuch as it likely enhances assimilation of the imbibed nutrients. This concoction is arguably the most important part of the diet insofar as it contains all requisite nutrients in adequate amounts. Essentially, nothing additional is needed to ensure adequate sustenance. The medicinal segment consists of slightly germinated (~24 hours) seeds of broccoli (*Brassica oleracea* L.). As shall be discussed later, broccoli seeds contain copious amounts of chemicals known to induce increased expression of detoxicant enzymes. Detoxification is a process explicitly promoted by the Amen Protocol. Other medicinal compounds, to be discussed later, are partaken prior to each exercise period, primarily to attenuate excessive oxidative stress. The saporal segment is simply intended to secure a state of satiety. As an integral part of an optimal diet, it is nonetheless important. Because variety is a superfluous concern (given that all essential nutrients are provided by the supplemental solution) it is important to select a staple that is, to

---

[1] The specific times are arbitrary. They are noted merely to stress the cyclicity of the regimen.

the greatest degree practicable, devoid of deleterious agents and, ideally, replete with ameliorative agents. To this end, I selected barley (*Hordeum vulgare* L.) as the staple of the Amen Diet. Barley is among the oldest of cultivated crops and for this reason one might expect it to be low in toxicants and high in nutrients, this being an intended goal of artificial agricultural selection. In keeping with the imperative of optimization, I treat the barley in such a way as to augment its nutritional and medicinal value. One such optimizing measure is germination. The barley grains are allowed to germinate for ~48-72 hours in an aqueous medium. The purpose of this treatment is to effect enzymatic conversion of complex storage nutrients in the grain into simpler compounds that are more easily assimilated. As I shall discuss further in the section describing the theoretical bases of the diet, I also expose the barley to a process intended to increase its production of protective antioxidants. The sprouted barley is thoroughly blended in a base of raw "soymilk"—an aqueous exudate of germinated soybeans (*Glycine max* L.)—and topped with raw, unfiltered honey. The blending is another measure aimed at heightening assimilation through chemical simplification. Blending, as it were, lyses the individual grains, liberating their constituent hydrolytic enzymes so as to yield a nutritious, mechanically masticated mixture. [Freshly baked whole-grain bread and fruit are partaken to occupy the balance of the 60-minute feeding period and to ensure sufficient satiety. Tea is typically imbibed after the evening meal to mitigate the effects of elevated glucose. This effect of tea shall be discussed in the following section.] Digestion and assimilation are permitted to proceed for 2-3 hours before nightly repose. Upon waking (~04:00 hours), an antioxidant preparation is partaken prior to the persistive (aerobic) exercise session. The cycle terminates with the ensuing evening meal. I shall now provide a more thorough analysis of the theoretical foundations of the Amen Protocol.

Elements of the Amen Fast

Apart from the known benefits of quantitative caloric restriction, temporal caloric restriction (i.e. fasting) exerts independent ameliorative effects on longevity and health. The most persuasive demonstration of this comes from intermittent feeding protocols. Such protocols provide experimental groups with unlimited quantities of food every other day. Strikingly, some of these subjects reportedly ingest twice as much food on feeding days as their freely fed counterparts consume daily. What is more, such temporal caloric restriction results in significant lifespan prolongation (Goodrick CL et al. 1990). These findings clearly suggest that certain physiological alterations induced by temporal caloric restriction replicate (to some degree) the anti-aging effects of quantitative caloric restriction. Impressive corroborative evidence has been amassed by Matthias Bauer and colleagues at the *Institut fuer Genetik* in Karlsruhe, Germany. These researchers investigated alterations in gene expression patterns under conditions of fasting and energy repletion and found suggestive resemblances between the fasted state and the calorie-restricted state. Such resemblances included indications of increased detoxification capacity, increased fat oxidation, increased protein catabolism (i.e. gluconeogenesis), decreased fat synthesis, decreased insulin/IGF I signaling, and decreased cell growth and proliferation (Bauer M et al. 2004). These findings accord with those of an earlier study published in the *Proceedings of the National Academy of Sciences* (*PNAS*), which analyzed alterations in gene expression following long-term and short-term quantitative CR. As with the fasting study, this study found increased expression of genes mediating detoxification, fat oxidation, and protein catabolism and decreased expression of genes mediating fat synthesis, insulin/IGF I signaling and cell growth and proliferation (Cao SX et al. 2001). Among other illuminating investigations, these two studies suggest, conservatively, that fasting may be an efficacious way of implementing caloric restriction. I favor a more speculative, though plausible, position that the particular fasting regimen prescribed by the Amen Protocol is additive in its ameliorative effects on health and longevity, additive to the established ameliorative effects of quantitative CR. Despite equivocal extant evidence, there are compelling reasons why one should expect to see synergism between quantitative and temporal caloric restriction, compelling reasons why the Amen Protocol is theoretically optimal. Briefly, the relevant processes encompass inhibition of glycation and adiposity and augmentation of genomic defense, neurologic defense, and autophagy.

Let us first consider glycation, a chemical correlate of age-related physiological decline. Intuitively, limiting the intake of calories should have the effect of reducing the extent of glycation-induced damage as less food would be converted into glucose—less glucose, less glycation. This has been experimentally established with impressive clarity by Edward J. Masoro and colleagues who demonstrated that CR resulted in significant suppression of glycation, an effect attributed to lifelong lessening of glucose levels (Masoro EJ et al. 1989). Nevertheless, the *duration* over which the body's tissues are exposed to glucose is undoubtedly of great importance—a longer period of exposure means a larger number of glycation reactions and more damage to tissues. Thus, the quantity of calories ingested is important but it seems reasonable to suppose that the *span of time* over which glucose circulates in the blood (at elevated post-prandial concentrations) is of greater import in averting glycation, all else being equal. Herein lies one of the distinctive benefits of the Amen Fast. Indeed, it is the fasting component of the regimen that arguably makes the Amen Protocol theoretically superior to quantitative caloric restriction alone. As noted previously, CR studies customarily employ methodologies wherein animals are given daily fractional quantities of food relative to a freely fed control population whereas the other frequently employed CR methodology effectuates caloric curtailment by restricting the feeding of experimental subjects to alternating days. In terms of anti-glycative potential, the former continuous CR protocol is less beneficial, theoretically, for it provides animals with a continuous (though calorie-restricted) allotment of food (for, say, an 8 to 12-hour duration) which would be expected to induce a continuous elevation of glucose (relative to fasted animals). In the case of intermittent CR protocols, animals are allowed to consume a quantity of food equivalent to that which 'libertine' animals ingest over a 1-day diurnal period or simply given free access to food on alternate days. Such animals are routinely allowed to feed over a period of 8-12 hours, every other day. Therefore, over a 2-day period, animals on a continuous CR protocol feed for a period of ~20 hours whereas those animals on an alternate day CR protocol feed for a period of ~10 hours. Clearly, the latter protocol should be superior in terms of glycative inhibition. Let us then compare this relatively superior, intermittent CR regimen to the Amen Protocol. In terms of absolute feeding time, animals subjected to standard intermittent CR protocols feed (discontinuously) for upwards of 12 hours over a 2-

day (48-hour) period. Conversely, over a 2-day period, the Amen Fast prescribes a feeding period of only 2 hours. Over a 1-week (168-hour) period, the absolute feeding time under standard intermittent CR conditions is upwards of 42 hours, whereas over a comparable 1-week period, an Amen adherent feeds for a mere 7 hours. Discrete instances of feeding also factor in this theoretical analysis. On a standard intermittent CR protocol, an animal can consume food on multiple occasions in the 8-12 hour interval over which feeding is permitted. On the Amen Fast, only 7 discrete feeding sessions ensue in the span of a week. The potential physiological consequences of this distinct divergence between standard CR and the Amen Protocol are apparent, the latter ostensibly effecting a greater attenuation of glycation. Theoretically, such a difference should result in less glycation-induced tissue damage and less precipitous aging. To reiterate, because food is ingested over an interval of only 1 hour each day on the Amen Protocol, the level of glucose circulating in the bloodstream is continually depressed and the potential for glycation-induced damage is commensurately reduced. Though quantitative CR is clearly efficacious in the mitigation of glycation, the Amen Protocol synergizes and maximizes this effect by tremendously truncating the time allotted for feeding. As previously mentioned, the Amen Protocol prescribes tea imbibition during the fasting phase. Green tea exhibits anti-glycative activity and this property has been attributed to its abundance of tannins and catechins (Yokozawa and Nakagawa 2004; Nakagawa T et al. 2002). In an interesting study published in the journal *Clinical and Experimental Pharmacology and Physiology*, Pon Babu and colleagues established the ability of green tea extract to inhibit the formation of advanced glycation end products, inhibit protein denaturation (as indicated by collagen cross-linkage), inhibit oxidative damage, and improve antioxidant status in animals with experimentally induced diabetes (Babu PV et al. 2006). Though this study did not investigate the mechanism(s) by which tea inhibited glycation and preserved protein integrity, it is worth noting that the researchers' administration of green tea extract was found to reduce plasma glucose concentration by more than 50%. Such substantial suppression of circulating glucose is undoubtedly an important factor in averting glycative damage. Similarly, the experimentally confirmed anti-glycative effect of ginseng (*P. quinquefolius*, specifically) is likely attributable to its suppression of serum glucose (Vuksan V et al. 2000 A; Vuksan V et al. 2000 B). This inhibitory effect on glycemia cannot be the sole mechanism via which ginseng attenuates glycation, however, as it has been demonstrated that ginseng disrupts glycation *in vitro*, under conditions wherein glucose concentration is invariant (Bae and Lee 2004). Hence, the tea component of the Amen Fast is efficacious in averting glycation in at least two distinct ways: by reducing glucose levels and by directly disrupting the interaction of glucose and proteins. At this juncture, it should be noted that a relationship exists between glycation and oxidation and that antioxidative mechanisms are implicated in the suppression of glucose-mediated protein damage. I shall have more to say about the relationship between glycation and oxidation and the mitigation thereof in the ensuing section on diet.

Caloric restriction has been found to exert a more marked inhibitory effect on insulin concentration than on glucose concentration. This insulin-inhibiting effect is thought to be an important factor in CR-mediated lifespan extension. Support for this supposition is supplied by studies involving genetic manipulation of insulin signaling. Of these studies, the one that entailed abolishment of insulin receptors on the surfaces of adipocytes is most intriguing.

Conducted by Matthias Blüher and colleagues, the study published in the journal *Science* found that selective extirpation of insulin receptors on murine adipocytes resulted in reduced bodyweight (15-25%), reduced body fat (50-70%), increased average lifespan (~20%) and increased maximum lifespan (~10%) (Blüher M et al. 2003). That this lengthening of lifespan occurred in the absence of appreciable caloric restriction is well worth noting for it would seem to reveal an independent ameliorative effect of hypoinsulinemia in attenuating aging and adiposity. As to the relationship between insulin and fat deposition, it should be recalled that insulin facilitates entry of glucose into adipocytes and this glucose serves as a substrate for the synthesis of fatty acids and glycerol, the chemical constituents of fat (Guyton and Hall 2000). The chief elicitor of insulin secretion is glucose and glucose is reduced to basal levels in the fasted state. The daily, durative fast prescribed by the Amen Protocol ensures minimal insulin availability, inhibits adiposity and may accordingly augment longevity independently of quantitative CR. Suppressed secretion of insulin may also attenuate aging by promoting enhanced *autophagy*. Autophagy is the process whereby cellular components—protienaceous and membranous—are degraded, yielding simpler macromolecules to be used in the synthesis of new cellular structures. The decline in this process likely eventuates in the accumulation of damaged, dysfunctional membranes and proteins—defining features of aging. Caloric restriction retards this process and the mechanism by which it does so involves inhibition of insulin. As to why this is so, it should be considered that a principle purpose of autophagy is to convert structural molecules into energy substrates during periods of prolonged food deprivation. Food deprivation depresses insulin secretion and, by so doing, augments autophagy. In an illuminative study conducted by researchers from Italy's *Universita di Pisà*, it was found that a single weekly bout of fasting, combined with a single weekly administration of an insulin-inhibiting, 'gluco-suppressant' drug (*3,5-dimethylpyrazole*, DMP), was sufficient to induce an autophagic response in rats comparable to the standard CR protocol of intermittent feeding (Donati A et al. 2004). Weekly fasting alone, however, was inefficacious in optimizing autophagy while cyclic, intermittent fasting was efficacious. This may point to the necessitation of a minimal requisite level of hypoinsulinemia/hypoglycemia above which autophagy will not be enhanced. The drug DMP apparently enhanced the insulin-inhibiting effect of weekly fasting in such a way that exceeded this threshold. Importantly, the attendant augmentation of autophagy occurred in the absence of appreciable caloric restriction and, as such, suggests an additional avenue conducive to selective synergy. That is, because the autophagic induction effectuated by CR is contingent upon curtailment of glucose and insulin, additional measures which modulate the levels of these molecules may augment autophagy even more and, accordingly, repress aging more robustly. Such measures include employment of insulin/gluco-suppressant agents and prolonged, cyclic phases of fasting of the sort prescribed by the Amen Protocol. Indeed, CR-mediated induction of autophagy was attributed to the protracted phases of fasting characteristic of quantitative CR. As explained by the Italian investigators:

> This report may indicate that both frequency and level of hypoinsulinemia may affect the rate of aging: the anti-aging effects of caloric restriction decreased with the decrease in the frequency of fasting, but were restored if level of lower-frequency hypoinsulinemia were further decreased by the administration of [DMP]. (Donati A et al. 2004: 1066)

Hypothetically, I posit that daily, cyclic fasting intervals (of the Amen ilk) ought to optimize autophagy beyond that induced by quantitative CR or intermittent CR. Moreover, the addition of 'gluco-suppressant' substances such as *Camellia senensis* and *Panax quinquefolius* should, theoretically, augment this autophagic effect even more appreciably.

Maintenance of genomic integrity is thought to be another important factor in CR-mediated lifespan extension. One mechanism by which genomic integrity is ensured is through a process termed silencing. In humans and other multicellular organisms, protein molecules called histones enmesh DNA in such a way as to render it inaccessible to polymerases and thereby transcriptionally "silent." Transcriptional silence is a state wherein a particular gene is not being transcribed, wherein a messenger RNA molecule is not being manufactured, wherein a protein product is not being produced. In any given cell, the vast majority of genes comprising the genome are not typically transcribed—that is, the majority of the genome is in a chemically quiescent, silent state. Silencing certain segments of the genome is indeed essential for cell specialization. The mechanism by which histones inhibit transcription involves structural modifications of the amino acid constituents of histone subunits that, in turn, modulate the manner in which histones link together and to DNA. When histone proteins are replete with *acetyl* groups they bind loosely to each other and to adjacent DNA segments. Conversely, when histone proteins are depleted of acetyl groups, they bind more tightly to each other, enmeshing DNA more thoroughly. Specific enzymes regulate genome silencing and activation by alternatively adding and removing acetyl groups from histones and accordingly altering histone binding affinity—respectively, histone acetyl transferases (HATs) and histone deacetylases (HDACs). While both are of obvious physiological import, it is the latter of the two that shall occupy our attention presently. The major point of the preceding introductory exposition is the following: HDACs lengthen lifespan by silencing segments of the genome and caloric restriction appreciably augments deacetylase activity and, as such, subserves silencing. In fact, it seems that significant, systematic silencing of the genome is essential for ensuring longevity. Before we consider the relevant scientific data, however, let us attempt to ascertain the theoretical underpinnings of this revelation. It should be noted that gene transcription is an energy intensive affair. The transcription of a messenger RNA molecule from a DNA template requires energy, as does the translation of a messenger RNA molecule into a protein product. Transcription of genes encoding unneeded proteins is therefore energetically wasteful and it seems reasonable to assume that processes which squander energy inevitably squander vitality and limit longevity. It should also be noted that DNA is subject to damage by oxidative, glycative and other genotoxic agents and the binding of histone proteins probably provides a measure of physical protection from these malevolent molecules. Finally, it should be appreciated that the very process of gene transcription inevitably results in the production of proteins that are deranged due to transcriptional error, due to non-erroneous transcription of genes that are themselves mutated, or due to mis-incorporation of amino acids during translational protein production. Thus, the more a gene is transcribed, the more likely it is to produce a dysfunctional protein product, and dysfunctional proteins are defining features of disease and degeneration. Ostensibly, errors in transcription and translation are especially deleterious to tissues (i.e. brain and muscle) whose cells are not routinely replicated and must be continually reconstituted through protein renewal. Perhaps tightly bound histone proteins protect the genome by inhibiting oxidative, glycative and genotoxic damage and by inhibiting unnecessary, energy-intensive production of proteins, a portion of which would be inevitably dysfunctional and therefore detrimental to the physiological integrity of the organism. Considering these points, we may be in a better position to understand the findings of several momentous investigations exemplifying the import of genome silencing in lifespan prolongation. In a seminal study of the sort, published in the journal *Nature*, it was found that an extra copy of the SIR2 gene significantly extended the lifespan of a multicellular eukaryotic organism, *Caenorhabditis elegans*, by 50% (Tissenbaum and Guarente 2001). SIR2 is one member of a family of genes that encode histone deacetylases (specifically *sirtuin* proteins), which augment histone-DNA binding affinity and consequently ensure genome silencing. Humans and other mammals reportedly possess seven distinct genes homologous to SIR2. Interestingly, these genes are common to all multicellular animals, yeast, and even bacteria, illustrating the ubiquity, antiquity, and centrality of this pathway to aging (Blander and Guarente 2004). Several studies indicate that caloric restriction increases the kinetic activity of sirtuin proteins (or <u>s</u>ilent <u>i</u>nformation <u>r</u>egulatory proteins, sir), thereby facilitating increased deacetylation of histone proteins and enhanced genome silencing (Masoro EJ 2004). Enhancement of histone binding is not, however, the only means by which histone deacetylase enzymes are thought to influence longevity. It has been experimentally established that sirtuins are able to avert adiposity by inhibiting the accumulation of fat by adipocytes. In a study published in *Nature*, it was found that a specific histone deacetylase expressed in mammals (sirt1) interferes with the differentiation of fibroblasts into adipocytes and inhibits adipogenesis (fat synthesis) by differentiated adipocytes (Picard F et al. 2004). The manner in which sirtuins exert this anti-adipogenic effect is by binding directly to regulatory regions of DNA that dictate fat deposition. One such adipogenic regulatory region is the *peroxisome proliferator-activated receptor gamma 2* (PPAR-γ 2), which stimulates differentiation of fat cells and modulates their metabolism of lipids (Tontonoz P et al. 1994). As it were, sirt1 binds to the same segment of DNA as PPAR-γ 2 but its effect is inhibitory instead of excitatory. Frédérick Picard and his colleagues conducted an *in vitro* experiment with murine fibroblast cells, which entailed genetic augmentation of sirtuin expression. They found that such cells exhibited far less fat accumulation. In a separate segment of their investigation, Picard's team exposed differentiated adipocytes to the sirtuin-stimulating substance, *resveratrol*. Resveratrol is a polyphenol phytoalexin present in peanuts, grapes, and other plants and its application to the fibroblast medium resulted in a significant increase in sirt1 and a consequent inhibition of adipogenesis. In yet another intriguing aspect of their investigation, they assessed the ability of food deprivation to alter sirtuin expression and adipocyte activity. After subjecting mice to an overnight fast, they found that the food-deprived mice exhibited robust binding of sirt1 to PPAR-γ 2 promoter sequences on the DNA molecule whereas non-fasted mice exhibited no such binding of sirt1. In effect, fasting specifically induced binding of sirtuins to DNA regulatory domains that, in turn, modulated fat metabolism. The synopsis of the investigators is as follows:

> As yeast Sir2 is important during calorie restriction, we assayed…the recruitment of Sirt1 to PPAR-γ-binding sites in the aP2 and PPAR-γ promoters in [adipose tissue] of mice that were either fed or fasted. In mice fed *ad libitum*, Sirt1 was not bound to aP2 or

PPAR-γ promoter sequences. However, Sirt1 was bound to these sequences after overnight food deprivation, showing that Sirt1 is recruited to PPAR-γ DNA-binding sites upon fasting. (Picard F et al. 2004: 773)

The most interesting aspect of this finding is its bimodal relationship to caloric restriction. It is bimodal in that both fasting and caloric restriction effectuate increased oxidation of fat and both fasting and caloric restriction increase sirtuin expression, activation, and/or binding and this effect, in turn, influences fat metabolism. There is, as previously cited, evidence that reduction of fat deposition in the body has a moderate, yet significant, positive effect on maximum lifespan (Blüher M et al. 2003). It was speculatively suggested that this might be attributable to the fact that fat is something of a toxic reservoir, enabling the accretion of carcinogenic chemicals and other noxious agents. Elimination of excess fat might therefore augment longevity by lessening exposure to life-threatening toxins. An alternative explanation is that fat may merely serve as a signal of energy repletion and that energy repletion, in turn, automatically abrogates myriad longevity-promoting processes in the body, including genome silencing. Determining the degree of fat deposition is not the only means by which the body assesses energy status however. Interestingly, NAD is reportedly an essential catalytic component of sirtuin proteins, which serves to increase the rapidity of the histone deacetylase reaction whereas NADH inhibits the kinetic activity thereof (Lin SJ et al. 2004). Thus, when energy is abundant, NADH abounds because copious quantities of hydrogen is extracted from food and channeled into the 'hydrogen harborer', NADH. Conversely, when energy is limited, NAD abounds because insufficient hydrogen is available to "reduce" and reconstitute NADH. Ultimately NAD activates and NADH inhibits genome silencing. This serves as another illuminating example of the manner in which energy deficiency (signaled in this instance by NAD) induces a physiological response that results in the preservation of physiological function and consequent augmentation of longevity. I shall reiterate the evolutionarily informed reasoning advanced previously that organisms seem to exhibit conserved mechanisms that conspire to preserve physiological functioning on a molecular level under conditions of food scarcity in order to maximize survival until such time as the prevailing caloric crisis subsides. NADH, a molecule sensitive to energy fluctuations, should be expected to serve as a metabolic signal. It is therefore not surprising that CR reduces NADH and therefore reduces the inhibitory effect of this molecule on sirtuin-mediated histone deacetylation (Lin SJ et al. 2004). Fasting also substantially suppresses NADH concentration and concomitantly increases sirtuin concentration. In an intriguing study published in the journal *Nature*, researchers from Johns Hopkins School of Medicine, in collaboration with scientists from Harvard Medical School, investigated alterations in sirtuin signaling in response to fasting. Upon subjecting mice to a 24-hour fast, hepatic NAD concentration was increased, NADH concentration was decreased, and the level of the sirtuin protein, sirt1, was elevated ~2.5 times relative to freely fed controls (Rodgers JT et al. 2005). When fasted animals were fed after their daylong bout of food deprivation, the level of sirtuin proteins produced by hepatocytes declined to libitum levels. This alternately inducing and repressing effect of fasting and feeding on hepatic histone deacetylase levels is mediated in part by glucose. The investigators found that elevated concentrations of glucose caused a marked decrease in sirtuin production. This illustrates the role of fasting in facilitating DNA defense through sirtuin-mediated genome silencing. Elevated glucose suppresses sirtuin synthesis similar to the way in which eating inhibits autophagy. It is interesting to note that the reduction in sirtuin production prompted by eating ensued over an interval of 24 hours—that is, animals were allowed to feed freely for a day, after which their concentration of sirt1 was assayed and found to be approximately equivalent to their continuously fed counterparts. This finding has implications for the Amen Protocol. Because the Amen Fast entails a 23-hour interval of food deprivation followed by a feeding interval of 1 hour, it is likely that sirtuin production remains substantially elevated without exhibiting a gradual reduction resulting from prolonged, multi-meal feeding as evidenced in the aforementioned experiment. It should also be stressed that the Amen Diet entails substantial caloric restriction and CR induces elevated sirtuin production even in the absence of complete food deprivation. This illustrates another instance of potential synergism—caloric restriction and cyclic fasting conceivably combine to cause copious production of sirtuin proteins.

Considering the centrality of complex cognition in human civilization, it is understandable why intellectual acumen is among the most coveted, quintessentially human, commodities. Intelligence is undoubtedly influenced by genetic endowment and by environmental conditions prevailing during neurological development. It is clear, moreover, that diet is an important factor influencing neurological function and mental acuity. It may seem superficially counterintuitive that dietary diminution can exert ameliorative effects on the brain—an organ so demanding of energy and metabolic resources—but the beneficial effects of caloric restriction on the brain are well documented (Mattson MP et al. 2003; Lee J et al. 2002; Dubey A et al. 1996; Gould TJ et al. 1995). We shall begin our discussion of CR-induced augmentation of neural function with an important study by Susumo Ando and colleagues. Before commencing with the explication and interpretation of this study, however, it is worth noting that neurons are primarily postmitotic, that once brain development ceases, new neurons are not normally generated. Thus, neurons must maintain their integrity throughout the lifespan of the individual. Considering, as we have, that the tissues of the body are incessantly bombarded with oxidative and glycative assaults, it is imperative that the brain possess some means by which to *renew*, if not replace, its neurons. Of particular importance to the maintenance of neural integrity is the renewal of neural membranes—membranes being the sites of synaptic synchronization. The study in question found that caloric restriction (70% of *ad libitum*) significantly accelerated the rate of renewal of protienaceous synaptic components as exemplified by analysis of a major synaptic protein, *synaptophysin* (Ando S et al. 2002). Synaptic membranes are sites of vigorous metabolic activity and, as such, are subject to more rampant, radical-induced damage. Hence, the principal means by which CR preserves cognitive capacity involve mitigation of membrane damage and rapid renewal of synaptic membranes to redress damage inevitably incurred. This finding comports with the consistently documented effect of CR on tissue renewal in other (non-neural) regions of the body (Spindler SR 2001). This study simply extends the renovative, rejuvenative effect of CR to the brain. Of particular importance is the demonstration that CR protects synapses from oxidative and 'toxicative' damage. This is indeed what Zhi Hong Guo and his colleagues found. Upon exposing restricted and replete rodents to oxidative and metabolic toxins—iron, *amyloid beta*, and *3-nitroproprionic acid*—the investigators noted the following:

> Cortical synaptosomes from [restricted] rats were more resistant to dysfunction caused by oxidative and metabolic insults than were synaptosomes from rats fed ad libitum…The mechanism whereby the three different insults impair [metabolic function] involves oxidative stress and membrane lipid peroxidation, suggesting that [CR] lessens the impact of such oxidative insults on synaptic function. (Guo Z et al. 2000: 319)

This effect of caloric restriction on synaptic membrane renewal also sheds some light on the efficacy of CR in the augmentation of mental acuity. It should be noted that impulse transmission in the brain is contingent upon release and recognition of neurotransmitters and that such recognition requires receptors. Receptors are embedded in neural membranes. Consequently, rapid renewal of synaptic membranes (and the receptors embedded therein) expectedly exerts an effect on neurotransmission and, by extension, on cognition. One type of receptor—the *NMDA receptor*—is especially important in the molecular mediation of memory. NMDA receptors modulate an electrochemical stimulatory sequence called *long-term potentiation* (LTP). The term "long term potentiation" is instructive because the particular pattern indicative thereof causes a stereotypic alteration of synaptic and neural function that persists from minutes to hours, modifying the cell's response to subsequent stimuli. From a cellular perspective, such a mechanism seems suited to the task of encoding memories and subserving learning—namely, a mechanism that modifies the behavior of neurons for a lengthy period and primes them for future activity. The matter is not purely speculative. Studies have demonstrated that chemical or electrical interventions that specifically inhibit LTP also inhibit memory formation (Davis S et al. 1992). What is more, aged animals with memory impairments have been shown to exhibit significant deficits in LTP and these deficits have been convincingly linked to reduced expression of NMDA receptors (Moore CI et al. 1993; Deupree DL et al. 1993). Clearly, LTP and the receptors which mediate it are operative in learning and memory. Interestingly, CR has been shown to attenuate both age-related deficits in memory and age-related declines in NMDA receptor expression (Eckles-Smith K et al. 2000). Whether or not LTP and NMDA reception are the principal molecular means by which learning and memory are modulated, they are of probable import and the heightened cognitive capacity of CR subjects may be partly attributable to selective modification of these specific mechanisms.

Another way in which CR might augment mental acuity is via selective elevation of *neurotrophic factors*. Neurotrophic factors are vital to the growth, survival, and maintenance of neurons in both the central and peripheral nervous system. Several intriguing studies have demonstrated that CR results in a significant increase in the genetic expression of such neurotrophic factors as *brain-derived neurotrophic factor* (BDNF), *glial-derived neurotrophic factor* (GDNF) and *neurotrophin-3* (NT-3). As stated previously, most regions of the adult brain are not capable of growth after the completion of differentiation. An important exception to this is a region of the *archaecortex* called the hippocampus. The hippocampus plays a central role in the storage, processing, and retrieval of memory and is accordingly operative in learning. Populations of neurons within the hippocampus are capable of growth and differentiation throughout the lifespan and these newly generated neurons are thought to play a crucial role in facilitating learning and memory formation, especially in response to novel experimental/environmental conditions. Investigators Jaewon Lee and colleagues give a lucid synopsis of this fascinating line of research in a paper presented in *The Journal of Neurochemistry*:

> The adult brain contains small populations of neural precursor cells (NPC) that can give rise to new neurons and glia (neural support cells), and may play important roles in learning and memory, and recovery from injury. Growth factors can influence the proliferation, differentiation and survival of NPC, and may mediate responses of NPC to injury and environmental stimuli such as enriched environments and physical activity. We now report that neurotrophin expression and neurogenesis can be modified by a change in diet. When adult mice are maintained on a dietary restriction (DR) feeding regimen, numbers of newly generated cells in...the hippocampus are increased, apparently as the result of increased cell survival. (Lee J et al. 2002: 539)

This study indicates that caloric restriction can alter the morphology of the adult brain by promoting the preservation of particular neurons, specifically in a region of the brain that plays a pivotal role in cognition. As the investigators correctly conjecture, the results of this study have important implications not only for the enhancement of learning but, more momentously, for the mitigation of memory-impairing neurological disorders.

Principal investigator Wenzhen Duan and colleagues carried out a striking demonstration of the protective effect of neurotrophin elevation. The researchers subjected a group of rodents to a 30-40% CR protocol for a period of only 3 months. This regimen, though brief, resulted in a substantial increase in BDNF in several regions of the brain—a 50% increase in the hippocampus, a 60% increase in the striatum, and a 40% increase in the cerebral cortex. They then subjected this experimental group of animals and a paired group of freely fed animals to intra-cranial injections of a highly toxic agent (*kanaic acid*) known to induce seizures and rampant destruction of nerve cells. They found that those animals subjected to the CR regimen exhibited far less neural loss (Duan W et al. 2001).

Aside from inducing neural proliferation in the hippocampus, neurotrophins exert a pronounced trophic effect on synapses and promote plasticity. An intriguing review by Kiyofumi Yamada and colleagues presented in the journal *Life Sciences* delineated the results of several studies establishing the efficacy of BDNF in synaptogenesis. Their synopsis is as follows:

> In addition to its actions on neuronal survival and differentiation, brain-derived neurotrophic factor (BDNF) has a role in the regulation of synaptic strength...BDNF also influences the development of patterned connections and the growth and complexity of dendrites in the cerebral cortex. These results suggest a role for BDNF in learning and memory processes, since memory acquisition is considered to involve both short-term changes in electrical properties and long-term structural alterations in synapses. Memory acquisition is associated with an increase in BDNF [expression]...(Yamada K et al. 2002: 735)

As this study indicates, BDNF plays a prominent role in dendrite ramification. Therefore, measures such as CR, which result in substantial elevation of BDNF and other neurotrophic factors, can be expected to result in increased dendritic ramification and, concomitantly, increased synaptic complexity. Synaptic complexity is thought to be a direct morphological correlate of intelligence and an increase in synaptic complexity as actuated by CR may be a proximate prelude to increased cognitive complexity. In keeping with the theme of selective synergism, it bears mentioning that neuroprotective effects attributed to CR occur with and without quantitative deficits in caloric intake. More explicitly, it has been found that intermittent CR (i.e., temporal caloric restriction) is efficacious in augmenting expression of neurotrophic factors, promoting proliferation of neural precursor cells, inhibiting neurotoxic insults and improving cognitive acuity (Lee J et al., 2002). This would seem to suggest that the state of dietary deprivation serves as a sort of signal, the reception of which elicits elaboration of neurotrophic agents. Support for this conjecture is provided by an important study published in *Nature Neuroscience*. The investigators found that a particular peptide—ghrelin—released by the gastrointestinal tract under fasting conditions, binds to receptors in the hippocampus and modulates the memory functions of this neurologic structure. In their well-reasoned discussion, investigator Sabrina Diano and colleagues offered the intuitive teleological idea that in a naturalistic context, hunger ought to encourage exploratory, food-seeking behavior—behavior that is buttressed by brain complexity and plasticity. In their words:

> ...[A] great number of cognitive tests on laboratory rodents and nonhuman primates are carried out after food deprivation or fasting, metabolic states that are paralleled by elevated levels of ghrelin. The notion that spatial learning and unfocused attention would be enhanced during fasting is...in line with the necessity of an animal that is in a negative energy balance to identify and locate energy sources in order to survive. (Diano S et al. 2006: 385)

Because ghrelin concentration correlates with the duration of dietary deprivation, the lengthy phases of fasting characteristic of the Amen Protocol ostensibly ensure high levels of this memory-modulating peptide. Conversely, because eating inhibits ghrelin release, feeding multiple times per day would seem to compromise cognitive function. Feeding, digestion, assimilation and evacuation are energy-intensive activities and to the extent that the Amen Protocol prescribes a single session of feeding, restricted to the nocturnal period, mental productivity is probably promoted thereby.

Elements of the Amen Diet

A theoretically formulated dietary protocol founded upon sound science and pursuant of optimal health and longevity must address itself to three important parameters—temporal, qualitative, and quantitative. That is, consideration must be given to the frequency with which feeding should ensue, the quantity of calories deemed nutritionally necessitous, and the qualitative character of the food so consumed. Having addressed the temporal factor, I am left to elucidate the latter two. I shall begin this segment by considering quality and end by considering quantity. Succinctly, the qualitative constitution of the diet is exclusively vegetal, low in fat and protein and replete with antioxidants, detoxicants and agents that ostensibly enhance genomic stability. The centrality of vegetation warrants some elaboration. In the book *Evolutionary Nutrition*, I delineate numerous deleterious consequences of meat consumption and argue that animal products must be excluded from any prudent human diet predicated on principles of optimal health (Amen-Ra N 2003). On the basis of certain considerations germane to the evolutionary origins of our species and the consequent phenotypic and physiological attributes molded thereby, I argue that *Homo sapiens* are constitutionally configured in such a way as to make habitual meat consumption detrimental to human health. I shall not recapitulate all of the arguments presented therein but I should like to reiterate (without exhaustive exposition) some salient corollaries of carnivory:

> Because meat is calorically dense (relative to vegetation), its consumption conduces to obesity, which in turn, is a facilitator of myriad maladies.

> Because meat is the *sole* source of exogenous (dietary) cholesterol and because cholesterol accretion is a predisposing factor in the etiology of such ailments as cardiovascular disease, cerebrovascular disease, and dementia (i.e. Alzheimer's disease), meat consumption potentiates these pathologies.

> Because ingested protein is toxic in excessive amounts (especially to the liver and kidneys), and because meat is relatively replete with protein, many disorders likely originate from the toxic effects of animal proteins on the body's major organs of detoxification and elimination.

> Because cooked foods generate harmful *glyco*toxins, because meat provides a better substrate for the generation of such toxins, and because meat, unlike vegetation, is invariably cooked, meat tends to toxify the body's tissues.

> Because cooked foods generate harmful *geno*toxins, because meat provides a better substrate for the generation of these toxins, and because meat, unlike vegetation, is invariably cooked, meat consumption can compromise the integrity of the genome (Cross AJ et al. 2005).

> Because the most deleterious toxins tend to be lipophylic and because animals abound in adipose, toxins tend to accumulate in the fatty tissues of animals. Ingesting the tissues and exudates (i.e. milk) of such toxin-tainted organisms may adversely affect human health.

> Because particular proteins predominant in meat elicit excessive acidification of the body's tissues and because constituents of muscle and bone are used to neutralize such acidic metabolites, consumption of animal products may promote progressive deterioration of the musculoskeletal system (Alpern and Sakhaee 1997).

> Because particular proteins predominant in meat elicit excessive production of the peptide insulin-like growth factor I (IGF-I), and because this agent is implicated in the pathogenesis of such scourges as cancer and cardiovascular disease, animal products are thereby implicated in their etiology (Allen NE et al. 2002).

> Because excessive secretion of bile is a predisposing factor in the etiology of colorectal cancer and because high-fat animal products are potent bile *secretagogues* (secretion-

inducing agents), consumption of animal products conduces to colorectal cancer (Amen-Ra N 2003).

Because consumption of animal products promotes excessive secretion of bile, because excessive bile facilitates heightened retention of steroidal sex hormones (e.g. estrogen and testosterone), and because excessive quantities of these hormones factor in the etiology of such malignancies as breast cancer, endometrial cancer, ovarian cancer, and prostate cancer, carnivory conduces to cancers of the female and male genital systems and accessory sex organs whose physiology is regulated by sex hormones (Amen-Ra N 2003).

Thus, meat consumption is dietetically incompatible with any conceivable optimal health regimen. Conversely, vegetal products have a nutritional/chemical profile that is diametrically different from that of meat. Consider the following:

Vegetation is calorically incopious and, consequently, less conducive to obesity.

Vegetation is comparatively low in protein and, consequently, does not tax the body's organs of detoxification to the same extent as animal products.

Vegetation is devoid of cardio-toxic cholesterol and, as such, less likely to precipitate angiopathy.

Plant products prominently featured in the Amen Diet (e.g. barley, soybean, ginseng, and green tea) inhibit hypercholesterolemia.

Specific vegetal products (e.g., barley) induce epigenetic modifications (i.e. I-compounds) that protect the genome from deleterious mutations, inhibit carcinogenesis and promote longevity. These protective epigenetic modifications are also induced by caloric restriction and, most appreciably, by fasting (Zhou GD et al. 1999; Li D et al. 1992; Randerath K et al. 1990).

Specific compounds in vegetal products (i.e. resveratrol and lunasin) induce alterations in the histone proteins associated with DNA. These alterations modify gene expression and subserve genome silencing. In some organisms, such histone-mediated alterations result in lifespan prolongation and inhibition of carcinogenesis.

Specific compounds in vegetal products (e.g., broccoli) induce increased expression of hepatic enzymes (i.e. Phase II or xenobiotic enzymes), which play pivotal roles in systemic detoxification.

Specific compounds in vegetal products (e.g., barley beta-glucan) augment immune function by modulating the manufacture or activity of protective immunologic agents (Yan J et al. 1999).

Thus, diets centered on vegetation are, in general, more compatible with caloric restriction and more facilitative of optimal health.

The issue of energetics is important in evaluating the anti-aging effects of caloric restriction. CR subjects exhibit physiological advantages compared to their freely fed counterparts. That these advantages, which eventuate in extended longevity, occur amidst energy restriction warrants reflection. To function better despite deficits in energy intake implies *improved efficiency*. A major consequence of such improved efficiency is the ability to allocate energy preferentially to processes that preserve physiologic integrity. As intimated earlier, it requires copious amounts of energy to degrade and renew proteins more rapidly, repair DNA damage more readily, produce abundant antioxidant and 'detoxicant' enzymes and augment neurological function via enhanced expression of neurotrophic factors—all effects ascribed to CR. Thus, if the calories one ingests remain constant amidst such ameliorative energy expenditures or if one's allotted rations are reduced, there must necessarily be some compensatory metabolic alteration, a sacrifice of something superfluous. Growth, body mass maintenance, proliferation of somatic cells, thermogenesis and sexual receptivity are all candidates for selective suppression due to their comparative superfluity under conditions of caloric curtailment. As noted previously, the manner in which organisms adapt metabolically to dietary deficits is complex and equivocal and studies have hitherto shed little light on the matter. In the absence of definitive data therefore, one must defer to theory and rationally based speculation. I have availed myself of these essential artifices in constructing my optimal dietary regimen. As such, a principle imperative of the Amen Diet is to promote energy efficiency by limiting metabolic waste. Central to this aim is the selection of dietary components that can be assimilated with the minimal practicable expenditure of energy—in short, the diet should be simplistic. It bears mentioning that the macromolecular constituents of food must be degraded before they can be assimilated and that digestive enzymes effect such degradation. Digestive enzymes are, however, energetically expensive. It seems reasonable to suppose that the synthesis, sequestration and secretion of pancreatic and enteric enzymes is metabolically demanding and that minimizing superfluous synthesis and secretion of these enzymes could conserve energy—energy that could alternatively be allotted to more pressing processes. Presumably, reducing the quantity of food consumed to a minimal requisite level eventuates in greater conservation of digestive enzymes. That is, by subjecting oneself to caloric restriction one may conserve digestive enzymes more appreciably. What is more, in addition to passively preserving digestive enzymes, caloric restriction actively augments assimilative capacity. This enhanced absorptive capacity induced by CR is attributable to increased enzymatic activity and elevated expression of intestinal digestive enzymes. CR-induced augmentation of assimilative enzymes enables more macromolecular nutrients to be metabolized more rapidly, more completely, and more efficiently. The increased activity of intestinal enzymes induced by CR is substantial. A study published in the *Journal of Gerontology* found enteric enzyme activity to be increased by as much as 300% by caloric restriction (Holt PR et al 1991). Evidently, caloric restriction also induces an increase in the expression of specific transport proteins that absorb nutrients from the lumenal surface of the intestines. Thus, not only are macromolecular nutrients degraded more completely and efficiently, these products are avariciously absorbed in energy-restricted states. An intriguing study published in *The American Journal of Physiology*, found that CR significantly enhanced intestinal nutrient absorption (Casirola DM et al 1996). Specifically, absorptive capacity for glucose, fructose and the amino acid proline was 80% greater in CR animals than freely fed subjects. The investigators interpreted this effect as follows:

Even though the supply of metabolizable energy is limiting for calorically restricted mice, these mice 'elect' to use whatever energy they have to adapt to caloric restriction by enhancing transport rate per unit intestinal tissue, perhaps to ensure that absorption of a limited amount of ingested nutrients is rapid and efficient. This adaptive method used by calorically restricted mice is relatively economical because it does not require synthesis of new tissue, only synthesis of more transporters inserted into similar amounts of tissue. (Casirola DM et al. 1996: G199)

It would seem that under conditions of chronic caloric restriction, a premium is placed on the ability to assimilate more of the nutrients embedded in the food one ingests. It is for this reason that the Amen Diet contains a supplemental component comprised of enzymatically hydrolyzed protein to which is added essential minerals, vitamins, fatty acids and simple sugars—all in a liquid solution. The simplicity and liquidity of the solution is intended to optimize uptake. It is plausible that increasing the area over which enzymes are resorbed increases assimilation of nutrients. Ensuring that the interior of the intestine is vacant between meals facilitates this effect. Thus, when ingested food is deposited in the small intestine, a clean lumen likely ensures that a maximal number of individual enterocytes are laden with enzymes (and their substrates) thereby facilitating absorption. An intermittent fasting phase of 23 hours ensures inter-digestive intestinal vacancy. It is also plausible that the inherent digestibility of particular foods determines the quantity of enzymes needed to effect digestion. Digestibility depends, quite probably, on the balance of enzymes and enzyme inhibitors contained in a particular food. Plants produce both enzymes and enzyme inhibitors. Presumably, the higher the ratio of enzymes to enzyme inhibitors, the more digestible a particular plant product will be, the less endogenous enzymes will be needed to effect digestion and the more energy will be conserved. The contribution of exogenous enzymes to the digestibility of particular foods may be moot however when cooked food is in question. Many enzymes incur inactivation and denaturation at cooking temperatures, loosing their catalytic capacity. Therefore, in order for vegetal enzymes to aid in the digestion of macromolecules present in plants, the vegetation must be consumed raw; hence the centrality of raw foods in the Amen Diet. Indeed, not only is the diet in consideration centered on vegetation, it is centered on germinated vegetation—that is, sprouts. The reasoning behind this is simple. We need only consider seeds. Seeds are, essentially, embryonic organisms within which concentrated proteins, carbohydrates, and fats are stored. These nutrients are embedded in seeds in order to support growth and maturation of the embryo during the initial stages of a plant's life. In the absence of water, seeds remain dormant and their stored nutrients exist in concentrated polymeric forms. Upon imbibition or exposure to water, the genome of the embryonic plant begins to actively transcribe genes necessary for the production of enzymes needed to hydrolyze polymeric molecules of protein, carbohydrate, and fat into simpler polypeptides, amino acids, sugars, and fatty acids. Germinating seeds therefore constitute a nutritious food source whose embedded nutrients are degraded into simple, easily assimilable forms. Seeds are, however, "designed" to be quiescent until conditions are suitable to support growth. This quiescence is ensured, in part, by the inactivity of genes necessary to specify the construction of hydrolytic enzymes and by various enzyme inhibitors embedded in seeds. Enzyme inhibitors ensure that enzymes do not catalyze the hydrolytic reactions necessary to initiate germination and growth until the time is right. Thus, seeds can remain quiescent for some time while maintaining their latent germinative potential. When conditions are conducive to growth, when moisture and temperature reach a requisite range, germination commences. During germination, the expression and activity of enzymes increase and greater quantities of complex nutrients are converted into their simpler precursors. The nutritional significance of this is that subsistence upon germinating plants, whose complement of enzymes have reduced their embedded nutrients into simplified forms, enables the preservation of one's own enzymes, thereby enabling the conservation of considerable quantities of energy.

The caloric cornerstone of the Amen Diet consists of barley—germinated and blended in a base of raw "soymilk". The soymilk is derived from soybeans sprouted for a 2-day period and thereafter pressed in an aqueous medium to produce a protienaceous extract. Perhaps because barley is the basis of the beer industry, its molecular machinations have been impressively elucidated for economic ends. Moreover, barley is arguably the eldest harvested grain. A paper published in the journal *Nature* provided evidence of the earliest human harvesting and processing of grain, that grain having been barley (Piperno DR et al. 2004). Because the process of artificial selection of barley ensued in the Upper Paleolithic Period (~20,000 years ago), one might expect this august grain to be benign, nutritious, and fecund—traits attractive to ancient human horticulturalists and moderns seeking a staple suitable for inclusion in an optimal human diet. Another attractive trait exhibited by barley is its inducible expression of antioxidant enzymes, especially upon exposure to oxidants. Before elaborating on this idea, I accept that the following claims are equivocal: (1) that CR increases expression of antioxidant enzymes and CR-mediated lifespan extension is partly attributable thereto and (2) that antioxidant enzymes expressed in plants can be effectively absorbed and utilized upon ingestion. Nevertheless, an important investigation illustrated the likely veracity of the former claim. The study, published in the journal *Science*, genetically altered mice in such a way that enabled them to express 50% more of the antioxidant enzyme catalase in peroxisomes, nuclei or mitochondria. This measure, they found, attenuated indices of oxidative damage and, more importantly, increased mean and maximum lifespan by ~20% (Schriner SE et al. 2005). That the amplification of a single gene product can increase mammalian lifespan to such an extent illustrates the importance of this enzyme. The leap from meticulously engineering increased expression of an antioxidant enzyme in particular organelles to increasing its amount in the body, nonspecifically, through oral intake is admittedly audacious. It is not untenable however. It has been shown that antioxidant enzymes can be appreciably absorbed, that their activity in the human body is maintained and that this activity attenuates oxidative damage. Though the efficacy of orally administered antioxidant enzymes has been evaluated and affirmed only in the case of superoxide dismutase, it is interesting to note that this enzyme was reportedly protected from proteolytic cleavage in the body by binding it to a gluten-like protein present in wheat (Vouldoukis I et al 2004). Such proteins are also present in barley and they may aid in the uptake of antioxidant enzymes. A study conducted by Jita Patra and Brahma Panda—botanists from India's Berhampur University—exposed germinating barley to hydrogen peroxide and found that it significantly increased its production of superoxide dismutase, peroxidase, catalase, glutathione, and glutathione reductase (Patra and Panda 1998). I employ a variation of this method, adding to the medium minerals known to be crucial cofactors of certain of the aforementioned enzyme isoforms. Daily ingestion of barley expressing elevated amounts of antioxidant enzymes synergizes CR-mediated suppression of free radical damage. This is what I suppositiously hypothesize.

As indicated above, the Amen Diet is centered upon *raw* vegetation. The reasons for this are manifold, though I presently intend to expound on only one—inhibition of glycation. Glycation was discussed previously in the context of fasting but it has relevance to feeding as well. Advanced glycation end products (AGEs) are formed in the body as a natural (though deleterious) consequence of circulating sugars interacting aberrantly with constitutive and catalytic proteins in the body. Of critical importance is the fact that glycation also occurs *ex vivo*, outside of the body. Cooking facilitates the formation of AGEs and it is for this reason that cooked foods ought not factor prominently in an optimal diet. Importantly, diet-derived AGEs bind to tissues in the body, exacerbating the effects of endogenous glycation. A study published in the *PNAS* found that people fed diets rich in AGEs retained a third thereof two days after ingestion (Koschinsky T et al. 1997). Clearly, the protracted presence of exogenous AGEs ensures their progressive accretion and undoubtedly inhibits the body's elimination of endogenously derived AGEs. This is indeed what was reported in a study published in the journal *Diabetes*. The investigators placed mice on two different diets, differing in AGE content by a factor of three. Over the course of four months, mice subsisting on the elevated AGE diet exhibited diminished insulin sensitivity and increased indices of diabetic damage (Hofmann SM et al. 2002). Interestingly, subjects subsisting on the elevated AGE diet exhibited increased bodyweight in the range of 10%. AGE-induced accretion of body mass occurred despite an equal intake of food between the groups. This clearly suggests sequestration of AGEs secondary to impaired detoxification and elimination. The most momentous study demonstating the deleterious nature of glycation was published in *The American Journal of Pathology*. In this experiment, investigators formulated two distinct diets, differing in detectable AGE content by a factor of two. Surprisingly, the method by which they manufactured the different diets involved a moderate manipulation of applied heat. Whereas the control diet consisted of conventional rodent chow prepared in the standard manner, the AGE-deficient chow was produced by modestly reducing the duration of heating during "pellet" production. Though composed of identical ingredients, the AGE-defficient diet had half as much glycotoxins as a result of reduced heating. Two groups of juvenile mice received equal amounts of either the standard rodent diet or the AGE-deficient diet for the duration of their lives. The result: AGE-deficient mice lived significantly longer, exhibiting a 15% increase in median lifespan and a 6% increase in maximum lifespan (Cai W et al. 2007). The significance of this study is considerable. While caloric restriction remains the most reproducible, most consistent conventional means by which to maximize mammalian lifespan, it is evidently no longer the sole means. And yet, this study, which did not entail caloric restriction, underscores the scientific utility of the CR paradigm. As indicated repeatedly, AGE inhibition is thought to be operavtive in CR-mediated lifespan prolongation. This investigation simply isolates an independent variable involved in dietetic modulation of senescence and establishes the acceleration of aging by AGEs. Additionally, this study accords with the imperatives of selective synergism. Because it is now known that AGE inhibition exerts an independent effect on longevity, a diet reduced in calories and AGEs may mitigate aging more appreciably than either intervention alone. Though this has not been experimentally established, it is theoretically plausible, practicable and prudent.

Another important consideration regarding dietary AGEs is their differential concentration in certain foods. Generally, animal-derived products contain higher concentrations of AGEs than vegetal products. One reason for this differential distribution of glycotoxins is attributable to the fact that the formation of AGEs entails interaction of aldehyde moieties in carbohydrate derivatives with nitrogenous moieties in proteins and polar lipids. Meat, being more replete with protein and fat, provides more molecules for attack by reactive aldehydes. A study published in the journal *Molecular Medicine* clearly demonstrated the greater glycative potential of animal products relative to vegetation. The investigators prepared foods of several types (e.g. beef, poultry, fish, vegetables, and pasta) under identical conditions and found substantially higher amounts of AGEs in animal-derived items. Moreover, in their *in vitro* analyses, they found that the animal-derived AGEs significantly increased indices of inflammation, catalyzed pervasive protein cross-links, and induced marked depletion of glutathione—a tripeptide instrumental in attenuating glycation (Cai W et al. 2002). Helen Vlassara and colleagues conducted a broader analysis of dietary glycotoxins. These investigators studied the effects of dietary AGEs in individuals with diabetes and noted the following:

> Based on testing of >200 common foods…several patterns emerged. Food from animal sources that were high in protein and lipid content (meat, cheese, and egg yolks) had the highest values of either CML or MG derivatives [indices of glycative potential] and the highest prooxidant, cell-activating potency. (Vlassara H et al. 2002: 15598)

The abundance of AGEs in flesh factors in my eschewal thereof and further necessitates its exclusion from a theoretically optimal diet. Conversely, certain plants contain chemicals that inhibit glycation. Among such anti-glycative agents is the aforementioned glutathione, a peptide present in barley. Importantly, barley's production of glutathione can be appreciably augmented by exposure to oxidants (Patra and Panda 1998). A clear demonstration of the efficacy of glutathione in inhibiting glycation is afforded by a study published in the *American Journal of Physiology: Cell Physiology*. The investigators incubated isolated, functional muscle tissue in glucose-rich media and observed its effects on measures of muscle contractility. They found that the glycative damage induced by elevated glucose diminished muscle motility and that this effect was altogether abolished by glutathione (Ramamurthy B et al. 2002). The experimental confirmation of glutathione's antiglycative potential factors in my inclusion of sprouted barley in the Amen Diet. It bears mentioning, however, that the Amen Diet is not entirely raw. Specifically, the saporal segment consists of baked bread, a product known to contain AGEs. To offset the potential dietary detriments of bread-borne AGEs, I add anti-glycative agents to the whole grain flour. As discussed previously, green tea and ginseng act as AGE inhibitors. Five grams of each powdered product are mixed with the dough before baking. This measure likely lessens the load of glycotoxins in bread, enhancing the nutritional profile of a perennial staple of the human diet.

Our bodies are continually exposed to environmental toxins that infiltrate our organs, tissues, cells, and molecules. Certainly, it is possible to lessen exposure to toxic agents by limiting one's consumption of foods and products known to contain noxious compounds. We are, however, exposed to toxins whose environmental ubiquity is such that they cannot be practically avoided. Such agents as industrial pollutants, airborne emissions from fuel combustion, and multifarious fertilizers, pesticides and herbicides foul the land, air, and water of the ecosphere. To what extent this incessant exposure to toxic chemicals contributes to disease and premature death we cannot be sure. We are, it seems, at the mercy of modernity. Yet, our apparent powerlessness in the face of industrial intransigence is not total. Fortunately, we possess chemical armamentaria exquisitely equipped to confer protection against exogenous environmental toxins that inevitably enter our bodies. The liver and its panoply of detoxifying enzymes is the body's principal protector against toxins of all types. It is the job of the liver to convert toxic chemical compounds into innocuous agents that can be effectively attenuated and excreted. However, the detoxifying capacity of the liver (and the excretory capacity of the kidneys) is limited. Toxins take their toll over time, eventually overcoming our innate defenses. This process, though ultimately ineluctable, is at least 'modulable'. Given what we know about the capacity of caloric restriction to augment longevity and preserve physiologic function, it is not entirely surprising that this restrictive regimen increases expression of hepatic detoxifying enzymes (Leakey JA 1989 A and B). This increased expression of detoxifying enzymes, also called Phase I and II enzymes, enables CR subjects to withstand substantially larger doses of toxins for prolonged periods. Quite probably, the documented cancer-preventing ability of CR is attributable largely to its enhancement of hepatic detoxification enzymes. In addition to CR, certain chemicals present in plants alter expression of detoxicant enzymes advantageously. One of the most potent natural inducers of Phase II enzymes is a class of chemicals called *isothiocyanates*. Plentiful in cruciferous vegetables such a broccoli, the parent compounds of isothiocyanates (*glucosinolates*) decrease during development such that sprouts (~3 days old) contain upwards of 100 times the amount of mature broccoli (Fahey JW et al. 1997). As it were, a particular enzyme—*myrosinase*—is responsible for converting the inert precursors in the immature plant into the active inducers, isothiocyanates. It has been shown that thorough mastication of broccoli sprouts greatly enhances this chemical conversion. As to the effects of broccoli-borne isothiocyanates, they have been found to suppress cell proliferation and inhibit carcinogenesis in addition to inducing increased expression of detoxicant enzymes as mentioned at the outset (Tang L et al. 2006). It is worth reiterating that CR exhibits these same effects. Thus, the addition of isothiocyanates to a calorie-restricted regimen replicates and reinforces the established anti-carcinogenic, anti-proliferative, anti-toxicant effects of CR. In this context, it is worth noting that barley expresses glutathione-S-transferase, an important phase II enzyme. If this enzyme is indeed bioavailable upon ingestion, it too can complement the aforementioned effects of CR. Another agent expressed in barley is evidently available and active upon ingestion. This peptide (also present in soybeans and wheat) is known as *lunasin* (de Lumen BO 2005; Jeong HJ et al. 2002). Lunasin acts as a histone deacetylase (HDAC). To recapitulate, HDACs such as sirtuins effect genome silencing and their experimental elevation has lead to lifespan prolongation. Caloric restriction reportedly increases expression of sirtuin proteins, which, via silencing of genome segments, apparently attenuate aging. Lunasin exhibits anti-carcinogenic and anti-proliferative effects in addition to its deacetylase activity. What is more, its pharmacokinetics is understood to some degree. Reportedly, it is appreciably absorbed in the gastrointestinal tract, detectable in serum and hepatic tissue within hours, and retains its chemical activity upon assay (de Lumen BO 2005). Thus, barley, soy and wheat—staples of the Amen Diet—conceivably complement CR-mediated genome silencing and CR-mediated suppression of carcinogenesis.

Because caloric paucity is central to the Amen Diet, it is imperative that we consider what prudent dietary diminution might entail from a human perspective and how this protocol can be effectively implemented. All studies of lifelong caloric restriction have been conducted in nonhuman animals. It is therefore necessary that we extrapolate data derived from CR studies in animals to humans. The concepts of *energetic equilibrium* and *metabolic rate* are important to evaluate in this regard. Simply stated, energetic equilibrium is the state wherein the amount of energy one ingests equals the amount of energy one expends, a state wherein energy intake equals energy expenditure. In such a state of energetic equilibrium, there will be no net weight gain or loss. Thus, in order to maintain a particular weight while subsisting upon a given customary quantity of calories, one must ensure a given daily expenditure of energy. Because every metabolic reaction in the body requires an expenditure of energy, calories are being combusted even while the body is in a state of relative repose. Indeed, for sedentary people who engage in little strenuous activity, the energy expended whilst at rest constitutes the largest fraction of spent energy. This energy expended at rest or whilst engaging in minimal exertion is called *basal energy expenditure* or resting energy expenditure (REE) and the rate with which energy is expended under such conditions is commonly called the *basal metabolic rate* (BMR). Normally, the principal physiological factors that determine one's basal metabolic rate are bodyweight and body composition. Generally, persons of a given size and body composition expend energy under basal conditions at a given rate—that is, a given basal metabolic rate. Body composition factors into metabolic rate determination because the chief nonaqueous components of the body—protienaceous tissue and fat tissue—expend energy at different rates. Fat, the chief role of which is to serve as a source of stored energy, is less metabolically active than skeletal muscle for instance. Under normal conditions, adult animals innately equilibrate their caloric consumption with their energy expenditure, thereby maintaining a stable bodyweight. Humans, though increasingly predisposed to obesity, also exhibit an impressive degree of energetic equilibration. Quite often, this homeostatic mechanism (modulated mainly by the hypothalamus) is ultimately unable to forestall the accretion of adipose that often accompanies aging. As one biochemistry text notes:

> Between the ages of 25 and 55, the average American male gains 20 pounds, corresponding to the ingestion over this 30-year period of a few tenths of a percent more calories per day than are expended. This is remarkably precise regulation! Nevertheless, the slight imbalance in favor of weight gain may be health-threatening. Life expectancy drops when adipose tissue becomes too large a fraction of overall body mass. (Nelson and Cox 2000: 896)

This natural tendency of humans to equilibrate energetically makes metabolic rate a suitable guideline for implementing a regimen of caloric restriction. Recall that CR studies are commonly conducted with a methodology that bases the magnitude of restriction on a reference population typically permitted to feed freely. No such reference population or "control group" exists for humans. However, invoking the idea of energy equilibration and metabolic rate, one can use oneself as a reference point or "control" of sorts. One need only determine one's basal metabolic rate at the time of initiation of CR, expressed as energy (calories) per day and consume a given percentage of this computed quantity. Over a period of time, one will expectedly experience a loss of bodyweight, yet the calculated BMR need not be re-computed to reflect this loss as the extent of restriction is to be based on one's initial state of energetic equilibrium. Given a moderate degree of restriction, say 25-30%, bodyweight will eventually stabilize. Practically, it is prudent to determine a given range of "normal" (non-obese) bodyweight and body composition (i.e. ratio of lean tissue to fat tissue) and modulate one's desired degree of restriction to maintain an idealized physique. To facilitate implementation of caloric restriction, one might consider beginning with 10% CR for the first month of the protocol and increasing by 5 or 10% each successive month until one's desired degree of restriction is reached. I shall use myself as an example of this approach. Before beginning CR, I allowed my bodyweight to stabilize at a weight of 95 kg (~210 lbs), consuming a quantity of calories comparable to the estimated energy output of a normal person of this body size. [This required no considerable effort but merely observation as I was indeed in a state of energetic equilibrium for many months thitherto.] In order to determine this energy estimate, I computed my basal metabolic rate, expressed in calories per day. This quantity I calculated to be ~2100 calories per day (C/d) and I made an effort (now conscious though previously unconscious) to consume this quantity of calories for a month. Thus, for the first month—let us call this initial month of intentional energy equilibration M_0—I consumed an amount of calories theoretically equivalent to my resting energetic output. Thus, for the first month of CR *proper* (M_1), I consumed ~1900 C/d; in M_2 ~1700 C/d; in M_3 ~1500 C/d; in M_4 ~1300 C/d, and in M_5 ~1100 C/d, eventuating in my goal of 50% CR. Instructive equations have been formulated to enable the estimation of energy expenditure under resting conditions. These equations are based upon analyses of metabolic rates of groups of people using various experimental apparatuses. The equations I employ are those developed by the World Health Organization (WHO) (WHO 1985). Because body composition (and hence metabolism) is influenced by age and sex, a single, species-specific equation would introduce too much inaccuracy to be of benefit for individual analyses. As such, the WHO developed different equations for males and females and contrived multiple chronological cohorts. Featured below are the REE equations specific for the cohort 18-30 years, females and males respectively:

Females: Calories/day=14.7(W)+496

and

Males: Calories/day=15.3(W)+679

[W is weight in kilograms; 1kg~2.2lbs.]

The Amen approach approximates the design of CR studies insofar as the extent of restriction is based upon an initial referent population of people or organisms assumed to be in energy equilibrium. Again, using my own initial bodyweight (~95 kg or 210 lbs) my computed REE was ~2100 C/d. We can conceive of this measurement as the quantity of calories needed by a person of my initial size to maintain a stable bodyweight under sedentary circumstances. I call it the *comparative caloric requirement* (CCR) in order to emphasize the idea that it reflects an estimation of one's caloric requirement compared to that of a random, representative reference population. Consider the fact that I sought to subject myself to a 50% CR regimen. Accordingly, I consistently consume ~1100 calories per day. Since initiating caloric restriction, I have lost 14 kg (~30 lbs). In terms of my present CCR (~1900 C/d), I consume little more than half the calories needed by an average person of comparable weight. Clearly, the only way one could maintain a stable weight whilst subsisting on half the calories needed by an average person of equivalent weight is to incur an increase in metabolic efficiency. As noted previously, it is unlikely that absolute reductions in metabolic rate underlie the anti-aging effects of CR. It is altogether probable, however, that alterations in energy allocation, enabled by increased energy efficiency, are operative in CR-mediated lifespan prolongation. Some insight into the molecular mechanisms involved in this enhanced energy efficiency can be gleaned from a study published in *The American Journal of Physiology Endocrinology and Metabolism*. Upon subjecting a group of animals to a 40% reduction in caloric intake initiated after weaning, the investigators analyzed various genes involved in metabolism, antioxidant defense, energy production, and molecular stress response. The regimen, imposed for a period of 36 weeks, resulted in a substantial elevation of enzymes involved in energy production. As the investigators explained in their discussion:

> ...Six genes involved in energy metabolism pathways...had increased transcript levels in the skeletal muscle of [CR] rats compared with muscle of control rats. These include genes associated with mitochondrial ATP production [i.e. components of the mitochondrial electron transport chain]...The upregulation of these genes could increase the capacity and efficiency of electron transport and oxidative phosphorylation in [CR] animals. Together, these alterations in the expression of genes involved in energy metabolism and mitochondrial function would be expected to increase the skeletal muscle capacity for ATP generation in these [CR] rats. (Bevilacqua L et al. 2005: E42)

Several elements of this investigation warrant consideration. First, the analysis was confined to skeletal muscle—this makes the findings particularly pertinent, as muscle metabolism comprises a substantial proportion of total metabolic rate. Secondly, the level of energy production (as reflected in ATP content) did not differ between CR animals and the freely fed animals to which they were compared, this despite the CR animals having an energy intake 60% that of freely fed rats and a 60% difference in bodyweight. What this means is that the restricted animals were able to convert the embedded energy of a fractional quantity of food into a quantity of metabolic energy (ATP) comparable to animals consuming 40% more food. This is a clear indication of improved energy efficiency. Finally, this regimen resulted in a substantial decrease in the level of a particular mitochondrial protein known as *mitochondrial uncoupling protein 3* (UCP-3). This protein predominates in the mitochondria of muscles and is thought to permit the efflux of electrons, thereby liberating heat. CR-induced reduction of this protein may be merely incidental or it may be responsible, in part, for the reduction in body temperature that commonly accompanies chronic CR and fasting. Suppression of electron efflux ostensibly enables more efficient production of ATP. Speculatively, CR may enhance energy efficiency by concomitantly reducing electron leakage (and therefore heat dissipation) and increasing expression of enzymes involved in energy production. Again, such improved efficiency is almost certainly an important factor in the anti-aging effect of CR, though there is much more to be learned.

It should be stressed that my chosen method of determining the extent of CR differs from those routinely employed in scientific studies. While I define caloric restriction by reference to basal metabolic rate, resting energy expenditure or comparative caloric requirement, it is more typically defined simply by reference to the amount of calories consumed by a "control" population of freely fed animals. Because the bodyweights and metabolic rates of animals or people on CR typically diminishes, the stated degree of dietary diminution does not clearly reflect the metabolic alteration effected by the regimen. By expressing the degree of CR in terms of one's own initial bodyweight and the calculated metabolic rate normally exhibited by persons of that bodyweight, a better sense is given of the magnitude of metabolic alteration. At this point, something should be said about the severity of restriction recommended. Studies have shown that restrictive regimens as marginal as 10% are efficacious in increasing maximum lifespan. Indeed, in one instructive study cited previously, experimenters subjected animals to 0%, 10%, 25%, and 40% CR and determined that the largest gain in longevity occurred between 0% CR (*ad libitum*) and 10% CR, with this moderate amount of restriction effectuating a 24% increase in proportional survival over freely fed control animals (Duffy PH et al. 2001). It is clear, however, that the greater the degree of restriction (up to a certain minimal requisite caloric intake) the greater the increase in maximum longevity. In a seminal study conducted by Richard Weindruch and colleagues, several different levels of caloric restriction were similarly assessed for their effect on longevity. Whereas 25% CR resulted in a 35% increase in maximum lifespan, 65% CR resulted in a *65% increase* in maximum lifespan (Weindruch R et al. 1986). Indeed, the longest-lived decile (10%) of the 65% CR group attained an age of nearly 4 ½ years, a lifespan exceeding that of any mouse specimen of any genetic strain theretofore known. Consider the fact that a 65% increase in human maximum lifespan (using 120 years as the reference) would mean a maximum lifespan of approximately *two centuries*. While doubt remains as to whether human practitioners of CR should expect such profound prolongation of lifespan, the ambition is not at all irrational.

There is yet an alternative to calorie counting. By diminishing the duration of the feeding interval (from say 3 hours to 1 hour), one can be certain that one is prudently practicing caloric restriction without having to meticulously count calories. Clearly, limiting one's feeding to a 1-hour interval each day ensures such a substantial dietary deficit that its efficacy is indubitable. In this regard, it is important to consider that temporal CR has been found to augment lifespan irrespective of quantitative caloric intake (Goodrick CL et al. 1990). It is also important to evaluate the significance of a previously cited study published in the journal *Physiology and Behavior*, which found that effecting a one quarter reduction in food intake relative to freely fed controls (i.e. 25% CR) required feeding times ranging from 2.75-4.0 hours (Nelson and Halberg 1986). While it is difficult to project these findings to humans, it is certainly reasonable to assume that a daily feeding period limited to a single hour necessarily entails substantial caloric restriction. What is more, restricting one's feeding in this manner ensures ease of estimation if, indeed, one wishes to precisely quantify calorie consumption. Additionally, it is rather difficult to overeat given a 1-hour "window of opportunity". I am aware of people who endeavor to implement CR regimens by simply reducing the size and caloric content of the food they ingest. Such people eat every day, several times per day, while attempting to avoid eating to the point of satiety. Practically speaking, there are reasons to doubt the efficacy of this approach to CR. The most glaring reason is that it is difficult to estimate and meticulously modulate one's caloric intake when multiple meals are ingested on a daily basis. One is inclined to wonder whether such persons are in fact practicing CR or merely avoiding gluttony. It should be considered that animals seem to have an innate behavioral propensity to eat to the point of satiation when food is abundant; and for most modern humans in affluent societies, food is always abundant, even if purposely limited. If at each of one's multiple daily meals one assiduously avoids indulging to the point of satiation, one is unnecessarily battling against one's biological proclivities. This is not inherently inane; it is simply unlikely to be sustained over a lifetime. Compare the Amen Diet. Because only one meal is partaken per day over a span of only 60 minutes, one may eat to the point of satiety while subsisting on a quantity of calories that is substantially reduced. To reiterate, it is veritably impossible (indeed, uncomfortable) to overeat at a single sitting in the span of an hour, especially when the meal is entirely vegetal. Admittedly, it requires some initial psychological conditioning to fast daily for 23 hours, but this exercise in austerity has it own rewards, psychological and philosophical in nature. One need not be an ascetic, however, to assent to the principles of the Amen Protocol. A small cadre of collaborators and I have adhered to the regimen for upwards of four years without encountering any adversities, neither physiological nor psychological. In my estimation, this serves as strong support for its sustainability. Finally, an important subjective element of the Amen Diet bears mentioning. Simply put, the brevity of feeding prescribed by the protocol so appreciably augments gustatory sensation and anticipation that feeding becomes far more festive, far more indulgent. Upon adopting the regimen, one may come to appreciate the fact that feeding, for most, is merely a source of entertainment, not sustainment. Psychologically and philosophically, moreover, it is edifying to know that one is not gorging oneself daily and hourly on abundant food while millions go hungry each passing day.

Elements of the Amen Exercise Regimen

The Amen Exercise Regimen consists of a *Persistence Phase* and a *Resistance Phase*. The Persistence Phase is aerobic in nature and is executed in the morning. It ranges in duration from 30-60 minutes. Among the most important effects of the Persistence Phase is depletion of stored glycogen. Glycogen is a polymer of glucose that is stored principally in the liver and in muscle tissue. It serves as a readily available source of energy during interdigestive intervals. If excess energy is ingested, appreciable amounts will be stored as glycogen. It is important to note that the body will preferentially use glycogen at the expense of fat and protein to spare these substrates. Engaging in a bout of morning exercise effectively depletes glycogen such that the body must necessarily rely on stored fat as an energy source throughout a fast. In individuals who have attained a certain level of leanness, appreciable adipose is unavailable for oxidation after glycogen is so depleted. The body is accordingly impelled to exploit protein as a source of fuel. While such catabolism is commonly considered deleterious, it is in fact advantageous. Consider that the solid portion of the body is composed primarily of protein. Each particular protein has a finite existence, after which it is deconstructed and, subsequently, replaced in a process termed autophagy. Thus, in a manner of thinking, each individual protein has a lifespan and the age of the aggregate *proteome* (the collective corpus of constituent proteins) determines the integrity and functional capacity of the organism. Avid catabolism and replacement of proteins therefore ensures optimal physiological integrity and juvenescence. As we shall see, however, protein comprising the contractile components of muscle tissue is preferentially preserved under conditions of chronic caloric curtailment. The Amen adherent is thus able to maintain muscle while benefiting from enhanced autophagy. Finally, it must be mentioned with all due discretion that morning aerobic exercise (combined with the additive effects of vegetal nutriture and prolonged fasting) encourages elimination of excrement. I maintain that the alimentary/evacuative apparatus ought to be veritably devoid of waste during the diurnal period. This hygienic ideal is both physiologically and aesthetically expedient as the rapid expurgation of excreta lessens the time over which toxic agents are available for absorption in the distal colon.

The Resistance Phase of the regimen consists of weightlifting. Exercises are executed in a gradual manner, with the intensity of the sessions progressively increasing in accordance with increased strength, muscularity, and endurance. The sessions range in duration from 30 to 60 minutes. Ideally, workouts are conducted on six successive days (E_1-E_6), with each major muscle group exercised at least once in a given week. Each exercise is performed to the point of momentary muscle failure or fatigue. Generally, three major muscle groups are exercised each day, with three different exercises executed per body part. Repetitions range from 3-9 per set, spanning 30-90 seconds. Each exercise is segmented into three sets; sets are separated by intervals of rest spanning 30-90 seconds. Executing three sets of three exercises for three major muscle groups typically takes ~30 minutes—the customary duration of my resistance workout. E_7 is reserved for prolonged stretching, relaxation and recuperation, or other recreational activities depending on the prerogatives of the practitioner. As shall be discussed below, arduous exercise engenders oxidative damage if the resulting radicals are not suppressed by antioxidants. To this end, antioxidants are ingested before engaging in exercise. The pre-workout antioxidant preparation consists principally of the following ingredients: resveratrol, *matcha* (powdered green tea), *N-acetylcysteine*, and ginseng. These items are infused in warm water to effect extraction of their active agents. While each of the aforementioned agents exhibit antioxidant effects, available evidence indicates their effectiveness in inhibiting glycation and inflammation and augmenting detoxification, fat oxidation and genomic integrity—all imperatives pursuant to the principles of the protocol.

Whereas the main physiological goals of the Amen Exercise Regimen are to promote the maintenance of muscle and the elimination of superfluous fat, the main psychological goal of the regimen is to impose repetitive stress upon the body and mind to which the individual is conditioned to respond, eventually, with calmness, detachment, and equanimity. Though exercises are ideally executed with a maximal amount of exertion, the practitioner is encouraged to limit outward expressions of strain or excessive respiration. The mind is to be directed not merely towards the act of executing repetitious movements, but to remaining relaxed while the body is being tremendously taxed. During the brief intervals between sets, the adherent endeavors to assume a state of 'ideational inanition'—a state wherein the mind is intentionally emptied of images, ideas, and impressions to the greatest extent practicable while the muscles recuperate from momentary overload. This stoic serenity amidst self-imposed duress I term the *Yoga of Resistance*. When successfully executed, its effects can be profitably extended to every facet of one's life and, ultimately, one's death. The ability to discipline and inure the mind by subjecting the body to physical austerities was appreciated by the Ancients and is embodied in the word "ascetic", the Greek root of which is *askein*, to exercise.

The Amen Exercise Regimen is reciprocal insofar as it complements the physiologic effects of caloric restriction and CR, in turn, facilitates the attainment of its aesthetic ends. However, because aestheticism is inherently subjective, one must cultivate or simply adopt an "aesthetic ideal". I shall therefore exposit an 'anatomic aesthetic', one that I have personally cultivated, in hopes that certain of the elements will resonate with my audience. Several principles inhere in my anatomic aesthetic. The first principle is functionality. The appearance of one's body should reflect an ability to function optimally on a daily basis and during duress. It should be able to perform rigorous physical tasks and withstand physical stresses of varying types and intensities. A premium is therefore placed on leanness, muscularity, endurance, and flexibility. Conversely, adiposity is expressly eschewed. Fat serves many useful, indeed indispensable, physiological functions in the body including its role as a substrate for the synthesis of various hormones, its role in insulating organs and its structural contribution to cellular membranes. However, its role as a repository for the storage of excess fuel is, in my opinion, marginal. Certainly, the storage of excess energy in the form of fat was once evolutionarily advantageous for the human species and adipose accretion remains vital for many other animals. In lean times the energy embodied in stored body fat can provide an organism with the fuel it needs to survive, especially under frigid conditions wherein the oxidation of fat yields precious heat. Fortunately, for most modern humans this fortuitous function of fat has outlived its utility. No longer must we accrete copious quantities of fat to forestall famine or frigidity. Not only is fat largely physiologically superfluous, it is, in excess, manifestly deleterious to human health. Excessive adiposity is associated with numerous chronic diseases including diabetes, cardiovascular disease and various cancers. What is more, there is evidence that adiposity promotes aging and, conversely, that its antagonism averts aging (Kloting and Bluher 2005). The manner in which excess fat deposition contributes to disease and premature death is not completely understood but considering the ineluctable premise that excess adipose results from excess energy intake and that caloric excess, in turn, eventuates in myriad maladies, it is evident that common mechanisms are involved. What is not commonly considered, however, is the previously described relationship between adiposity, toxicity and 'lipophilicity'. That is, many of the toxic chemicals and environmental pollutants to which we are repeatedly exposed are fat-soluble (lipophilic), meaning that these noxious chemicals deposit preferentially in adipose and the more fat one has, the more toxic chemicals one is able to accumulate. Because toxins can damage the body in myriad ways and impair the organ (i.e. the liver) principally responsible for the elimination of such toxins, it is imperative that measures be taken to lessen the accumulation of toxins. This can be accomplished, in part, by lessening the accumulation of fat. [As argued previously, it is also imperative to avoid *ingesting* animal fat for the same reason.]

To be sure, there is a philosophical element to the desirability of diminishing deposits of fat. Exorbitant amounts of adipose symbolize self-indulgence and, to the extent that obese individuals unsuccessfully endeavor to rid themselves of superfluous fat, it communicates a dearth of discipline. It must be stressed that there is but one way to accrete excess fat—to ingest more energy than one expends. Conversely, there is but one way to eliminate excess fat—to expend more energy than one ingests. There is, therefore, little ambiguity as to the origin of obesity. The chief barrier to the eradication of excessive adipose is arguably an unwillingness to subject oneself to the requisite restraint and discipline necessitated to induce a state of negative energy balance. Superficially, this sounds snobbish. It is admittedly absurd to evaluate an individual's internal psychological state on mere appearance and repugnant to asses someone's worth thereupon. I am, however, espousing *an* anatomic aesthetic ideal, not *the* ideal. Moreover, my attempt is to explicitly identify the underlying bases for unarticulated aesthetic ideals that often lie latent in the minds of many. A final caveat to consider is that the rapidity with which one oxidizes energy is dictated, in part, by biologically-based variables that are, by their very nature, resistant to modulation. Indeed, because humans evolved in an environment that featured frequent food shortages, we have acquired evolutionarily conferred mechanisms by which to avidly accrete excess energy in the form of adipose. As such, continual availability of calorie-rich food, consumed to the point of satiety multiple times daily, veritably ensures excessive adiposity. It is entirely natural to satiate one's appetite with palatable food. However, the evolutionarily dictated consequence of such incessant indulgence is obesity. This simply illustrates the obliviousness of Nature to our immediate, individual interests and impresses upon us the incompatibility of our animalistic appetition and the promotion of prudence.

Another compelling aesthetic/philosophic indictment against adiposity and, indeed, excessive robusticity (massiveness) concerns the apparent dualistic nature of Being. In a manner of speaking, the ultimate essence of an individual is embodied by his mind. The mind is an immaterial entity, I avow. It is endowed with ideas, affects, and aspirations—endowments decidedly nonphysical in nature. On the other hand, the mind undoubtedly requires the nominally material substance of the brain and body to exist. There is, however, a sense in which the body is subordinate to the mind and, therefore, somewhat superfluous and superficial. Consider the intuitive veracity of the phrase 'The mind is *me*, the body is mine.' In a sense, you are your mind whereas you simply possess your body. To accentuate the mind, the intellect, the psyche, over the body is therefore to uphold an aesthetic ideal of considerable gravity. How does one accentuate the immaterial essence of his being, given the indispensability of the material body? By assuming a state wherein the proportions and composition of the body are exquisitely fashioned to facilitate optimal functioning of the mind and the physiological machinations vital to existence. Simply stated, one does this by incorporating the minimum amount of matter (equivalently, energy) necessitated to subserve or support optimum mental and physical activity. Ingestion of energy in excess of this quantity, this 'metabolic modicum', results in the incorporation of inert matter into the very substance of one's being. This is inimical to the ideals of the Amen aesthetic. These statements are speculative and subjective and, admittedly, it is not intellectually edifying to suppose that Nature is inherently dichotomous, woven of interrelated immaterial and material entities. Alas, it seems we have no empirical basis for dethroning Descartes and dispensing with Dualism.

In contrast to adipose, muscle is a functional tissue. It is lean, contractile and kinetic, enabling the execution of movement. It takes concerted exertion to accrete or maintain muscle mass, whereas inertia and indulgence inevitably eventuate in the accumulation of excess adipose. The predomination of active skeletal muscle over inert adipose therefore communicates activity and vitality. Muscularity is, accordingly, a central element of the Amen aesthetic ideal. Succinctly, the regimen seeks to promote muscle retention, facilitate fat depletion and eliminate excess poundage. We shall see how CR and fasting optimize bodyweight and promote the predomination of muscle over fat, resulting in a lean, athletic physique. We shall then discuss the principles of the Amen Exercise Regimen in detail, focusing on the underlying mechanisms whereby the essential elements of the protocol facilitate the attainment and maintenance of muscularity.

Customarily, caloric restriction results in substantial loss of bodyweight. What is more notable about the loss of excess weight is its *compositional selectivity*. CR seems to selectively suppress fat mass while effecting comparatively marginal losses of lean body tissue. Let us consider a study cited previously, where a population of primates (rhesus monkeys, *Macaca mulatta*) were subjected to a regimen of 30% CR (Blanc S et al. 2003). The study involved 30 juvenile animals ranging from 8 to 14 years old and lasted for 11 years. At the end of the study, the CR animals weighed 26% less than the control animals whose diet contained 28% more calories. Though lean body mass differed by only 12% between CR and control animals, CR animals had *56%* less body fat than controls. The investigators highlighted the significance of this finding, stressing that "Expressed as a percentage of body weight, fat mass was 41% lower in the DR group" (Blanc S et al 2003: 18). Teleologically speaking, why should caloric restriction result in such compositional selectivity, why should it induce a metabolic state wherein fat is selectively suppressed while muscle protein is selectively salvaged? The answer may lie in energy efficiency. The energy embedded in carbohydrates (such as the glycogen stored in the liver) amounts to ~4 Calories per gram. Similarly, the energy embedded in protein (such as that stored in muscle) amounts to ~4 Calories per gram. Conversely, the energy embedded in fat amounts to ~9 Calories per gram, twice the energy density of carbohydrates and protein. What is more, due to its chemical compaction and inherent inertness, considerably greater amounts of adipose tissue can be stored in/upon the body. It is therefore a more replete reservoir of energy. There is a more crucial factor to consider in the preference for fat over muscle as an energy source under CR conditions. The proteins constitutive of muscle exist as polymers of amino acids. These amino acids are, in turn, constituted by both carbonaceous moieties and nitrogenous moieties. While the carbonaceous moiety can readily serve as a substrate for carbohydrate construction and, ultimately, energy production, the nitrogenous moiety is, essentially, a waste product. What is more, this nitrogenous amino moiety takes the form of ammonia, a toxic chemical capable of wreaking woe on the organs of the body, especially the all-important brain. As such, ammonia must be detoxified via chemical conversion. It is ultimately converted into urea by the liver and excreted from the body by the kidneys in the medium of urine. The liver and kidneys, however, have a limited capacity to catabolize protein and detoxify its metabolite, ammonia. It is estimated that the energetic cost of detoxifying one gram of ammonium-derived nitrogen amounts to over 10,000 Calories (Whiten and Widdowson 1992). Clearly, it would be excessively wasteful were the body to rely on the protein contained in muscle tissue for its energy during dietary deprivation. In such a state, the body is compelled to preferentially preserve protein at the expense of fat. The pronounced alteration of body composition conduced by CR is consonant with the stated aesthetic imperative of reducing body fat while maintaining lean body tissue. Let us now consider some of the molecular mechanisms involved in CR-induced reduction of body fat and concomitant preservation of muscle tissue as well as the augmentation of these mechanisms by fasting. Summarily, these mechanisms involve suppression of insulin and glucose, elevation of cortisol and glucagon, induction of growth hormone release and alteration of enzymes involved in fat and protein metabolism.

We have noted on several occasions that caloric restriction consistently causes substantial suppression of circulating insulin. Indeed, in a seminal study on the effects of CR on glucose and insulin responsiveness of muscle tissue, it was found that a 30% decrease in caloric intake resulted in a 50-70% reduction in circulating concentrations of insulin (Gazdag A et al. 1999). This effect is due, in large measure, to the reduction in circulating glucose induced by fasting and CR which, in the cited study, declined by ~25-30%. In a previous section of this chapter, it was mentioned that insulin is a *mitogen*, which promotes proliferation of cells, and that excessive cell proliferation is a cancer catalyst. Thus, the anti-neoplastic effect of CR is partly attributable to its antagonistic effect on insulin release. Moreover, insulin acts as a catalyst for free radicals and experimental investigations indicate that exogenously applied insulin actually abrogates or attenuates some of the beneficial physiological effects induced by CR, such as protection against mitochondrial membrane peroxidation (Lambert AJ et al. 2004). Germane to our present discussion, however, is the role of insulin in effecting fat deposition in adipose cells. As explained in Guyton and Hall's highly informative *Textbook of Medical Physiology*:

> Insulin has several effects that lead to fat storage in adipose tissue. First, insulin increases the utilization of glucose by most of the body's tissues, which automatically decreases the utilization of fat, thus functioning as a fat sparer...[I]nsulin also promotes fatty acid synthesis. This is especially true when more carbohydrates are ingested than can be used for immediate energy, thus providing the substrate for fat synthesis. Almost all this synthesis occurs in the liver cells, and the fatty acids are then transported form the liver...to the adipose cells to be stored. (Guyton and Hall 2000: 888)

Delving into a deeper level of specificity, insulin exerts an antagonistic effect on fat utilization by inhibiting the enzyme *hormone-sensitive lipase*. This chemical catalyzes the initial step in fat hydrolysis, causing fat to be mobilized from adipocytes. Furthermore, insulin facilitates the uptake of glucose by adipose cells and this glucose not only serves as a substrate for fatty acid synthesis but results in the formation of large quantities of the glycolytic intermediate *α–glycerol phosphate*. Recall that fat is stored in the form of triacylglycerol, this molecule consisting of three chains of fatty acids attached to a 3-carbon glycerol moiety. α-Glycerol phosphate, derived from glucose, supplies the glycerol that ultimately combines with fatty acids to form triacylglycerol (triglyceride), the storage form of fat. In the absence of appreciable insulin, as occurs in the intervals between meals, fat, instead of glucose, serves as the body's principal source of fuel. The longer the lapse of time between meals and the fewer the calories ingested during meals, the less insulin is secreted and the more fat is mobilized to serve as a substrate for energy production. Thus, the Amen Fast, entailing and inter-digestive phase of 23 hours, concomitant with considerable caloric curtailment, has a potent synergistic effect, resulting in enhanced elimination of body fat.

Caloric restriction routinely results in elevated concentrations of plasma cortisol (Masoro EJ 1998). Cortisol is a so-called "stress hormone" produced by the adrenal cortex in response to various stressful stimuli as well as certain dietary conditions, especially starvation. Cortisol has myriad physiological effects in the body but I should like to focus primarily on its effects upon fat. Essentially, cortisol has precisely the opposite effect of insulin on adipose cells. As the *Textbook of Medical Physiology* states, cortisol:

> ...promotes mobilization of fatty acids from adipose tissue. This increases the concentration of free fatty acids in the plasma, which also increases their utilization for energy. Cortisol seems also to have a direct effect to enhance the oxidation of fatty acids in the cells. (Guyton and Hall 2000: 876)

One of the mechanisms by which cortisol mediates mobilization of fat from adipose cells is by simply opposing the uptake of glucose by adipocytes. As explained above, adipocytes use the glucose metabolite α-glycerol phosphate to synthesize fat and under conditions of elevated cortisol, less glucose gets into fat cells, less α-glycerol phosphate is produced, less fat is synthesized and stored and more fat is mobilized. In this way, cortisol acts as a major metabolic modulator. As Guyton and Hall explain:

> The increased mobilization of fats by cortisol, combined with increased oxidation of fatty acids in the cells, helps shift the metabolic systems of the cells in times of starvation or other stresses [e.g. fasting and CR] from utilization of glucose for energy to utilization of fatty acids. This cortisol mechanism...requires several hours to become fully developed...(Guyton and Hall 2000: 876)

The Amen Fast provides ample time for the "cortisol mechanism" to develop, synergizing the cortisol-elevating effect of CR and facilitating a more robust mobilization of fat from adipose tissue. In addition to promoting fat oxidation, cortisol promotes efflux of protein from tissues and augments gluconeogenesis—the conversion of amino acids from tissue proteins into glucose. As we are concerned with the enhancement of muscle development and maintenance, this effect may seem decidedly detrimental to our designs. After all, deposition of protein in muscle augments muscularity while the converse diminishes the same. Cortisol, however, promotes catabolism of more expendable proteins while preserving vital neurological and contractile proteins:

> Cortisol usually does not mobilize the basic functional proteins of the cells, such as the muscle contractile proteins and the proteins of the neurons, until almost all other proteins have been released. This preferential effect of cortisol in mobilizing labile proteins could

make amino acids available to needy cells to synthesize substances essential to life. (Guyton and Hall 2000: 877)

What is more, cortisol, by increasing catabolism of labile cellular proteins, increases the pool of amino acids available for renewed protein synthesis, thereby contributing to tissue juvenescence. The liver, a principal site of protein production is central in this process:

> Coincidentally with the reduced proteins elsewhere in the body, the liver proteins become enhanced. Furthermore, the plasma proteins (which are produced by the liver and then released into the blood) are also increased. These increases are exceptions to the protein depletion that occurs elsewhere in the body…[T]his difference results from a possible effect of cortisol to enhance amino acid transport into liver cells (but not into most other cells) and to enhance the liver enzymes required for protein synthesis. (Guyton and Hall 2000: 876)

Thus, cortisol increases catabolism of non-neuromuscular proteins, increases influx of amino acids into the liver, increases synthesis of liver proteins and inhibits deposition of fat into adipose tissue. On a molecular level, all these effects accord amicably with the Amen aesthetic.

Another hormone that acts obversely to insulin upon adipose is glucagon. As insulin is produced by the beta cells of the pancreas in response to *rising* plasma glucose, glucagon is produced by the alpha cells of the pancreas in response to *falling* plasma glucose. Moreover, just as insulin facilitates cellular *influx* of glucose, glucagon facilitates cellular *efflux* of glucose. Accordingly, glucagon inhibits deposition of fat in adipose cells and promotes its effluence and hydrolysis. Glucagon acts as a "fasting hormone" that enhances exploitation of fat between meals when glucose levels drop, an inductive effect similar to that of cortisol. The proximate mechanism by which glucagon facilitates fat utilization is as follows:

> …[G]lucagon *activates adipose cell lipase* [a fat hydrolyzing enzyme], making increased quantities of fatty acids available to the energy systems of the body. It also inhibits the storage of triglycerides in the liver, which prevents the liver from removing fatty acids from the blood; this also helps make additional amounts of fatty acids available for the other tissues of the body [to use as energy]. (Guyton and Hall 2000: 892)

Though this section is focused on the capacity of CR and fasting to augment muscularity and enhance aesthetic appeal, there is compelling evidence that the lypolytic action of CR is, in itself, partly responsible for longevity-enhancement or that reducing the amount of stored body fat actually promotes longevity. The supporting study was cited previously but it is so momentous that it warrants recapitulation. It will be recalled that the investigators genetically engineered a strain of mice devoid of insulin receptors on their adipose cells. The reader is reminded that the pancreatic hormone, insulin, binds to specific receptors on the surface of cells and by so doing, enables the influx of glucose. The glucose so absorbed thereupon serves as a substrate for fat synthesis. The mutated mice were therefore deprived of their capacity for fat synthesis, sequestration and accumulation. As such, this genetic manipulation resulted in a substantial reduction in the rodents' body fat depots:

Starting at 3 months of age, [genetically altered] mice maintained 15 to 25% lower body weights and a 50 to 70% reduction in fat mass throughout life. The reduction in adiposity was…apparent in all fat depots and was also reflected by a reduction of 25% in total-body triglyceride content. (Blüher M et al 2003: 572)

This degree of body weight reduction and body fat loss is comparable to that observed in the primate study cited earlier in this section. Note that the body weight/fat reduction in the study in question was effectuated through genetic manipulation whereas the body weight/fat reduction in the primate study was effectuated through caloric restriction, suggesting that CR-induced fat loss is similarly mediated via alteration of gene expression. These murine mutants were not only leaner and healthier than their control counterparts but lived substantially longer:

The median life-span of most laboratory mice is…30 months. Consistent with this we found that 45 to 54% of the mice in the control groups lived to 30 months of age. By contrast about 80% of the [genetically altered] mice were alive at this age…Complete survival curves revealed that the mean life-span was increased by…18%. The median life-span in [genetically altered] mice was extended by ~5 months. At 36 months, all mice in the control groups had died, whereas ~25% of the [mutated] mice were still alive…[E]xtended longevity in [genetically altered] mice is associated with both a shift in the age at which the 'age-dependent increase in mortality risk' becomes appreciable and a decreased rate of age-related mortality…(Blüher M et al 2003: 572-573)

This study has several intriguing implications, two of which were intimated earlier: (1) the longevity-enhancing effects of CR may be partly attributable to its suppression of fat deposition (2) reduction of body fat depots may augment longevity through mechanisms analogous to caloric restriction (3) alteration/inhibition of insulin signaling is an operative mechanism by which longevity is enhanced and (4) excess body fat is not only superfluous, it conceivably compromises longevity—both average and maximal longevity. Indeed, a study published in the *International Journal of Obesity and Related Metabolic Disorders* directly compared the effects of bodyweight reduction and caloric restriction on mortality in murine subjects. Though the study found CR to be far more efficacious in augmenting longevity, bodyweight reduction was found to exert an independent effect on mortality. As I indicate in *Evolutionary Nutrition*, it is plausible that adipose serves as a sort of molecular signal of energy/nutrient repletion, which the genome meticulously monitors in its modulation of aging. It should be noted that growth, sexual maturation and reproductive receptivity are all augmented by appreciable adiposity and that these variables are *inversely* correlated with species-specific maximum lifespan. Stated more succinctly, fat promotes rapid growth, rapid sexual development and heightened fecundity and each of these physiological features is associated with shorter species lifespan.

Though fat loss comprises a disproportionate fraction of CR-mediated weight loss, lean body tissue is also inevitably lost. CR, however, promotes preferential preservation of muscle tissue. To reiterate, this effect—enhanced elimination of adipose concomitant with preferential preservation of muscle—is central to our aesthetic imperative. Caloric restriction and fasting promote muscularity via multiple mechanisms:

1) By concomitantly increasing the *efflux* of protein from the liver and increasing the *influx* of amino acids into muscle cells
2) By increasing the contractile capacity of muscle fibers
3) By augmenting energy availability to muscles (thereby increasing muscle endurance)
4) By lessening acid-induced muscle fatigue
5) By lessening free radical-induced muscle fatigue
6) By increasing the rapidity with which muscle proteins are synthesized upon protein ingestion
7) By increasing the rapidity with which muscle proteins are renewed and recycled

Each of these effects of CR and fasting enable muscles to respond more adaptively to the stress imposed by endurance and resistance training, thereby permitting more intense bouts of exercise and further facilitating aesthetic augmentation. Let us see how.

The augmented influx of amino acids into *myocytes* is aided by accelerated efflux of amino acids from the liver. It will be recalled that when protein is ingested, it is degraded into peptides and amino acids by pancreatic and intestinal enzymes, absorbed by the enterocytes of the small intestine and ultimately transported to the liver via the *portal vein*. Nutrient-rich serum converges on the liver whose principal task is to apportion adequate amounts to the tissues of the body. CR affects the physiology of the liver in myriad ways. Most germane to our present discussion, however, is that caloric restriction significantly increases the synthesis of hepatic (liver) proteins and concomitantly increases the rate with which proteins are extruded from the liver into the bloodstream to be made available to the body's cells. A study published in the journal *Biochemical and Biophysical Research Communications* found that CR increased the rate of release of some hepatic proteins by as much as 250% (Dhahbi JM et al 2001). Not only does this CR-induced acceleration of hepatic protein efflux augment muscle protein repletion, it helps to accelerate the rate with which all tissue proteins are renewed, thereby contributing to the pronounced juvenilizing effect of caloric restriction.

It is perhaps counterintuitive that one of the most potent inducers of growth hormone (GH) secretion is fasting. Whereas normal concentrations of GH range from ~1.5 to 3 nanograms per milliliter, fasting can induce a 30-fold increase in GH concentration (Guyton and Hall 2000). Why, it might be asked, should chronic deficits in energy intake engender heightened release of a hormone whose principal role is to effect enhanced growth? The role of *somatotropin* (growth hormone) in muscle protein preservation renders its responsiveness to fasting more intelligible. The reader will recall my reasoning that energy deficits compel the body to utilize its most efficiently exploitable energy reserve (i.e. fat) while selectively preserving protein, a comparatively inferior substrate for energy extraction. Increased production of GH enables just such compositional selectivity, enabling a fasting person to preserve precious protein at the expense of expendable adipose. One of the mechanisms whereby GH ensures selective protein preservation is by simply making more fatty acids available for the body's immediate energy needs. As explained in Guyton and Hall's *Textbook of Medical Physiology*:

Growth hormone has a specific effect in causing release of fatty acids form adipose tissue and, therefore, increasing the concentration of fatty acids in the body fluids. In addition, in tissues of the body, it enhances the conversion of fatty acids to acetyl coenzyme A (acetyl CoA) and subsequent utilization of this for energy. Therefore, under the influence of growth hormone, fat is used for energy in preference to use of both carbohydrates and proteins. Growth hormone's effect to promote fat utilization, together with its protein anabolic effect, causes an increase in lean body mass. (Guyton and Hall 2000: 849)

This "protein anabolic effect", which results in selective salvaging of lean body mass is attributable, in turn, to two GH-mediated effects:

Growth hormone directly enhances transport of at least some and perhaps most amino acids through the cell membranes to the interior of the cells. This increases the concentrations of the amino acids in the cells and is presumed to be at least partly responsible for the increased protein synthesis. This control of amino acid transport is similar to the effect of insulin in controlling glucose transport through the membrane...(Guyton and Hall 2000: 849)

Secondly:

Over more prolonged periods (24 to 48 hours), growth hormone also stimulates the transcription of DNA in the nucleus, causing formation of increased quantities of RNA. This in turn promotes more protein synthesis and promotes growth if sufficient energy, amino acids, vitamins, and other necessities for growth are available. (Guyton and Hall 2000: 849)

Note the latency of growth hormone's transcription-enhancing effect—24 to 48 hours. The Amen Protocol is particularly efficacious in exploiting this anabolic induction. Throughout the course of the 23-hour Amen Fast, levels of growth hormone increase. The Amen Exercise Regimen is executed at the end of the day (contemporaneous with the 22nd hour of the fast). Aside from fasting, strenuous exercise is the most potent inducer of growth hormone secretion, eliciting plasma concentrations as high as 30 ng/mL—a concentration 20 times greater than the basal level (Guyton and Hall 2000). After executing the strenuous resistance regimen, the amino acid-rich, enzyme-incubated protein beverage is immediately imbibed. Due to the combined effects of elevated GH and enhanced insulin receptivity, these amino acids, peptides and proteins are avidly assimilated by the body (an effect that is further enhanced by CR-induced increases in intestinal absorptive capacity). Finally, it bears mentioning that another potent elicitor of GH secretion is slumber. Within the first hours of sleep, levels of growth hormone rise to concentrations greater than 10 times above basal levels (Guyton and Hall 2000). Thus, after fasting-induced elevations of GH, exercise-induced elevations of GH, post-exercise provisionment of protein, and sleep-induced elevations of GH, a concatenation of physiological factors conspire to concomitantly oppose adipose accretion, promote muscle protein production and facilitate recuperation from the intense Amen Exercise Regimen.

Growth hormone does not act alone in exerting its anabolic, protein-preserving effects; it is aided in this respect by a class of peptides known collectively as somato*medins*, so named because they *mediate* the effects of somato*tropin* (GH). After being released by the pituitary gland, GH flows freely in the blood. Upon interacting with the requisite receptors in the liver, somatotropin ultimately elicits hepatic release of somatomedins. The chief somatomedin operative in muscle hypertrophy is insulin-like growth factor I (IGF-I). In order to appreciate the role of this peptide in modulating muscle physiology it is worth considering the molecular basis of muscle hypertrophy. As mentioned previously, three conditions can cause compensatory muscle hypertrophy (growth): electrical-chemical-neural stimulation, muscle contraction and muscle elongation (stretching). The proximate means by which these stimuli induce growth are believed to be dependent upon *satellite cells*. Recall that muscle cells are post-mitotic, lacking the capacity for cell division after differentiation. Thus, under normal circumstances, muscle cells can undergo hyper*trophy* (volumetric accretion) but not hyper*plasia* (numerical accretion). Muscle hypertrophy is dependent upon infiltration of satellite cells—immature, progenitive stem cells that intervene between individual muscle cells and abut the membranes of myocytes. When sufficiently stimulated by one of the three means mentioned above, satellite cells proliferate and fuse with muscle fibers. In this fusive process, satellite cells proffer additional nuclei to multinucleated myocytes, magnifying the morphology of muscles. IGF-I is instrumental in inducing proliferation of satellite cells and therefore plays a crucial role in regulating muscle growth. The reader will recall that CR reduces circulating IGF-I and that suppression of this mitogenic molecule is thought to be partly responsible for the anti-cancer character of caloric curtailment. However, CR concomitantly causes suppression of circulating IGF-I and elevation of IGF-I *receptors*. This effect apparently enables enhanced IGF-I receptivity, especially when its levels are acutely elevated—such elevations as are elicited upon increased GH secretion. A study published in the journal *Mechanisms of Ageing and Development* found levels of IGF-I receptors to be increased by as much as 100% in response to CR (D'Costa AP et al. 1993). Consonant with the speculative reasoning advanced above, the study found that though IGF-I levels were reduced ~40% by their regimen of 40% CR, protein synthesis increased by as much as 70%, illustrating the importance of receptor repletion over elevated chemical concentration in this case. It is conceivable that CR-mediated reductions in IGF-I and a concomitant increase in its receptor is an ameliorative adaptation aimed at conserving energy while simultaneously increasing cellular sensitivity to this important mitogenic molecule. It may be more energetically efficient (and physiologically favorable) under conditions of caloric curtailment to maintain more receptors for IGF-I than to maintain normal basal levels of this peptide. Furthermore, reducing the circulating concentration of IGF-I—an excess of which is implicated in the etiology of cancer—may have the effect of reducing exposure of the body's tissues to the mitogenic, proliferative effects of this agent.

Several intriguing studies have yielded valuable insights into the effects of CR and fasting on the response of muscle to strenuous exercise. One such study, which clearly establishes the ameliorative interactivity of diet and exercise on muscle mechanics, appeared in *The American Journal of Physiology*. In this investigation, four groups of experimental animals were employed. Group I was sedentary and allowed to feed *ad libitum*—this group served as the control group; group II was likewise fed freely but permitted to engage in exercise using a wheel attached to their cages; group III was energy restricted, receiving 30% less calories than the *ad libitum* groups; and group IV was likewise energy restricted but also permitted to engage in exercise (Horska A et al. 1999). Thus, there were two exercise groups and two sedentary groups, two CR groups and two freely fed groups. The investigators compared the groups on the basis of several physiological parameters, including the relative force with which their muscles contracted upon stimulation, the duration over which their muscles were able to sustain contraction, the acidity of their muscle tissue secondary to contractile activity, and the concentration of certain enzymes operative in the biochemical pathway known as the *tricarboxylic acid* (TCA) *cycle*. What they found is as follows. First, the weight reduction commonly associated with exercise and the weight reduction consistently observed in animals on CR was *additive*, resulting in a 25% difference in bodyweight relative to the free-fed exercise group and, identically, a 25% difference in bodyweight relative to the sedentary CR group. The difference in bodyweight between the sedentary free-fed group and the restricted exercise group amounted to ~37%, the latter having bodyweights less than two thirds that of the former. Secondly, the animals subjected to CR engaged in far more voluntary exercise than the freely fed group provisioned with an exercise apparatus in their cages. Indeed, the daily distance ran by the CR exercise group was over 40% greater than the free-fed exercise group. This finding is particularly illuminating in that it serves as an empirical index of a subjective phenomenon—something we might call vitality or simply "energy". Presumably, the fact that the energy-restricted group voluntarily engaged in more exertive exercise is indicative of increased levels of *perceived* energy. This subjective sensation of increased energy or vitality is something that many diets claim to induce but in this experiment, we have what seems to be a demonstration of the capacity of energy restriction to induce a perceived elevation in energy. The investigators also found that the CR exercise group exhibited a superior degree of what might be termed 'biomechanical energy transduction'. Applying two successive bouts of electrical stimulation to the lower legs of the animals—stimulation sufficient to induce complete muscle contraction—they measured the resultant force with which their muscles contracted as well as the 'temporal evolution of the contraction' and noted the following:

> At the beginning of the second stimulation, the average relative force levels were highest in the [energy restricted exercise group]. In addition, relative force was better maintained throughout the second stimulation period in this group; at the end of the second stimulation, relative force decreased by ~40% in [groups I, II, and III] but by only 18% in [group IV, the CR exercise group]. (Horska A et al 1999: E769)

This finding is intriguing. It indicates that chronic restriction of energy intake can eventuate in a substantial alteration of muscle physiology, enabling enhanced energy transduction, enhanced mechanical force production, enhanced maintenance of muscle contractile force and enhanced resistance to muscle fatigue (i.e. increased muscle endurance). The investigators found two interesting chemical correlates of this CR-induced muscular modification: (1) the muscles of the CR exercise group exhibited less acidosis than the other groups and (2) the muscles of the CR exercise group had higher concentrations of the TCA enzyme *citrate synthase*. Let us consider the significance of these chemical correlates. First, it should be noted that actively contracting muscles derive a plentiful portion of their available energy from glycogen, a polymer of glucose stored principally in hepatocytes and myocytes. The stockpile of polymeric sugar serves to supplement muscles' initial source of energy during intense exertion—this initial energy source is *phosphocreatine*. Essentially, phosphocreatine replenishes the phosphate pool present in muscle, thereby enabling reconstitution of ATP. The contraction of muscles is dependent upon the binding of two types of protein fibers—*actin* and *myosin*. Binding of these filamentous fibers is, in turn, dependent upon provisionment of a high-energy phosphate moiety from adenosine triphosphate (ATP). The concentration of ATP in active muscle is too marginal, however, to meet the metabolic demands of concerted contraction:

> The concentration of ATP in the muscle fiber, about 4 millimolar, is sufficient to maintain full contraction for only 1 to 2 seconds at most. After this, ATP is split to form ADP...[T]he ADP is rephosphorylated to form new ATP within another fraction of a second, which allows the muscle to continue its contraction. (Guyton and Hall 2000: 74)

Rephosphorylation is effectuated by phosphocreatine. In the process of proffering phosphate to replenish the ATP pool, protons [H^+] are produced. This increases the acidity of muscle tissue and inhibits contraction via mechanisms that are incompletely understood. Phosphocreatine is not the only contributor to elevated acidosis in muscle. Anaerobic utilization of glucose yields additional acid. This mechanism mobilizes when phosphocreatine wanes due to depletion:

> [T]he total amount of phosphocreatine in the muscle fiber is also very little—only about five times as great as ATP. Therefore, the combined energy of both the stored ATP and the phosphocreatine in the muscle is capable of causing maximal muscle contraction for only 5 to 8 seconds. (Guyton and Hall 2000: 74)

Enter glycolysis:

> Rapid enzymatic breakdown of the glycogen to pyruvic acid and lactic acid liberates energy that is used to convert ADP to ATP, and the ATP can then be used directly to energize muscle contraction or to re-form the stores of phosphocreatine...Unfortunately, however, so many end products of glycolysis accumulate in the muscle cells that glycolysis also loses its capability to sustain maximum muscle contraction after about 1 minute. (Guyton and Hall 2000: 74)

The acidic "end product", lactic acid, inhibits continued muscle contraction and is responsible for the burning sensation associated with muscle fatigue. Exercise is impeded when the acute accretion of lactic acid exhausts the capacity of muscle to expurgate the inhibitory metabolite. This expurgatory mechanism involves diffusion of lactic acid from muscles into the bloodstream where the metabolite is transported to the liver to be reconverted into glucose and thereupon returned to the muscle. The sequence is known in biochemical parlance as the Cori cycle and its efficiency determines the functional capacity of muscle. It is therefore significant that CR has been shown to augment the efficiency of the Cori cycle. One of the principal mechanisms by which CR effects this augmentation is via increased activity of the enzyme *lactate dehydrogenase*. This enzyme catalyzes the first step in the conversion of lactic acid to glucose in the liver and its induction by energy restriction is an important factor in CR-mediated exercise enhancement. In a study published in the journal *Metabolism*, it was found that a brief bout of CR (6 weeks) resulted in a ~50% increase in the enzymatic activity of lactate dehydrogenase (Lambert K et al. 2003). What is more, this increased activity was reportedly accompanied by a concomitant decrease in lactic acid concentration within muscle and an increase in its concentration in the bloodstream. Thus, CR caused enhanced *efflux* of lactic acid from muscle and enhanced *influx* of lactic acid into the liver. Efficient lactic acid efflux/influx is important because it provides a critical source of energy during exercise. Whereas the phosphocreatine mechanism provides more ATP to muscles per unit time than the glucose/lactic acid mechanism (4 moles per minute versus 2.5 moles per minute), the latter mechanism can provide this energy over a longer interval (1.5 minutes versus several seconds) (Guyton and Hall 2000). The lactic acid mechanism is therefore uniquely suited to provide energy during rigorous resistance exercise. Succinctly, CR accelerates removal of lactic acid from muscle, increases its uptake by the liver and increases its conversion into glucose. Glucose does not diffuse passively into muscles however. Its influx is effected by integral transport proteins embedded in the membranes of muscles. One such transport protein is *GLUT-4*, the most abundantly expressed glucose transporter in muscle tissue. An intriguing study published in *The American Journal of Physiology* found that a brief bout (20 days) of moderate caloric restriction resulted in a significant increase in the translocation of GLUT-4 transporters on the surfaces of muscle cells (Dean DJ et al 1998). Interestingly, the study found no absolute increase in the amount of GLUT-4 contained in the muscle cells of CR subjects but found instead that upon exposure to insulin, the CR animals "transolcated" more glucose transporters to the surfaces of their cells, thereby augmenting influx of glucose.

Considering the fact that endogenous muscle ATP is only able to supply energy for 1 to 2 seconds, phosphocreatine for only 5 to 8 seconds, and glycogen-derived glucose for only 1 minute during maximal muscle contraction, alternative metabolic mechanisms are necessitated to support sustained muscle activity. These mechanisms are, in turn, dependent upon two processes: (1) efflux of lactic acid to the liver where it is thereupon reconverted into glucose and ultimately returned to muscle and (2) funneling of pyruvate into muscle mitochondria where its constituents ultimately serve as substrates for ATP production via the TCA cycle and, subsequently, oxidative phosphorylation via the mitochondrial electron transport chain (ETC). This oxidative mechanism supplies more than 95% of the energy used by muscle during intense exercise (Guyton and Hall 2000). Importantly, the rate with which ATP is produced via the TCA/ETC pathway is dependent upon the first step in the pathway. This step is catalyzed by the enzyme *citrate synthase*. This is precisely the enzyme elevated by the combined effects of exercise and energy restriction in the study cited previously. Presumably, increased quantities of this enzyme enable a greater amount of ATP to be produced, thereby replenishing the phosphate pools of muscles. This replenishment provides the necessary substrates for prolonged muscle contraction and would seem to enable muscles to contract more forcefully and more efficiently for a longer period.

Muscle contraction is contingent not only upon the availability of ATP but on the activity of membrane-bound receptors. Certain of these receptors control calcium influx and efflux, the proximate causes of muscle depolarization, re-polarization and contraction. As explained in Guyton and Hall's *Textbook of Medical Physiology*:

The action potential depolarizes the muscle membrane, and much of the action potential electricity also travels deeply within the muscle fiber. Here it causes the sarcoplasmic reticulum [a specialized muscle organelle] to release large quantities of calcium ions that have been stored within this reticulum. The calcium ions initiate attractive forces between the actin and myosin filaments, causing them to slide alongside each other, which is the contractile process. (Guyton and Hall 2000: 69)

The contracted muscle must thereafter be re-polarized and *de*-contracted:

After a fraction of a second, the calcium ions are pumped back into the sarcoplasmic reticulum by a [Ca^{2+}] membrane pump, and they remain stored until a new muscle action potential comes along: this removal of the calcium ions from the myofibrils causes muscle contraction to cease. (Guyton and Hall 2000: 69)

Two receptors are operative in this molecular mediation of contraction—the *dihydropyridine receptor* (DHPR) and the *ryanodine receptor* (RyR1)—and the levels of both are reportedly increased by CR. As to the respective roles of these receptors in controlling calcium concentration in muscle, the ensuing excerpt explains:

The DHPR is a voltage-gated Ca^{2+} channel and its activation by...membrane depolarization evokes Ca^{2+} release from sarcoplasmic reticulum through RyR1 into the myoplasm [muscle cell cytoplasm]. Contractile proteins on binding Ca^{2+} initiate muscle contraction and force development. Hence, DHPR and RyR1 play a central role in the mechanism of excitation-contraction coupling in skeletal muscle. (Renganathan and Delbono 1998: 349)

In a study published in the journal *Biochemistry and Biophysics Research Communications*, CR-induced increases in DHPR and RyR1 resulted in substantially greater muscle contractile force upon stimulation and greater muscle "tetanic tension" relative to freely fed control animals (Mayhew M et al. 1998). Moreover, CR has been found to avert age-related losses of these receptors, thereby resisting reductions in muscle mass and muscle strength that commonly accompany aging. This effect of CR was documented by Renganathan and Delbono in a study published in the journal of the *Federation of European Biochemical Societies*:

In this study, young (8-month), middle-aged (18-month) and old (33-month)...rats were examined to determine whether age-related changes in the number of DHPR, RyR1 and DHPR/RyR1 ratio can be prevented or delayed by calorie restriction...We report that restricting the calorie intake of the rats to 60% of the control ad libitum fed group from 16 weeks of age *prevents* the decline in the number of DHPR, RyR1 and DHPR/RyR1 ratio in aged skeletal muscles. These results may be functionally relevant for age-associated muscle weakness. [emphasis mine] (Renganathan and Delbono 1998: 346)

Interestingly, it has been found that IGF-I is partly responsible for inducing enhanced expression of DHPR and we have already seen that CR reportedly augments IGF-I signaling by effecting an increase in the expression of IGF-I receptors (Delbono O 2000). Thus, enhancement of IGF-I signaling may be the proximate modality via which CR increases contraction-regulating receptors.

The reader will recall that over 95% of the energy needed to fuel muscle contraction is provided through oxidative mechanisms. Such metabolic processes proceed in the mitochondria of muscles and inevitably eventuate in some degree of oxidative damage to muscles. There is evidence that oxidative damage due to exhaustive exercise imposes a physiological limit to the endurance of the exercising subject—that is, free radicals resulting from exercise inhibit further exertion, thereby leading to cessation of contraction, muscle fatigue, prolongation of the time necessitated for recuperation and (potentially) lasting damage to muscle tissue. This exercise-induced oxidative damage is insidious as it impairs the organelle primarily responsible for energy provisionment during exercise—the mitochondrion. We have seen that CR attenuates free radical damage through multiple mechanisms. Particularly relevant to our present discussion is the localization of CR-mediated radical repression to the mitochondrion—the focal point of exercise-induced oxidative damage. In an intriguing study published in the journal *Free Radical Biology and Medicine*, experimenters sought to determine the effectiveness of CR in reducing oxidative damage to mitochondria, with particular attention focused on the diminution of such damage as animals advanced in age. They used various technical indices of mitochondrial damage, including the presence and prevalence of such products as *thiobarbituric acid-reactive substances* (TBARS), *sulfhydryl* and *carbonyl* moieties and assessed the extent of free radical production in groups of CR and freely fed, *ad libitum* (AL) subjects. Caloric restriction was found to significantly suppress the extent of mitochondrial damage, completely preventing the age-associated increase in certain indices of oxidative damage:

> Mitochondrial carbonyl content [indicative of protein damage] in the AL mice, measured from 7 to 29 months of age, remained at relatively the same level between 6 and 12 months of age, but increased steadily thereafter [eventuating in a relative increase of] ~150% at 29 months of age. In contrast, during a comparable range of age, mitochondria from the CR mice exhibited no discernible increase in carbonyl content...Mitochondrial protein sulfhydryl content in the AL mice decreased steadily by about 50% between 3 and 18 months of age [indicative of pathophysiolgical protein degradation]...whereas no demonstrable age-associated loss occurred in the CR mice. The concentration of TBARS in the mitochondrial homogenates from the AL mice showed a sigmoidal increase with age [indicative of oxidative damage to mitochondrial membranes]. The rapid increase (~2.5-fold) was observed between 12 and 14 months of age...In sharp contrast, the concentration of TBARS in mitochondria from the CR group remained virtually unaltered during a comparable period of the life span. (Lass A et al. 1998: 1092-1093)

As for free radical 'generativity' they found that...

> The rate of [superoxide free radical] generation...was 41% higher in the 20-month-old AL mice as compared to the 4-month-old AL mice, however, no significant differences were observed between the 20-month-old CR and 4 month-old AL mice. (Lass A 1998: 1093)

Considering the above results, it is conceivable that the enhanced adaptability of CR subjects to physical exertion is partly attributable to an augmented ability to avert mitochondrial free radical damage. Particularly interesting was the virtual elimination of age-associated increases in mitochondrial damage and free radical 'generativity'. As the above excerpt indicates, the extent of free radical generation of middle-aged CR animals was comparable to that of adolescent *ad libitum* animals. The significance of this finding is heightened when one considers the contribution of muscle tissue to the net generation of free radicals over time. It is largely the aberrant affixation of electrons to oxygen during oxidative phosphorylation that engenders free radicals. This pathophysiological process is likely accelerated in actively contracting muscle and its effective inhibition by CR probably spares the body substantial oxidative insults over the course of a lifespan. Because exercise induces such profligate production of free radicals, the benefits thereof must be weighed against its potential perils. It is for this reason that the Amen Protocol prescribes that antioxidants be partaken before exercise. As enumerated earlier, the following antioxidant agents are indicated: resveratrol, N-acetylcysteine, matcha, and ginseng. Ingestion of these substances serves as an added measure of protection against exercise-induced oxidative stress, potentially nullifying the negative effects of intense exertion.

Another mechanism efficacious in the preservation of muscle integrity is the rapid renewal of protein prompted by CR. As indicated previously, this is effect extends to all protienaceous tissues of the body and is arguably the most important attribute responsible for the rejuvenative effect of CR. It has the potential to exert an especially ameliorative effect on skeletal muscle simply because this tissue is so replete with protein, 80% of which consists of contractile myofibrillar protein (Husom AD et al. 2004). The proximate mechanism whereby CR accelerates the renewal of bodily proteins is via increased expression of enzymes operative in protein degradation. Specifically, it is the *proteasome* that is responsible for the degradation of damaged proteins. The proteasome is a cytoplasmic enzyme complex, whose constituent catalytic proteins interact specifically with oxidatively damaged proteins, effecting their removal from the body. Importantly, damaged proteins are known to accumulate gradually with age. The centrality of proteins in mediating multifarious physiological functions makes their age-associated derangement a particularly pernicious problem—one that is strongly implicated in the molecular etiology of aging itself. In a study that appeared in the *Archives of Biochemistry and Biophysics*, it was found that the pronounced age-associated loss of muscle mass is associated with a reduction in the specific enzymatic activity of proteasome proteins (Husom AD et al. 2004). Conversely, as documented in a study published in the *Annals of the New York Academy of Sciences*, caloric restriction was found to be efficacious in increasing proteasome activity and this effect was associated with increased replacement and rejuvenation of proteins (Goto S et al 2002). Though the study was limited to analysis of the liver proteasome, it is probably operative in muscle tissue and conceivably acts to avert senescence-associated *sarcopenia* (muscle atrophy). Another mechanism by which CR suppresses sarcopenia is by maintaining muscle innervation. As it were, muscle fibers are innervated by *motor* neurons originating in the anterior region of the spinal cord. Electro-chemical discharge of these neurons stimulates muscles to contract and loss of such stimulatory neurons accompanies and/or causes age-associated atrophy of muscles. In a study published in the journal *Microscopy Research and*

Technique it was determined that lifelong CR promoted the preservation of motor neurons (Kanda K 2002). This maintenance of muscle innervation enabled more muscle fibers to be recruited in response to sufficient stimuli, thereby permitting muscles to produce greater contractile force. The suggestion that the loss of motor neurons is a causative factor in the etiology of sarcopenia is based on the fact that muscle innervation has a *trophic* role; that is, innervation maintains the structure and function of muscle fibers. As Guyton and Hall's *Textbook of Medical Physiology* explains:

> When a muscle loses its nerve supply, it no linger receives the contractile signals that are required to maintain normal muscle size. Therefore, atrophy begins almost immediately. After about 2 months, degenerative changes also begin to appear in the muscle fibers themselves. If the nerve supply grows back rapidly to the muscle, full return of function usually occurs in about 3 months, but from that time onward, the capability of functional return becomes less and less, with no further return of function after 1 to 2 years. (Guyton and Hall 2000: 78)

The age-associated extirpation of neurons is methodic and progressive, as is the atrophy it induces. These interrelated pathological processes commence in early adulthood, resulting in reductions in muscle mass in the range of 30%-40% from the third to ninth decades of life (Mourad LA 1998). What is more, remaining muscle is often aberrantly altered in such a way that considerably compromises contractile capacity and the cytologic vacancy left by atrophied muscle is filled by fat and other fibrous tissue. Guyton and Hall explain this phenomenon thusly:

> In the final stage of denervation atrophy, most of the muscle fibers are destroyed and replaced by fibrous and fatty tissue. The fibers that do remain are composed of a long cell membrane with a line-up of muscle cell nuclei but with no contractile properties and no capability of regenerating myofibrils if a nerve regrows. The fibrous tissue that replaces the muscle fibers during denervation atrophy has a tendency to continue shortening...(Guyton and Hall 2000: 78)

The replacement of functional contractile tissue with inert, fatty, fibrous tissue calls to mind the image of "bodybuilders" who at their zenith accrete massive muscles only to have them waste away with the passage of time into unsightly flab.

Caloric restriction attenuates age-associated atrophy of muscles via multiple mechanisms. In a study published in the journal of the *Federation of American Societies for Experimental Biology*, it was found that CR resulted in a substantial suppression of muscle atrophy and complete preservation of muscle fibers. Whereas free-fed rats lost as much as half of their muscle fibers as they advanced in age, calorie-restricted subjects showed no such change (McKiernan S et al. 2004). Another way in which CR averts atrophy is by mitigating muscle *apoptosis*—a programmed process of cellular suicide prompted when cells incur various toxic, metabolic and oxidative insults. An interesting study published in the journal *Free Radical Biology and Medicine* found that apoptosis accelerated in the skeletal muscles of aged animals and that CR significantly reduced the rapidity and severity of apoptotic cell death in muscle tissue (Dirks and Leeuwenburgh 2004). The investigators attributed this anti-apoptotic effect to the suppression of certain regulatory proteins that promote apoptosis. They summarized their findings as follows:

> [T]his study shows that the apoptotic potential is increased in aged skeletal muscle and that [it] is reduced in calorie-restricted rats compared with their age-matched controls. The pro-apoptotic proteins…are all elevated with age…[S]lowing the aging process by lifelong calorie restriction appears to attenuate potential apoptotic stimuli, such as mitochondrial oxidant production (hydrogen peroxide) and DNA damage…In this study the levels of [pro-apoptotic proteins] were reduced significantly with calorie restriction and this reduced the potential for skeletal muscle apoptosis which may result in a reduction in the incidence and severity of sarcopenia through the preservation of muscle mass and muscle function and a slowing of myofiber loss with age. (Dirks and Leeuwenburgh 2004: 28)

Interestingly, the aged animals in this study exhibited such substantial preservation of muscle tissue that their ratios of muscle mass to bodyweight were higher than freely fed animals less than half their age.

As the aforementioned experiments indicate, the quantitative constitution of the diet exerts an important influence on the physiology of muscle. It is evident, however, that the qualitative constitution of the diet influences musculoskeletal physiology as well. In *Evolutionary Nutrition*, I relate evidence that the preponderance of sulfur-containing amino acids in meat—specifically cysteine and methionine which yield sulfuric acid as a product—elevates the acidity of the body such that it induces a compensatory mechanism eliciting efflux of amino acids from muscle. As the following excerpt explains:

> Metabolic acidosis stimulates catabolism of skeletal muscle proteins but not their synthesis. Nitrogen end products increase and muscle mass decreases during experimentally induced metabolic acidosis. This effect may be a homeostatic mechanism that maintains acid-base balance: catabolism of skeletal muscle provides glutamine, which the kidney extracts to produce the base ammonia, for the excretion of acid (as ammonium)…Thus, skeletal muscle, like bone, may serve as a reservoir of base that is gradually depleted to maintain acid-base balance. Chronic depletion of skeletal muscle could lead to weakness and a greater number of falls, both factors in hip fracture. (Sellmeyer et al. 2001: 121)

Habitual consumption of meat can consequently exacerbate age-associated muscle atrophy and is evidently an etiological factor in osteoporosis and bone fracture (Amen-Ra N 2003). Conversely, the preponderance of basic (alkaline) compounds common in vegetal products likely opposes muscle atrophy. Thus, the vegetal constitution of the Amen Diet may provide added protection against muscle deterioration, complementing the sarcopenia-suppressing effect of CR.

Conclusion

Aging is a complex, multi-faceted phenomenon. Any intervention aimed at reducing its rapidity must accordingly be multi-faceted (if not commensurately complex). As such, the protocol presented in this chapter amalgamates multifarious, theoretically substantive, anti-aging interventions with the only experimentally validated methodology known to consistently maximize mammalian lifespan—caloric restriction. I have defined my intellectual approach as selective synergism—an approach predicated upon identifying the manner in which caloric restriction modulates the molecular milieu of the body so as to synergize these self-same variables in an effort to augment the assumptive anti-aging effects thereof. The resulting regimen is admittedly austere and I am duly sympathetic to the anticipated objections of less disciplined dissenters. It is important, however, not to conflate and confuse matters of theory with matters of practicality. Science has afforded moderns the informational means with which to maximize individual longevity. What individuals endeavor to do with this momentous knowledge is a matter of personal judgment, a matter of practicality. I haven't the hubris to pretend that this is the final, definitive word in theoretical Biogerontology but the phylogenetic generality of CR suggests that all roads to that ever-elusive elixir of life is linked to caloric curtailment—whether quantitative or temporal. It is undoubtedly unpalatable to some that longevity and vitality should be so inextricably linked to restriction and restraint. Others appreciate, as do I, the ancient aphorism that 'All things worth wielding require discipline to attain'. One need not adopt asceticism in order to assent to the Amen Protocol, assent being a purely intellectual affair. Death, however, is a serious matter and the likelihood that it can be forestalled lends a greater degree of gravity to what would otherwise be entirely academic. It is for this reason that the protocol is, in part, experientially based. It is intellectually incongruous, I aver, to covet life and health on one hand and, on the other, to neglect knowledge as to the manner in which they can be cultivated, sustained, and prolonged. As such, I subject myself to the principles inherent in the Amen Protocol and I have presented them herein for the benefit of all inclined to do likewise.

References

Aiello, LC and Wells, JCK. Energetics and the evolution of the genus Homo. *Annual Review of Anthropology* 2002 31, 323-338.

Allen, NE; Apple, PN; Davey, GK; Kaaks, R; Rinaldi, S; and Key, TJ. The associations of diet with serum insulin-like growth factor I and its main binding proteins in 292 women meat-eaters, vegetarians, and vegans. *Cancer Epidemiology, Biomarkers and Prevention.* 2002 11, 1441-1448.

Alpern, RJ and Sakhaee, K. The clinical spectrum of chronic metabolic acidosis: homeostatic mechanisms produce significant morbidity. *American Journal of Kidney Diseases* 1997 29, 291-302.

Aly, KB; Pipkin, JL; Hinson, WG; Feuers, RJ; Duffy, PH; Lyn-Cook, L; and Hart, RW. Chronic caloric restriction induces stress proteins in the hypothalamus of rats. *Mechanisms of Ageing and Development* 1994 76, 11-23.

Amen-Ra, N. How dietary restriction catalyzed the evolution of the human brain: An exposition of the nutritional neurotrophic neoteny theory. *Medical Hypotheses* 2007 doi:10.1016/j.mehy.2007.02.035.

Amen-Ra, N. Humans are evolutionarily adapted to caloric restriction resulting from ecologically dictated dietary deprivation imposed during the Plio-Pleistocene period. *Medical Hypotheses* 2006 66, 978-984.

Amen-Ra, N. Evolutionary Nutrition: The Scientific and Theoretical Validation of Veganism. Damascus, MD: Amenta Press; 2003.

Ando, S; Tanaka, Y; Toyoda nee Ono, Y; Kon, K; and Kawashima, S. Turnover of synaptic membranes: age-related changes and modulation by dietary restriction. *Journal of Neuroscience Research* 2002 70, 290-297.

Anson, RM; Guo, Z; de Cabo, R; Iyun, T; Rios, M; Hagepanos, A; Ingram, DK; Lane, MA; and Mattson, MP. Intermittent fasting dissociates beneficial effects of dietary restriction on glucose metabolism and neuronal resistance to injury from calorie intake. *Proceedings of the National Academy of Sciences* (USA) 2003 100, 6216-6220.

Arumugam, TV; Gleichmann, M; Tang, SC; and Mattson, MP. Hormesis/preconditioning mechanisms, the nervous system and aging. *Ageing Research Reviews* 2006 5, 165-178.

Babu, PV; Sabitha, KE; and Shyamaladevi, CS. Therapeutic effect of green tea extract on advanced glycation and cross-linking of collagen in the aorta of streptozotocin diabetic rats. *Clinical and Experimental Pharmacology and Physiology* 2006 33, 351-357.

Bae, JW and Lee, MH. Effect and putative mechanism of action of ginseng on the formation of glycated hemoglobin in vitro. *Journal of Ethnopharmacology* 2004 91, 137-140.

Barbieri, M; Bonafe, M; Franceschi, C; and Paolisso, G. Insulin/IGF-I-signaling pathway: an evolutionarily conserved mechanism of longevity from yeast to humans. *American Journal of Physiology: Endocrinology and Metabolism* 2003 285, E1064-E1071.

Bauer, M; Hamm, AC; Bonaus, M; Jacob, A; Jaekel, J; Schorle, H; Pankratz, MJ; and Katzenberger, JD. Starvation response in mouse liver shows strong correlation with life-span-prolonging processes. *Physiological Genomics*, 2004 17, 230-244.

Bevilacqua, L; Ramsey, JJ; Hagopian, K; Weindruch, R; and Harper, ME. Long-term caloric restriction increases UCP3 content but decreases proton leak and reactive oxygen species production in rat skeletal muscle mitochondria. *American Journal of Physiology: Endocrinology and Metabolism* 2005 289, E429-E438.

Blanc, S; Schoeller, D; Kemnitz, J; Weindruch, R; Colman, R; Newton, W; Wink, K; Baum, S; and Ramsey, J. Energy expenditure of rhesus monkeys subjected to 11 years of dietary restriction. *The Journal of Clinical Endocrinology and Metabolism* 2003 88, 16-23.

Blander, G and Guarente, L. The Sir2 family of protein deacetylases. *Annual Review of Biochemistry* 2004 73, 417-435.

Blüher, M; Kahn, BB; and Kahn, CR. Extended longevity in mice lacking the insulin receptor in adipose tissue. *Science*, 2003 299, 572-574.

Cabelof, DC; Yanamadala, S; Raffoul, JJ; Guo, Z; Soofi, A; and Heydari, AR. Caloric restriction promotes genomic stability by induction of base excision repair and reversal of its age-related decline. *DNA Repair* 2003 2, 295-307.

Cai, W; He, JC; Zhu, L; C, Xue; Wallenstein, S; Striker, GE; and Vlassara, H. Reduced oxidant stress and extended lifespan in mice exposed to a low glycotoxin diet: Association with increased AGER1 expression. *The American Journal of Pathology*, 2007 doi: 102353/ajpath.2007.061281.

Cai, W; Gao, QD; Zhu, L; Peppa, M; He, C; and Vlassara, H. Oxidative stress-inducing carbonyl compounds from common foods: novel mediators of cellular dysfunction. *Molecular Medicine* 2002 8, 337-346.

Cao, SX; Dhahbi, JM; Mote, PL; and Spindler, SR. Genomic profiling of short- and long-term caloric restriction effects in the liver of aging mice. *Proceedings of the National Academy of Sciences, USA*, 2001 98, 10630-106305.

Casirola, DM; Rifkin, B; Tsai, W; and Ferraris, RP. Adaptations of intestinal nutrient transport to chronic caloric restriction in mice. *American Journal of Physiology* 1996 271, G192-G200.

Cross, AJ; Peters, U; Kirsh, VA; Andriole, GL; Reding, D; Hayes, RB; Sinha, R. A prospective study of meat mutagens and prostate cancer risk. *Cancer Research* 2005 62, 11779-11784.

Davis, S; Butcher, SP; and Morris, RG. The NMDA receptor antagonist D-2-amino-5-phosphonopentanoate (D-AP5) impairs spatial learning and LTP in vivo at intracerebral concentration comparable to those that block LTP in vitro. *The Journal of Neuroscience* 1992 12, 21-34.

D'Costa, AP; Lenham, JE; Ingram, RL; and Sonntag, WE. Moderate caloric restriction increases type 1 IGF receptors and protein synthesis in aging rats. *Mechanisms of Ageing and Development* 1993 71, 59-71.

Dean, DJ; Broznick, JT; Samuel, WC; and Cartee, GD. Calorie restriction increases cell surface GLUT-4 in insulin-stimulated skeletal muscle. *American Journal of Physiology* 1998 275, E957-E964.

Delbono, O. Regulation of excitation contraction coupling by insulin-like growth factor-1 in aging skeletal muscle. *Journal of Nutrition, Health and Aging* 2000 4, 162-164.

De Lumen, BO. Lunasin: a cancer-preventive soy peptide. *Nutrition Reviews* 2005 63, 16-21.

Deupree, DL; Bradley, J; and Turner, DA. Age-related alteration in potentiation in the CA1 region in F344 rats. *Neurobiology of Aging* 1993 249-258.

Dhahbi, JM; Cao, SX; Tillman, JB; Mote, PL; Madore, M; Walford, RL; and Spindler, SR. Chaperone-mediated regulation of hepatic protein secretion by caloric restriction. *Biochemical and Biophysical Research Reviews* 2001 284, 335-339.

Diano, S; Farr, SA; Benoit, SC; McNay, EC; daSilva, I; Horvath, B; Gaskin, FS; Nonakam, N; Jaeger, LB; Banks, WA; Morley, JE; Pinto, S; Sherwin, RS; Xu, L; and Yamada, KA; Sleeman, MW; Tschop, MH; Horvath, TL. Ghrelin controls hippocampal spine synapse density and memory performance. *Nature Neuroscience* 2006 9, 381-388.

Dirks, AJ and Leeuwenburgh, C. Aging and lifelong calorie restriction result in adaptations of skeletal muscle apoptosis repressor, apoptosis-inducing factor, x-linked inhibitor of apoptosis, caspase-3, and caspase-12. *Free Radical Biology and Medicine* 2004 36, 27-39.

Diskin, MG; Mackey, DR; Roche, JF; and Sreenan, JM. Effects of nutrition and metabolic status on circulating hormones and ovarian follicle development in cattle. *Animal Reproductive Science* 2003 78, 345-370.

Donati, A; Cavallini, G; Carresi, C; Gori, Z; and Parentini, I; Bergamini, E. Anti-aging effects of anti-lypolytic drugs. *Experimental Gerontology* 2004 39, 1061-1067.

Duan, W; Guo, Z; and Mattson, MP. Brain-derived neurotrophic factor mediates an excitoprotective effect of dietary restriction in mice. *Journal of Neurochemistry* 2001 76, 619-626.

Dubey, A; Forster, MJ; Lal, H; and Sohal, RS. Effect of age and caloric intake on protein oxidation in different brain regions and on behavioral function of the mouse. *Archives of Biochemistry and Biophysics* 1996 333, 189-197.

Duffy, PH; Seng, JE; and Lewis, SM; Mayhugh, MA; Aidoo, A; Hattan, DG; Casciano, DA; Feuers, RJ. The effects of different levels of dietary restriction on aging and survival in the Sprague-Dawley rat: implications for chronic studies. *Aging (Milano)* 2001 13, 263-272.

Eckles-Smith, K; Clayton, D; Bickford, P; and Browning, MD. Caloric restriction prevents age-related deficits in LTP and in NMDA receptor expression. *Brain Research: Molecular Brain Research* 2000 78, 154-162.

Fahey, JW; Zhang, Y; and Talalay, P. Broccoli sprouts: an exceptionally rich source of inducers of enzymes that protect against chemical carcinogens. *Proceedings of the National Academy of Sciences (USA)* 1997 94, 10367-10372.

Feuers, RJ; Weindruch, R; and Hart, RW. Caloric restriction, aging, and antioxidant enzymes. *Mutation Research* 1993 295, 191-200.

Gazdag, AC; Dumke, CL; Kahn, CR; and Cartee, GD. Calorie restriction increases insulin-stimulated glucose transport in skeletal muscle from IRS-1 knockout mice. *Diabetes* 1999 48, 1930-1936.

Goodrick, CL; Ingram, DK; Reynolds, MA; Freeman, JR; and Cider, N. Effects of intermittent feeding upon body weight and lifespan in inbred mice: interaction of genotype and age. *Mechanisms of Ageing and Development* 1990 55, 69-87.

Goto, S; Takahashi, R; Araki, S; and Nakamoto, H. Dietary restriction initiated in late adulthood can reverse age-related alterations in protein and protein metabolism. *Annals of the New York Academy of Sciences* 2002 959, 50-56.

Gould, TJ; Bowenkamp, KE; Larson, G; Zahniser, NR; and Bickford, PC. Effects of dietary restriction on motor learning and cerebellar noradrenergic dysfunction in aged F344 rats. *Brain Research* 1995 684, 150-158.

Greenberg, JA and Boozer, CN. Metabolic mass, metabolic rate, caloric restriction, and aging in male Fischer 344 rats. *Mechanisms of Ageing and Development* 2000 113, 37-48.

Guo, Z; Ersoz, A; Butterfield, DA; and Mattson, MP. Beneficial effects of dietary restriction on cerebral cortical synaptic terminals: preservation of glucose and glutamate transport and mitochondrial function after exposure to amyloid beta-peptide, iron, and 3-nitropropionic acid. *Journal of Neurochemistry* 2000 75, 314-320.

Guyton, AC and Hall, JE. *Textbook of Medical Physiology* (10th edition). Philadelphia, PA: Saunders; 2000.

Guzman, M and Blazquez, C. Ketone body synthesis in the brain: possible neuroprotective effects. *Prostaglandins, Leukotrienes and Essential Fatty Acids* 2004 70, 287-292.

Hagopian, K; Ramsey, JJ; and Weindruch R. Caloric restriction increases gluconeogenic and transaminase enzyme activities in mouse liver. *Experimental Gerontology* 2003 38, 267-278.

Hart, RW; Leakey, JE; Chou, M; Duffy, PH; Allaben, WT; and Feuers, RJ. Modulation of chemical toxicity by modulation of caloric intake. *Advances in Experimental Medicine and Biology* 1992 322, 73-81.

Hodgson, E. Introduction to Toxicology. In: Hodgson E, Editor. *A Textbook of Modern Toxicology* (3rd edition). Hoboken, NJ: John Wiley and Sons; 2004; 1-12.

Hofmann, SM; Dong, HJ; Li, Z; Cai, W; Altomonte, J; Thung, SN; Zeng, F; Fisher, EA; and Vlassara, H. Improved insulin sensitivity is associated with restricted intake of dietary glycoxidation products in the db/db mouse. *Diabetes* 2002 51, 2082-2089.

Holt, PR; and Heller, TD; Richardson, AG. Food restriction retards age-related biochemical changes in rat small intestine. *Journal of Gerontology* 1991 46, B89-B94.

Horska, A; Brant, LJ; and Ingram, DK; Hansford, RG; Roth, GS; Spencer, RG. Effect of long-term caloric restriction and exercise on muscle bioenergetics and force development in rats. *American Journal of Physiology* 1999 276, E766-E773.

Husom, AD; Peters, EA; Kolling, EA; Fugere, NA; Thompson, LV; and Ferrington, DA. Altered proteasome function and subunit composition in aged muscle. *Archives of Biochemistry and Biophysics* 2004 421, 67-76.

Jeong, HJ; Lam, Y; and de Lumen, BO. Barley lunasin suppresses ras-induced colony formation and inhibits core histone acetylation in mammalian cells. *Journal of Agricultural and Food Chemistry* 2002 50, 5903-5908.

Kanda K. Effects of food restriction on motoneuronal loss with advancing age in the rat. *Microscopy Research and Technique* 2002 59, 301-305.

Kloting, N and Bluher, M. Extended longevity and insulin signaling in adipose tissue. *Experimental Gerontology* 2005 40, 878-883.

Koizumi, A; Masuda, H; Wada, Y; Tsukada, M; Kawamura, K; Kamiyama, S; and Walford, RL. Caloric restriction perturbs the pituitary-ovarian axis and inhibits mouse mammary tumor virus production in a high-spontaneous-mammary-tumor-incidence mouse strain (C3H/SHN). *Mechanisms of Ageing and Development* 1989 49, 93-104.

Koschinsky, T; He, CJ; Mitsuhashi, T; Bucala, R; Liu, C; Buenting, C; Heitmann, K; and Vlassara, H. Orally absorbed reactive glycation products (glycotoxins): an environmental risk factor in diabetic nephropathy. *Proceedings of the National Academy of Sciences (USA)* 1997 94, 6474-6479.

Lambert, K; Py, G; Eydoux, N; Matecki, S; Ramonatxo, M; Prefaut, C; and Mercier, J. Effect of food restriction on lactate sarcolemmal transport. *Metabolism* 2003 52, 322-327.

Lambert, AJ; Wang, B; and Merry, BJ. Exogenous insulin can reverse the effects of caloric restriction on mitochondria. *Biochemical and Biophysical Research Communications* 2004 316, 1196-1201.

Lamming, DW; Wood, JG; and Sinclair, DA. Small molecules that regulate lifespan: evidence for xenohormesis. *Molecular Microbiology* 2004 53, 1003-1009.

Lass A, Sohal BH, Weindruch R, Forrster MJ, and Sohal RS. Caloric restriction prevents age-associated accrual of oxidative damage to mouse skeletal muscle mitochondria. *Free Radical Biology and Medicine* 1998 25, 1089-1097.

Leakey, JA; Cunny, HC; Bazare, J; Webb, PJ; Feuers, RJ; Duffy, PH; and Hart, RW. Effects of aging and caloric restriction on hepatic drug metabolizing enzymes in the Fischer 344 rat. I: The cytochrome P-450 dependent monooxygenase system. *Mechanisms of Ageing and Development* 1989 A 48, 145-155.

Leakey, JA; Cunny, HC; Bazare, J; Webb, PJ; Lipscomb, JC; Slikker, W; Feuers, RJ; Duffy, PH; and Hart, RW. Effects of aging and caloric restriction on hepatic drug metabolizing enzymes in the Fischer 344 rat. II: Effects on conjugating enzymes. *Mechanisms of Ageing and Development* 1989 B 48, 157-166.

Lee, J; Duan, W; and Mattson, MP. Evidence that brain-derived neurotrophic factor is required for basal neurogenesis and mediates, in part, the enhancement of neurogenesis by dietary restriction in the hippocampus of adult mice. *Journal of Neurochemistry* 2002 82, 1367-1375.

Lee, J; and Seroogy, KB; Mattson, MP. Dietary restriction enhances neurotrophin expression in the hippocampus of adult mice. *Journal of Neurochemistry* 2002 80, 539-547.

Leite, M; Frizzo, JK; Nardin, P; Almeida, LM; Tramontina, F; Gottfried, C; and Goncalves, CA. Beta-hydroxy-butyrate alters the extracellular content of S100B in astrocyte cultures. *Brain Research Bulletin* 2004 64, 139-143.

Li, D; Chen, S; Randerath, E; and Randerath, K. Oat lipids-induced covalent DNA modifications (I-compounds) in female Sprague-Dawley rats, as determined by P32-postlabeling. *Chemico-Biological Interactions* 1992 84, 229-242.

Lin, SJ; Ford, E; Haigis, M; Liszt, G; and Guarente, L. Calorie restriction extends yeast life span by lowering the level of NADH. *Genes and Development* 2004 18, 12-16.

Masoro, EJ. Dietary restriction-induced life extension: a broadly based biological phenomenon. *Biogerontology* 2006 7, 153-155.

Masoro, EJ. Role of sirtuin proteins in life extension by caloric restriction. *Mechanisms of Ageing and Development* 2004 125, 591-594.

Masoro, EJ. Hormesis and the antiaging action of dietary restriction. *Experimental Gerontology* 1998 33, 61-66.

Masoro, EJ; Katz, MS; and McMahan, CA. Evidence for the glycation hypothesis of aging from the food-restricted rodent model. *Journal of Gerontology* 1989 44, B20-B22.

Masoro, EJ; McCarter, RJ; Katz, MS; and McMahan, CA. Dietary restriction alters characteristics of glucose fuel use. *Journal of Gerontology* 1992 47, B202-B208.

Massieu, L; Haces, ML; Montiel, T; and Hernandez-Fonseca, K. Acetoacetate protects hippocampal neurons against glutamate-mediated neuronal damage during glycolysis inhibition. *Neuroscience* 2003 120, 365-378.

Maswood, N; Young, J; Tilmont, E; Zhang, Z; Gash, DM; Gerhardt, GA; Grondin, R; Roth, GS; Mattison, J; Lane, MA; Carson, RE; Cohen, RM; Mouton, PR; Quigley, C; Mattson, MP; and Ingram, DK. Caloric restriction increases neurotrophic factor levels and attenuates neurochemical and behavioral deficits in a primate model of Parkinson's disease. *Proceedings of the National Academy of Sciences (USA)* 2004 101, 18171-18176.

Mattson, MP; Duan, W; and Guo, Z. Meal size and frequency affect neuronal plasticity and vulnerability to disease: cellular and molecular mechanisms. *Journal of Neurochemistry* 2003 84, 417-431.

Mayhew, M; Renganathan, M; Delbono, O. Effectiveness of caloric restriction in preventing age-related changes in rat skeletal muscle. *Biochemical and Biophysical Research Communications* 1998 251, 95-99.

McKiernan, S; Bua, E; McGorray, J; and Aiken, J. Early-onset calorie-restriction conserves fiber number in aging rat skeletal muscle. *The FASEB Journal* 2004 18, 580-581.

Moore, CI; Browning, MD; and Rose, GM. Hippocampal plasticity induced by primed burst, but not long-term potentiation, stimulation is impaired in area CA1 of aged Fischer 344 rats. *Hippocampus* 1993 3, 57-66.

Mourad, LA. Structure and Function of the Musculoskeletal System. In: McCance, KL and Huether, SE editors. Pathophysiology: The Biologic Basis for Disease in Adults and Children (3rd edition). St. Louis, MO: Mosby; 1998; 1405-1432.

Nakagawa, T; Yokozawa, T; Terasawa, K; Shu, S; and Juneja, LR. Protective activity of green tea against free radical- and glucose-mediated protein damage. *Journal of Agricultural and Food Chemistry* 2002 50, 2418-2422.

Nelson, DL and Cox, MM. *Lehninger Principles of Biochemistry* (3rd edition). New York, NY: Worth Publishers; 2000.

Nelson, W and Halberg, F. Schedule-shifts, circadian rhythms and lifespan of freely-feeding and meal-fed mice. *Physiology and Behavior* 1986 38, 781-788.

Oftedal OT. The nutritional consequences of foraging in primates: the relationship of nutrient intakes to nutrient requirements. *Philosophical Transactions of the Royal Society of London. Series B, Biological Sciences* 1991 334, 161-169.

Osborne, TB; Mendel, LB; and Ferry, EL. The effect of retardation of growth upon the breeding period and duration of life in rats. *Science,* 1917 45, 294-295.

Patra, J and Panda, B. A comparison of biochemical responses to oxidative and metal stress in seedlings of barley, Hordeum vulgare L. *Environmental Pollution* 1998 101, 99-105.

Picard, F; Kurtev, M; Chung, N; Topark-Ngarm, A; Senawong, T; Machado de Oliveira, R; Leid, M; McBurney, MW; and Guarente, L. Sirt1 promotes fat mobilization in white adipocytes by repressin PPAR-gamma. *Nature* 2004 429, 771-776.

Piperno, DR; Weiss, E; Holst, I; and Nadel, D. Processing of wild cereal grains in the Upper Paleolithic revealed by starch grain analysis. *Nature* 2004 430, 670-673.

Radak, Z; Takahashi, R; Kumiyama, A; Nakamoto, H; Ohno, H; Ookawara, T; and Goto, S. Effect of aging and late onset dietary restriction on antioxidant enzymes and proteasome activities, and protein carbonylation of rat skeletal muscle and tendon. *Experimental Gerontology* 2002 37, 1423-1430.

Ramamurthy, B; Jones, DA; and Larsson, L. Glutathione reverses early effects of glycation on myosin function. *American Journal of Physiology: Cell Physiology* 2002 285, C419-C424.

Randerath, K; Randerath, E; and Danna, TF. Lack of I-compounds in DNA from a spectrum of Morris hepatomas. *Carcinogenesis* 1990 11, 1041-1044.

Ravelo, AC; Andreasen, DH; Lyle, M; Lyle, AO; and Wara, MW. Regional climate shifts caused by gradual global cooling in the Pliocene epoch. *Nature* 429, 263-267.

Reed, KE. Early hominid evolution and ecological change through the African Plio-Pleistocene. *Journal of Human Evolution* 1997 32, 289-322.

Renganathan, M and Delbono, O. Caloric restriction prevents age-related decline in skeletal muscle dihydropyridine receptor and ryanodine receptor expression. *FEBS Letters* (the journal of the Federation of European Biochemical Societies) 1998 434, 346-350.

Rodgers, JT; Lerin, C; Haas, W; Gygi, SP; Spiegelman, BM; and Puigserver, P. Nutrient control of glucose homeostasis through a complex of PGC-1 alpha and SIRT1. *Nature* 2005 434, 113-118.

Schriner, SE; Linford, NJ; Martin, GM; Treuting, P; Ogburn, CE; Emond, M; Coskun, PE; Ladiges, W; Van Remmen, H; Wallace, DC; and Rabinovitch, PS. Extension of murine life span by overexpression of catalase targeted to mitochondria. *Science* 2005 308, 1909-1911.

Sellmeyer, DE; Stone, KL; and Sebastian, A; Cummings, SR. A high ratio of dietary animal to vegetable protein increases the rate of bone loss and the risk of fracture in postmenopausal women. Study of Osteoporotic Fractures Research Group. *American Journal of Clinical Nutrition* 2001 73, 118-122.

Sohal, RS. Role of oxidative stress and protein oxidation in the aging process. *Free Radical Biology and Medicine* 2002 33, 37-44.

Sohal, RS and Weindruch, RL. Oxidative stress, caloric restriction, and aging. *Science* 1996 273, 59-63.

Soti, C and Csermely, P. Chaperones come of age. *Cell Stress and Chaperones* 2002 7, 186-190.

Speakman, JR; Selman, C; McLaren, JS; and Harper, EJ. Living fast, dying when? The link between aging and energetics. *The Journal of Nutrition* 132 (6 Suppl 2), 1583S-1597S.

Spindler, SR. Calorie restriction enhances the expression of key metabolic enzymes associated with protein renewal during aging. *Annals of the New York Academy of Sciences* 2001 928, 296-304.

Strassmann, BI. The evolution of endometrial cycles and menstruation. *The Quarterly Review of Biology* 1996 71, 181-220.

Tang, L; Zhang, Y; Jobson, HE; Li, J; Stephenson, KK; Wade, KL; and Fahey, JW. Potent activation of mitochondria-mediated apoptosis and arrest in S and M phases of cancer cells by a broccoli sprout extract. *Molecular Cancer Therapeutics* 2006 5, 935-944.

Tissenbaum, HA and Guarente, L. Increased dosage of a sir-2 gene extends lifespan in Caenorhabditis elegans. *Nature* 2001 410, 227-230.

Tontonoz, P; Hu, E; and Spiegelman, BM. Stimulation of adipogenesis in fibroblasts by PPAR-gamma 2, a lipid-activated transcription factor. *Cell* 1994 79, 1147-1156.

Vuksan, V; Sievenpiper, JL; Koo, VY; Francis, T; Beljan-Zdravkovic, U; Xu, Z; and Vidgen, E. American ginseng (Panax quinquefolius L) reduces postprandial glycemia in nondiabetic subjects and subjects with type 2 diabetes mellitus. *Archives of Internal Medicine*, 2000 A 160, 1009-1013.

Vlassara, H; Cai, W; Crandall, J; Goldberg, T; Oberstein, R; Dardaine, V; Peppa, M; and Rayfield, EJ. Inflammatory mediators are induced by dietary glycotoxins, a major risk factor for diabetic angiopathy. *Proceedings of the National Academy of Sciences (USA)* 99, 15596-15601.

Vouldoukis, I; Conti, M; Krauss, P; Kamate, C; Blazquez, S; Tefit, M; Mazier, D; Calenda, A; and Dugas, B. Supplementation with gliadin-combined plant superoxide dismutase extract promotes antioxidant defenses and protects against oxidative stress. *Phytotherapy Research* 2004 18, 957-962.

Vuksan, V; Stavro, MP; Sievenpiper, JL; Koo, VY; Wong, E; Beljan-Zdrakovic, U; Francis, T; Jenkins, AL; Leiter, LA; Josse, RG; and Xu, Z. American ginseng improves glycemia in individuals with normal glucose tolerance: effect of dose and time escalation. *Journal of the American College of Nutrition*, 2000 B 19, 738-744.

Weindruch, R; Gottesman, SR; and Walford, RL. Modification of age-related immune decline in mice dietarily restricted from or after midadulthood. *Proceedings of the National Academy of Sciences (USA)* 1982 79, 898-902.

Weindruch, R and Walford, RL. *The Retardation of Aging and Disease by Dietary Restriction*. Springfield, Il: Charles C. Thomas; 1988.

Weindruch, R and Walford, RL. Dietary restriction in mice beginning at 1 year of age: effect on life-span and spontaneous cancer incidence. *Science* 1982 215, 1415-1418.

Weindruch, R; Walford, RL; Fligiel, S; and Guthrie, D. The retardation of aging in mice by dietary restriction: longevity, cancer, immunity and lifetime energy intake. *The Journal of Nutrition* 1986 116, 641-654.

Whiten, A and Widdowson, EM eds. *Foraging Strategies and Natural Diet of Monkeys, Apes, and Humans*. New York, NY: Oxford University Press; 1992.

WHO (World Health Organization). *Energy and Protein Requirements*. Report of a Joint FAO/WHO/UNU Expert Consultation. Technical Report Series 724. World Health Organization, Geneva; 1985.

Wu, A; Wan, F; Sun, X; and Liu, Y. Effects of dietary restriction on growth, neurobehavior, and reproduction in developing Kunmin mice. *Toxicological Sciences,* 2002 70, 238-244.

Yamada, K; Mizuno, M; and Nabeshima, T. Role for brain-derived neurotrophic factor in learning and memory. *Life Sciences,* 2002 70, 735-744.

Yan, J; Vetvicka, V; Xia, Y; Coxon, A; Carroll, MC; Mayadas, TN; and Ross, GD. Beta-glucan a "specific" biologic response modifier that uses antibodies to target tumors for cytotoxic recognition by leukocyte complement receptor type 3 (CD11b/CD18). *Journal of Immunology,* 1999 163, 3045-3052.

Yokozawa, T and Nakagawa, T. Inhibitory effects of Loubuma tea and its components against glucose-mediated protein damage. *Journal of Agricultural and Food Chemistry* 2004 42, 975-981.

Yu, BP; Masoro, EJ; and McMahan, CA. Nutritional influences on aging of Fischer 344 rats: I. Physical, metabolic, and longevity characteristics. *Journal of Gerontology,* 1985 40, 657-670.

Zhou, GD; Hernandez, NS; Randerath, E; and Randerath, K. Acute elevation by short-term DR or food deprivation of type I I-compound levels in rat liver DNA. *Nutrition and Cancer,* 1999 35, 87-95.

In: Handbook on Longevity: Genetics, Diet and Disease ISBN 978-1-60741-075-1
Editors: Jennifer V. Bentely and Mary Ann Keller © 2009 Nova Science Publishers, Inc.

Chapter IX

Protective Effect of Calorie Restriction on Age-Induced Fibrosis

E. Chiarpotto[1], L. Castello[1], E. Bergamini[2], and G. Poli[1]

[1]Department of Clinical and Biological Sciences, University of Torino, Regione Gonzole 10, 10043 Orbassano (TO), Italy.
[2]Research Center on the Biology and Pathology of Aging, Department of Experimental Pathology, University of Pisa, Via Roma 55, 56123 Pisa, Italy.

Abstract

Starting from research by McCay et al., several studies have demonstrated that controlled calorie restriction (CR) exerts an anti-ageing effect in different organisms, from invertebrates to mammals. Observational studies suggest that CR also has beneficial effects on human longevity. However, the anti-aging mechanisms of CR are still not clearly understood. One mechanism might be protection against the age-associated increase of oxidative stress and consequent cellular damage.

In parallel, a role of oxidative stress in fibrosis induction and progression has been demonstrated in many human diseases, such as pneumoconiosis, interstitial pulmonary fibrosis, cystic fibrosis, cirrhosis, neurodegenerative diseases and atherosclerosis.

In fibrosis, fibroblasts or fibroblast-like cells are activated by various cytokines, among which transforming growth factor β1 (TGFβ1) is prominent, to proliferate and produce high levels of extracellular matrix and collagen. High TGFβ1 levels have been found in human diseases of different organs all characterized by excessive ECM deposition and marked fibrosis (cirrhosis, chronic hepatitis, glomerulonephritis, diabetic nephropathy, atherosclerosis, sclerodermia, pulmonary fibrosis). Fibrosis is also a constant distinctive feature in tissue aging.

TGFβ1 exerts its multiple biological activities through interaction with type I and type II receptors. Signaling to the nucleus is principally through cytoplasmic proteins of the Smad family, but in various cell types TGFβ1 also activates mitogen activated protein kinase (MAPK) pathways, i.e. extracellular regulated kinase 1 and 2 (ERK1/2), c-Jun N-terminal kinase (JNK) and p38, leading to collagen type I synthesis through activation of the transcription factor activator protein 1 (AP-1).

In this context, it is of interest to study the possible protective effect of CR against the onset of fibrosis in the frame of tissue and soma aging.

In this connection, our group has shown that, with aging, there is an increase of oxidative stress in rat aorta, with a progressive hoarding of biologically-active end-products, in particular 4-hydroxy-2,3-nonenal (HNE). Moreover, the increase of oxidative stress with aging is accompanied by increased fibrosis in terms of TGFβ1 and collagen levels. CR protects against both phenomena.

With regard to possible protective mechanisms of CR against fibrosclerosis, we believe they may be closely connected to the reduction of oxidative stress: by decreasing HNE levels in older rat aortae, CR significantly decreases JNK and p38 activity. Since JNK is central for AP-1 activation, by negatively modulating JNK, CR also prevents AP-1 activation and consequently down-regulates transcription of AP-1-dependent genes, including TGFβ1, vimentin and collagen.

The possibility of controlling the fibrogenesis process by modifying dietary habits opens new nutritional horizons in the prevention and treatment of several pathological processes characterized by excessive fibrosis. However, since it seems difficult to transpose animal CR model as such to man, interest in natural and/or pharmacological CR mimetic molecules is increasing.

Introduction

Aging is a multifactorial process that affects nearly all organisms, and which is believed to be produced by intrinsic (developmental-genetic) (Atzmon et al., 2005; Novelli et al., 2008) and extrinsic (stochastic-environmental) causes (Burhans & Weinberger, 2007; Passos et al., 2007). These are not mutually exclusive, and both are important. Observations have been accumulating on both the genetic determinants of aging and the major cellular mechanisms involved in this process (e.g. free radicals, mitochondrial dysfunction and oxidative stress, autophagy, insulin-like growth factor/growth hormone signaling, cholesterol and glucose metabolism, telomere shortening, etc.).

Since we cannot act on our genetic background, any intervention on the environmental factors becomes extremely important as an anti-aging strategy.

One of the most enduring theories to explain aging is the free radical theory initially proposed by Harman in the 1950s (Harman, 1956) which implicates free radicals and other reactive molecules derived from oxygen (reactive oxygen species, ROS) as mediators of age-dependent cell decline. Oxidants are normal by-products of cellular metabolism, most being generated in the mitochondria along the electron transport chain during cellular respiration (for a review, see Poli et al., 2004). Mitochondria are not only the primary producers of ROS, they are also highly susceptible to oxidant-induced damage because of the proximity of ROS, and because mitochondrial DNA cannot be repaired (Grishko et al., 2005). This has led to the formulation of the mitochondrial theory of aging (Miquel et al., 1980; Trifunovic & Larsson, 2008) that suggests senescence is the result of damage caused by ROS to the mitochondrial genome in post mitotic cells. Once mitochondria become injured, they become less efficient at producing energy and produce larger amounts of ROS. In young cells, damaged mitochondria, as well as unwanted or redundant cell membranes and organelles, may be removed via autophagy (Bergamini et al., 2007; Kurz et al., 2007) and in this perspective autophagy may well be considered as an anti-aging mechanism (Donati, 2006).

Oxidative Stress, Lipid Peroxidation and Fibrogenesis

The term fibrosis is used to define the excessive accumulation of connective tissue in parenchymal organs. Regardless of the underlying etiology, the process shows common features in terms of induction mechanisms, cells involved in the overproduction of extracellular matrix (ECM) components and the frequent progression to sclerosis. A central and essential role is played by macrophages and by ECM producing cells (hepatic stellate cells, smooth muscle cells, mesangial cells, myofibroblasts) which become the mediators of this process through the production of a complex network of growth factors, cytokines, chemoattractants and other reactive molecules (Wynn, 2008). Among these, transforming growth factor β1 (TGFβ1) is prominent (Branton & Kopp, 1999; Wynn, 2008). TGFβ1 is the most potent direct stimulator of collagen production, and it induces the transcription and synthesis of various other components of the ECM, such as fibronectin, glycosaminoglycans and proteoglycans (Verrecchia & Mauviel, 2002). In addition it stabilizes the newly formed ECM proteins by inhibiting their degradation (Hall et al., 2003). Thus, TGF-β1 is associated with fibrosis in a number of human diseases of different organs (including the lung, heart, liver, kidney, skin, artery) (Blobe et al., 2000; Bartram & Speer, 2004; Sharma et al., 2006). Moreover, fibrosis is a constant distinctive feature of tissue aging (Abrass, 2000; de Souza, 2002).

In parallel, a role of ROS and of lipid peroxidation in fibrosis induction and progression is now generally acknowledged in many human diseases, such as pneumoconiosis, interstitial pulmonary fibrosis, cystic fibrosis, cirrhosis, neurodegenerative diseases and atherosclerosis (Poli & Parola, 1997; Poli, 2000; Chiarpotto et al., 2005). In this connection, at physiopathological doses 4-hydroxy-2,3-nonenal (HNE), the major aldehyde deriving from the peroxidative breakdown of membrane phospholipids, has been shown to stimulate TGFβ1 expression and synthesis (Leonarduzzi et al., 1997) and the binding to DNA of the nuclear transcription factor AP-1 (Leonarduzzi et al., 1997; Chiarpotto et al., 2005), responsible for the activation of several genes, among which TGFβ1 itself, procollagen type I and vimentin (Armendariz et al., 1994; Kim et al., 1989; Rittling et al., 1989).

In most cell types, intracellular signaling of TGFβ1 occurs via two receptor serine/threonine kinases. The active form of TGFβ1 binds to specific type II receptors, which trigger recruitment of type I receptors to form tetrameric complexes that become phosphorylated (Massaguè & Chen, 2000). This propagates the signal intracellularly downstream to the nucleus through the phosphorylation of cytoplasmic proteins of the Smad family, Smad2 and Smad3, which form complexes with Smad4. The complex finally translocates to the nucleus, where it may activate target genes (Massaguè & Chen, 2000). However, in recent years alternate modes of TGFβ1 signaling have been described, particularly the mitogen activated protein kinase (MAPK) pathways, i.e. extracellular regulated kinase 1 and 2 (ERK1/2), c-Jun N-terminal kinase (JNK) and p38 (Mulder, 2000). Subsequent to the activation of MAPKs by TGFβ1, transcriptional responses mediated by activator protein 1 (AP-1) can lead to type I collagen synthesis (Cheon et al., 2002; Sato et al., 2002).

Anti-Aging Effect of Calorie Restriction

Starting from research by McCay et al. in the 1930s (McCay et al., 1935), diet restriction has been shown to extend median and maximum life span in all animal species tested thus far, from invertebrates to larger mammals like dogs (Sohal & Weindruch, 1996). Studies on the effects of diet restriction have been extended to primates, and the results thus far obtained are positive (Ramsey et al., 2000; Mattison et al., 2007). Importantly, indices of risk for cardiovascular disease and diabetes, such as blood pressure, blood lipids, glucose tolerance, and insulin sensitivity, have been reported to improve in monkeys on calorie restriction (CR) and also in humans who practice CR (Fontana et al., 2004; Meyer et al., 2006; Holloszy & Fontana, 2007). Reduced body weight and adiposity are other common changes in body composition that are similar among different mammalian species subjected to CR. On the basis of the relationship in humans between body weight and adiposity on one hand, and general mortality and morbidity on the other (Shiner & Uehlinger, 2001; Samaras et al., 2002), these data indicate that CR should also enhance longevity in man. Additionally, other metabolic and hormonal indices, such as reduced body temperature, triiodothyronine (T3) and insulin, that are predictive of increased survival, have been reported in rodents and rhesus monkeys on CR (Mattison et al., 2003; Roth et al., 2004), and also in humans in the CALERIE study (Redman et al., 2008). Scientific evidence also supports the view that lower calorie diets in humans may decrease the incidence of many age-related diseases, including cardiovascular disease, diabetes, cancer and neurodegenerative disorders, such as Alzheimer's and Parkinson's diseases (Mattson, 2005; Roberts & Barnard, 2005) .

Despite the plethora of scientific studies on the anti-aging effect of CR, the underlying mechanism/s have not yet been fully clarified. A comprehensive review on the numerous hypotheses on this topics was attempted by Chiarpotto et al. (2006). One theory that still remains popular is that CR protects against the age-related increase of oxidative damage (Merry, 2004).

Even if CR regimens applied to man are not so restrictive (about 1700 Kcal/day) (Meyer et al., 2006), it is difficult for most individuals to practice CR. Increasing interest is thus now being shown for the search for organic or inorganic compounds that mime the biological effects of CR, often called "CR mimetics".

In this context, it is of considerable importance to improve the caloric restriction approach, in view of its positive interference with most important mechanisms that lead to aging of the organism.

Molecular Mechanisms of Calorie Restriction's Protection Against Age-Induced Fibrosis

Aging is generally characterized by increased fibrotic tissue deposition in many organs; hence fibrosis/sclerosis is considered to be a significant index of tissue aging. It is thus of interest to study the possible protective effect of CR against the onset of fibrosis, in the framework of tissue and soma aging.

In this connection, we have shown that, with aging, oxidative stress increases in the rat aorta, with a progressive hoarding of biologically-active end-products, in particular 4-hydroxy-2,3-nonenal (HNE) (Table 1). Moreover, the increase with aging of oxidative stress is accompanied by increased fibrosis in terms of collagen and TGFβ1 levels (Figure 1). It is conceivable that HNE is involved in the pathogenesis of sclerotic diseases through the up-regulation of pro-inflammatory and pro-fibrotic genes (Nitti et al., 2002; Leonarduzzi et al., 2005; Uchida, 2008).

Table 1. Effect of calorie restriction (CR) on oxidative stress markers in rat aorta homogenates during aging

Dietary Treatment	HNE-protein adducts (Arbitrary Fluorescence Units/mg protein)	
	YR	OR
AL	127.6 ± 14.9	156.6 ± 28.0[a]
EOD	133.0 ± 15.5	81.0 ± 22.0[b]
	MDA-protein adducts (Arbitrary Fluorescence Units/mg protein)	
	YR	OR
AL	89.9 ± 18.6	122.7 ± 19.8[a]
EOD	80.6 ± 9.1	77.2 ± 24.4[b]

Data are means ± SD of 5 animals per group.
AL: rats fed ad libitum; EOD: rats starved every other day from 2 months of age.
YR: 6 months of age; OR: 24 months of age.
[a] Significantly different from AL YR, $p < 0.01$
[b] Significantly different from AL OR, $p < 0.05$

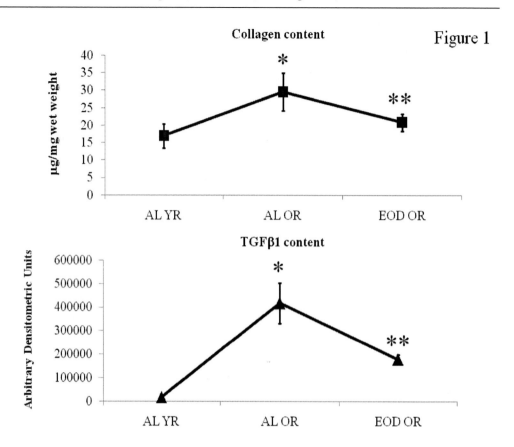

Figure 1. Effect of calorie restriction on fibrosis markers in homogenates of aortas from rats of different ages. Collagen content is expressed as μg/mg wet weight; TGFβ1 content is expressed as Arbitrary Densitometric Units. Data are means ± SD of 5 animals per group. * Significantly different from AL YR $p < 0.001$. ** Significantly different from AL OR $p < 0.001$. AL YR: rats aged 6 months fed ad libitum; AL OR: rats aged 24 months fed ad libitum; EOD OR: rats aged 24 months starved every other day from 2 months of age.

CR, achieved by feeding animals a standard diet on alternate days (EOD), protects against both oxidative stress and fibrosis (Table 1 and Figure 1). Possible protective mechanism/s of CR against fibrosclerosis might be closely connected to the reduction of oxidative stress: we observed increased JNK and p38 activation in rat aorta with age, both decreased by CR (Figure 2), while ERK1/2 are not influenced either by aging or by CR (data not shown). Moreover, AP-1 DNA binding is also increased in older rats and, as a consequence, the transcription of AP-1-dependent genes is also up-regulated, among which TGFβ1, collagen and vimentin (Figures 1, 3). CR is preventive against increased AP-1 activation and increased vimentin content (Figure 3); it may thus be assumed that, by decreasing HNE levels in older rat aortas, CR significantly decreases JNK and p38 activity. Since AP-1 activation is related to JNK activation (Karin & Gallagher, 2005), by down-regulating JNK, CR might prevent the age-related increase of AP-1 activation and consequently the transcription of AP-1-dependent genes, including TGFβ1, collagen and vimentin. Consistently, in the kidney, aging increases c-Fos and c-Jun levels and induces c-Jun phosphorylation, resulting in increased AP-1 activity, and CR prevents AP-1 activation by suppressing nuclear levels of c-Fos and c-Jun (Kim et al., 2002). Moreover, Bhattacharya et al. (2006) reported significant inhibition of NF-kB (p65/p50) and AP-1 (c-Fos/c-Jun) activities in splenocytes from WT/CR mice compared to WT/AL mice, suggesting that CR inhibits the redox-sensitive NF-kB and AP-1-dependent inflammatory responses. In this connection, CR has also been found to modulate activity and expression of several pro-inflammatory cytokines including TNF-α, IL-1β and IL-6, and to limit synthesis of other pro-inflammatory mediators (Chung et al., 2002; Chung et al., 2006). Moreover, inflammation markers are reduced in the plasma of animals and human volunteers subjected to CR (Ugochukwu & Figgers, 2007; Holloszy & Fontana, 2007; Johnson et al., 2007).

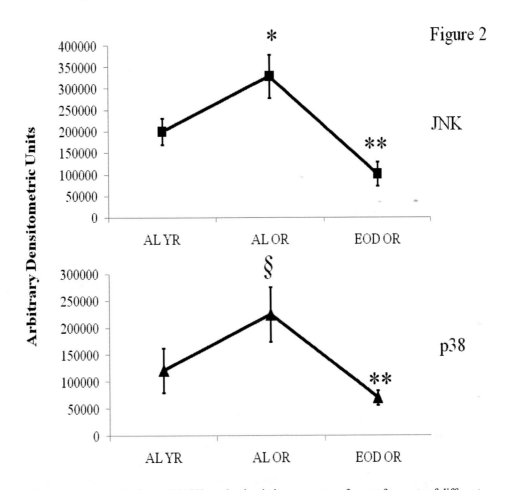

Figure 2. Effect of calorie restriction on MAPKs activation in homogenates of aortas from rats of different ages. Data are expressed as Arbitrary Densitometric Units and are means ± SD of 5 animals per group. * Significantly different from AL YR p < 0.001. § Significantly different from AL YR p < 0.05. ** Significantly different from AL OR p < 0.001. AL YR: rats aged 6 months fed ad libitum; AL OR: rats aged 24 months fed ad libitum; EOD OR: rats aged 24 months starved every other day from 2 months of age.

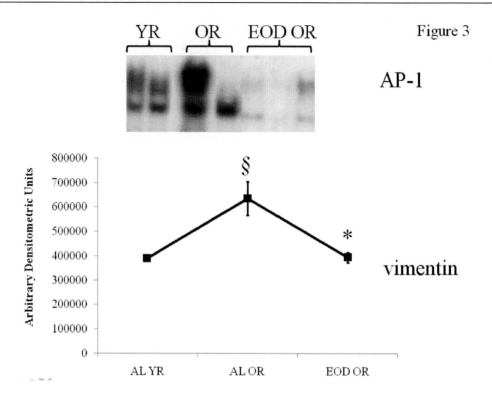

Figure 3. Effect of calorie restriction on AP-1 DNA binding activity (upper panel) and on vimentin levels (lower panel) in homogenates of aortas from rats of different ages. Data are expressed as Arbitrary Densitometric Units and are means ± SD of 5 animals per group. § Significantly different from AL YR p < 0.01. * Significantly different from AL OR p < 0.001. AL YR: rats aged 6 months fed ad libitum; AL OR: rats aged 24 months fed ad libitum; EOD OR: rats aged 24 months starved every other day from 2 months of age.

Conclusion

The free radical theory of aging proposed by Harman (1956) asserts that radicals endogenously produced during aerobic metabolism or induced by exogenous stimuli (irradiation, smoking, environmental pollution, dietary components) are major factors that contribute to aging. Oxidative damage to cells and tissues may be directly related to ROS and/or to final products of oxidative modifications of biological macromolecules, in particular lipids. Of these, lipid peroxidation-derived aldehydes (HNE) play a key role in the initiation and progression of fibrosis in various organs.

Among the several mechanisms proposed for the anti-aging action of CR, protection against oxidative damage is one of the most convincing.

In connection with fibrosclerosis, which is a constant and distinctive feature of tissue aging, CR decreases oxidative stress, with consequent reduction of the levels of HNE. CR may thereby also reduce fibrosis markers, TGFβ1 and collagen, most probably by reducing JNK and AP-1 activation. Acting on ROS and oxidative stress, CR may also influence the inflammatory environment by down-modulating inflammatory mediators (Figure 4).

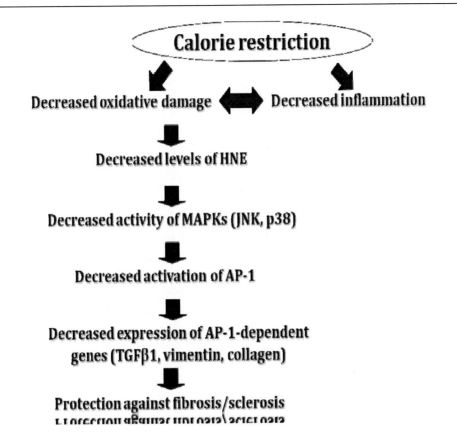

Figure 4. Possible model for the protective mechanism of calorie restriction against fibrosclerosis during aging.

The possibility of interfering in the fibrogenesis process by modifying dietary habits opens new nutritional horizons in the prevention and treatment of several pathological processes characterized by excessive fibrosis. The pharmacological or nutritional manipulation of endogenous cellular mechanisms is conceivably an innovative approach to therapeutic intervention in diseases causing tissue damage; this suggests potential novel therapeutic strategies relying upon the simultaneous activation of cytoprotective genes of the cell life program and down-regulation of pro-inflammatory and pro-oxidative genes. In light of the poor adherence of subjects to continuous low calorie restricted diets, studies are increasingly aimed at determining the feasibility and efficacy of natural and/or pharmacological CR mimetic molecules.

Acknowledgments

This work was supported by grants from the University of Turin, the Piedmont Regional Government, and the Italian Ministry for the Education, University and Research, PRIN 2007, Italy.

References

Abrass, C. K. (2000). The nature of chronic progressive nephropathy in aging rats. *Adv. Ren. Replace Ther., 7*, 4-10.

Armendariz-Borunda, J., Simkevitch, C. P., Roy, N., Raghow, R., Kang, A. H.& Seyer, J. M. (1994). Activation of Ito cells involves regulation of AP-1 binding proteins and induction of type I collagen gene expression. *Biochem. J., 304*, 817-824.

Atzmon, G., Rincon, M., Rabizadeh, P. & Barzilai, N. (2005). Biological evidence for inheritance of exceptional longevity. *Mech Ageing Dev., 126,* 341-345.

Bartram, U. & Speer, C. P. (2004). The role of transforming growth factor β in lung development and disease. *Chest, 125,* 754-765.

Bhattacharya, A., Chandrasekar. B., Rahman, M. M., Banu, J., Kang, J. X. & Fernandes, G. (2006). Inhibition of inflammatory response in transgenic fat-1 mice on a calorie-restricted diet. *Biochem. Biophys. Res. Commun., 349*, 925-930.

Bergamini, E., Cavallini, G., Donati, A. & Gori, Z. (2007). The role of autophagy in aging: its essential part in the anti-aging mechanism of caloric restriction. *Ann. N. Y. Acad. Sci., 1114,* 69-78.

Blobe, G. C., Schiemann, W. P. & Lodish, H.F. (2000). Role of TGFβ in human diseases. *N. Engl. J. Med., 342,* 1350-1358.

Branton, M. H. & Kopp, J. B. (1999). TGF-β and fibrosis. *Microbes and Infection, 1,* 1349-1365.

Burhans, W. C. & Weinberger, M. (2007). DNA replication stress, genome instability and aging. *Nucleic Acids Res., 35,* 7545-7556.

Cheon, H., Yu, S. J., Yoo, D. H., Chae, I. J., Song, G. G. & Sohn, J. (2002). Increased expression of pro-inflammatory cytokines and metalloproteinase-1 by TGF-beta1 in synovial fibroblasts from rheumatoid arthritis and normal individuals. *J. Clin. Exp. Immunol., 127,* 547-552.

Chiarpotto, E., Castello, L., Leonarduzzi, G., Biasi, F. & Poli, G. (2005). Role of 4-hydroxy-2,3-nonenal in the pathogenesis of fibrosis. *Biofactors, 24,* 229-236.

Chiarpotto, E., Bergamini, E. & Poli, G. (2006). Molecular mechanisms of calorie restriction's protection against age-related sclerosis. *IUBMB Life, 58,* 695-702.

Chung, H. Y., Kim, H. J., Kim, K. W., Choi, J. S. & Yu, B. P. (2002). Molecular inflammation hypothesis of aging based on the anti-aging mechanism of calorie restriction. *Micr. Res. Tech., 59,* 264-272.

Chung, H. Y., Sung, B., Jun, K. J., Zou, Y. & Yu, B. P. (2006). The molecular inflammatory process in aging. *Antioxid. Redox Signal., 8,* 572-581.

de Souza, R. R. (2002). Aging of myocardial collagen. *Biogerontology, 3,* 325-335.

Donati, A. (2006). The involvement of macroautophagy in aging and anti-aging interventions. *Mol. Aspects Med., 27,* 455-470.

Fontana, L., Meyer, T. E., Klein, S. & Holloszy, J. O. (2004). Long-term calorie restriction is highly effective in reducing the risk for atherosclerosis in humans. *Proc. Natl. Acad. Sci. U S A, 101,* 6659-6663.

Grishko, V. I., Rachek, L. I., Spitz, D. R., Wilson, G. L. & LeDoux, S.P. (2005). Contribution of mitochondrial DNA repair to cell resistance from oxidative stress. *J. Biol. Chem., 280,* 8901-8905.

Hall, M. C., Young, D. A., Waters, J. G., Rowan, A. D., Chantry, A., Edwards, D. R. & Clark, I. M. (2003). The comparative role of activator protein 1 and Smad factors in the regulation of Timp-1 and MMP-1 gene expression by transforming growth factor-beta 1. *J. Biol. Chem., 278,* 10304-10313.

Harman, D. (1956). Aging: a theory based on free radical and radiation chemistry. *J. Gerontol., 11,* 298-300.

Holloszy, J. O. & Fontana, L. (2007). Caloric restriction in humans. *Exp. Gerontol., 42,* 709-712.

Johnson, J. B., Summer, W., Cutler, R. G., Martin, B., Hyun, D. H., Dixit, V. D., Pearson, M., Nassar, M., Telljohann, R., Maudsley, S., Carlson, O., John, S., Laub, D. R. & Mattson, M. P. (2007). Alternate day calorie restriction improves clinical findings and reduces markers of oxidative stress and inflammation in overweight adults with moderate asthma. *Free Radic. Biol. Med., 42,* 665-674.

Karin, M. & Gallagher, E. (2005). From JNK to pay dirt: jun kinases, their biochemistry, physiology and clinical importance. *IUBMB Life, 57,* 283-295.

Kim, S. J., Dehnez, F., Kim, K. Y., Holt, J. T., Sporn, M. B. & Roberts, A. B. (1989). Activation of the second promoter of the transforming growth factor-β1 gene by transforming growth factor-β1 and phorbol ester occurs through the same target sequences. *J. Biol. Chem., 264,* 19373-19378.

Kim, H. J., Jung, K. J., Yu, B. P., Cho, C. G., Choi, J. S. & Chung, H. Y. (2002). Modulation of redox-sensitive transcription factors by calorie restriction during aging. *Mech. Ageing Dev., 123,* 1589–1595.

Kurz, T., Terman, A. & Brunk, U. T. (2007). Autophagy, ageing and apoptosis: the role of oxidative stress and lysosomal iron. *Arch. Biochem. Biophys., 462,* 220-230.

Leonarduzzi., G., Scavazza, A., Biasi, F., Chiarpotto, E., Camandola, S., Vogel, S., Dargel, R. & Poli, G. (1997). The lipid peroxidation end product 4-hydroxy-2,3-nonenal up-regulates transforming growth factor β1 expression in the macrophage lineage: a link between oxidative injury and fibrosclerosis. *FASEB J., 11,* 851-857.

Leonarduzzi., G., Chiarpotto, E., Biasi, F., & Poli, G. (2005). 4-Hydroxynonenal and cholesterol oxidation products in atherosclerosis. *Mol. Nutr. Food Res., 49,* 1044-1049.

Massagué, J. & Chen, Y.-G. (2000). Controlling TGF-beta signalling. *Genes Dev., 14,* 627-644.

Mattison, J. A., Lane, M. A., Roth, G. S.& Ingram, D. K. (2003). Calorie restriction in rhesus monkeys. *Exp. Gerontol., 38,* 35-46.

Mattison, J. A., Roth, G. S., Lane, M. A. & Ingram, D. K. (2007). Dietary restriction in aging nonhuman primates. *Interdiscip. Top. Gerontol., 35,* 137-158.

Mattson, M. P. (2005). Energy intake, meal frequency, and health: a neurobiological perspective. *Annu. Rev. Nutr., 25,* 237-260.

McCay, C. M., Crowell, M. F. & Maynard, L. A. (1935).The effect of retarded growth upon the length of lifespan and upon the ultimate body size. *J. Nutr., 10,* 63-69.

Merry, B. J. (2004). Oxidative stress and mitochondrial function with aging– the effects of calorie restriction. *Aging Cell, 3*, 7-12.

Meyer, T. E., Kovàcs, S. J., Ehsani, A. A., Klein, S., Holloszy, J. O. & Fontana, L. (2006). Long-term caloric restriction ameliorates the decline in diastolic function in humans. *J. Am. Coll. Cardiol., 47*, 398-402.

Miquel, J., Economos, A. C., Fleming, J. & Johnson, J. E. Jr. (1980). Mitochondrial role in cell aging. *Exp. Gerontol., 15*, 575-591.

Mulder, K. (2000). Role of Ras and Mapks in TGFbeta signalling. *Cytokine & Growth Factor Rev., 11*, 23-35.

Nitti, M., Domenicotti, C., D'Abramo, C., Assereto, S., Cottalasso, D., Melloni, E., Poli, G., Biasi, F., Marinari, U. M. & Pronzato, M. A. (2002). Activation of PKC-beta isoforms mediates HNE-induced MCP-1 release by macrophages. *Biochem. Biophys. Res. Commun., 294*, 547-552.

Novelli, V., Viviani Anselmi, C., Roncarati, R., Guffanti, G., Malovini, A., Piluso, G. & Puca, A. A. (2008). Lack of replication of genetic associations with human longevity. *Biogerontology, 9*, 85-92.

Passos, J. F., Saretzki, G., Ahmed, S., Nelson, G., Richter, T., Peters, H., Wappler, I., Birket, M. J., Harold, G., Schaeuble, K., Birch-Machin, M. A., Kirkwood, T. B. & von Zglinicki, T. (2007). Mitochondrial dysfunction accounts for the stochastic heterogeneity in telomere-dependent senescence. *PLoS Biol., 5*, 1138-1151.

Poli, G. & Parola, M. (1997). Oxidative damage and fibrogenesis. *Free Radic. Biol. Med., 22*, 287-305.

Poli, G. (2000). Pathogenesis of liver fibrosis: role of oxidative stress, *Mol. Aspects Med., 21*, 49-98.

Poli, G., Leonarduzzi, G., Biasi, F. & Chiarpotto, E. (2004). Oxidative stress and cell signalling. *Curr. Med. Chem., 11*, 1163-1182.

Ramsey, J. J., Colman, R J., Binkley, N. C., Christensen, J. D., Gresl, T. A., Kemnitz, J. W. & Weindruch, R. (2000). Dietary restriction and aging in rhesus monkeys: the University of Wisconsin study. *Exp. Gerontol., 35*, 1131-1149.

Redman, L. M., Martin, C. K., Williamson, D. A. & Ravussin, E. (2008). Effect of caloric restriction in non-obese humans on physiological, psychological and behavioral outcomes. *Physiol. Behav., 94*, 643-648.

Rittling, S. R., Coutinho, L., Amram, T. & Kolbe, M. (1989). AP-1/jun binding sites mediate serum inducibility of the human vimentin promotor. *Nucleic Acid Res., 17*, 1619-1633.

Roberts, C. K. & Barnard, R.J. (2005). Effects of exercise and diet on chronic disease. *J. Appl. Physiol., 98*, 3-30.

Roth, G. S., Mattison, J. A., Ottinger, M. A., Chachich, M., Lane, M. A. & Ingram, D. K. (2004). Aging in rhesus monkeys: relevance to human health interventions. *Science, 305*, 1423-1426.

Samaras, T. T., Storms, L. H. & Elrick, H. (2002). Longevity, mortality and body weight. *Ageing Res. Rev., 1*, 673-691.

Sato, M., Shegogue, D., Gore, E. A., Smith, E. A., McDermott, P. J. & Trojanowska, M. (2002). Role of p38 MAPK in transforming growth factor-beta stimulation of collagen production by scleroderma and healthy dermal fibroblasts. *J. Invest. Dermatol., 118*, 704-711.

Sharma, R., Sharma, M., Reddy, S., Savin, V. J., Nagaria, A. M. & Wiegmann, T. B. (2006). Chronically increased intrarenal angiotensin II causes nephropathy in an animal model of type 2 diabetes. *Front. Biosci., 11*, 968-976.

Shiner, J. S. & Uehlinger, D. E. (2001). Body mass index: a measure for longevity. *Med. Hypotheses, 57*, 780-783.

Sohal, R. S. & Weindruch, R. (1996). Oxidative stress, caloric restriction, and aging. *Science, 273*, 59-63.

Trifunovic, A., & Larsson, N.-G. (2008). Mitochondrial dysfunction as a cause of ageing. *J. Intern. Med., 263*, 167-178.

Uchida, K. (2008). A lipid-derived endogenous inducer of COX-2: a bridge between inflammation and oxidative stress. *Mol. Cells, 25*, 347-351.

Ugochukwu, N. H. & Figgers, C. L. (2007). Caloric restriction inhibits up-regulation of inflammatory cytokines and TNF-alpha, and activates IL-10 and haptoglobin in the plasma of streptozotocin-induced diabetic rats. *J. Nutr. Biochem., 18*, 120-126.

Verrecchia, F. & Mauviel, A. (2002). Transforming Growth Factor-β Signaling Through the Smad Pathway: Role in Extracellular Matrix Gene Expression and Regulation. *J. Invest. Dermatol., 118*, 211-215.

Wynn, T.A. (2008). Cellular and molecular mechanisms of fibrosis. *J. Pathol., 214*, 199-210.

In: Handbook on Longevity: Genetics, Diet and Disease   ISBN 978-1-60741-075-1
Editors: Jennifer V. Bentely and Mary Ann Keller   © 2009 Nova Science Publishers, Inc.

Chapter X

Engineered Natural Longevity-Enhancing Interventions

Arkadi F. Prokopov[1] and Tamara N. Voronina[2]
[1] Integrative Medicine, Mallorca, Spain
Email: ark1860@gmail.com
[2] (Ukraine)
12C Portman Mansions, Chiltern Street, London, W1U 6NU
Email: info@tvrejuvenation.com

Abstract

Currently developing engineered biogerontological interventions promise to radically extend healthy life span. Nevertheless, the exploration of natural strategies that underlie longevity and resistance to age-related diseases in exceptionally long-living mammals, such as the bowhead whale (BW, *Balena mysticetus*) and naked mole rat (NMR, *Heterocephalus glaber*) is also rational.

This paper is an attempt to analyze the advantages and limitations of these strategies, and to elucidate their existing derived applications, as well as to estimate their future prospects in the practice of biogerontology.

Two natural longevity-modulating strategies (intermittent calorie/nutrient restriction—ICR, and intermittent oxygen restriction—IOR) utilize the universal development-and adaptational genetic programs, evolutionary "preinstalled" in all aerobic organisms. ICR and IOR synergistically diminish the basal level of mitochondria-dependent oxidative stress that is supposed to be the key factor, modulating life span and resistance to age-related diseases in aerobes.

ICR and IOR employ a common mitochondria-rejuvenating pathway, *mitoptosis*—a selective elimination of excessively ROS-producing mitochondria in the cells. Mitoptosis is a natural process that maintains the "quality" of mitochondria in the female germinal cells during early embryogenesis, and can be stimulated and maintained by IOR and ICR also in the postmitotic cells of adult organisms. Behaviorally induced continuous mitoptosis seems to be the key mechanism responsible for exceptional longevity and resistance to age-related diseases in BW and NMR.

Additionally, ICR and IOR influence the longevity and tempo of development of age-related diseases via several mitochondria-independent pathways, such as suppressed protein glycation, enhanced DNA repair, accelerated protein turnover, stimulation of EPO, GH, HSP70 and other functional proteins. In addition, IOR distinctively intensifies stem-cell-dependent tissue repair.

The unified positive effect of IOR and ICR on the cells and organisms manifests in enhanced genome stability and increased non-specific resistance to multiple stressors.

Various forms of ICR and IOR have an impressively positive account of empiric and evidence-based use in the health-improving practices of various human cultures. Recently developed engineered techniques, such as short-termed, or alternate-day fasting (ADF, derivative of ICR) and intermittent hypoxic training/therapy (IHT, derivative of IOR) induce measurable mitochondrial and systemic rejuvenation.

The vitamin-nutriceutical supplementation synergistically enhances the efficiency of IOR and ICR.

Further development of engineered ICR and IOR protocols should facilitate their advanced clinical implementation and user-friendly, self-help applications.

Keywords: adaptation, autophagy, cancer, hypoxic preconditioning, intermittent hypoxic therapy, life span, mitochondria, mitoptosis

Introduction

This paper aims to elucidate two natural mitochondria-rejuvenative strategies and to outline their current derivative applications in clinic. The authors explore the evolutionary strategies and pathways that underlie the extraordinary longevity of some mammals. On the other hand, we make it known that the corresponding engineered life-extending natural interventions have already been successfully used in clinic. This article is neither a systemic review nor a summary of controlled double-blind clinical interventions; it is more an unfolding reflection and analysis of both authors' ideas and experiences during nearly two decades of practical application of described regenerative interventions.

It is agreed that any efficient prophylactic and therapeutic strategy that aims to increase healthy lifespan, retard the aging process and suppress age-related pathology shall address superior preservation and continuous rejuvenation of mitochondria in the postmitotic cells [1].

Mitochondria carry out multiple functions other than ATP production [2]. Among these are participation in apoptosis and cellular proliferation, generation and transmission of a transmembrane potential, oxygen sensing, regulation of the cellular redox state and the level of second messengers, heme and steroid syntheses, calcium storage and release, detoxification and heat production. In the majority of the listed functions, ROS and RNS modulate vitally important non-destructive cellular activities; hence the importance of integrity of mtDNA.

On the other hand, the oxidative mutational damage to the nuclear genome (nuDNA) and, particularly, to the mitochondrial genome (mtDNA) are believed to be the culprit of aging-related genomic instability that is associated with degenerative disease and frailty. Reactive oxygen and nitrogen species (ROS and RNS) are abundantly produced in oxidative phosphorylation (OXPHOS) in the mitochondria, inducing mutational deletions in mtDNA [3]. Modulation of lifespan by mitochondrial ROS production was shown in numerous studies on different species [4, 5].

Currently used mitochondria-supportive interventions are largely limited to slowing down ROS- and RNS-induced damage either by dietary supplementation of antioxidants [6], or by engineered overexpression of genes encoding antioxidant enzymes (e.g., SOD, catalase, glutathion-peroxidase). However, the antioxidative supplementation shows controversial results [7], while the engineered enhancement of antioxidant enzymes-encoding genes is still far from practical use.

Perhaps the most proficient bioengineered intervention that is currently under clinical testing employs the SkQ—a completely new type of synthetic mitochondria-targeting antioxidant based on mitochondrial membrane-penetrating ions [8]. This radically new approach promises to dramatically alleviate the burden of age-related diseases, as well as probably extend the healthy life span in humans in the observable future.

In the meantime, the analysis of the exceptional longevity phenomenon found in some mammals is also important if we are to evaluate practical interventions designed to postpone or alleviate aging when begun late in life. Elucidation of constituting pathways may help to synergistically increase the effectiveness of current and prospective, straightforwardly pharmaceutical, and/or genomic therapies.

The Challenge of Bowhead Whales and Naked Mole Rats

The extraordinary longevity of two mammals: bowhead whales (BW, *Balena mysticetus)* and naked mole rats (NMR, *Heterocephalus glaber*), as well as their remarkable resistance to cancer, attracted attention recently. These enormously different animals seem to have at least two key denominators in common: 1) they both occupy ecological niches in rather unproductive environments that offer season-dependent nutrition and have relatively few predators (killer whales and humans in BW and snakes in NMR); 2) both animals regularly experience significant oscillations of cellular O_2 and CO_2 tensions (diving in BW and burrowing in NMR), combined with seasonal (winter months in BW and dry season in NMR) severe calorie restriction or fasting.

Diving in BW, and living in underground, poorly-ventilated burrowing tunnels in NMR creates in both animals the intermittent hypoxic-hypercapnic state, which is interspersed by periods of normoxia and normocapnia. Earlier it was elucidated in detail [9] how these conditions may result in diminished mtDNA mutations and continuous elimination of mutated mtDNA in somatic cells, in increased autophagy, improved genome stability, increased allocation of stem cells for tissue maintenance and, ultimately, in the expression of a neotenic, life-span-enhanced and neoplasia-resistant phenotype in both animals.

Enhanced Longevity and Low Cancer Morbidity

George et al. [10] conducted aspartic acid racemization measurements of the eye lenses of 48 BW harvested between 1978 and 1996 to estimate the whale's age at the time of death. It was found that four animals were older than 100 y.o., and one was estimated to be 211 y.o. (the method has an accuracy range of about 16 %, which means this whale could have been from 177 to 245 y.o.). Amazingly, one of 100 + males was killed during mating.

The oldest living person with a birth certificate was a 122 y.o. French woman who died in 1997. Elephants have lived to 70 years in captivity, so bowheads appear to hold "the longevity record" for mammals.

Of 130 harvested BW examined between 1980 and 1989, only one exemplar had a benign tumor, found in the liver. According to Philo et al. [11], "It is unlikely that tumors are major contributors to bowhead whale morbidity or mortality."

In general, the necropsy studies of numerous baleen whales and odontocetes, harvested during decades of industrial whale hunting in the North and Antarctic regions, or stranded on the shores, show inexplicably low cancer morbidity compared to humans or terrestrial mammals. Thus: "A single cancer was found in over 1,800 other cetaceans examined, and tumors were not found in approximately 50 beluga examined in the Canadian Arctic" [12].

A single benign tumor was observed in 55 slaughtered pilot whales in Newfoundland [13], and only two benign tumors (0.1%) were reported in 2000 baleen whales hunted in South African waters [14]. Only three cases of cancers (0.7%) were found during the postmortem examination of 422 odontocetes from British waters [15]. Among few cancerous tumors ever discovered in baleen whales there were no metastatic ones and those found were small and encapsulated [16].

Naked mole rats can live more than 28 years in captivity, which is about nine times longer than similarly sized mice. There was neither a single cancer reported in the large 25 year-old captive colony [17], nor there are known NMR cancer cases described by other researchers.

What biological mechanisms provide such an extraordinary combination of increased cancer-resistance and enhanced longevity?

Peculiarities of BW Physiology

Bowhead whales live in water temperature near 0°C and feed while diving up to 33 minutes long. Diving hypoxia (that is essentially intermittent and accompanied by hypercapnia) is common to all diving mammals and birds.

According to George et al. [18], because of very thick blubber, BW may experience a "heat load" even at rest. However, the mean deep body temperature measured in 30 killed BW was 33.6 +/- 0.82°C. This is significantly lower than reported for other large cetaceans (baleen whales maintain a core body temperature between 36.6 and 37.2°C) and for other non-hibernating mammals.

We did not find neither published studies evaluating oxidative damage and mitochondrial functions in BW; however, a comparison of their known physiological and biochemical parameters with those of other baleen whales reveals no significant differences, except notably lower core body temperature in BW.

Peculiarities of NMR Physiology

In their natural environment in Kenyan and Ethiopian plains, NMR live in hypoxic, hypercapnic, subterranean burrows [19]. Their lungs are minimally developed [20], and, alike to fetal hemoglobins, their hemoglobin has high oxygen affinity [21]. NMRs basal metabolic rate is near 0.70 ml O2/g-h, which is extremely low for their body mass [22]. Under food restriction, NMR metabolic rate further decreased by 25% [23,24].

There is evidence that NMR´s maintain and remodel bone structure with much higher efficacy compared with similar- sized mice [25].

It was also found that NMR retain a youthful vascular function and protective cellular oxidant/antioxidant balance much longer than shorter-living rats; which indicates that NMR are better protected against aging-induced oxidative stress [26].

Physiological Pathways Common in the BW and NMR

What unifying factors, common in the both extremely dissimilar mammals permit so much greater longevity and cancer-resistance compared with animals about the same size (at least in the case of NMR) and similar living conditions? As oddly as it may seem, in general - it is the oscillations of tension of O_2 and CO_2 in their cells and their patterns of oxygen metabolism.

In their natural habitats both NMR and BW continuously undergo the *intermittent oxygen restriction* (IOR), characterized by hypercapnic hypoxia that all mammals normally exposed to during embryonic and prenatal period. IOR is dubbed to emphasize its deep relationship with the established term: *intermittent calorie restriction* (ICR). The behavioral IOR in BW and in NMR induces and maintains a universal phenotypic adaptation to hypoxia, or a life-long phenomenon of hypoxic preconditioning that is well known to reduce and/or prevent apoptic and necrotic damage caused by acute hypoxia-reoxygenation [27, 28].

It is obvious that IOR and ICR governed phylogenesis of both animals in their particular environmental niches.

Life Span, Cancer and Mitochondria

All metazoan face the problem of controlling cancer, which is by-product of one of the major evolutionary events, the advent of multicellularity [29]. The chance of malignant transformation is proportional to the number of cells multiplied on the lifespan of the organism [30]. So humans have much higher cancer-control capacity then mice (about 2/3 of wild mice, kept in a laboratory setting naturally die from cancer). Prevention and suppression of malignancy in constantly proliferating tissues (epithelial, liver, bone marrow) becomes progressively more difficult as body size increases, requiring the accelerated recruitment of additional controls that supposed to operate efficiently during initiation, promotion and progression—at all three levels of cancerous genome evolution in the host. Therefore BW that can weight 2000 times more and live twice longer than humans, obviously have much better cancer control. The same relates to the NMR, which have body mass equal to mice but live without cancer a magnitude longer.

It is recognized that malignous cells and tumors in an organism are products of multistage evolution of instable copies of the "selfish" mutated genome that escape immune surveillance and apoptosis [31]. Characteristically, most of these events are mediated by mitochondria-produced ROS and RNS.

On the other hand, it is assumed that each somatic cell initially contains a pool of mtDNA copies, having various degrees of oxidative/mutational deletions (*heteroplasmy*). It was found that under normal, affluent in fuel and oxygen, stabile metabolic conditions the damaged, partially deleted mtDNA copies acquire replicative advantage and increase their number more rapidly than intact and less damaged ones, thus progressively escalating accumulative ROS burden [32].

Genomocentristic Viewpoint

In contrast to often-prevailing cellulocentristic image of an organism, the following argumentation employs the evolutionary-based genomocentristic viewpoint. We believe that bodies, cells and cellular organelles can be logically viewed as molecular machines that are designed, assembled, and used by their genomes with the single purpose to enable transferring derivative genome copies into the next generations [33]. According to Dawkins' "Selfish Gene" theory, adaptations are the phenotypic tools through which genes secure their propagation.

The interactions among nuclear and mitochondrial genomes in mammalian cells, the mutual cooperation of both genomes is similar to that one, which exists between a shepherd and his cattle. Both benefit from each other, but it is the shepherd who governs his herd and controls the cattle's quantity and quality.

Since uncorrected accumulation of mtDNA mutations would within a very small number of generations become incompatible with survival, there should exist some common mechanisms for preservation of innate, wild-type mtDNA and selection against harmful, ROS-enhancing mtDNA deletions.

Evolutionary Maintenance of mtDNA

According to Allen [34], the *mtDNA evolutionary maintenance mechanism* relies on the repressed oxidative function of female germline mitochondria (*promitochondria*). The obligatory matrilineal mitochondria inheritance is found in the vast majority of species. This mechanism conserves germline promitochondria, preventing them from entering postmitotic oxidative phosphorylation, which is followed by oxidative mutational damage. The irreversible differentiation of promitochondria into fully functional mitochondria of somatic cell results in increased ATP production that is necessary for a multitude of developmental events.

Degradation of Somatic Mitochondria

MtDNA of functional mitochondria is more vulnerable to oxidative damage than nuclear DNA because it is not protected by histones and mitochondria are the primary sites of ROS generation. [35] This leads to mutations of mtDNA, involving the genes coding for respiratory chain proteins and also may disturb the continuous fission and fusion of mitochondria, resulting in their enlargement. Larger mitochondria are less autophagocytosed and undergo further oxidative damage, as well as produce more ROS [36]. As the oxidative mtDNA damage gradually progresses, and heteroplasmy—the proportion of deleted mtDNA to wild-type mtDNA, increases [37]. Critically damaged mitochondria undergo *mitoptosis* (self-destruction of mutated and "worn out" mitochondria) [38,44] and mitophagy; whereas the *less damaged mtDNAs multiply continuously and more rapidly than wild-type mtDNAs, thus achieving selective replicative advantage* [39].

Furthermore, it was suggested that *microheteroplasmy* (accumulation of acquired mutations in mitochondria of somatic and germinal cells that begins already in early embryonic period) is the primary cause of the exhaustion of the tissue renewal capacity in advanced age [40].

Another mechanism underlying cellular senescence is telomere attrition [41]. It is also found that a high level of oxidative stress shortens telomeres and triggers the senescence [42].

Functional activity stimulates mitochondrial biogenesis in the postmitotic cells. The primary messenger NO, thyroid and steroid hormones and mitochondria-specific nutrients and cofactors (L-carnitine, alpha-lipoic acid, taurine, coenzyme Q10, etc.) stimulate and support mitochondrial proliferation non-specifically, irrespectively of the degree of mutational burden presented in a particular clone of mtDNA.

Natural Selection of Better Quality Mitochondria

The *mtDNA selection and purification mechanism* is presented by the follicular atresia [43]. This mechanism selects for germline mtDNA quality in vertebrates. Follicular atresia (apoptic and/or necrotic elimination of about 90% of germinal cells in the ovaries of early female embryos) is an efficient "quality control" tool [44]. It eliminates the majority of ROS – producing mitochondria in the female germinal cell lines, thus preventing them from entering future generations, which could reduce offspring evolutionary fitness.

The clonal expansion of mutated and partially deleted mtDNA copies that occupy more intensively ROS-producing mitochondria correlates with advance of senescence and aging. It is found that with *ad libitum* available nutrition and with uninterrupted supply of sea level O_2

(21%, 160 torr), the damaged mtDNA enjoy replicative advantage over wild-type (non-mutated) mtDNA, which ultimately accelerates senescence [32, 39]. This pathway employs the chemo-kinetic advantages for shorter mtDNA molecules replication during mitochondria reproduction cycle.

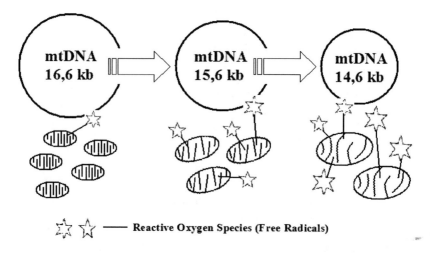

Figure 1. Some mtDNA mutations/deletions produce less efficient and more polluting mitochondria. MtDNA (ring-shaped molecule, approximate size in kb.) suffers about a magnitude higher oxidative mutational damage, compared to nuDNA. During insufficient self-repair the mutated segment of mtDNA ring would be excised/deleted and free ends fused together. The mtDNA looses information, its ring molecule becomes smaller and the mutated mitochondrion turns to be less efficient and more polluting. Wild-type mitochondria are small and dense; they move and fuse easily into the mitochondrial network. The mutated mitochondria are inefficient, large, and sluggish; they do not fuse together and produce increased amounts of ROS.

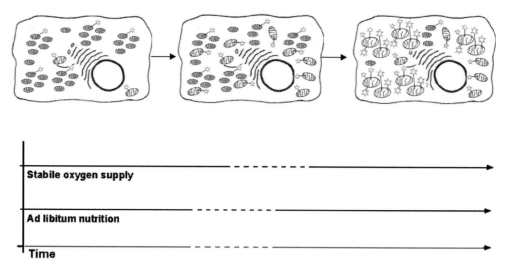

Figure 2. Affluent and uninterrupted supply of oxygen and nutrients (calories) accelerates mitochondrial decay and cellular senescence. With stabile oxygen delivery and ad libitum nutrition the mutated mitochondria out compete wild-type mitochondria for room and resources. They multiply faster, because their deleted mtDNA molecules are shorter. This vicious circle brings up the basal ROS output, which accelerates cellular senescence and the development of age-related pathology.

However, there is evidence that nuclear genome can indirectly preserve higher quality mtDNA also in somatic cells of adult animals, which may significantly increase their life span and delay the onset of age-related diseases. This would be typically achieved as a "side effect" of behavioral adaptational strategies, described by Dawkins [45] as the "extended phenotype". Such evolutionary conserved strategies as adaptation to IOR and ICR provide survival in environments characterized by rhythmic fluctuations in the availability of oxygen and nutrients, which is the apparent case in BW and NMR.

Intermittent Oxygen Restriction (IOR)

Combined hypoxia-hypercapnia is a primary physiological state in a developing mammalian embryo, and is essential to support its growth [46, 49]. The corresponding redox potential of embryonic tissues differs significantly from that of newborn and adult, and is a necessary condition for growth and development [47]. On the other hand, the gradual increase of cellular oxygen tension during the later phases of fetal development induces differentiation and maturation of tissues and organs [48, 50]. However, even the first observations of life under increased oxygen partial pressure revealed that "Oxygen might burn the candle of life too quickly, and soon exhaust the animal power within" (J. Priestley, 1775).

One possible strategy to slow down the ongoing oxidative mtDNA damage in somatic cells could employ maintaining and/or constantly returning, back to more economical, embryonic-type pattern of oxidative metabolism with its hypoxia-resistance and more youthful, chronologically earlier gene expression profile. This type of metabolism is known to protect both germinal and somatic cells from excessive mutational damage and to support their proliferation [51, 52].

A complementary strategy, useful in qualitative selection of mtDNA would be a periodical exposure of a pool of heteroplasmic mitochondria in somatic cells to a critical functional load; such as increased energy demand combined with limited availability of fuel and/or oxygen. For instance, by exposing an adult organism to a controlled multiple ischemia-hypoxia-reoxygenation episodes, which yet remain under threshold of a massive apoptic damage. Such O_2 oscillations boost mitochondrial ROS production that consequently stimulates enhanced enzymatic antioxidative defense in healthy mitochondria [53], while destroying mutated mitochondria via *mitoptosis* [38]. Mitoptosis is not only a key mechanism of germinal follicles atresia [54], but also plays an important role in the erythrocyte maturation cycle [55] and underlies apoptic remodeling in normal tissue development and healing.

One can hypothesize that mitoptosis, being repeatedly induced by IOR in an adult organism, could purify mitochondrial populations of postmitotic somatic cells from the constantly appearing, oxidatively damaged, ROS-producing mtDNA copies. This should bring replicative advantage for the wild-type, non-mutated mtDNA's that are significantly less ROS-producing, but multiply slower than mutated mtDNA copies [37, 39, 56].

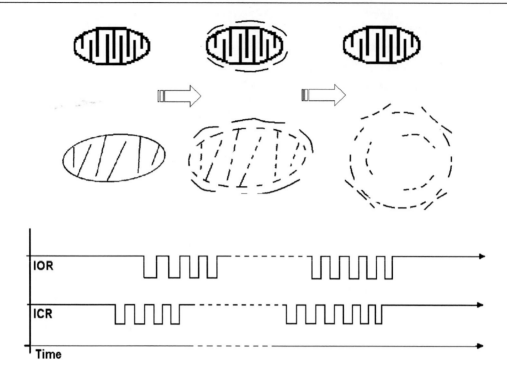

Figure 3. Mitoptosis is a physiological response to hypoxia-reoxygenation and calorie restriction. Oscillations of oxygen and nutrients (intermittent oxygen restriction—IOR and intermittent calorie restriction —ICR) stimulate impulse ROS production in mitochondria, consequently overloading mitochondrial antioxidative defense. Wild-type mitochondria (above) respond by increased production of antioxidative enzymes and survive. Mutated mitochondria (below) are much more sensitive to oxidative stress; they would be selectively eliminated in mitoptosis.

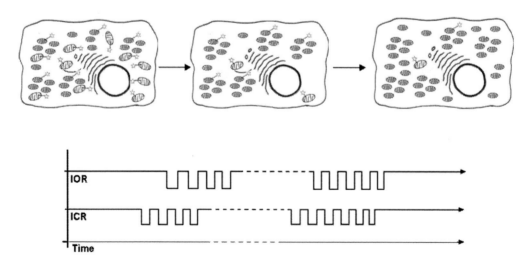

Figure 4. Oscillations of oxygen and fuel supply selectively eliminate ROS-producing mitochondria. Multiple oscillations of O_2 and nutrients purify postmitotic cells from mutated mitochondria via mitoptosis. In the absence of competition from deleted mitochondria, wild-type mitochondria quickly repopulate cells.

The IOR Stimulates Multiple Genome-Stabilizing Mechanisms

It is recognized that within the physiological range hypoxia is a universal challenge rapidly triggering multiple compensatory strategies that support genome integrity [57, 62].

Most eukaryotic cells maintain biological functions under hypoxia by switching energy source from fat acids to glucose and shutting down mitochondria. The switch is virtually instant and occurs simultaneously at the level of enzyme activity and gene expression [57]. The first-line antioxidative defense is triggered by hypoxia-induced mitochondrial ROS production and employs the glucose metabolism alteration. Underlying mechanism is based on a redirection of the metabolic flux from glycolysis to the pentose phosphate pathway, altering the redox equilibrium of the cytoplasmic NADP(H) pool [58]. The reversion to hypoaerobic metabolism is not limited to bioenergetic pathways, it stimulates expression of multiple genes and their products; numerous systems integrate to provide improved oxygen absorption, transportation and utilization.

Generally, it is found that under lower oxygen tension the mitochondrial ROS production is suppressed significantly, OXPHOS is more efficient and the maintenance energy is reduced because of notably lesser proton leak [59].

However, the IOR in form of physiological intermittent hypoxia evokes particularly beneficial adaptations, not seen in continuous hypoxia. On the other hand, the obstructive sleep apnea (OSA) presents a pathological IOR pattern.

Adaptation to IOR elicits upregulation of cytoglobins (myoglobin and neuroglobin), which function as intracellular O_2 buffer and provide protection against RNS [60].

IOR stimulates insulin-independent glucose transport and accumulation of glycogen in the oxygen-sensitive cells, including cardiomyocytes and neurons; thus increasing instantly available intracellular energy reserves [61].

IOR is more efficient than chronic hypoxia in stimulating activator protein-1 and HIF-1, the master proteins, responsible for numerous adaptational pathways [63].

IOR efficiently stimulates erythropoetin (EPO) production [63]. EPO is not only the main regulator of erythropoesis, but also provides multiple adaptogenic and protective effects, particularly in the CNS [64].

HSP70, one of the majors in the chaperons family, is also stimulated by IOR [65]. It was demonstrated recently, that lifelong overexpression of HSP70 in skeletal muscle provided protection against injury and facilitated successful recovery after damage in muscles of old mice [66].

IOR is shown to stimulate growth hormone and IGF-1 release, while chronic hypoxia suppresses both [67].

IOR stimulates increased production of endogenous antioxidative enzymes [68].

IOR modulates humoral and cellular immunity [69, 70].

IOR stimulates brain-derived growth factor (BDGF) and glial cells-derived growth factor (GDNF) that provide neuronal protection and regeneration [71].

Hypoxia Facilitates Stem Cell-Based Tissue Repair

Remarkably that IOR modulates production and release of not only hematopoetic, but also stromal stem cells. Stromal, or mesenchimal stem cells (MSC) are known to convert into specialized postmitotic cells (neurons, cardiomyocytes, chondrocytes and osteocytes) in damaged tissues [72]. Normal autoreparative processes in the body seem to be highly dependent on MSC. Thus, progeria particularly affects stem cells, reducing their resistance to oxidative stress and preventing stem-cells-dependent repair of tissues damaged with age [73].

Physiological hypoxia universally protects SC and stimulates release and homing of MSC [74]. It is found that MSC reside not only in the bone marrow, but also in perivascular tissues [75]; thus their activation by IOR seems to be a part of natural tissue-repair mechanism.

At least in some occasions, MSC can donate wild-type mtDNA by fusion with alternated cells without actually transforming into them [76]. In all variants, the IOR opens opportunity for enhanced MSC - dependent mitochondrial rejuvenation of damaged, non-replaceable cells (myocytes, cardiomyocytes, neurons, hormone-producing cells).

Protective Hypercapnia vs. Harmful Hypocapnia

In diving animals IOR is accompanied by simultaneous intermittent hypercapnia. Compared to humans, diving mammals have increased basal CO_2 values, but similar upper hypercapnia tolerance limit (37–60 torr vs. 45–60 torr, respectively) [77].

Physiological hypercapnia in vivo prevents damaging effects of ischemia or extreme hypoxia, which is widely used in clinic [78]. Several mechanisms may explain the protective role of CO_2 in vivo. One of the most significant appears to be the stabilization of the iron-transferrin complex, which prevents the involvement of iron ions in the initiation of free radical reactions [79].

It is found that even moderately elevated pCO_2 directly suppresses mitochondrial ROS production [80]. It was shown in human blood phagocytes and alveolar macrophages, in the cells of the liver, brain, myocardium, lungs, kidneys, stomach, and skeletal muscle, as well as in mice tissue phagocytes and liver mitochondria. Generation of ROS was measured in the cell cultures and biopsies using different methods after exposure of cells and whole body to hypercapnia. CO_2 at a tension close to that observed in the blood (37.0 torr) and higher (60 or 146 torr) is a potent inhibitor of mitochondrial ROS generation. The mechanism of CO_2 effect appears to depend, partially, on the inhibition of the NADPH-oxidase activity [80].

In addition, increased CO_2 efficiently scavenges peroxynitrite, which diminishes or prevents relevant nitration and oxidative damage, particularly in neurons [81].

In contrast to hypercapnic IOR in diving mammals, the continuous altitude hypoxia (such as in high mountains) is coupled with persistent hypocapnia caused by altitude hyperventilation. Furthermore, compared to consistently intermittent diving hypoxia, the constant altitude hypoxia poses on the body significantly higher "price of adaptation" due to combined hypocapnia, hypohydration, UV rays, low temperatures and insufficient rest, additionally aggravated by nutritional deficiencies, typical in mountains. It was shown that many mountain-climbers that completed Everest trail without supplementary oxygen suffer long-term CNS damage. The extent of this damage was proportional to degree of altitude hypocapnia [82, 83]. It is found that continuous hypoxia caused accelerated mitochondrial damage, seen as lisosomal mitochondrial "junk" – lipofuscin [84].

Compared to beneficial effects of IOR the continuous exposure to high altitude hypoxia, combined with hypocapnia accelerates development of age-related pathology in humans, as it was demonstrated in a study focused on the relationship linking human aging and altitude [85].

The author examined cardiovascular, respiratory, neurological, immune and endocrine systems of the subjects at different altitudes. Study showed that memory (in particular, short-term memory) declined with altitude. The age of memory loss at high altitude began several years earlier than that of the subjects in lowland areas. The altitude also negatively influenced cardiac functions. The lung function of middle and old aged subjects living at altitude and then moving to lowland areas for 4–7 years were still lower than those of resident subjects in lowland areas. Their immune and endocrine functions were suppressed as well. These changes indicated that environmental stresses such as chronic hypoxia, hypocapnia, ultraviolet irradiation and cold exposure result in more rapid aging at high altitude.

The underlying molecular mechanisms have been elucidated in the study of Jefferson et al. [86]. The authors verified that oxidative stress is increased following both acute exposures to high altitude without exercise and with chronic residence at high altitude. The limit of human altitude hypoxia adaptability is believed to be located around 3500–4000 m.

Summarizing, these data indicate that a radical deviation from the evolutionary shaped intermittent hypoxia/hypercapnia pattern, found in normal embryonic development might cause oxidative distress, disadaptation, functional overload of mitochondria and their accelerated structural degradation.

IOR in Non-Diving and Non-Burrowing Mammals

Whereas longevity-inducing and health-benefiting effects of ICR have been extensively demonstrated in numerous studies and in diverse species, there is also growing data on similar effects of IOR. Experiments show that beneficial adaptations and prolongation of life span may be induced by IOR in species that habitually live in normoxic and normocapnic atmosphere.

Honda [87] has shown that in *C. elegans*, changes in the generation and destruction of free radicals are implicated in life span modulations. The life spans under high and low oxygen concentrations were shorter and longer, respectively, than those under normoxic conditions. Short-term exposure to high and low oxygen concentration lengthens the life span. This is considered to be the result of an increase in antioxidant defense induced by short-term oxidative stress.

Since the pioneer publication of Meerson et al. [88] multiple aspects of adaptation to IOR were elucidated. Recently, the IOR was shown to directly prevent mtDNA deletions and mitochondrial structure damage in ischemia-reperfusion in vivo [89].

An important study of Milano et al. [90] focused on the difference in adaptation to continuous, compared with intermittent hypoxia. Authors tested the hypothesis that repeated brief reoxygenation episodes during chronic hypoxia improve myocardial tolerance to hypoxia-induced dysfunction. Three groups of male rats were exposed for two weeks to chronic hypoxia (10% O_2 and 90% N_2), intermittent hypoxia (same as chronic hypoxia, but 1 hr/day exposure to room air), or remained in normoxia (room air, 21% O_2). To evaluate myocardial tolerance to reperfusion, hearts of sacrificed animals were isolated and perfused for 30 min.; initially with hypoxic and then with hyperoxic medium. Exposure to either chronic hypoxia or intermittent hypoxia increased hematocrit, hemoglobin concentration, and erythrocytes count. Hypoxia decreased food and water intake with respect to normoxia. As a result, normoxic rats experienced net weight gain in two weeks. In contrast, chronically hypoxic rats underwent weight loss, whereas intermittent hypoxia rats neither gained nor lost weight. As the energy expenditure in caged rats can be assumed to be the same in all animals, the efficiency in food assimilation should have been greater in intermittent hypoxia group. In normoxia and especially in intermittent hypoxia group, the deleterious effect of reperfusion stress was apparently less than in continuous hypoxia group. Thus, despite differing only for 1 hr daily exposure to room air, chronic and intermittent hypoxia induced different responses in animal homeostasis, markers of oxidative stress, and myocardial tolerance to reoxygenation. Authors conclude that the protection in rats exposed to intermittent hypoxia appears conferred by the hypoxic preconditioning due to the repetitive reoxygenation, rather than by hypoxia per se.

A number of animal studies show that beneficial effects of IOR can be achieved during short and/or multiple hypoxic exposures, varying from half an hour to several hours a day [91, 92].

The Difference between Sanogenic and Pathogenic IOR

There are contrasting differences in physiological outcomes of various intermittent hypoxic regiments and protocols. Persistent hypertension is a common disorder found in patients and animals exposed to a severe, brief IOR, as occurs in obstructive sleep apnea (OSA) [93]. Alternatively, the adaptation to mild, physiological, normo - or hypobaric IOR has been repeatedly demonstrated to prevent development of experimental hypertension, and reduce blood pressure of hypertensive animals and patients [94].

The main reason for this discrepancy is that the cardiovascular and cellular response to IOR greatly depends on the parameters of hypoxic intervention. Experimental protocols vary greatly in duration and intensity of hypoxia. Thus, protocols that simulate OSA, inducing systemic hypertension and impairing endothelium-dependent vasorelaxation generally employ brief, repetitive, severe hypoxia episodes for prolonged periods. For instance, the inspiration of 2–3% O_2 for 6 sec. at 30 sec. intervals, several hours per day for 4–7 weeks, or inspiration of 10% O_2 for 1 min. at 4 min. intervals, 12 h per day, for 14 days.

In contrast, the protocols that stimulate beneficial long-termed adaptation to hypoxia (hypoxic preconditioning) are based on the physiological IOR; for instance an intermittent inspiration of 9–12% O_2 for one hour a day during 3–12 weeks. Such treatments prevent development of endothelial dysfunction and abolish rise of blood pressure in spontaneously hypertensive rats [94].

The physiological justification of the most efficient intermittent hypoxia protocols stems from the study of naturally occurring IOR (hypoxic cycles) in non-pregnant and pregnant mammalian uterus by Chizov et al. [95, 96]. The authors discovered series of rhythmical plummeting of oxygen tension in the uterus (- 4 ± 2 torr from 6–8 pO_2 torr baseline, duration for 3–5 min.) with subsequent return to baseline that appeared several times a day, and continued for about an hour in each series. It is suggested that these oscillations serve as an evolutionary conserved cellular "hypoxic training" mechanism that assists embryogenesis, development and maturation of embryo's enzymatic antioxidative defense. Logically, one can presume that these O_2 oscillations, caused by rhythmical spasms of uterine arteries may serve as an instrument of mitoptosis execution in follicular atresia. Similar spontaneous pO_2 oscillations were also found in the various tissues of adult mammals [97, 98]. The IOR protocols based on this discovery are currently known under the name of "The Intermittent Hypoxic Training/Therapy" (IHT) and used in clinic, as well as serve to enhance athletic training [99]. The IHT efficiently induces hypoxic preconditioning, or long-term adaptation to hypoxia in oxygen-sensitive organs [100, 101].

Hypoxic preconditioning (hypoxia adaptation) presents a common physiological pathway that involves adaptive genexpression and synthesis of corresponding proteins; it modulates multitude of cellular functions both in health and disease. The mitochondria-produced ROS and RNS triggering the adaptation in hypoxic preconditioning [102].

Messenger nitric oxide (NO) seems to play a central role in hypoxia adaptation. The NO-dependent protective mechanisms activated by IHT include stimulation of NO synthesis, as well as restriction of NO overproduction. The availability of NO precursors and donors (arginine and ornitine) and negative feedback of NO synthesis may optimize NO production. The adaptive enhancement of NO synthesis activates other protective factors, such as heat shock proteins, enzymatic antioxidants and prostaglandins, making the adaptation to hypoxia multilevel and sustained [103].

The unified positive effect of physiological IOR on the body is called cross-adaptation (induction of non-specific resistance to multiple stressors) and is a highly conserved characteristic that employs fundamental regulatory pathways that were established at the beginning of evolution of aerobes [88].

Intermittent Calorie Restriction (ICR)

Back to bowhead whales, who are the only baleen whales that spend their entire lives near polar ice edge; they do not migrate to temperate or tropical waters to calve. BWs are well adapted for living in cold waters—they have very thick, up to 0.5 m. blubber, which provides insulation and energy storage. Nutritional, and-energy balance in BW is characterized by deep excursions into stored nutrients during winter months, followed by summer periods of great abundance. This pattern of ICR makes BWs fully dependent on the affluent nutrients buildup in summer, while their survival throughout winter months under extreme fasting relies on autophagy (especially in pregnant and nursing females). The autophagy is a well recognized tissue-rejuvenating and cancer-suppressing strategy [104, 105, 106].

As all baleen whales, BWs thrive on fat-and protein-rich zooplankton. Fat-based OXPHOS has distinctive advantages compared to glucose-dependent OXPHOS (the latter prevails in mitochondrial energy pathways in some terrestrial herbivores). Marine mammals do not drink seawater; instead they produce it metabolically (oxidation of 1g fat gives 1.07 g. water).

Remarkably that in summer periods of affluent nutrition, as well as during fasting months the blood glucose in BW corresponds to the levels found in terrestrial animals [107].

Due to absence of carbohydrates in their food, glucose in BW is synthesized from glycerin, amino acids and lactate in gluconeogenesis, thus providing mitochondria with optimal amount of essential energy substrate and important metabolic precursor.

However, under starvation-induced hypoglycemia, mitochondria switch to metabolizing fat-derived ketones for energy production. This is a highly conserved adaptation to fasting and prolonged food restriction that evolved to enhance survival and maintain adequate functions while sparing proteins [108, 109, 110].

Ketone bodies, consisting of acetoacetate and β-hydroxybutirate are derived from fat in the liver and their concentration in blood is inversely related to that of glucose. Ketone bodies are more energetically efficient than either pyruvate or fatty acids because they are more reduced (greater hydrogen/carbon ratio) than pyruvate and do not uncouple the mitochondrial proton gradient as occurs with fatty acid metabolism [111]. In contrast to glucose, ketone bodies bypass cytoplasmic glycolysis and directly enter the mitochondria where they are oxidized to acetyl-CoA. The amount of acetyl-CoA formed from ketone body metabolism is also greater than that formed from glucose metabolism [112], which increases ATP production. Remarkably, the ketone body-induced boost in the ATP production is also accomplished using less oxygen [113].

In addition to increasing ATP production while sinking oxygen consumption, ketone metabolism also lessens production of free radicals, which diminishes tissue inflammation provoked by ROS [111, 112, 113]. Noteworthy that compared to oxidation of fat acids and ketones, glucose oxidation in mitochondria results in significantly higher ROS production [114].

Conversely, physiological hypoglycemia selectively induces mitochondria-triggered apoptosis of malignant cells, while mitochondria of normal cells easily tolerate even deeper hypoglycemia [115]. Thus, fat-derived ketone bodies are not only a more efficient metabolic fuel than glucose, but also provide anti-inflammatory and anti-neoplastic effects.

Bowheads grow to about 8 m during their first year; then grow very slowly after weaning.

Affluent, protein and fat-rich nutrition during weaning and growing period, followed by a life-long, rhythmically predictable, season-dependent ICR results in downregulation of longevity-modulating genes daf-2 and daf-16 [116, 117]—a highly conserved genomic response found in yeasts, C. elegans, mice and men. Hsu et al. have found that in adulthood only daf-2-deficient C. elegans are both longer-lived and resistant to oxidative stress [116]. Noteworthy that ICR can induce daf-2 product deficiency.

In nature, foraging of NMR is severely restricted throughout dry seasons. Animals cannot search extensively for new food sources unless the ground has been sufficiently moistened by rainfall [118]. During brief periods after rain, NMR dig intensively to find enough food to sustain them through the long, irregular droughts. Such foraging pattern may maintain the ICR in wild NMR. The NMR colonies feed on plant roots and tubers rich with carbohydrates, but relatively poor in proteins and fats. NMR practice coprophagy that allows "fair distribution" of scarce nutritional recourses and contributes to digestive efficiency, as well as reinoculates NMR with endosymbionts that supply an additional source of protein and energy from digestion of the microbes themselves [119]. Endosymbionts ferment indigestible cellulose and fibers into short-chain fatty acids and other nutrients, which supply a significant fraction of basal energetic rations, and also may offer precursors that provide increased cellular/mitochondrial membrane resistance to oxidative damage. NMR also drink no water, receiving it exclusively from food.

Why Do Normoxic and Ad-Libidum-Fed NMRs Still Express Longevity and Cancer-Resistant Phenotype?

The study of oxidative damage in lipids, DNA and proteins in ad-libitum fed captive or laboratory-born NMR, which in contrast to wild NMR live in normoxic and normocapnic conditions, showed greatly increased oxidative stress markers compared to mice [120]. The level of isoprostanes in the urine was 10 times higher, the level of malondialdehyde in liver tissue was twice as high and isoprostane levels in heart tissue in the NMR was 2.5 times higher then in mice. It was also found significantly more DNA and protein damage in their kidney, liver and in the heart. Nevertheless, captive NMR live an order of magnitude longer than predicted based on their body size and suffer no cancer. What mechanisms may explain these striking findings?

According to Buffenstein [121]

In preliminary studies we have found that NMR cells are more resistant to neoplastic transformation. We hypothesize that NMRs have both more efficient DNA repair, and reduced mutagenesis leading to genomic stability.

Remarkably, that the blueprint of protective pathways and mechanisms, synergistically integrated by IOR and ICR evolutionary-shaped genotype, provides expression of the longevity and cancer-resistant phenotype even at increased basal level of oxidative stress. The question arises, if the naturally occurring in captive NMR spontaneous IOR and ICR episodes may be responsible for the expression of innate, unique NMR phenotype in an affluent, pro-oxidative laboratory conditions?

The laboratory studies of the interaction between sleep and thermoregulation in NMR revealed functional poikilothermia for the period of the REM bout [122,123]. It is known that the functional hypometabolic states induce relaxation response and mitigate stress in mammals. It cannot be excluded that captive NMR are still capable maintaining in an affluent environment their natural behavioral pattern and circadian rhythm. For instance, a typical in NMR resting-sleeping pattern (when many animals huddle in the sleeping chamber) can facilitate in their bodies temporary state of physiological hypoventilation, hypoxia-hypercapnia and hypometabolism that stimulate cellular regeneration. Such "rejuvenative hypoxic-hypothermic naps" may represent the naturally occurring IOR episodes. So, the intermittent periods of behavioral hypoxia-hypercapnia, hypometabolism and hypothermia may still be incorporated in their daily life cycle in normoxic atmosphere.

On the other hand, there is a recent parallel finding in the knockout Glutathione peroxidase 4-deficient mice that shown higher level of basal oxidative stress, but paradoxally, had longer median life span than wild-type mice [124]. It was found that the Gpx4-deficient mice have significantly increased sensitivity to oxidative stress-induced apoptosis. Authors conclude that lifelong reduction in Gpx4 increased life span and reduced/retarded age-related pathology most likely through alterations in apoptic sensitivity of tissues, which supports the IOR-dependent mitoptosis pathway hypothesis.

Additionally, both wild and captive NMR are naturally low in vitamin D3; this condition is known to evoke metabolic deficiency, similar to caloric restriction [125] and in ad libitum fed NMR it can act as a natural CR-inductor.

The other protective mechanism may involve the microbial symbionts-produced volatile fatty acids, proteins and lipids, which can significantly impact the life span and cancer resistance in NMR. Among them the butyric acid and its derivates are known to offer antineoplastic and life span-prolonging properties [126, 127].

And at last, remembering that mitochondrial and bacterial lipids belong to the same family, one can deduce that digested bacterial endosymbionts may supply valuable precursors, supporting mitochondrial biogenesis in NMR.

The IOR in Clinic

The IOR, optimised as designed protocols that vary in periodicity, duration and intensity of hypoxic challenge, is used for a long time to accomplish particular aims, such as preacclimatize to high altitude and improve athletic performance [128].

It is demonstrated that the intermittent hypoxic therapy/training (IHT) as the most "engineered" and particularly mitochondria-targeting among various IOR protocols, presents a feasible, compliant intervention, which is effective in prevention, treatment and rehabilitation of numerous chronic degenerative diseases [129, 130, 131].

The IHT technology has been gradually developing during the last decades [99]. It belongs to the tools of evolutionary medicine [132], which harnesses the process of adaptation to challenging environmental conditions or physical stimuli and evokes innate genetic potential to withstand these challenges. A completed and sustained adaptation to IHT may bring multiple health-benefits and alleviation or cure in numerous chronic degenerative diseases [129,130].

Technically, an IHT session consists of 6–10 repeated, 2–6 min. duration intervals of hypoxic (9–12% O_2) air inhalation, interspersed with 3–6 min. duration inhalations of normoxic or hyperoxic air. Optimally, such daily sessions shall be consequently repeated 3 to 6 days a week. Throughout each session a patient experiences controlled multiple hypoxia-reoxygenation episodes that in the course of 2–6 weeks of treatment gradually induce a systemic, long-termed hypoxia adaptation.

The Summary of IHT Experience

During the last three decades the IHT gradually progressed as a non-medication treatment, and revealed its notable preventative, curative and rehabilitative potential. While theoretical basis of IHT has been consolidating via several decades of academic research, the practical knowledge of curative power of moderately hypoxic "mountain air", as well as familiarity with breathing techniques that induce a temperate hypoxia-hypercapnia, accounts for millennia and runs through various cultures and civilizations. Current technology advancement catalyzed the evolution and development of hypoxic treatment from esoteric concepts and costly mountain sanatoriums to molecular-biological insights and high-tech, user-friendly equipment that supports individualized treatment protocols.

The IHT centers in Russia and CIS, Europe and USA, China, Japan, Australia and New Zealand accumulated nearly three decades of physiological, sport medicine-and clinical research in this modality. Up to date, only in Russia clinical scientific research in IHT resulted in hundreds of dissertations, as well as numerous publications and presentations at international conferences [133]. In the light of accumulated evidence, it is hard questioning the effectiveness and safety of IHT. The statistics of treatment of 46,723 patients (incl. 4716 children) revealed good and satisfactory results in 75–95% of cases treated during a standard 2- to 3-week cure [134].

Contraindications to IHT include acute infections, intoxications, exacerbations of chronic inflammatory diseases, fever, acute somatic conditions and trauma (shock syndrome, myocardial infarction, stroke, asthma attack, etc.), and decompensated chronic conditions.

A Multiple-Modality Rejuvenative Intervention

The IHT modulates several underlying mechanisms of aging, such as: expression of p53 and p66 proteins that modulate apoptosis and inflammation, as well as DNA maintenance and tissue repair [64-69, 135]. These pathways underlie the pathogenesis of aging and also function as the key players in a host of common degenerative or "civilization" diseases. Those include atherosclerosis and its main manifestations (cardiovascular disease, myocardial infarction, stroke), as well as diabetes type 2, arterial hypertension, inflammatory diseases of joints and respiratory ways, allergy, gastrointestinal problems and autoimmune conditions, cancer and neurodegenerative diseases.

The potential of IHT in rejuvenative therapies is recognised [136]. However, up till now we have found only one paper aimed to evaluate effects of IHT on various biomarkers of aging. In this study, using the biochemical parameters (levels of ROS, POL and antioxidative enzymes) and psychometric tests, researchers demonstrated that in average, a single completed course of IHT results in reversal of selected markers of aging on 3 to 5 years [137].

The ICR in the Clinic

While a life long caloric restriction remains a golden standard in life–extending interventions, it is recently demonstrated that various forms of the intermittent caloric restriction (ICR) can have similar or even higher efficiency in inducing favorable gene-expression changes and corresponding health benefits.

A study of Anson et al. [138] compared intermittent fasting and continuous calorie restriction in mice. A control group was fed ad libitum; another group was fed 60% of the calories that the control group consumed. A third group was fasted for 24 hours, and then permitted to free-feed. The intermittently fasting mice didn't cut total calories at the beginning and the end of the observation period, and only slightly cut calories in between. A fourth group was fed the average daily intake of the fasting mice every day. Both the fasting mice and those on a restricted diet had significantly lower blood sugar and insulin levels than the free-fed controls. Kainic acid, a toxin that damages neurons, was injected into the dorsal hippocampus of all mice. Hippocampal damage is associated with Alzheimer's. Interestingly, less damage was found in the brains of the intermittently fasting mice than in those that were on a restricted diet, and most damage in mice with an unrestricted diet. But the control group, which ate the average daily intake of the fasting mice, also showed less damage than the mice with restricted diet.

ICR decreases incidence and increases latency of mammary tumors in mice to a greater extent than does chronic caloric restriction [139].

Human studies confirm the efficiency of ICR. A six-month caloric restriction protocol resulted in improvement of biomarkers of longevity and oxidative stress in overweight subjects [140].

Similar results were obtained by Skrha et al. in obese diabetic patients [141]. Johnson et al. investigated the efficiency of alternate day calorie restriction (ADCR) protocol in asthma patients [142]. The study aimed to determine if overweight asthma patients would adhere to this dietary regimen, and to establish the effects of the protocol on their symptoms, pulmonary function, markers of oxidative stress, and inflammation. Ten subjects with BMI>30 were maintained for 8 weeks on a dietary regimen in which they ate ad libitum every other day, while consuming less than 20% of their normal calorie intake on the intervening days. Nine of the subjects adhered to the diet and lost an average of 8% of their initial weight during the study. Their asthma-related symptoms, asthma control, and quality of life improved significantly, within two weeks of diet initiation; these changes persisted for the duration of the study. Levels of serum beta-hydroxybutyrate were increased and levels of leptin were decreased on CR days, indicating a shift in energy metabolism toward utilization of fatty acids and confirming compliance with the diet. The improved clinical findings were associated with decreased levels of serum cholesterol and triglycerides, notable reductions in markers of oxidative stress (8-isoprostane, nitrotyrosine, protein carbonyls, and 4-hydroxynonenal adducts), and increased levels of the endogenous antioxidant uric acid. Indicators of inflammation, including serum tumor necrosis factor-alpha were also significantly decreased by ADCR. Compliance with the ADCR diet was high, symptoms and pulmonary function improved, and oxidative stress and inflammation declined.

In the human calorie restriction study by Civitarese et al. [143] mitochondrial DNA content increased by 35% ± 5% in the CR group and 21% ± 4% in the CR+ exercise group, with no change in the control group. The authors demonstrated that in overweight nonobese humans, short-term calorie restriction lowers whole-body energy expenditure and oxygen consumption in parallel with an induction of mitochondrial biogenesis, PPARGC1A and SIRT1 mRNA, and a decrease in DNA damage with a tendency toward lower SOD activity. Authors conclude that caloric restriction directly stimulates biogenesis of more efficient mitochondria in human skeletal muscle, which diminishes basal oxidative stress.

Spindler [144] have found that acute CR partially or completely reverses age-related alterations of liver, brain and heart proteins. CR also rapidly and reversibly mitigates biomarkers of aging in adult rhesus macaques and humans. He concludes that: "...highly conserved mechanisms for the rapid and reversible enhancement of life-and health-span exist for mitotic and postmitotic tissues."

Synergism of IHT and ICR

The IOR and ICR synergistically modulate OXPHOS in the mitochondria and stimulate mitochondrial turnover and biogenesis [89, 143]. Similarly to ICR, the short-termed IOR (as intermittent exposure to mountain altitude) induced clinical improvements in patients with metabolic syndrome and related conditions [145].

Current research together with earlier observations, clearly indicate a spectacular similarity in outcomes of adaptation to ICR and IOR and justify concomitant use of both. In our practice we have found that a combination of modified IHT and Extended Morning Fasting (EMF) shows synergism in the accelerated recovery of diabetes type 2 patients and in other degenerative diseases. Previous research demonstrated the possibility of increasing the number of insulin receptors in cellular membranes and their enhanced sensitivity to insulin after ICR [146].

It was also shown that the sensitivity to insulin and the number of pancreatic beta cells increases, following IHT application [147]. Physiological hypoxia upregulates the activity of the glucose transporter GLUT1 by opening the K-ATP channels for glucose transport activity [148]. The pancreatic ATP- sensitive potassium (K-ATP) channel is a critical regulator of beta-cell insulin secretion and glucose metabolism [149, 150, 151]. This information provided ground for introducing IHT in combination with ICR and other integrative modalities in the treatment of patients with diabetes type 2.

Our earlier clinical research [152] has demonstrated that ICR in 5 - 7 days clinical setting induces a significant improvement in diabetes type 2 patients. We also found that outpatients could be more conveniently treated with a partial (early daytime) fasting regime, which we dubbed Extended Morning Fasting, EMF. Eight diabetes type 2 patients (duration of illness from 3 to 12 years) were subjected to ICR (fasting during the day lasting 16/18 hours out of 24 (the first food consumption took place at approximately 14.00–16.00 and the second at 19.00–20.00). All patients (five of theme were obese) arrived at the clinic in a state of decompensated diabetes. Before treatment with ICR-IHT protocol, four of patients received regular insulin injections, and three with oral hypoglicemic medication. One patient partially controlled diabetes by diet. The basic condition for starting the IHT element of our therapy was normoglycaemia, which was achieved by a low-calorie diet and oral medication, or insulin injections. During the first 2–3 days of IHT treatment the oral medication or/and insulin dosage were decreased gradually.

As a result of the two to three weeks' daily treatment in four patients on insulin injections, the diabetes was compensated by diet and lower doses of insulin (reduction, respectively from 180 to 30 units; from 100 to 20 units; from 70 to 40 units and from 64 to 40 units). The three patients formerly on oral hypoglycaemics were compensated with diet alone after the IHT treatment. One patient with mild diabetes achieved stable compensation on the diet as well. Patients were observed for from five months to five years. Regular morning fasting and hypoglycaemic diet maintained the achieved improvements indefinitely.

We hypothesise that IHT with concomitant glucose deprivation via EMF protocol helps overcome the cellular glucose/insulin resistance, probably as a result of synergistic upregulating effect on the membrane and nuclear binding sites such as the peroxisome proliferator-activated receptors. These candidate receptors mediate insulin-sensitivity. We believe that the effect of ionic K-ATP channel activation upregulates metabolic activity generally and also the overexpression of the glucose transporter GLUT1 participate in the total therapeutic effect.

**Table 1. The results of treatment (individualized ICR-IOR protocols) of
102 patients in 1998–2006**

Diseases and conditions		Outcome		
Nr. of patients		Improvement or cure	No effect	Worsening
Cardiovascular disease	8	6	1	1
Arterial hypertension	12	11	1	0
Type 2 diabetes	16	15	1	0
Burnout syndrome	4	4	0	0
Depression	2	2	0	0
Bronchial asthma	7	7	0	0
Emphysema	2	1	1	0
Multiple sclerosis	3	2	1	0
Neuroborreliosis	3	2	1	0
Epilepsy	1	1	0	0
Premenstrual syndrome	12	10	2	0
Postmenopausal syndrome	9	9	0	0
Infertility	4	2	2	0
Hypothyroids	11	10	1	0
Irritable bowel syndrome	5	5	0	0
Wound healing	3	3	0	0
Total	102	90	11	1
	100%	88,2%	10,8%	0,98%

To achieve the optimum results from this intervention, it is necessary to individualise the correct intensity, dose, frequency and timing between the applications of hypoxic stimuli and also monitor the patient response. Fluctuations of blood oxygen saturation (SpO2) during an IHT session serve as a valuable indicator of sensitivity to treatment.

Authors's practical experience with the IHT and our clinical outcomes in general corresponds to the published results of other researchers. A summary table below shows the results of synergistic application of IOR and ICR. As both authors are privately practicing holistic physicians, we use the reasonable evaluation criteria of evidence-based medicine and do not apply controlled randomized double-blind experimental clinical study design.

Discussion

Aging bears the general characteristics of gradual depletion of functional and structural reserves at the cellular level. Aging is also associated with the lowered ability of an organism to respond to stress and maintain homeostatic regulation when given a challenge, thereby decreasing the organism's capacity to resist detrimental changes occurring in adult life. Consequently, increased resistance to degenerative disease, as well as extended life span depend on the capacity and plasticity of intracellular structural – and energy reserves.

At the molecular level, any physiological activity induces some degree of functional damage and depletion of reserves, which should be repaired and, under certain conditions may be consequently (over) compensated, thus increasing amount of available cellular reserves. The same pathways and same cellular energy-and structural reserves participate in normal aging; they may decline if they are not used and do not go through continuous functional repair. On the other hand, they degrade if overused and chronically under repaired. In both cases, mitochondria-modulated oxidative stress seems to be the culprit.

Currently, the ultimate test of mitochondrial-oxidative stress theory of aging is underway in the Skulachev project [153]. Mitochondria-specific antioxidant SkQ, which selectively accumulates in mitochondria, applied in nanogram concentrations inhibited development of such age-related conditions as osteoporosis, involution of thymus, cataract, retinopathy, tumors, etc. SkQ1 has a strong therapeutic action on some already developed retinopathies, in particular, congenital retinal dysplasia. With drops containing SkQ1, vision is recovered in 50 of 66 animals that became blind because of retinopathy. SkQ1-containing drops instilled in the early stage of the disease prevent the loss of sight in rabbits with experimental uveitis and restore vision to animals that had already become blind. Alleviation is also achieved in experimental glaucoma in rabbits. Further, the pretreatment of rats with SkQ1 significantly decreases the H_2O_2-induced arrhythmia of the isolated heart. SkQ1 strongly reduces the damaged area in myocardial infarction or stroke and prevents the death of animals from kidney infarction. In p53-deficient mice, SkQ1 decreases the ROS level in the spleen cells and inhibits appearance of lymphomas, which are the main cause of death of such animals. These data support the main postulates of the mitochondrial-oxidative stress theory of aging.

According to the theory of stress-induced premature senescence [154], sublethal doses of various stressor agents (such as environmental and behavioral stress, H_2O_2, hypoxia and hyperoxia, ionizing irradiation, UV light, etc.) lead to the exhaustion of the replicative potential of the proliferative normal cell types and the accumulation of senescent cells, which might be responsible for the creation of a micro-inflammatory state, thereby participating in tissue ageing.

On the other hand, the same agents and interventions being applied in proper doses and timing may induce increased non-specific resistance to multiple stressors and increase life span in various species via hormetic effect [155]. This is fully applicable to both IOR and ICR and their synergistic combination.

ICR is common in the nature and is more beneficial for survival compared with continuous calorie restriction, because a chronic restriction of availability of energy –and structural resources in the extreme and fluctuating, or low-productive natural environments diminishes adaptational potential. Calorie-restricted and chronically hypoxic animals and humans are more sensitive to cold, susceptible to viral infections and food intoxications; they also have decreased endurance.

On the other hand, the predictably oscillating availability of oxygen and nutrients activates multiple (from intracellular to behavioral level) "saving" strategies, which are not only free from these limitations, but induce increased genome stability and extend life span in diverse species. Both IOR and ICR synergistically stimulate multiple genome-stabilizing pathways. Concomitant application of IOR and ICR seem to significantly intensify DNA-and tissue repair.

ICR also may efficiently minimize latent threats that are presented by constantly appearing mutated genome copies, such as cancerous cellular clones. Under a severe calorie restriction or fasting first the alternated and mutated cells undergo apoptosis and autophagy, while survived healthy cells recover and proliferate in feasting times. It is found that tumors that have lost their self-eliminatory apoptic mechanisms still can undergo immune attacks, and if not destroyed by them, they would be encapsulated and stay dormant [156, 157]. These processes seem to be strongly facilitated by ICR.

Observing appropriate recovery and repair intervals in contrast to constant, uninterrupted functional load—drastically lowers risk of pathological outcomes. Thus, interval physical training in general is significantly safer and more efficient than continuous training [158, 159].

The oscillating character of the IOR and ICR, as well as their synergism seems to be crucial for observed effects. Species adapted to a rhythmic, oscillating pattern of accumulation and depletion of structural and energy reserves constantly exercise their storage and mobilization mechanisms, according to the universal principle "Use it, or loose it." Exercising energy-extracting and energy-storing systems, as well as continuous training of endogenous cellular antioxidative defense network provides a specific maintenance-and repair tool to slowing down aging process.

Conclusion

Exercising physiological functions, building up and regularly emptying the bodily reserves is a widely-known recommendation, which becomes more difficult to follow with each passing year of an individual's life, particularly when a person has no previous experience of regular exercising. Certainly, there is a constant demand for cost-efficient, naturally-based rejuvenative interventions that could be used in clinical settings, as well as incorporated into the most demanding and time-deficient lifestyles. The engineered derivatives of IOR and ICR seem to fulfill this requirement.

Nature offers a universal mitochondria-rejuvenating and tissue-regenerative strategy that modulates life span in evolutionary distanced species such as *C. elegans*, the naked mole rat and the bowhead whale, in correspondence with the cyclic availability of O_2 and nutrients. This natural strategy incorporates an affluent nutrition during postnatal development, followed by continuous ICR and IOR in adulthood. The underlying mechanisms and pathways synergistically modulate oxygen absorption, transportation and utilization, resulting in improved mitochondrial efficiency and reduction of basal oxidative stress. This in turn brings improved genome stability, postponed senescence and retarded development of age-related pathology, which ultimately increases healthy lifespan. While the underlying conserved evolutionary pathways have been found at all levels of biological organization, there is little doubt that the same strategy is equally efficient in humans. Historically, different forms of ICR and IOR have an impressive account of empiric and evidence-based use in health and spiritual practices of various human cultures.

The efficient mitochondria-rejuvenating intervention in the form of IOR and ICR derivates IHT and ADF/EMF is already used successfully in clinical settings. It brings measurable reversal of biomarkers of aging, aging signs and age-related pathology, improved homeostatic and hormonal regulation, balanced humoral and cellular immunity, reduced chronic inflammation and markedly augmented non-specific stress resistance. The synergistic application of such protocols, accompanied by an individualized nutriceutical supple-mentation program, brings multiple anti-aging benefits and alleviation or cure in numerous chronic degenerative and age-related diseases.

Abbreviations

ADF	alternate day fasting
ADCR	alternate day calorie restriction
ATP	adenosine triphosphat
BW	bowhead whale (*Balena mysticetus*)
BMI	body mass index
CNS	central nervous system
EMF	extended morning fasting
EPO	erythropoetin
GH	growth hormone
HIF-1	Hypoxia inducible factor -1
ICR	intermittent caloric restriction
IHT	intermittent hypoxic therapy/training
IOR	intermittent oxygen restriction
MSC	mesenchymal stem cells
mtDNA	mitochondrial DNA

NMR	naked mole rat (*Heterocephalus glaber*)
NO	nitric oxide
nuDNA	nuclear DNA
OXPHOS	oxidative phosphorylation
OSA	obstructive sleep apnea
ROS	reactive oxygen species
RNS	reactive nitrogen species
SC	stem cells
SOD	superoxiddismutase

References

[1] de Grey AD. Inter-species therapeutic cloning: the looming problem of mitochondrial DNA and two possible solutions. *Rejuvenation Res.* 2004;7(2):95-98.

[2] Zorov DB, Krasnikov BF, Kuzminova AE, Vysokikh M, and Zorova LD. Mitochondria revisited. Alternative functions of mitochondria. *Bioscience Reports*, Volume 17, Number 6, December 1997: 507-520.

[3] Lacza Z, Kozlov AV, Pankotai E, Csordás A, Wolf G, Redl H, Kollai M, Szabó C (Csaba), Busija DW, and Horn TF. Mitochondria produce reactive nitrogen species via an arginine-independent pathway. *Free Radic Res.* 2006; 40: 369-78.

[4] Skulachev V, and Longo V. Aging as a mitochondria-mediated atavistic program: Can aging be switched off? *Ann NY Acad Sci.* 2005; 1057: 145-164.

[5] Gredilla R, and Barja G. Minireview: The Role of Oxidative Stress in Relation to Caloric Restriction and Longevity. *Endocrinology*, 2005. Vol. 146, No. 9; 3713-3717

[6] Liu J, and Ames B. Reducing mitochondrial decay with mitochondrial nutrients to delay and treat cognitive dysfunction, Alzheimer's disease, and Parkinson's disease. *Nutritional Neuroscience*, Volume 8, Number 2, April, 2005: 67 - 89.

[7] Gomez-Cabrera MC, Domenech E, Romagnoli M, Arduini A, Borras C, Pallardo FV, Sastre J, and Viña J. Oral administration of vitamin C decreases muscle mitochondrial biogenesis and hampers training-induced adaptations in endurance performance. *American Journal of Clinical Nutrition*, January 2008. Vol. 87, No. 1: 142-149,

[8] Skulachev VP. A biochemical approach to the problem of aging: "megaproject" on membrane-penetrating ions. *Biochemistry* (Mosc), 2007; 72: 1385-96.

[9] Prokopov A. Exploring overlooked natural mitochondria - rejuvenative intervention. The puzzle of bowhead whales and naked mole rats. *Rejuvenation Research,* 2007. V.10. N 4: 543-559.

[10] George J C, Bada J L, Zeh J, Scott J, Brown S, O'Hara T, and Suydam R. Age and growth estimates of bowhead whales (Balaena mysticetus) via aspartic acid racemization. *Can. J. Zool.* 1999; 77: 571-580.

[11] Philo L M, Shotts EB, and George J C. Morbidity and mortality. In Burns J J, Montague J J, and Cowles C J (Editors). The bowhead whale. *Soc. Mar. Mamm.* Spec. Publ; 1993; 2: 275-312.

[12] De Guise S, Lagacé A, and Béland P. Tumors in St. Lawrence beluga whales (*Delphinapterus leucas*). *Vet Pathol.* 1994; 31:444–449

[13] Cowan DF. Pathology of the pilot whale. *Globicephala melaena.* A comparative survey. *Arch Pathol.* 1966; 82:178–189

[14] Uys CJ and Best PB. Pathology of lesions observed in whales flensed at Saldanha Bay, South Africa. *J Comp Pathol.* 1966; 76:407–412

[15] Kirkwood JK, Bennett PM, Jepson PD, Kuiken T, Simpson VR, and Baker JR. Entanglement in fishing gear and other causes of death in cetaceans stranded on the coasts of England and Wales. *Vet Rec.* 1997;141: 94–98

[16] Geraci JR, Palmer NC and St Aubin DJ. Tumors in cetaceans: analysis and new findings. *Can J Fish Aquat Sci.* 1987; 44:1289-1300.

[17] Buffenstein R. The Naked Mole-Rat: A new long-living model for human aging research. *The Journals of Gerontology Series A*: Biological Sciences and Medical Sciences. 2005; 60:1369-1377.

[18] George JC, Goering D, Sturm M, Elsner R, and Follmann E. Energetic adaptations of the bowhead whales. Abstracts of 14th Marine Mammal Biennial Conference. 28 November - 3 December 2001. Vancouver, Canada.

[19] Jarvis JUM and Bennett NC. Ecology and behavior of the family Bathyergidae. In: The biology of the naked mole-rat (P. W. Sherman, J. U. M. Jarvis, and R. D. Alexander, Eds.). Princeton University Press, New Jersey. 1991. Pp. 66–96.

[20] Maina J N, Maloiy G M O and Makanya A N. Morphology and morphometry of the lungs of two East African mole-rats, *Tachyoryctes splendens* and *Heterocephalus glaber.* Zoomorphology. 1992; 112:167–179.

[21] Johansen K, Lykkeboe G, Weber R E, and Maloiy G M O. 1976. Blood respiratory properties in the naked mole-rat *Heterocephalus glaber*, a mammal of low body temperature. *Respiratory Physiology*; 28:303–314.

[22] Mc Nab B K. The influence of body size on the energetics and distribution of fossorial and burrowing mammals. *Ecology,* 1979; 60:1010–1021.

[23] Buffenstein R, Woodley R, Thomadakis C, Daly JM, and Gray DA. Cold-induced changes in thyroid function in a poikilothermic mammal, the naked mole-rat. *Am J Physiol Regul Integr Comp Physiol.* 2001; 280: R149-R155.

[24] Goldman B D, Goldman S L, Lanzt T, Magaurin A., and Maurice A. Factors influencing metabolic rate in naked mole-rats (*Heterocephalus glaber*). *Physiology and Behavior*, 1999; 66:447–459.

[25] Kramer Y, Courtland H, Terranova C, Jepsen K, and Buffenstein R. Age-related changes in bone in the longest-living rodent, the naked mole-rat. Abstr. 35.3 APS Intersociety Conference Comparative Physiology "Integrating Diversity." 2006: October 8 -11, Virginia Beach, VA, USA.

[26] Csiszar A, Labinskyy N, Orosz Z, Buffenstein R, and Ungvari Z. Vascular aging in the longest-living rodent, the naked mole-rat. *The FASEB Journal*, 2007;21:743.5

[27] Meerson FZ, Gomzakov OA and Shimkovich MV. Adaptation to high altitude hypoxia as a factor preventing development of myocardial ischemic necrosis. *Am J Cardiol.* 1973; 31:30–34.

[28] Ruscher K, Isaev N, Trendelenburg G, Weih M, Iurato L, Meisel A, and Dimagl U. Induction of hypoxia inducible factor 1 by oxygen glucose deprivation is attenuated by hypoxic preconditioning in rat cultured neurons. *Neurosci. Lett.* 1998; 254:117–120.

[29] Maynard Smith J and Szathmary E. The major transitions in evolution. 1995. Oxford: Freeman.

[30] Peto R. Epidemiology, multistage models, and short-term mutagenicity tests. In The origins of human cancer (ed. H. H. Hiatt, J. D. Watson & J. A. Winsten), Cold Spring Harbor Conferences on Cell Proliferation, 1977 vol. 4. NY: Cold Spring Harbor Laboratory Press. pp.1403-1428.

[31] Nunney L. Lineage selection and the evolution of multistage carcinogenesis. *Proc. R. Soc.* Lond. 1999; 266: 493-498.

[32] Moraes CT, Kenyon L and H.Hao. Mechanisms of human mitochondrial DNA maintenance: the determining role of primary sequence and length over function. *Mol. Biol. Cell*, 1999;10: 3345–3356.

[33] Dawkins R. *The Selfish Gene*. 1976. Oxford University Press. Oxford.

[34] Allen J F. Separate Sexes and the Mitochondrial Theory of Ageing. *J Theor Biol.* 1996. 180. 135 - 140.

[35] Wallace DC. Mitochondrial DNA in Aging and Disease. Scientific American. August 1997.; 40-47

[36] Terman A, Dalen H, Eaton JW, Neuzil J, and Brunk UT. Mitochondrial recycling and aging of cardiac myocytes: the role of autophagocytosis. *Experimental gerontology*, 2003, vol. 38; 8; 863-876

[37] Khrapko K, Nekhaeva E, Kraytsberg Y, and Kunz W. Clonal expansions of mitochondrial genomes: implications for in vivo mutational spectra. *Mutat Res.* 2003 Jan 28; 522 (1-2):9-13.

[38] Skulachev V P. *Mol. Aspects Med.* 1999; 20:139-184.

[39] Taylor D, Zeyl C and Cooke E. Conflicting levels of selection in the accumulation of mitochondrial defects in Saccharomyces cerevisiae. *PNAS*, March 19, 2002 vol. 99 no. 6: 3690–3694.

[40] Smigrodzki RM and Khan SM. Mitochondrial microheteroplasmy and a theory of aging and age-related disease. *Rejuvenation Res.* 2005;8 (3):172-98.

[41] Harley CB, Futcher AB, and Greider CW. Telomeres shorten during ageing of human fibroblasts. *Nature,* 1990;345:458-60.

[42] von Zglinicki T. Oxidative stress shortens telomeres. *Trends Biochem Sci.* 2002 Jul;27(7):339-44.

[43] de Bruin J.P, Dorlandb M, Spekc E R, Posthumad G, van Haaftena M, Loomane CWN, and te Veldef E R. Ultrastructure of the Resting Ovarian Follicle Pool in Healthy Young Women. *Biology of Reproduction,* 2002; 66: 1151-1160.

[44] Krakauer D C, and Mira A. Mitochondria and germ cell death. *Nature*, 1999; 400: 125–126.

[45] Dawkins R. The Extended Phenotype. 1982. Oxford University Press, Oxford.

[46] Fischer B, and Bavister B D. Oxygen tension in the oviduct and uterus of rhesus monkeys, hamsters and rabbits. *J. Reprod. Fertil.* 1993;99:673-679.

[47] Singer D. Neonatal tolerance to hypoxia: a comparative-physiological approach. Comparative Biochemistry and Physiology 1999. Part A; 123: 221–234.

[48] Huckabee W, Metcalfe J, Prystowsky H, and Barron D.H. Blood flow and oxygen consumption of the pregnant uterus. *Am J Physiol.* 1961; 200: 274-278.

[49] Jauniaux E, Watson A, and Ozturk O. In-vivo measurement of intrauterine gases and acid-base values early in human pregnancy. *Hum Reprod.* 1999;14:2901–2904.

[50] Gassmann M, Fandrey J, Bichet S, Wartenberg M, Marti H, Bauer C, Wenger R, and Acker H. Oxygen supply and oxygen-dependent gene expression in differentiating embryonic stem cells. *Proc. Natl. Acad. Sci. USA*, 1996; 93:2867-2872.

[51] Danet GH, Pan Y, and Luongo JL. Expansion of human SCID-repopulating cells under hypoxic conditions. *J Clin Invest.* 2003;112:126–135.

[52] Ahmad S, Ahmad A, Gerasimovskaya E, Stenmark K, Allen C, and White C. Hypoxia protects human lung microvascular endothelial and epithelial-like cells against oxygen toxicity. Role of Phosphatidylinositol 3-Kinase. *Am. J. Respir. Cell Mol. Biol.* 2003. Vol. 28: 179–187.

[53] Bell EL, Klimova TA, Eisenbart J, Schumacker PT, and Chandel NS. Mitochondrial ROS trigger HIF-dependent extension of replicative lifespan during hypoxia. Mol Cell Biol. 2007 Aug;27(16):5737-45.

[54] Krysko D, Mussche S, Leybaert L D, and Herde K. Gap junctional communication and connexin 43 expression in relation to apoptotic cell death and survival of granulosa cells. *J Histochem Cytochem.* 2004; 52:1199 – 207.

[55] Géminard C, de Gassart A and Vidal M. Reticulocyte maturation: mitoptosis and exosome release. *Biocell*; 2002 (26): 205-15.

[56] Yoneda M, Chomyn A, Martinuzzi A, Hurko O, and Attardi G. Marked replicative advantage of human mtDNA carrying a point mutation that causes the MELAS encephalomyopathy. *Proc Nat Acad Sci USA*, 1992; 89:11164-11168.

[57] Bickler PE and Donohoe PH. Adaptive responses of vertebrate neurons to hypoxia. *The Journal of Experimental Biology,* 2002; 205: 3579-3586.

[58] Breitenbach M, Lehrach H and Krobitsch S. Dynamic rerouting of the carbohydrate flux is key to counteracting oxidative stress. *Journal of Biology*, 2007, 6:10 (doi:10.1186/jbiol6

[59] Gnaiger E, Méndez G and Hand SC. High phosphorylation efficiency and depression of uncoupled respiration in mitochondria under hypoxia. *Proc Natl Acad Sci U S A,* 2000 September 26; 97(20): 11080-11085.

[60] Sun Y, Jin K and Mao XO. Neuroglobin is up-regulated by and protects neurons from hypoxic-ischaemic injury. *Proc Natl Acad Sci USA*, 2001, 98:15306-15311.

[61] Brucklachera RM, Vannuccia RC and Vannucci SJ. Hypoxic preconditioning increases brain glycogen and delays energy depletion from hypoxia-ischemia in the immature rat. Developmental *Neuroscience*, 2002;24:411-417.

[62] Prabhakar N. Physiological and genomic consequences of intermittent hypoxia. Invited review: oxygen sensing during intermittent hypoxia: cellular and molecular mechanisms. *J Appl Physiol.* 2001; 90:1986–1994.

[63] Heinicke K, Cajigal J, Viola T, Behn C, and Schmidt W. Long-term exposure to intermittent hypoxia results in increased hemoglobin mass, reduced plasma volume,

and elevated erythropoietin plasma levels in man. *European Journal of Applied Physiology,* 2003 Volume 88, 6: 535-543.

[64] Erbayraktar S, Yilmaz O, Gökmen N and Brines M. Erythropoetin is a multifunctional tissue-protective cytokine. *Current Hematology Reports*, 2003; 2:465-470.

[65] Zhong N, Zhang Yi, Fang Q, and Zhou Z. Intermittent hypoxia exposure-induced heat-shock protein 70 expression increases resistance of rat heart to ischemic injury. Zhōngguó yàoli xuébào 2000, vol. 21, N5: 467-472.

[66] Broome C S, Kayani A C, Palomero J, Dillmann W H, Mestril R, Jackson M J, and McArdle A. Effect of lifelong overexpression of HSP70 in skeletal muscle on age-related oxidative stress and adaptation after nondamaging contractile activity. *The FASEB Journal,* 2006;20:1549-1551.

[67] Wang X, Deng J, Boyle D, Zhong J, and Lee W. Potential role of IGF-I in hypoxia tolerance using a rat hypoxic-ischemic model: activation of hypoxia-inducible factor 1{alpha}. *Pediatric Research,* 2004; 55:385-394.

[68] Zhuang J and Zhou Z. Protective effects of intermittent hypoxic adaptation on myocardium and its mechanisms, *Biol Signals Recept.* 1999 Jul-Oct;8(4-5):316-322.

[69] Kotlyarova L.A., Stepanova E.N., Tkatchouk E.N., Ehrenbourg I.V., Kondrykinskaya I.I., and Gorbatchenkov A.A. The immune state of the patients with rheumatoid arthritis in the interval hypoxic training. *Hyp. Med. J.* 1994.V. 2. N 4. P.11-12.

[70] Geppe N.A., Kurchatova T.V., Dairova R.A., Tkatchouk E.N., and Farobina E.G. Interval hypoxic training in bronchial asthma in children//Hyp.Med.J. 1995. N 3. P.11-14.

[71] Gidday JM. Cerebral preconditioning and ischaemic tolerance. Nature Reviews. *Neuroscience,* Vol.7. June 2006.; 437- 448

[72] Krause DS, Theise ND, Collector MI, Henegariu O, Hwang S, and Gardner R. Multi-organ, multi-lineage engraftment by a single bone marrow-derived stem cell. *Cell,* 2001; 105: 369–377.

[73] Halaschek-Wiener J and Brooks-Wilson A. Progeria of stem cells: stem cell exhaustion in Hutchinson-Gilford progeria syndrome. *The journals of gerontology series A: Biological sciences and medical sciences*, 2007; 62:3-8

[74] Rochefort GY, Delorme B, Lopez A, Hérault O, Bonnet P, Charbord P, Eder V, and Domenech J. Multipotential mesenchymal stem cells are mobilized into peripheral blood by hypoxia. *Stem Cells*, October 2006. Vol. 24 No. 10: 2202-2208.

[75] da Silva-Meirelles L, Chagastelles PC and Nardi NB. Mesenchymal stem cells reside in virtually all post-natal organs and tissues. *Journal of Cell Science*, 2006; 119: 2204-2213.

[76] Spees JL, Olson SD, Whitney MJ, and Prockop DJ. Mitochondrial transfer among cells can rescue aerobic respiration. *Proc Natl Acad Sci USA*, 2006;103:1283–1288.

[77] Butler P J and Jones D R. Physiology of diving of birds and mammals. *Physiol. Rev.* 1997; 77: 837–899.

[78] Laffey J, Motoschi T and Engelberts D. Therapeutic hypercapnia reduces pulmonary and systemic injury following in vivo lung reperfusion. *Am. J. Respir. Crit. Care Med.* December 2000, Volume 162, Number 6:2287-2294.

[79] Vesela A, and Wilhelm J. The role of carbon dioxide in free radical reactions of the organism. *Physiol. Res.* 2002; 51: 335-339.

[80] Kogan A Kh, Grachev SV, Eliseeva SV, and Bolevich S. Carbon dioxide - a universal inhibitor of the generation of active oxygen forms by cells. Izv Akad Nauk Ser Biol. 1997 Mar-Apr; (2): 204-17.

[81] Vanucci RC, Towfigi J, Heitjan DF, and Brucklacher RM. Carbon dioxide protects the perinatal brain from hypoxic-ischemic damage: an experimental study in the immature rat. *Pediatrics*, 1995; 95: 868-874.

[82] West JB. Do climbs to extreme altitudes cause brain damage? *Lancet.* 1986;2:387

[83] Garrido E, Castello A, and Ventura J L. Cortical atrophy and other brain magnetic resonance imaging (MRI) changes after extremely high-altitude climbs without oxygen. *Int. J. Sport Med.* 1993; 14: 232–23.

[84] Hoppeler H, Kleinert E, Schlegel C, Claassen H, Howald H, Kayar SR, and Cerretelli P. Morphological adaptations of human skeletal muscle to chronic hypoxia. *Int J Sports Med.* 1990, 11, suppl. 1, S3–S9.

[85] Chu Yi-De. High altitude and aging. In: High altitude medicine and biology. VI World Congress on Mountain Medicine & High Altitude Physiology, Xining, Qinghai, and Lhasa, Tibet, August 12-18, 2004. *High Alt Med Biol.* 2004. Volume 5, Number 2; 350.

[86] Jefferson J, Ashley J, Simoni J, Escudero E, Hurtado M E, Swenson E R, Wesson D E, Schreiner J F, Schoene R B, Johnson R J, and Hurtado A. Increased oxidative stress following acute and chronic high altitude exposure. *High Alt. Med. Biol.* 2004; 5:61–69.

[87] Honda Y and Honda S. Oxidative stress and life span determination in the nematode Caenorhabditis Elegans. *Ann N Y Acad Sci.* 2002 Apr; 959:466-74.

[88] Meerson FZ. Mechanism of phenotypic adaptation and the principles of its use for prevention of cardiovascular disorders. *Kardiologiia,* 1978; 18 (10):18–29.

[89] Ning Z, Yi Z, Hai-Feng Z, and Zhao-Nian Z. Intermittent hypoxia exposure prevents mtDNA deletion and mitochondrial structure damage produced by ischemia/reperfusion injury. *Acta Physiologica Sinica*, Oct. 2000; 52 (5): 375-380.

[90] Milano G, Corno A, Lippa S, von Segesser L, and Samaja M. Chronic and intermittent hypoxia induce different degrees of myocardial tolerance to hypoxia-induced dysfunction *Exp Biol Med.* 2002; Vol. 227(6):389–397.

[91] Sazontova T.G., Arkhipenko Yu.V., and Lukyanova L.D. Comparative study of the effect of adaptation to intermittent hypoxia on active oxygen related systems in brain and liver of rats with different resistance to oxygen deficiency. In *Adaptation Biology and Medicine, Vol.1: Subcellular Basis*. B.K. Sharma, N. Takeda, N.K. Ganguly, and P.K. Singal, eds. 1997. Narosa Publishing House, New Dehli, India,:260–266.

[92] Neubauer JA. Physiological and pathophysiological responses to intermittent hypoxia. *J Appl Physiol.* 2001. 90:1593–1599.

[93] Foster GE, Poulin MJ and Hanly PJ. Intermittent hypoxia and vascular function: implications for obstructive sleep apnoea. *Exp Physiol.* 92: 51–65, 2007.

[94] Serebrovskaya T, Manukhina EB, Smith ML, Downey HF, and Mallet R. Intermittent Hypoxia: Cause of or Therapy for Systemic Hypertension? *Exp Biol Med.* 233:627–650, 2008.

[95] Chizov A I, Filimonov V G, Karash Y M, and Strelkov RB. On oxygen tension biorhythm in the tissues of uterus and fetus. Bulletin of experimental biology and medicine. 1981; 10: 392-392 (Article in Russian).

[96] Chizov A.I. Physiologic bases of the method to increase nonspecific resistance of the organism by adaptation to intermittent normobaric hypoxia. *Fiziol. Zh.* 1992. 38(5):13–17.

[97] Grechin.V. B. and Krauz. E. I. Spontaneous fluctuations of oxygen tension in human brain structures. Bulletin of Experimental Biology and Medicine.Volume 75, Number 3. March, 1973: 240-242.

[98] Kunze K. Spontaneous oscillations of pO2 in muscle tissue. *Adv Exp Med Biol.* 1976; 75:631-637.

[99] Serebrovskaya T V. Intermittent hypoxia research in the former Soviet Union and the Commonwealth of Independent States: History and review of the concept and selected applications. *High Alt Med Biol.* 2002; 3:205–221.

[100] Zhuang J, and Zhou Z. Protective effects of intermittent hypoxic adaptation on myocardium and its mechanisms, *Biol Signals Recept.* 1999 Jul-Oct;8(4-5):316-22.

[101] Yellon DM, and Downey JM. Preconditioning the myocardium: from cellular physiology to clinical cardiology. *Physiol Rev.* 2003; 83: 1113–1151.

[102] Vanden Hoek T, Becker L, Shao Z, Li C, and Schumacker T. Reactive Oxygen Species Released from Mitochondria during Brief Hypoxia Induce Preconditioning in Cardiomyocytes. *The Journal of biological chemistry*, 1998. Vol. 273, No. 29, Issue of July 17 :18092–18098.

[103] Manukhina E.B, Downey F.H, and Mallet R.T. Role of Nitric Oxide in Cardiovascular Adaptation to Intermittent Hypoxia. *Exp Biol Med.* 2006; 231:343–365,

[104] Ogier-Denis E, and Codogno P. Autophagy: a barrier or an adaptive response to cancer. *Biochimica et Biophysica Acta,* 2003; 1603: 113 – 128.

[105] Dhahbi J, Kim HJ, Mote PL, Beaver RJ, and Spindler SR. Temporal linkage between the phenotypic and genomic responses to caloric restriction. *PNAS*, April 13, 2004. Vol. 101 No. 15: 5524-5529.

[106] Lemaster JJ. Selective mitochondrial autophagy, or mitophagy, as a targeted defense against oxidative stress, mitochondrial dysfunction and aging. *Rejuvenation Res.* 2005;8:3–5.

[107] Heidel JR, Philo LM, Albert TF, Andreasen CB, and Stang BV. Serum chemistry of bowhead whales (Balaena mysticetus). *Journal of Wildlife Diseases*, 1996; 32 (1): 75-79.

[108] Cahill GF, Jr. Starvation in man. *N Engl J Med.* 1970, 282:668-675.

[109] Owen OE, Morgan AP, Kemp HG, Sullivan JM, Herrera MG, and Cahill GF, Jr. Brain metabolism during fasting. *J Clin Invest.* 1967;46:1589-1595.

[110] Morris AA. Cerebral ketone body metabolism. *J Inherit Metab Dis.* 2005; 28:109-121.

[111] Veech RL. The therapeutic implications of ketone bodies: the effects of ketone bodies in pathological conditions, ketosis, ketogenic diet, redox states, insulin resistance, and mitochondrial metabolism. *Prostaglandins Leukot Essent Fatty Acids*, 2004, 70:309-319.

[112] Sato K, Kashiwaya Y, Keon CA, Tsuchiya N, King MT, Radda GK, Chance B, Clarke K, Veech RL. Insulin, ketone bodies, and mitochondrial energy transduction. *Faseb J.* 1995; 9:651-658.

[113] Evans JL, Goldfine ID, Maddux BA, and Grodsky GM. Ketones metabolism increases the reduced form of glutathione thus facilitating destruction of hydrogen peroxide. *Endocr. Rev.* 2002; 23: 599–622.

[114] Russell J W, Golovoy D, Vincent A M, Mahendru P, Olzmann J A, Mentzer A, and Feldman E L. High glucose-induced oxidative stress and mitochondrial dysfunction in neurons. *The FASEB Journal,* 2002;16:1738-1748.

[115] Jelluma N, Yang X, Stokoe D, Evan G I, Dansen T B, and Haas-Kogan D A. Glucose withdrawal induces oxidative stress followed by apoptosis in glioblastoma cells but not in normal human astrocytes. *Molecular Cancer Research*, 2006; 4:319-330.

[116] Hsu AL, Murphy CT, and Kenyon C. Regulation of aging and age-related disease by DAF-16 and heat-shock factor. *Science*, 2003; 300:1142–1145.

[117] Gami MS and Wolkow CA. Studies of Caenorhabditis elegans DAF-2/insulin signaling reveal targets for pharmacological manipulation of lifespan. *Aging Cell*, 2006 February; 5(1): 31–37.

[118] Jarvis J U M, O'Riain M J, Bennett N C, and Sherman P W. Mammalian eusociality: a family affair. *Trends in Ecology and Evolution*;1994. 9:47–51.

[119] Buffenstein R. Ecophysiological responses of subterranean rodents to underground habitats. in *Life underground: the biology of subterranean rodents* (E. A. Lacey, J. L. Patton, and G. N. Cameron, Eds.). 2000. University of Chicago Press, Illinois. Pp. 62–110.

[120] Hulbert A, Faulks S, and Buffenstein R. Oxidation-resistant membrane phospholipids can explain longevity differences among the longest-living rodents and similarly-sized mice. *The Journals of Gerontology*, 2006. Series A: Biological Sciences and Medical Sciences; 61:1009-1018.

[121] Buffenstein R. Genomic Stability in the Naked Mole-Rat: A Role for Cancer Resistance and Extended Longevity. *Senior Scholar Award in Aging*, 2006. http://www.ellisonfoundation.org/awrd.jsp?id=508.

[122] Herold N, Spray S, Horn T, and Henriksen SJ. Activity and temperature rhythms of the naked mole-rat. *Sleep Research,* 1997; 26:175.

[123] Withers PC, and Jarvis JUM. The effect of huddling on thermoregulation and oxygen consumption for the Naked Mole-Rat. *Comparative Biochemistry and Physiology*, 1980; 66A: 215-219

[124] Ran Q, Liang H, Ikeno Y, Qi W, Prolla TA, Roberts LJ, Wolf N, VanRemmen H, and Richardson A. Reduction in Glutathione Peroxidase 4 Increases Life Span Through Increased Sensitivity to Apoptosis. The Journals of Gerontology Series A: *Biological Sciences and Medical Sciences*, 2007; 62:932-942.

[125] Yahav S, and Buffenstein R. Cholecalciferol supplementation alters gut function and improves digestibility in an underground inhabitant, the naked mole rat. *British Journal of Nutrition,* 1993; 69: 233-241

[126] Rephaeli A, Rabizadeh E, Aviram A, Shaklai M, Ruse M, and Nudelman A. Derivatives of butyric acid as potential anti-neoplastic agents. *Int J Cancer*. 1991 Aug 19;49(1):66-72.

[127] Kang HL, Benzer S and Min KT. Life extension in Drosophila by feeding a drug. *Proc. Natl. Acad. Sci. U.S.A.* 2002; 99: 838-843.

[128] Hamlin MJ and Hellemans J. Effect of intermittent normobaric hypoxic exposure at rest on haematological, physiological, and performance parameters in multi-sport athletes. *Journal of Sports Sciences*, 2007; 25(4): 431 – 441.

[129] Tkatchouk EN, Gorbatchenkov AA, Kolchinskaya AZ, Ehrenbourg IV, and Kondrykinskaya II. Adaptation to interval hypoxia for the purpose of prophylaxis and treatment. In: Meerson FZ, Ed. Esentials of Adaptive Medicine: Protective Effects of Adaptation. 1994 Moscow: *Hypoxia Medical LTD*, 200–221.

[130] Kolchinskaya AZ, Tsyganova TN and Ostapenko LA. *Normobaric Interval Hypoxic Training in Medicine and Sports* [in Russian]. Moscow: Meditsina, 2003.

[131] Burtscher M, Pachinger O, Ehrenbourg I, Mitterbauer G, Faulhaber M, Puhringer R, and Tkatchouk E. Intermittent hypoxia increases exercise tolerance in elderly men with and without coronary artery disease. *Int J Cardiol.* 2004. 96:247–254,

[132] Trevathan, WR. Evolutionary Medicine. *Annual Review of Anthropology,* 2007.Vol. 36: 139-154.

[133] http://www.hypoxia.ru/en-journal.htm?PHPSESSID=88deaaded3ef07b9db6a98637a0f3d2d

[134] Information Brief of Federal Center of Prophylactics of Russian Health Ministry Nr. 048 from 04.07.1996. (in Russian).

[135] Bianchi G, Di Giulio C, Rapino C, Rapino M, Antonucci A, and Cataldi A. p53 and p66 Proteins Compete for Hypoxia-Inducible Factor 1 Alpha Stabilization in Young and Old Rat Hearts Exposed to Intermittent Hypoxia. *Gerontology,* 2006;52(1):17-23.

[136] Kotliar I, and Prokopov A. The perspectives of hypoxic treatment in the anti - aging medicine. In: The fourth international conference "Hypoxia in medicine". 26-28 Sept. 2001. Geneva. Switzerland. *Hypoxia Med J.* 2001. Nr.3: 37.

[137] Golikov M.A. Health, endurance, longevity: the role of hypoxic stimulation. In: Intermittent normobaric hypoxytherapy. Annals of International Academy of problems of hypoxia. Vol. IV. Editor R.B.Strelkov. Moscow. "Bumaznaja Galereja", 2005. (In Russian, Engl. abstracts):164-200.

[138] Anson RM, Guo Z, de Cabo R, Iyun T, Rios M, Hagepanos A, Ingram DK, Lane MA, and Mattson MP. Intermittent fasting dissociates beneficial effects of dietary restriction on glucose metabolism and neuronal resistance to injury from calorie intake. *PNAS.* 2003, Vol. 100, Nr. 10: 6216-6220.

[139] Cleary MP, Jacobson MK, Phillips FC, Getzin SC, Grande JP, and Maihle NJ: Weight-cycling decreases incidence and increases latency of mammary tumors to a greater extent than does chronic caloric restriction in mouse mammary tumor virus-transforming growth factor-alpha female mice. *Cancer Epidemiol Biomarkers Prev.* 2002, 11:836-843.

[140] Heilbronn LK, de Jonge L, Frisard MI, DeLany JP, Larson-Meyer DE, Rood J, Nguyen T, Martin CK, Volaufova J, Most MM, Greenway FL, Smith SR, Deutsch WA,

Williamson DA, Ravussin E, and Pennington CT. Effect of 6-month calorie restriction on biomarkers of longevity, metabolic adaptation, and oxidative stress in overweight individuals: a randomized controlled trial. *JAMA,* 2006. 295: 1539–1548,

[141] Skrha J, Kunesova M, Hilgertova J, Weiserova H, Krizova J, and Kotrlikova E. Short-term very low calorie diet reduces oxidative stress in obese type-2 diabetic patients. Physiol Res. 2005;54(1):33-9.

[142] Johnson JB, Summer W, Cutler RG, Martin B, Hyun DH, Dixit VD, Pearson M, Nassar M, Tellejohan R, Maudsley S, Carlson O, John S, Laub DR, and Mattson MP. Alternate day calorie restriction improves clinical findings and reduces markers of oxidative stress and inflammation in overweight adults with moderate asthma. *Free Radic Biol Med.* 2007 Mar 1;42(5):665-74.

[143] Civitarese AE, Carling S, Heilbronn LK, Hulver MH, Ukropcova B, Deutsch WA, Smith SR, and Ravussin E. Calorie restriction increases muscle mitochondrial biogenesis in healthy humans. PLoS Med 2007. 4(3): e76 doi:10.1371/journal.pmed.0040076

[144] Spindler S. Rapid and reversible induction of the longevity, anticancer and genomic effects of caloric restriction. *Mech Ageing Dev.* 2005;126(9):960-966.

[145] Lee, Wen-Chih, Jin-Jong Chen, Hsin-Yi Ho, Chien-Wen Hou, Ming-Pen Liang, Yih-Wen Shen, and Chia-Hua Kuo. Short-term altitude mountain living improves glycemic control. *High Alt Med Biol.* 2003.4:81–91

[146] Balobolkin M. I., Nedosugova L. V., Gavriluk L. I., and Gingerman L. E. The influence of fasting on the interaction between insulin and insulin receptors in diabetic patients. *Therapeutic Archive,* 1983. No 9 :136–140 (article in Russian).

[147] Kolesnik Y. M., Kadjaryan V. G., Zhulinsky V. A., and Abramov A. V. The new approaches to diabetes mellitus treatment. From a collection of scientific works Zaporozhye state medical university, 1998: 223-229 (article in Russian).

[148] Ouiddir A, Planès C, Fernandes I, VanHesse A,. Hypoxia Upregulates Activity and Expression of the Glucose Transporter GLUT1 in Alveolar Epithelial Cells. *Am. J. Respir. Cell Mol. Biol.,* December, 1999 Volume 21; 6:710-718.

[149] Babenko A.P., Kazantseva S.T., Romanova Yu.V., Samoilov V.O. The Mechanisms of Activation Of the ATP-Sensitive Potassium Channels of the Sarcolemma Of Cardiomyocytes In Hypoxia. Materials of the VII All-Russian Symposium on Ecological and Physiological Problems of Adaptation, Moscow 1994. p. 24,

[150] de Deux A P, Tarasov A, Dusonchet J, and Ashcroft F. The Beta-Cell ATP-Sensitive K+ Channels Metabolic Regulation of the Pancreatic Beta-Cell ATP-Sensitive K+ Channel. *Diabetes,* 2004; 53:S113-S122.

[151] Hattersley A T. Molecular genetics goes to the diabetes clinic. *Clin. Med.* 2005;476-81.

[152] Voronina T N. Fasting therapy in the treatment of diabetes. In: Fasting therapy in the treatment of internal disease. From a collection of scientific works. ed. Volgarev M N and Maximov V A. Ministry of Health of the Russian Federation. Institute of Nutrition of Russian Academy of Medical Science. Moscow; 1993: 94 (article in Russian).

[153] Skulachev VP. A biochemical approach to the problem of aging: "megaproject" on membrane-penetrating ions. *Biochemistry,* (Mosc) 2007; 72: 1385-96.

[154] Chen J, and Patschan S, Goligorsky MS. Stress-induced premature senescence of endothelial cells. *J Nephrol.* 2008 May-Jun;21(3):337-44.

[155] Rattan S. Hormetic Interventions in Aging. American Journal of Pharmacology and *Toxicology,* 2008. 3(1): 27-40

[156] Kappauf HW. Unexpected benign course and spontaneous recovery in malignant disease. *Onkologie.* 1991. Vol 14; Suppl. 1: 32-35.

[157] Chang WY. Complete spontaneous regression of cancer; four case reports, review of literature, and discussion of possible mechanisms. *Hawaii Med J.* 2000 Oct;59(10):379-87

[158] Meyer K, Foster C, Georgakopoulos N, Hajric R, Westbrook S, Ellestad A, Tilman K, Fitzgerald D, Young H, Weinstein H, and Roskamm H. Comparison of left ventricular function during interval versus steady-state exercise training in patients with chronic congestive heart failure. *The American journal of cardiology,* 1998, vol. 82, no11, pp. 1382-1387.

[159] Wisløff U, Støylen A, Loennechen Jan P., Bruvold M, Rognmo O, Haram PM, Tjønna A E, Helgerud J, Slørdahl SA, Lee SJ, Videm V, Bye A, Smith GL, Najjar SM, Ellingsen O, and Skjærpe T. Superior Cardiovascular Effect of Aerobic Interval Training Versus Moderate Continuous Training in Heart Failure Patients: A Randomized Study. *Circulation, Jun.* 2007; 115: 3086 – 3094.

In: Handbook on Longevity: Genetics, Diet and Disease   ISBN 978-1-60741-075-1
Editors: Jennifer V. Bentely and Mary Ann Keller   © 2009 Nova Science Publishers, Inc.

Chapter XI

Be Young in Mind - Against Aging and Alzheimer's Disease

Kun Zou[1,2]

Department of Neuroscience, School of Pharmacy, Iwate Medical University, 2-1-1
Nishitokuda, Yahaba, Iwate 028-3694, Japan.
Tel: 81 19 698 1820; Fax: 81 19 698 1864; Email: kunzou@iwate-med.ac.jp
Department of Alzheimer's Disease Research, National Institute for Longevity Sciences,
NCGG, 36-3 Gengo, Morioka, Obu, Aichi 474-8522, Japan

Abstract

Life expectancy around the world has increased steadily for nearly 200 years. The continuing increase in life expectancy has made us face age-related diseases that we overlooked in the nineteenth and early twentieth centuries. Age is by far the biggest risk factor for a wide range of clinical conditions that are prevalent today. Although cardiovascular diseases and cancers still remain the leading causes of death for both men and women among age-related diseases, Alzheimer's disease has been in the spotlight recently because the number of its patients is increasing at an unexpected speed. Onset of Alzheimer's disease begins with short-term memory loss in its early stage and gradually the sufferer loses minor, and then major bodily functions, until death occurs. Unlike cardiovascular diseases and cancers, current knowledge of the processes leading to Alzheimer's disease is still limited, and very few effective treatments are available. Many treatment strategies have reached the clinical trial stage and some hopeful clinical trials failed to improve the survival or the cognitive ability of Alzheimer's patients. Up to now, clinically validated treatments for Alzheimer's disease remain confined to symptomatic interventions and recent studies suggest that frequent cognitive activity in old age has been associated with reduced risk of Alzheimer's disease. Thus, preventive strategies have become important in our daily life against aging and Alzheimer's disease.

How Long Can Most People Live?

Two thousand and two hundred years ago, the first emperor of China feared death and sought a way to live forever. He sent an islander, Xu Fu, with hundreds of young men and women to Japan to look for the elixir of life from the Eight Immortals who lived on Penglai Mountain (Fuji Mountain). Xu never returned from this trip. The *Records of the Grand Historian* of China says he came to a place with "flat plains and wide swamps" (possibly Kyushu of Japan) and proclaimed himself to be king, never to return, a view that many Chinese and Japanese people are familiar with today.

Although the Bible lists people with far greater life spans, the *2002 Guinness Book of World Records* says that the age of the oldest person who ever lived was 122 years and 164 days. The oldest man in the world now in 2008 is living in Japan, Tomoji Tanabe, 114 years old, and the oldest woman is an American woman, Edna Parker, 115 years old. It is not clear that how long Japanese people could live two thousand years ago; however, the life expectancy in Japan has kept increasing after the Second World War and has been the longest in the world since 1986 according to the World Health Organization (WHO) list of average life expectancy. Japan life expectancy hit record highs of 79 years for males, 86 years for females and 83 years as an average for both sexes in 2006. More interestingly, the WHO also has another table of the average healthy life in each country. This table shows the average age to which people can expect to stay healthy and socially active, which is called healthy life expectancy. Japan again is at the top of this at an average age of 75 years for both sexes. For other developed countries, for example, the U.S., the life expectancy of males is 75 years and that of females is 80 years old. Developing countries also have had a great increase in the life expectancy. China increased 5 years from 68 years in 1990 to 73 years in 2006 for both sexes and Brazil increased from 67 years to 72 years (World Health Statistics 2008, WHO).

Why Do We Age?

Humans reach a peak of growth and development around the time of their mid 20s. Starting at what is commonly referred to as "middle age", the operations of the body become more susceptible to damage, and there is a general decline in physical and possibly mental performance. During the latter half of life, an individual is more prone to experiencing problems with a range of bodily functions and to developing various chronic or fatal diseases. "Why we age" or "why the aging body loses functional capacity" has been debated for nearly 150 years and remains a mystery. Is aging the result of fundamental limitations that apply to all living things, or are organisms designed by nature to age because a limited life span conveys some advantage?

Some important theories of aging were proposed from more than a century ago. The "Wear and tear" theory was proposed by Dr. August Weismann, a German biologist, in 1881. According to this theory, the body and its cells are worn down by toxins in our diet and environment; by the excessive consumption of fat, sugar, caffeine, alcohol and nicotine; by the ultra-violet rays of the sun; and by the many other chemical, physical and emotional stresses to which we are routinely exposed (1). One of the most popular theories of aging is the "free radical theory", first proposed by Dr. Denham Harman in 1956. This theory postulates that aging results from the gradual accumulation of cellular damage caused by reactions with highly reactive molecules known as "free radicals". Free radicals (or reactive oxygen or nitrogen species) are produced endogenously via normal metabolic processes or upon exposure to numerous exogenous agents, including ionizing radiation and cigarette smoke (2). Another popular theory is "telomerase theory of aging", which was proposed in 1996. Evidence clearly indicates a critical role for telomerase, a protein that maintains the caps of chromosome ends, in dictating replicative life span (3). Recently, comparing young and old C. elegans nematode worms, researchers at the Stanford University School of Medicine found that shifts in levels of three transcription factors--the molecular switches that turn genes on and off--appeared to trigger genetic pathways that age the worms. This finding suggests that aging may be part of the genetic plan, called the "genetic control theory of aging", not the result of wear-and-tear on the body and gives hope that science eventually may find a way to stop or reverse the aging process (4).

Human Society is Aging

It is believed that the main reasons for people's longevity are the many advances in medical science. For developed countries, the most elderly (over 85 years old) is the fastest growing segment of the population, and the increase results mainly from a reduction in mortality rates among the most elderly (5). Old-age has increased since 1950 for female octogenarians in Sweden, England, France, Iceland, Japan and the United States. Japan, with the world's longest expectancy and lowest levels of mortality at older ages, has been a leader in the quickening pace of increase in old-age survival. Since the early 1970s female death rates in Japan have declined at annual rates of about 3% for octogenarians and 2% for nonagenarians. Mortality among octogenarians and nonagenarians has been the low in the United States. The reasons for the U.S. advantage and the recent loss of this advantage to Japan and France are not well understood.

While more and more Japanese elders enjoy watching their great-grandchildren grow up, the Japanese government has issued a white paper on Japan's aging society. The white paper says nearly 20 percent of the total population was 65 years old or older as of October 2003. The figure is estimated to exceed 35 percent by 2050. In other words, one out of three people will be 65 years old or older in 2050, compared with one out of five in 2003. At the same time, the percentage of people 100 years old or older has almost doubled since 1998. Japanese society has been aging because of the declining birthrate and death rate as well as increasing life expectancy. This trend was mirrored in all industrial nations. The G7 countries (Canada, France, Germany, Italy, Japan, the United Kingdom, and the United States) showed that mortality in all these nations declined exponentially and at a roughly constant rate from 1950 to 1994. In 1930, life expectancy at birth in the United States was 58 for men and 62 for women. By 2006, the average U.S. life expectancy was 75 for men and 80 for women. French men live an average of 77 years, while French women average 84 years. The people of Japan and other developed countries began to worry that the population decrease, the aging of the general population and workforce, and the decline in birthrate may progress to the point of dampening economic activity, escalating the load on the social security system, and sapping the vigor of society as a whole. At the same time, however, the maturing of society has made them less concerned about satisfying their material needs and more interested in mental and spiritual enrichment, a long life that is also healthy, safety and peace of mind, and the opportunity to follow their own personal values and choose from among a variety of life styles. The governments are responding to these population issues with various initiatives aimed at increasing the birthrate and overcoming problems concerning the elderly.

What Are Age-Related Diseases?

Although a lot of people live extremely long lives, more and more people are suffering from various problems regarding age-related diseases at the same time. Late-life loss of independence in daily living is a central concern for the aging individual and for society. This can come about through deterioration of eyesight and hearing, which can make it hard to get around and to interact with people. As people get older, the cardiovascular, digestive, excretory, nervous, reproductive and urinary systems are particularly vulnerable. The prevalence of disease increase and the common age-related ailments include cancer, heart disease, stroke, arthritis, diabetes and osteoporosis. Recently, a worrying prospect for anyone approaching old-age is the possibility of getting Alzheimer's disease (AD) which has no current cure.

The U.S. center for disease control reported that rates for 14 of the top 15 causes of death fell in 2006. While AD, the most common form of dementia, become No. 6 on the list of leading cause of death, killing 72,914 Americans in 2006, diabetes fell to No. 7 on the list. A Japanese government report shows that cancer remains the leading cause of death for both men and women in Japan, followed by heart disease and stroke in 2004. Although the mortality probability of the three leading causes of death accounts for over 50 percent for both sexes, a surprising increase in the number of AD patients was reported in 2006. Trends in the rates of estimated inpatients/outpatients per 100,000 population (per day) by diseases referred to "The New Health Frontier Strategy", total AD patients increased 67% from 2002 to 2006, in which inpatients increased 53% and outpatients increased about 100%. In contrast, other age-related disease patients did not show such a great increase or even declined. For example, total malignant neoplasm increased about 10%, cerebrovascular disease was unchanged and ischemic heart disease even declined by 6% from 2002 to 2006 in Japan. In the U.S., people dying from AD increased 32.8% from 2000 to 2004, whereas those from heart disease and stroke decreased 8% and 10.4%, respectively (Center for Disease Control and Prevention, National Vital Statistics Reports).

What is Alzheimer's Disease?

Alzheimer's disease (AD) is a progressive neurodegenerative disease named for the German physician Alois Alzheimer, who first described it in 1906. He reported the first AD patient, a 55-year-old woman. Her symptoms had begun at the age of 51 with an unreasonable jealousy of her husband. As her illness progressed, the woman endured a rapid decline in memory, paranoid delusions, auditory hallucinations, and finally, complete dementia. Within 4 and half years after the onset of symptoms, the woman died at age 56. Alzheimer described the senile plaques, and neurofibrillary tangles (NFTs), coiled fibers within the cytoplasm of the cerebral cortical neurons.

AD can affect different people in different ways, but the most common symptom pattern begins with gradually worsening difficulty remembering new information. This is because disruption of brain cells usually begins in regions involved in forming new memories. As damage spreads, AD not only causes problems with memory, but also with thinking and behavior, which are severe enough to affect work, lifelong hobbies or social life. AD gets worse over time, and it is fatal. AD affects 5 million Americans and around 25 million people worldwide, and this number is increasing rapidly. By 2050, the number of individuals with AD could range from 11.3 to 16 million in the U.S. (6,7). From a social and economic view, the explosion of AD cases is now a big concern for the developed countries. By 2010, AD care will cost Medicare about $160 billion a year in the U.S. alone. By 2035, it could overtake the defense budget. One analysis has estimated that by 2050, AD will cost Medicare more than $1 trillion annually. Those numbers do not include privately insured and uninsured costs.

Pathogenesis and Therapeutic Strategies of AD

There is much disagreement even among AD specialists about the basic nature of the disease and how the disease is initiated at the molecular level. Most of the AD investigators consider that the abnormal deposition of amyloid beta-protein (Aβ), a major component of senile plaques, or the Aβ oligomer in the brain is crucial to AD pathogenesis, which is called the "amyloid hypothesis". Aβ is constantly secreted by many types of cell and are normally found in body fluids, including cerebrospinal fluid (CSF) and the monomeric Aβ is nontoxic or even protective (8). The amyloid hypothesis is centered on the overproduction, or inadequate clearance, in the brain of Aβ. The strongest evidence for the crucial role played by Aβ in AD pathogenesis has been the mutations that underlie familial early onset cases of the disease. All of these inherited mutations affect the processing and accumulation of Aβ. Aβ is generated from the amyloid precursor protein (APP) by the proteolytic activities of β- and γ-secretase (9,10). It is known that transmembrane proteins presenilin 1 (PS1) and presenilin 2 (PS2) are essential for intramembranous proteolytic γ–cleavage of APP (11). Familial Alzheimer's disease (FAD) is associated with point mutations in APP in regions that are involved in the proteolytic processing of Aβ (12,13) and with point mutations in presenilins (PSs) 1 and 2. Mutations in either PS or APP consistently increase the relative ratio between the long (Aβ1-42) and short (Aβ1-40) Aβ peptides (14,15) (Figure 1). In addition to these FAD, it is suggested that the trisomy of choromosome 21, where the APP gene is localized, causes the overexpression of APP and the formation of Aβ deposits in Down syndrome (16).

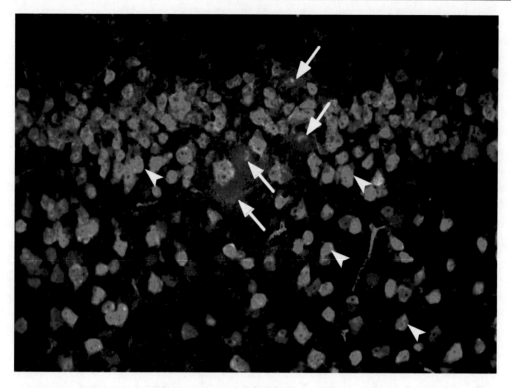

Figure1. Immunostaining of amyloid plaques and neuronal cells in the brain cortex.

Brain sections of aged Swedish mutant APP transgenic mice (Tg2576) were stained with anti-Aβ1-42 antibody (red) and anti-NeuN antibody (green). The overexpression of human familial AD APP gene in mice induced extensive Alzheimer disease-like amyloid depositions in the brain, which are shown as red plaques (arrows). The green cells indicate the NeuN-positive mature neuronal cells (arrowheads).

A rival idea of the "amyloid hypothesis" is called the "tau hypothesis". Aβ generally aggregates outside brain cells, the protein tau aggregates into fibrous structures, called neurofibrillary tangles (NFTs), inside the neurons. NFTs consist of intracellular nonmembrane-bound bundles of abnormal fibers that ultrastructurally appear as pairs of filaments wound into helices (paired helical filaments or PHF). PHFs are composed of the microtubuleassociate protein tau in its hyperphosphorylated form (17). For many years no causal link between Aβ and tau has been evident and researchers in the field of AD have become subdivided into two warring camps, called "βaptists" and "tauists" according to their, sometimes ideological, belief concerning the main, primarily affected molecular species. In later studies, however, both in vitro and in vivo studies strongly suggest that exposure of neurons to Aβ transforms tau in a phosphorylated condition and may provoke the assembly of PHF-like tau filaments (18,19). Because of these findings, the "amyloid hypothesis" gains an advantage in the recent strategies for the development of AD therapies.

There is not yet any treatment that can delay or stop the deterioration of brain cells in AD. The U.S. Food and Drug Administration (FDA) has so far approved five drugs that temporarily slow worsening of symptoms for about 6 to 12 months. Based on the "amyloid hypothesis", many treatment strategies have been proposed and conducted in clinical trials, aiming at stopping the deterioration of brain cells. Drugs used for lowering the Aβ level include Aβ secretase inhibitors or modulators, which inhibit the Aβ secretion or modulate Aβ secretion by shifting the toxic longer form of Aβ to a nontoxic short form, and Aβ immunization reagents, by which antibodies to Aβ decrease cerebral levels of the peptide by promoting microglial clearance or by redistributing the peptide from the brain to the systemic circulation. Small peptide which binds to Aβ and inhibits its aggregation has been also conducted in clinical trials. Other drugs include anti-inflammatory drugs, cholesterol-lowering drugs, metal chelators and neuroprotective drugs, such as antioxidants and neurotrophins. Cholesterol-lowering drugs have been shown to reduce the risk of AD and Aβ deposition in APP transgenic mice and metal chelators may prevent Aβ deposition in the brain (20-22). Epidemiological studies have shown that nonsteroidal anti-inflammatory drugs (NSAIDs) reduce the risk of AD (23,24).

Unfortunately, some therapeutic strategies that entered the clinical trials were reported to have no effects on improving the survival or the cognitive ability of Alzheimer's patients. One of the most hopeful strategies has been the active immunization against Aβ42, a toxic longer form of Aβ. British researchers reported a 6-year prospective follow-up study, which examined 80 patients with mild to moderate dementia who had been immunized with AN1792, a drug which acts to clear amyloid plaques from the brain. As expected, cortical Aβ loads were lower in patients who were immunized than in the control group and patients with the biggest antibody response had more extensive Aβ removal. Unexpectedly, however, there was no evidence of improved survival or of an improvement in the time to severe dementia, even in patients with high antibody titers compared with non-immunized control patients (25). In addition, a phase III clinical trial that involved 1684 patients reported that Flurizan, a selective Aβ42-Lowering agent failed to improve cognitive functioning or activities of daily living. Another Aβ generation inhibitor, Alzhemed, showed the similar result. These studies will undoubtedly evoke concern that anti-amyloid therapies will be ineffectual and the previous consensus among AD researchers that removing amyloid plaques is a key to defeating Alzheimer's may need to be reconsidered.

Many other clinical trials did not show optimistic results either. In the American Academy of Neurology's annual meeting in Chicago, April 2008, Dr. Howard Feldman and coworkers showed that Lipitor, the best-selling cholesterol-lowering statin drug, has no significant benefits on the symptoms of mild to moderate AD patients. For the anti-inflammatory drugs, there has been retrospective evidence that they might have some protective effects in AD (23,24); however, in contrast to results expected from epidemiological studies, a report found that the drugs did not improve cognitive function in elderly individuals with a family history of AD (26).

Interestingly, some drugs that do not target Aβ have shown a protective effect against AD. In July 2008, at the annual meeting of the Alzheimer's Association, researchers presented data about the discovery of two drugs that might help prevent cognitive decline. One is called methylene blue, which selectively inhibited tau-aggregation, and slowed the progression of AD by 81% as compared to placebo. Another is developed by Russian scientists, called Dimebon. It significantly improved the clinical course of patients with mild-to-moderate AD. Previous reports showed that Dimebon has antihistamine properties, inhibitory effects on acetylcholinesterase and N-methyl-D-aspartate (NMDA) receptors.

These combined effects are considered to be beneficial for AD patients (27). In 2008, a summary issued by America's Pharmaceutical research companies reported that there are still 89 drugs for dementias, including AD, which are under phase I to III clinical trials, and of these, 15 are in the phase III. Whether an effective treatment for AD can be achieved by these drugs is still unknown.

The major problem today for AD therapy is that the causes of AD are not fully understood, making development of ways to treat it problematic. Without knowing the main cause of a disease it is hard to develop effective treatments. It has been 101 years since Alzheimer's disease was first theorized, and billions of dollars have been spent for research on it. Because the clinical trials based on the "amyloid hypothesis" or "tau hypothesis" are not successful so far, it is still debatable whether amyloid plaques and tau tangles are causes of AD or results of neuroprotection. There is also considerable evidence indicating that amyloid deposition and tau tangles are byproducts of protective mechanisms (8,28,29) and it is clearly recognized that amyloid depositions in the brain parenchyma and blood vessels are common in nondemented individuals of advanced age (30,31).

Healthy Life and to be Young in Mind

More and more AD investigators agree that AD, like other common, chronic conditions, likely develops as a result of multiple factors rather than a single cause. A tiny percentage of AD is caused by rare genetic variations found in a few hundred families worldwide. In these inherited forms of AD, the disease tends to develop before age 65, sometimes in individuals as young as 30. However, for the sporadic type AD, the most common case, the greatest risk factor by far is advancing age. Most individuals with AD are age 65 or older. Other risk factors for the late-onset AD include the genetic risk factors, apolipoprotein E4 and angiotensin-converting enzyme I allele, and other age-related disorders induced by high fat diets and sedentary lifestyles, such as obesity, diabetes, hyperlipidemia, hypertension, atherosclerosis, etc (32). A 20-year-long longitudinal study conducted by Sweden researchers showed that environmental factors, life habits, social factors and medication are all related to the risk of dementia and AD. Having manual work as the lifetime principal work, and work involving goods production in particular, was found to be related to a significantly increased risk of AD and all types of dementia. A low level of education and malnutrition were also found related to increased risk of AD in this study (33). U.S. researchers also demonstrated that extensive social networks are related to high cognitive ability and reduced AD pathology .In general, in addition to improving one's life style to prevent obesity, hyperlipidemia and hypertension, it is important for old people to participate in activities which are mentally as well as socially and physically stimulating. Such an active life may postpone the onset of AD.

Among industrial nations, despite high levels of stress, tobacco, pollution and alcohol, how do Japanese people keep the longest healthy life expectancy and stay healthy and socially active? The long healthy life expectancy suggests less or late-onset of age-related diseases, such as cancer, heart disease, stroke and AD. Again, there seem to be multiple answers; healthcare level, food, life style, social factors and environmental factors can be taken into account. However, smoking and drinking alcohol are very common among

Japanese men (especially) and they often lead to a stressful, competitive lifestyle, epitomizing the "work hard, play hard" image. Then how do they remain active and healthy into old age? The traditional Japanese diet is said to be one of the healthiest in the world. When Sushi restaurants are burgeoning around the world, people often neglect the attitude of Japanese people towards health. In Japan, the enthusiasm for health is very high in the whole nation. For example, Japanese children need to go to school by walking and by themselves. Going to school in their parent's car is not encouraged, and they need to get up at 6 o'clock during their summer holidays and gather outside to do radio exercises together. These may be unthinkable in other developed countries. In addition, products for measuring how healthy you are or maintaining one's health are everywhere in Japan. For example, the city halls and the ward offices are usually equipped with blood-pressure meters in the waiting area for free-use; people living in the urban area can buy an electric horse which mimics the movement of horse-riding; a weight scale can tell your fat percentage and body-mass index and whether you are in a normal range; and the "health slippers" incorporate interesting but painful spikes in them for stimulating the nerves and blood circulation of the foot. Most interestingly, when Japanese people realized that AD had become one major problem for the aging society in recent years, brain-training games and software emerged quickly and have become a boom for middle-age and aged people. The same brain-training games boom is also spreading in the U.S. and their sales reached more than 200 million dollars in 2007.

Nowadays, more and more old Japanese people are isolated and live alone and this will undoubtedly reduce their social activities and increase the risk for AD. Those who have become bedridden, demented, and/or frail because of specific age-related diseases such as early-stage dementia and cerebrovascular disorders will need long-term care supported by the society. The Japanese government has established a long-term care insurance system which responds to society's major concern about aging, the care problem, whereby people can be assured that they will receive care and be supported by society as a whole. However, there are still many efforts needed to be put into an earlier stage to prevent aging. For example, having old people in periodic contact with young people, especially their children, may be very important in helping them maintain a young mind. In addition, to increase the social activities among old people would be also very helpful for keeping young in mind, for example, studying painting and gardening together. Another good example is that like Japanese children gathering together in the morning of summer holidays to do radio exercises, the old people in China get together every morning to do Tai Chi Chuan, to talk with each other or to play chess.

Before we are able to have effective drugs to stop the progression of AD, developing preventive therapies for it may be a better way, that is, to be young in mind. With a young mind one may fight against most of the age-related diseases and AD. As proposed by the Japanese Society of Anti-Aging Medicine, "Anti-Aging medicine is not confined solely to detecting and treating age-related diseases. It is also about preventing disease and maintaining well-being as we age, thus improving the quality of life for all. It promotes a new paradigm of healthy and energetic people who can actively participate in society and enjoy a happy and fruitful life."

References

[1] Kirkwood, T. B., and Cremer, T. (1982) *Hum Genet.* 60, 101-121.

[2] Harman, D. (1956) *J Gerontol.* 11, 298-300.

[3] Holt, S. E., Shay, J. W., and Wright, W. E. (1996) *Nat Biotechnol.* 14, 836-839.

[4] Budovskaya, Y. V., Wu, K., Southworth, L. K., Jiang, M., Tedesco, P., Johnson, T. E., and Kim, S. K. (2008) *Cell,* 134, 291-303.

[5] Vaupel, J. W., Carey, J. R., Christensen, K., Johnson, T. E., Yashin, A. I., Holm, N. V., Iachine, I. A., Kannisto, V., Khazaeli, A. A., Liedo, P., Longo, V. D., Zeng, Y., Manton, K. G., and Curtsinger, J. W. (1998) *Science,* 280, 855-860.

[6] Hebert, L. E., Scherr, P. A., Bienias, J. L., Bennett, D. A., and Evans, D. A. (2003) *Arch Neurol* 60, 1119-1122.

[7] Ferri, C. P., Prince, M., Brayne, C., Brodaty, H., Fratiglioni, L., Ganguli, M., Hall, K., Hasegawa, K., Hendrie, H., Huang, Y., Jorm, A., Mathers, C., Menezes, P. R., Rimmer, E., and Scazufca, M. (2005) *Lancet,* 366, 2112-2117.

[8] Zou, K., Gong, J. S., Yanagisawa, K., and Michikawa, M. (2002) *J Neurosci* 22, 4833-4841.

[9] Masters, C. L., Simms, G., Weinman, N. A., Multhaup, G., McDonald, B. L., and Beyreuther, K. (1985) *Proc Natl Acad Sci. U S A,* 82, 4245-4249.

[10] Kang, J., Lemaire, H. G., Unterbeck, A., Salbaum, J. M., Masters, C. L., Grzeschik, K. H., Multhaup, G., Beyreuther, K., and Muller-Hill, B. (1987) *Nature,* 325, 733-736.

[11] De Strooper, B., Saftig, P., Craessaerts, K., Vanderstichele, H., Guhde, G., Annaert, W., Von Figura, K., and Van Leuven, F. (1998) *Nature,* 391, 387-390.

[12] Goate, A., Chartier-Harlin, M. C., Mullan, M., Brown, J., Crawford, F., Fidani, L., Giuffra, L., Haynes, A., Irving, N., James, L., and et al. (1991) *Nature,* 349, 704-706.

[13] Lendon, C. L., Ashall, F., and Goate, A. M. (1997) *Jama,* 277, 825-831.

[14] Borchelt, D. R., Thinakaran, G., Eckman, C. B., Lee, M. K., Davenport, F., Ratovitsky, T., Prada, C. M., Kim, G., Seekins, S., Yager, D., Slunt, H. H., Wang, R., Seeger, M., Levey, A. I., Gandy, S. E., Copeland, N. G., Jenkins, N. A., Price, D. L., Younkin, S. G., and Sisodia, S. S. (1996) *Neuron.* 17, 1005-1013.

[15] Scheuner, D., Eckman, C., Jensen, M., Song, X., Citron, M., Suzuki, N., Bird, T. D., Hardy, J., Hutton, M., Kukull, W., Larson, E., Levy-Lahad, E., Viitanen, M., Peskind, E., Poorkaj, P., Schellenberg, G., Tanzi, R., Wasco, W., Lannfelt, L., Selkoe, D., and Younkin, S. (1996) *Nat Med.* 2, 864-870.

[16] Patterson, D., Gardiner, K., Kao, F. T., Tanzi, R., Watkins, P., and Gusella, J. F. (1988) *Proc Natl Acad Sci U S A.* 85, 8266-8270.

[17] Grundke-Iqbal, I., Iqbal, K., Tung, Y. C., Quinlan, M., Wisniewski, H. M., and Binder, L. I. (1986) *Proc Natl Acad Sci U S A,* 83, 4913-4917.

[18] Busciglio, J., Lorenzo, A., Yeh, J., and Yankner, B. A. (1995) *Neuron.* 14, 879-888

[19] Sturchler-Pierrat, C., Abramowski, D., Duke, M., Wiederhold, K. H., Mistl, C., Rothacher, S., Ledermann, B., Burki, K., Frey, P., Paganetti, P. A., Waridel, C., Calhoun, M. E., Jucker, M., Probst, A., Staufenbiel, M., and Sommer, B. (1997) *Proc Natl Acad Sci U S A.* 94, 13287-13292.

[20] Cherny, R. A., Atwood, C. S., Xilinas, M. E., Gray, D. N., Jones, W. D., McLean, C. A., Barnham, K. J., Volitakis, I., Fraser, F. W., Kim, Y., Huang, X., Goldstein, L. E., Moir, R. D., Lim, J. T., Beyreuther, K., Zheng, H., Tanzi, R. E., Masters, C. L., and Bush, A. I. (2001) *Neuron.* 30, 665-676.

[21] Jick, H., Zornberg, G. L., Jick, S. S., Seshadri, S., and Drachman, D. A. (2000) *Lancet,* 356, 1627-1631.

[22] Refolo, L. M., Pappolla, M. A., LaFrancois, J., Malester, B., Schmidt, S. D., Thomas-Bryant, T., Tint, G. S., Wang, R., Mercken, M., Petanceska, S. S., and Duff, K. E. (2001) *Neurobiol Dis.* 8, 890-899.

[23] Vlad, S. C., Miller, D. R., Kowall, N. W., and Felson, D. T. (2008) *Neurology,* 70, 1672-1677

[24] in t' Veld, B. A., Ruitenberg, A., Hofman, A., Launer, L. J., van Duijn, C. M., Stijnen, T., Breteler, M. M., and Stricker, B. H. (2001) *N Engl J Med.* 345, 1515-1521.

[25] Holmes, C., Boche, D., Wilkinson, D., Yadegarfar, G., Hopkins, V., Bayer, A., Jones, R. W., Bullock, R., Love, S., Neal, J. W., Zotova, E., and Nicoll, J. A. (2008) *Lancet,* 372, 216-223.

[26] Martin, B. K., Szekely, C., Brandt, J., Piantadosi, S., Breitner, J. C., Craft, S., Evans, D., Green, R., and Mullan, M. (2008) *Arch Neurol.* 65, 896-905.

[27] Doody, R. S., Gavrilova, S. I., Sano, M., Thomas, R. G., Aisen, P. S., Bachurin, S. O., Seely, L., and Hung, D. (2008) *Lancet,* 372, 207-215.

[28] Lee, H. G., Zhu, X., Castellani, R. J., Nunomura, A., Perry, G., and Smith, M. A. (2007) *J Pharmacol Exp Ther.* 321, 823-829.

[29] Castellani, R. J., Nunomura, A., Lee, H. G., Perry, G., and Smith, M. A. (2008) *J Alzheimers Dis.* 14, 377-383.

[30] Mann, D. M., Jones, D., South, P. W., Snowden, J. S., and Neary, D. (1992) *Acta Neuropathol (Berl)* 83, 415-419.

[31] Schmitt, F. A., Davis, D. G., Wekstein, D. R., Smith, C. D., Ashford, J. W., and Markesbery, W. R. (2000) *Neurology,* 55, 370-376.

[32] Martins, I. J., Hone, E., Foster, J. K., Sunram-Lea, S. I., Gnjec, A., Fuller, S. J., Nolan, D., Gandy, S. E., and Martins, R. N. (2006) *Mol Psychiatry,* 11, 721-736.

[33] Fratiglioni, L., Winblad, B., and von Strauss, E. (2007) *Physiol Behav.* 92, 98-104.

In: Handbook on Longevity: Genetics, Diet and Disease   ISBN 978-1-60741-075-1
Editors: Jennifer V. Bentely and Mary Ann Keller   © 2009 Nova Science Publishers, Inc.

Chapter XII

Understanding Aging: Prejudices and Misconceptions

Carles Zafon

Division of Endocrinology, Hospital General Vall d'Hebron
Barcelona (Spain).

Abstract

Current evolutionary biology has rejected any theory that supports a selective purpose for aging. However, recent findings have forced a reconsideration of this concept and an effort to update old statements that have been made. In accordance, several evolutionary propositions have been suggested to justify the broad presence of aging in the animal kingdom and the wide range of longevity. Nevertheless, many of these alternative hypotheses have been dismissed using a small set of arguments that have been systematically repeated without, in some cases, any compelling proof of evidence. Moreover, there exists a variety of preconceptions and biases that could hinder the progression in theoretical thought about aging and longevity. The aim of this "author comment" is to expose some of these preconceptions to generate a productive debate which can enrich the progress in the field of evolutionary biology of aging. In particular, I will discuss three critical points that have not usually been considered in related papers. The first point is the "emotional bias" observed when authors argue the purpose of aging. The second point (When does aging begin?) pertains to the beginning of aging. The third topic (The old watchmaker) discusses the meaning of the aging process from an evolutionary perspective, and the evolutionary origin of the aging strategy.

Introduction

In recent decades, experimental data from molecular biology have revealed the existence of genes, manipulations of which can alter longevity. This discovery has been used by some researchers that defend aging as a genetic program, at the same level, for example, as embryogenesis or puberty. Thus, the debate between supporters and detractors of a "programmed senescence" has been reopened, especially in the field of evolutionary biology. Since the classic propositions from Medawar [1], Williams [2], and Kirkwood [3], the current position is that aging is a non-adaptive process because it is far form the scope of natural selection. During the last half century, the main argument to justify this notion has been "copied and pasted" without, as it has been stated, any appropriate update [4,5]. The aim of this article is to bring out some concepts that, in my opinion, make difficult the exact comprehension and hamper the progress in the amazing range of the evolutionary theories of aging. In particular, I discuss three points that often bias the scientific approach to this unsolved problem of biology.

1. Emotional Bias

Sexual cannibalism describes a special form of cannibalism in which a female kills and consumes her conspecific male before, during or after copulation. This behaviour is commonly related with the praying mantis. Benefits to the female are clear, she gains valuable reproductive resources and it has been demonstrated that she produces a greater number of offspring. In contrast, the possibility that males may also benefit from sexual cannibalism remains controversial [6]. Let us imagine that the praying mantis males were able to think about this behaviour; it seems reasonable that they would not find any advantage to this strategy. Fortunately, our species does not practice sexual cannibalism, and our most natural form of death is a result of growing old. However, our opinion about the process of aging is as negative as the opinion of the male mantis about sexual cannibalism. We have the experience that aging is a deleterious process, associated with discomfort, diseases, and death. Moreover, scientists who have defined aging have used the same negative approach. Thus, for example, Maynard Smith stated that the "aging processes may be defined as those which render individuals more susceptible as they grow older to the various factors, intrinsic or extrinsic, which may cause death" [7].

Aging has focused important attention and during the last century many evolutionary hypotheses have been proposed to explain the ultimate reason for this near-universal feature in the animal kingdom. However, the vast majority of propositions initiate the reasoning with this aforementioned preconception, the idea that growing old is "bad business," which is the same preconception a male mantis would start with in analyzing cannibalism. Thus, it is not surprising that these theories conclude that the phenomenon can not be the result of natural selection, and for that, the notion that senescence is a strategy actively selected has been systematically rejected. Mitteldorf has written "the idea that aging is a genetic program shaped over evolutionary time and selected for its own sake, is anathema to evolutionary theory" [8]. It is noteworthy to remember that, 50 years ago, Williams claimed that "senescence is a widespread phenomenon, but it has been largely neglected by non-medical biologists. This neglect may be attributed to a number of causes," and he continued "Another (cause), perhaps, is an emotional difficulty associated with aging" [2].

It is possible that we can apply to the aging concept the same idea that Kovacs has brought to the concept of health, i.e., "biological notion of health expresses how efficiently the body and the mind of an individual can be 'used' by the genes for their own multiplication, the cultural notion of health expresses how efficiently the body and mind can be used as tools to realise certain preferred ways of living, values, and standards, desired by given culture or individual" [9]. Thus, it is possible that we judge aging under a cultural or humanistic point of view, not under a strictly biological focus. Milne has written that "Attribution of aging to the adverse element is no more than a self-interested value judgement by a thinking soma" [10].

2. When Does Aging Begin?

Current evolutionary biology rejects selected aging according to a few different arguments. The main thrust of these arguments has been extensively used and can be summarised in the words of Kirkwood as "mortality in the wild populations is usually so great that individuals rarely live long enough to show clear signs of senescence" [11]. This asseveration has been interpreted as follows: aging does not exist in nature. However, it is interesting to note that the fact that animals do not die old does not mean that they do not age. Aging and dying is not the same thing [7]. The objection is really important; if animals in the wild (and humans along their history) do not practise aging, it appears comprehensible that natural selection has not been able to plan it. However, this reiterative argument appears so inconsistent. Effectively, papers that express this principle do not prove it. The argument must be justified only after answering two previous questions: When does aging begin? And, afterwards, do animals die before aging begins? It is obvious that the answer to the first question is mandatory, and till now nobody has been able to do it. The problem has been hardly discussed. In 1984, Hayflick proposed different possibilities; aging begins before conception, after conception, and after sexual maturation, but he confessed that "the lack of a precise definition for biological aging precludes a definitive answer to when the phenomenon begins" [12]. Finally, his personal point of view was that "aging begins when longevity assurance genes cease to be expressed" [12]. On the other hand, Milne, in a recent report, has pointed that whether the onset of aging must be in coincidence with the nadir of mortality, nowadays in developed nations the nadir lies at 5 – 9 years, predating fertility at a mean of 12 – 13 years [10].

Generally, aging is defined as a "continuous process" that starts at conception and continues until death [13]. According with this time-dependent concept, the visible phenotypic expression of the process is not the same in relation with the moment we evaluate it. Nowadays, we are familiar with a characteristic picture of very old people (and pet animals). However, several centuries ago, as well as in the case of wild animals, external signs of aging would be more subtle, by the fact they did not reach the same older age, but, in any case, it does not mean that they did not age. Finally, there is a generalized consensus that we do not have biological aging markers sensitive enough to characterise the phenomenon with the precision desired. In summary, the argument of a lack of aging in nature seems so poor to support the negation of a selected strategy.

3. The Old Watchmaker

The "blind watchmaker" was the most famous creationist argument exposed by the eighteenth-century theologian, William Paley. He exposed that just as a watch is too complicated and too functional to have sprung into existence by accident, so too must all living things, with their far greater complexity, be purposefully designed. Paley also compared the eye with a telescope, to conclude that "there is precisely the same proof that the eye was made for vision, as there is that the telescope was made for assisting it" [14]. One century later, Richard Dawkins used the same argument precisely to rebate the anti-Darwinian proposition in a book entitled "The blind watchmaker". Dawkins defined that "a complicated thing is one whose existence we do not feel inclined to take for granted, because it is too "improbable" [14]. Afterwards, he wrote that the explanation to the existence of a complex thing (like the eye) is "the gradual step by step transformation from simple beginnings, from primordial entities sufficiently simple to have come into existence by chance. Each successive change in the gradual evolutionary process was simple enough, relative to its predecessor, to have arisen by chance. But the whole sequence of cumulative steps constitutes anything but a chance process" [14]. In the same manner, aging appears to be a feature so complex that its existence seems difficult to be explained. Researchers have failed to find a unique theory able to state the cause of the senescence. Nevertheless, as in the case of the eye, a probable aging genotype should be understood as the consequence of a step by step transformation, an evolutionary process evolved from a primordial and simple nucleus. Over this initial nucleus, other changes have been added to reach the current characteristic of what we can define as aging. Present-day senescence is not a compact, well-structured, genetic program, nor a random stochastic process. Both conceptions do not have in mind the dynamic and evolutionary aspect of any living process.

On the other hand, to understand the gradual notion in the evolution of any feature, it is necessary to know the time elapsed since the first of all these steps. Generally, it has been believed that the first organisms did not age, and that aging evolved only after the origin of eukaryotes. However, recent studies have reported aging in bacteria. For example, Stewart et al have shown that an old pole of *Escherichia coli* exhibits multiple phenotypes associated with aging, namely, decreased metabolic efficiency, reduced offspring biomass production, and an increased chance of death [15]. Moreover, it has been proposed that reproduction by asymmetric division is a prerequisite for aging [16].

Conclusion

Prior to undertaking the task of postulating any evolutionary hypothesis to explain aging, it is mandatory to define several previous rules. First, it is necessary to eradicate all emotional biases and we must treat senescence as any other biological feature. Second, we must refuse any asseveration that has not been convincingly demonstrated. Third, we must consider that aging has evolved following the same principles accepted for other physiologic traits. Fourth, we must take into account what could be the target of the process and what could be the variable submitted to natural selection. And, finally, our theoretical propositions must be confronted with experimental advances and, when needed, update and revise old conceptions. Solely following all these steps we will be able, perhaps, to understand this "unsolved problem of biology".

References

[1]   Medawar, P. An unsolved problem in biology. 1952. H.K.Lewis: London.

[2]   Williams, G. Pleiotropy, natural selection, and the evolution of senescence. *Evolution*, 1957; 11: 398-411. 1957.

[3]   Kirkwood, T. Evolution of aging. *Nature*, 1977; 270: 301-304.

[4]   Nesse, T. Life table tests of evolutionary theories of senescence. *Exp Gerontol.* 1988; 23: 445-453.

[5]   Promislow, D, and Pletcher S. Advice to an aging scientist. *Mech Ageing Dev.* 2002; 123: 841-850.

[6]   Lelito, J. and Brown, W. Complicity or conflict over sexual canibalism? Male risk taking in the praying mantis *Tenodera aridifolia sinensis*. *Am Nat.* 2006; 168: 263-269.

[7]   Maynard Smith, J. The causes of ageing. *Rev Lect Senescence*, 1962;115-127.

[8]   Mitteldorf, J. How evolutionary thinking affects people's ideas about aging interventions. *Rejuvenation Res.* 2006; 9: 346-350.

[9]   Kovács, J. The concept of health and disease. *Med Health Care Philos.* 1998; 1: 31-39.

[10]   Milne, E. When does ageing begin? *Mech Ageing Dev.* 2006; 127: 290-297.

[11]   Kirkwood, T. The origins of human ageing. *Phil Trans R Soc Lond B,* 1997; 352: 1765-1772.

[12]   Hayflick, L. When does aging begin? *Res Aging,* 1984; 6: 99-103.

[13]   Balcombe, N. Ageing: definitions, mechanisms and the magnitude of the problem. *Best Pract Res Clin Gastroenterol.* 2001; 15: 835-849.

[14]   Dawkins, R. The Blind watchmaker. Penguin Books London, 6. 2000.

[15]   Stewart, E., Madden, R., Paul, G., and Taddei, F. Aging and death in an organism that reproduces by morphologically symmetric division. *PLoS Biol,* 2005; 3: 295-300.

[16]   Stearns, S. Life history evolution: successes, limitations, and prospects. *Naturwissenschaften,* 2000; 87: 476-486.

In: Handbook on Longevity: Genetics, Diet and Disease   ISBN 978-1-60741-075-1
Editors: Jennifer V. Bentely and Mary Ann Keller   © 2009 Nova Science Publishers, Inc.

Chapter XIII

Longevity: Genetics, Diet and Disease

E. Naumova, I. Atanasova, M. Ivanova and G. Pawelec
Central Laboratory of Clinical Immunology,
University Hospital, Bulgaria

Abstract

The aging process is very complex. Human longevity is a multifactorial trait which is determined by genetic and environmental factors and the interaction of "disease" processes with "intrinsic" ageing processes. Twin and family studies imply that up to 25% of human lifespan is heritable and increases in long-lived people to 36-40%. Longevity is a complex phenotype associated with different genes and gene polymorphisms, some of which are involved in metabolic pathways and endocrine system functioning, which affect diet-related health risks. For example, about 10 loci in the human genome have now been found that seem to confer susceptibility to type 1 diabetes mellitus, where insulin deficiency is due to autoimmune beta cell destruction. Nutrition is one of the hypothetical disease-triggering factors and low and special carbohydrate diet is obligatory for disease control. The best studied longevity pathway involves the genes regulating insulin and insulin-like growth factor-1 (IGF-1) signaling, as well as environmental effects on gene expression. Some of these genes are responsible also for oxidative stress, inflammation and tumor suppression. Another conventional group of genes currently under intense investigation are those involved in innate and adaptive immune responses. The pathogenesis of some of the most frequent human age-related diseases, like metabolic syndrome, diabetes mellitus type 2, and atherosclerosis is associated with a change in the circulating levels of C-reactive protein, tumor necrosis factor-α, interleukin-6, leptin, resistin, adiponectin, omentin, visfatin, and expression of CD40, - CD40 ligand, E-selectin, ICAM-1, and VCAM-1. Some of these genes may be responsible for mediating the beneficial effects of caloric restriction by regulating energy balance as well as stress resistance and oxidative damage. Additionally, other genes such as those encoding TLR, CCR5, KIR and MBL2 have also been associated with different age-related diseases and therefore with human longevity.

There are rare monogenic human diseases which are models for accelerated aging and progeria. Others are caused by inborn errors of metabolism: inherited traits that are due to a mutation in a metabolic enzyme, mutations in regulatory proteins and in transport mechanisms. Some metabolic disorders are due to structural chromosome aberrations and genomic imprinting, such as life-threatening obesity in Prader-Willi and Angelman syndrome.

In conclusion, this review will summarize current information on genome-wide dietary target genes, regulatory pathways affecting human homeostasis and diseases, and the role of immune response genes and particularly genes of innate immunity with an impact on lifespan.

Introduction

Longevity, i.e., the possibility of being long-lived, is limited by the ageing process. Life expectancy in the US increased from 49 years in 1900 to about 76 in 1998, with centenarians the fastest growing population segment. This increase was likely due to several factors, but perhaps the most important were the improvements in sanitation, hygiene, and public health from 1900 to 1998. However, other elements of modern life emerged as strong influences on lifespan, such as diet, exercise, and socioeconomic status. Age-related diseases affect a large proportion of older people including diabetes mellitus, obesity, cancer, cardiovascular diseases, osteoarthritis, osteoporosis, Alzheimer disease, etc. Obviously it is of great importance to understand factors that affect human longevity and ways to improve quality of life which motivate longevity research. Human longevity is at least partly heritable, and the progeroid syndromes of accelerated aging certainly have a genetic basis (1,2). A strong genetic component of longevity has become apparent from studies with a variety of organisms, from yeast to humans. Genetic screening efforts with invertebrates have unraveled multiple genetic pathways that suggest longevity is promoted through the manipulation of metabolism and resistance to oxidative stress. To some extent, these same mechanisms appear to act in mammals also, despite considerable divergence during evolution.

The genetic contribution to longevity is under an intensive investigation. Different studies contribute to answering the tantalizing question: "Whether genetics really does play a role in longevity?" Twin studies revealed the magnitude of the genetic influence on lifespan while centenarian studies lead scientists to longevity genes. Twin and family studies showed that somewhere between 15 and 30% of lifespan is controlled by our genes (3, 4). Gavrilova and Gavrilov (5) carried out a pilot search of prospective data resources related to familial occurrence of longevity using genealogical databases, published family history data, available scientific data resources, data sets on long-lived people and centenarians, concluding that millions of familial longevity records are available for research but so far underused. McGue et al. studied 2872 pairs of Danish twins born between 1870 and 1900, and found that lifespan is "only moderately heritable" (6, 7, 8). How long we live depends to a great extent on environmental and chance factors like random genetic alteration (epigenetics) that takes place during a lifetime. Studies on centenarians, on the other hand, suggest that they owe their good fortune to their inheritance of a small number of powerfully acting longevity genes. Such genes might for example allow centenarians to stave off the inflammation that exacerbates many of the diseases of old age. Furthermore the siblings of centenarians have a dramatically higher likelihood of becoming centenarians themselves, compared with the general population. The sisters and brothers of those over 100 were between 8 and 19 times more likely to reach that age than "the average person" born in the same area. These data suggest a strong role for heredity in making centenarians what they are (9).

In addition to survival data, genetic marker data are available for twins. How can these data be used in genetic studies for longevity? Genetic markers can be considered as observed covariates. The influence of these covariates on survival can be estimated by standard techniques that involve a Cox-type proportional hazards model and its extensions specified for univariate or multivariate survival analyses. The main advantage of the multivariate analysis is that it allows one to determine the location of longevity genes at the chromosome, even in the case of linkage equilibrium, because different methods for linkage analysis can be applied, such as regression models and maximization of likelihood (10,11).

What is the difference between genes increasing susceptibility or resistance to disease and those acting on aging? Current studies in humans are focusing on the growing number of centenarians among us. There is evidence for genetic differences between centenarians and the general population. The (sex-specific) association of longevity with alleles or haplotypes of several genes related to risk factors for a variety of diseases (cardiovascular diseases, cancer) including HLA alleles and haplotypes is not unexpected on the basis of studies on the genetics of longevity in centenarians. Further, evidence from population-based studies with humans suggests the importance of genes involved in cardiovascular disease as crucial determinants of longevity. This is in line with an earlier study showing that activity levels of a key enzyme which reacts to DNA damage within minutes of a stress correlate with mammalian species lifespan, longer-lived species having higher levels(15,16,17,18). Thus it appears, at least in this case, that the same genetic factor can contribute to differences in life span between and within species.

Why do humans live so long - if it is evolutionarily programmed, it must be genetics? There is a wealth of evidence that genes play a crucial role in the ageing process. The obvious fact that different species have different lifespan indicates that the genes are important factors affecting the ageing. Further, in different inbred animals held in identical environmental conditions lifespan differences were observed. The obtained results from recent studies on simple organisms like fruit flies and nematodes have revealed some gene mutations that significantly affect the lifespan. Furthermore, infectious diseases have been pervasive factors for longevity throughout evolution and have played a major role in the survival of human beings in the rigorous conditions under which we evolved. Longevity is associated with a positive or negative selection of alleles (or haplotypes) that respectively confer resistance or susceptibility to disease during different periods of the life span, via peptide presentation or via antigen non-specific control of immune responses. This association may be gender-related, but this is not unexpected on the basis of data available on the genetics of longevity, showing that on several occasions, the association of longevity with particular alleles has been found only in one gender, as in the case of tyrosine hydroxylase and of mitochondrial DNA. As a whole, these results might be interpreted under the perspective of a well known evolutionary theory of ageing, i.e antagonistic pleiotropy (12).

This theory predicts that the same gene (or allele or haplotype) can have different roles (positive or negative) in different period of the lifespan.

In this review we will summarize current information on genome-wide dietary target genes, regulatory pathways affecting human homeostasis and diseases, and the role of immune response genes and particularly genes of innate immunity with an impact on lifespan.

Longevity Genes, Age Related Physiological Changes in Metabolism

The genetic contribution of longevity is under an intense investigation. Different methodological approaches /study designs/ contribute to the answer of the following questions:

- Are there longevity genes in humans and are they similar to diverse species, making it possible to relate findings to human age-related physiological changes, in particular concerning metabolism, nutrition and diet related health risks?
- Which genes predispose to age related metabolic and endocrine diseases, and are there "resistance" genes; which, mechanisms and pathways shorten or increase lifespan?

Aging, Genetics and Metabolism Among Species

The rate of aging and lifespan vary greatly among species, and therefore must be under genetic control (13, 14). The Longevity Associated Gene (LAG)Initiative identified longevity genes across species finding similar mechanisms and pathways among them (Table 1). The Age-1 nematode gene is related to human PI3-kinase /glucose metabolism/, nematode daf-2 to human insulin-like receptor, daf16 to human HNF3 /transcription factor/, catalase and WRN genes are found in both species. Mutations in several genes have been found to markedly increase lifespan in nematode worms (C. elegans), fruit flies (Drosophila), and mice by slowing the aging process (15, 18). These genes functionally affect stress resistance and oxidative damage as mutations in daf-2 and age-1 increased resistance to reactive oxygen and heavy metals. Their human homologues are the genes for insulin and insulin-like growth factor-1 receptor /IGF-1 receptor/ and PI3K which codes for phosphatidylinositol-3 kinase participating in metabolism and endocrine system functioning. A relation between stress resistance and longevity has been observed in mammals. Analyses of cells from a variety of different species from hamsters to humans have shown good correlations between resistance to cytotoxic stress and maximal life span (19).There is enough data to believe that understanding these "longevity genes" will be useful in studying human aging and lifespan. These results support the idea that the evolution of long-lived species required metabolic pathways to resist and repair different forms of intracellular damage. These systems for conditional differentiation may then have been adopted for developmental control pathways by more advanced organisms, including the precursors of mammals. The genes and proteins involved in regulating stress resistance in humans have not been fully characterized. There is substantial interest in superoxide dismutases, which regulates the metabolism of reactive oxygen species. Although mutations in these genes have been associated with atherosclerosis, cardiovascular diseases, metabolic syndrome, type 2 diabetes, cancer, neurological diseases like amyotrophic lateral sclerosis (20), their effects on longevity are still under investigation. Another group of longevity genes related to metabolism and currently attracting great interest are those that mediate the effects of caloric restriction. There is enough data in mice, rats, fruit flies, worms, and yeast showing that one of the most effective environmental factors to increase lifespan is caloric restriction (21, 23). Caloric restriction appears to operate by slowing the aging process and the onset of diseases and disorders that are associated with advancing age, perhaps by reducing the lifelong production of harmful reactive oxygen metabolites (24,25)   Initial experimental results with monkeys suggest that the same phenomenon will also apply to non-human primates (26, 27) The effects of caloric restriction in humans remain to be determined. The responses to caloric restriction and other forms of cellular stress trigger mechanisms, including activation of the sirtuin pathways, that may protect cells. Sirtuins are deacetylases, enzymes that regulate (silence) gene expression. The beneficial effects of caloric restriction in yeast require an intact sirtuin pathway (28, 29) and overexpression of sir2 increases lifespan in C. Elegans (30). Resveratrol, a polyphenol compound found in red wine that activates sir2 in yeast, mimics the effects of caloric restriction. Yeast sir2 has a human homologue (SIRT1); the effects of mutations in SIRT1 and related genes on human lifespan are not known. However, SIRT1 may have adverse effects in human cells on p53, a tumor suppressor, because it functions as an NAD-dependent p53 deacetylase (31).

Table 1. Some longevity genes related to metabolism among species and their human analogues

Species	Human
Age-1 (nematode)	PI3-kinase (glucose metabolism)
daf-2 (nematode)	HNF3 (transcription factor)
catalase	catalase
WRN	WRN
sir2 (yeast)	SIRT1
IGF-1 receptor (mice)	IGF-1 receptor

Perhaps the best ontogenetically studied longevity and metabolic pathway includes genes that regulate signaling by insulin and insulin-like growth factor-1 (IGF-1)-like molecules (32) Reduced function of this pathway is associated with lifespan extension in several species (29) In C. elegans, for example, a reduction-in-function mutation in daf-2, the homologue of the mammalian insulin and IGF-1 receptors, doubles lifespan and slows tissue aging (33, 34, 35) Mutations in many of the downstream signaling elements in this pathway, including age-1, PDK1, daf-18, akt , and daf-16 also affect longevity. These same genes are also involved in the response to oxidative stress , including the upregulation of heat shock proteins, as well as tumor suppression (36, 37) apparently similarly in mammals. Mice with heterozygous deletions of the IGF-1 receptor have longer lifespans (38) and mice without an insulin receptor in adipose tissue live about 20% longer than controls (39) Thus, decreased insulin signaling in certain tissues may extend life. In humans, insulin resistance, which results in increased insulin signaling, leads to obesity, diabetes mellitus and shortened lifespan (40, 41, 42, 43). An association between a SNP in the IGF-1 receptor gene which was associated with lower circulating levels of IGF-1 and human longevity has been identified (44) Protein tyrosine phosphatase 1B (PTP1B) protein is a ubiquitously expressed phosphatase that dephosphorylates phosphotyrosine residues of the active insulin receptor, disrupting the insulin signaling pathway (45, 46) PTPIB-deficient mice show increased insulin sensitivity and resistance to diet-induced obesity (47,48) Both - function and genomic location are consistent with a role in type 2 diabetes, possibly mediated through a contribution to insulin resistance. Thus, PTPN1 represents a promising positional candidate gene for analysis in type 2 diabetes and associated phenotypes.

Mutations in two of the genes involved in the metabolism and repair of DNA, and in nuclear structure and function, cause clinical syndromes that have features suggestive of "accelerated aging" (49, 50, 51, 52, 53). Werner's syndrome is caused by several different mutations of the WRN gene (54) which encodes a protein belonging to the RecQ helicase family. The mutations result in a truncation of the normal WRN protein. It is not known how this shortening causes the clinical manifestations of the syndrome, which include lack of an adolescent growth spurt, alopecia or graying of hair, sclerotic skin, cataracts, type 2 diabetes, hypogonadism, atherosclerosis, osteoporosis, and certain forms of cancer (55, 56). The median age of death is the late 40s, primarily from myocardial infarction and cancer. Hutchinson-Gilford progeria is caused by a mutation of LMNA (57), a gene that codes for a group of proteins (lamins) that are part of the filamentous network located along the inner membrane of the nuclear envelope. These proteins are believed to affect nuclear morphology, chromatin structure, DNA synthesis, and gene expression. Patients with the syndrome typically exhibit growth retardation within the first few months of life and have accelerated degenerative changes in the cutaneous, musculoskeletal, and cardiovascular systems. The median age of death is 13.5 years, due to rapidly progressive atherosclerosis (58).

Aging, Genetics, Metabolism Among Humans

Research on longevity genes in humans is more complicated than in experimental animals, since scientists cannot experimentally control genes to test their effects on longevity. Therefore, genetic studies of human longevity require a more observational approach. Nowadays it is accepted that human longevity is a result of the combined effect of many genes and environmental factors, part of which are nutrition and eating disorders. Little is known about genes that control human longevity. Are there "good" genes which assure longevity and/or "bad' genes which shorten life span?

Recent advances in genomics enable genome-wide association studies (GWAS), an approach in which a substantial fraction of common genetic variation is tested for a role in determining phenotypic variation (59) These advances include a map of the correlation structure for approximately 4 million common genetic variants (minor allele frequency >5%) and whole-genome genotyping technologies capable of assaying 100,000–500,000 single nucleotide polymorphisms (SNPs) in an individual (60). Utilizing a fixed genotyping marker set such as the Affymetrix 100K GeneChip in an association study can test a substantial fraction of the genome in Caucasians, ~30–45% in some estimates (61) GWAS has been successfully applied to identify novel genetic loci related to several clinical phenotypes including age-related diseases. Heritability estimates for the lipid phenotypes in 1087 Framingham Heart Study Offspring cohort participants were obtained from extended families with at least two members by variance-components methods using the Sequential Oligogenic Linkage Analysis Routines (SOLAR) package (62, 63). Using a 100K genome-wide scan, they have generated a set of putative associations for common sequence variants and lipid phenotypes and heritabilities of MeanLDL-C, MeanHDL-C, and MeanTG. These were 0.66, 0.69, and 0.58, respectively, and the highest heritability estimate was that for lipoprotein (a) at 0.90. They failed to identify any novel loci related to blood lipids.Due to a lack of SNPs in the Affymetrix 100K GeneChip correlated with previously reported variants (at $r^2 > 0.5$ threshold) in the APOE, PCSK9, CETP, LIPC, and APOA5 genes, they were unable to confirm these other previously reported associations but using the Affymetrix 500 K array the glucokinase regulatory protein (GCKR) was identified as a novel locus associated with TG (64).

Type 2 diabetes, obesity and metabolic syndrome are heterogeneous diseases and genetic susceptibility plays a substantial role in their pathogenesis (65,66,67,68,69) but nutrition, quality of life, lack of physical activity and stress are important etiological factors too. Such genes have proven hard to detect using linkage-based approaches, although recent rapid advances in genetic association methodologies have led to some successes. The P12A polymorphism in the gene encoding the peroxisome proliferator-activated receptor-γ (PPARG) (66), the E23K polymorphism in the gene encoding the islet ATP-dependent potassium channel Kir6.2 (ABCC8-KCNJ11) (70,71,72) and common variants in the gene encoding the transcription factor 7-like 2 gene (TCF7L2) (73,74) were all found using well-powered association mapping, and all have been reproducibly associated with diabetes in diverse samples at highly significant p-values. Current gene discovery strategies have focused on coding regions, but regulatory variants also influence disease (75, 76) A comprehensive picture of diabetes genetics will require a wide and adequately dense search across coding and conserved non-coding genomic regions using an association analysis approach, where power is superior to linkage analysis when seeking common variants of modest effect (77). Resources are now becoming available to perform such genome-wide association studies of type 2 diabetes. The Framingham Heart Study (FHS) includes a genome-wide association study resource for type 2 diabetes, which is population-based (not diabetes proband-based), studies two generations, and has decades of longitudinal, standardized, detailed follow-up (78). They have used 100K SNPs in an *in silico* replication analysis that tests the hypothesis that SNPs in LD with published causal variants in PPARG, ABCC8, TCF7L2, CAPN10, and HNFa are associated with diabetes and related quantitative traits. The trial included 1,345 subjects of which 1,087 were offsprings. The three insulin traits are fasting insulin, homeostasis model-assessed insulin resistance (HOMA-IR), and Gutt's 0–120 min insulin sensitivity index (ISI_0-120). In addition to glucose and insulin traits, levels of adiponectin and resistin are available in the FHS dbGaP resource. About 0.3%–0.6% of SNPs in the 100K array with MAF > 10% are associated at p < 0.001 with six diabetes-related quantitative traits or with incident type 2 diabetes. A similar proportion of SNPs in the array (0.21%) is associated with multiple related diabetes traits. These several hundred SNPs likely contain more false positive than true positive associations with diabetes and related traits. However, they offer logical next targets for the follow-up replication studies in independent samples necessary to resolve true diabetes risk genes. The FHS 100K data replicate the otherwise widely-replicated TCF7L2 association with diabetes (79,80,81, 82,83,84,85,86,87,88). In an association analysis of genetic markers, Price et al. (89) identified three regions of type 2 diabetes susceptibility. Within one of these type 2 diabetes– associated regions is a positional candidate gene, PTPN1, chr 20q12–13.1, that codes for the protein tyrosine phosphatase 1B (PTP1B) protein. It dephosphorylates phosphotyrosine residues of the active insulin receptor, disrupting the insulin signaling pathway. To examine the association of PTPN1 variants with type 2 diabetes, Bento et al (90) performed a genetic analysis with 23 single nucleotide polymorphisms (SNPs) covering the 161-kb region encoding PTPN1 and the 5_ and 3_ genomic sequences. Evidence for association of these polymorphisms with type 2 diabetes was assessed in two independently ascertained case-control populations. The results show that PTPN1 polymorphisms and haplotypes are associated with Si, a measure of insulin sensitivity, and fasting glucose and is a significant contributor to diabetes. This is an interesting systematic approach in several populations, investigating both diabetes and metabolic traits.

Age-Related Lifespan-Shortening Metabolic Disease Genes

Most common age-related diseases which shorten lifespan are metabolic diseases which are increasing in frequency epidemically in most countries. This is demonstrated by the significant link between obesity, cardiovascular diseases, diabetes mellitus type 2 and certain cancers. A research team from the Division of Geriatrics and Nutritional Sciences of Washington University School of Medicine have identified five common genetic variations in CD36 gene, chr.7, that increase the risk of metabolic syndrome, highly associated with coronary heart disease and type 2 diabetes and a variant which appeared to be protective /91/.

In people, longevity-promoting genes might act by slowing the rate of age-related changes in cells, increase resistance to environmental stress-induced diseases, and reduce the risk of many age-related conditions. Several genetic pathways appear to be involved in the aging process and longevity, including genes involved in the progeroid syndromes, telomeres and telomerase, caloric restriction, stress resistance and oxidative damage, mitochondrial DNA, insulin signaling, and inflammation (92). It seems that at least part of them are involved in the pathogenesis of most common age-related diseases which are the result of or at least exacerbated by low grade chronic metabolic imbalances related to diet. Regulation of metabolism is under the control of many genes and disease predisposition or resistance is a result of the gene-gene interactions of allelic variants /gene polymorphisms/ whiles the gene-environment interactions are important for the etiology and prophylaxis of these diseases. Defining an adequate diet is a great challenge for nutrition research. While the more rare monogenic inborn errors of metabolism due to a mutation in a metabolic enzyme, regulatory proteins or transport mechanisms can be controlled nowadays by nutrient substitution, the monogenic human diseases which are models for accelerated aging and progeria cannot be. Some of them are inborn errors of metabolism: inherited traits like adrenoleicodystrophy /ALD gene, transporter protein expression/, Gaucher disease /metabolic glucocerebrosidase enzyme mutation/, glucose galactose malabsorpsion /SGLT1 gene in chromosome 22, defect in glucose and galactose intestinal transport/, Lesch-Nyhan syndrome / mutation in HPRT1 gene on X chromosome, accumulation of uric acid/, maple syrup urine disease /mutation in one of the six genes for branched- chain alpha-ketoacid dehydrogenase complex including three catalytic components and two regulatory enzymes for three essential for the diet aminoacids- valine, leucine and isoleucine/, phenylketonuria / autosomal recessive disease due to mutations phenylalanine hydroxylase gene on chromosome 12/, etc.

Some metabolic disorders are due to structural chromosome aberrations and genomic imprinting like the life-threatening obesity in Prader-Willi and Angelman syndrome /deletion in the paternally derived 15q11-13 in Prader- Willy syndrome or Angelman syndrome when the deletion is maternally derived/.

Genes Involved in Innate and Acquired Immunity

There is an emerging consensus that many aspects of senescence in humans are characterized by increase baseline inflammatory status, leading to extended tissue damage. Chronic inflammation, as manifested by high circulating levels of factors and cytokines like C-reactive protein, tumor necrosis factor, and interleukin-6, have been associated with several age-related diseases, including atherosclerosis, obesity, type 2 diabetes and cancer (93,94,95,96) The inflammatory response may be a prime example of antagonistic pleiotropy (97), in which genes that are required to increase the inflammatory response to infectious organisms in early life are also associated with harmful effects, such as atherosclerosis in the post-reproductive period. The extent to which these changes depend on the genetic background needs to be established. Family segregation analysis has shown that CD4, CD8 and e CD4/CD8 ratio are under genetic control (98, 99) . Longitudinal studies of the very elderly have documented an "immune risk profile", a cluster of immune parameters predicting 2-8 yr mortality, and characterized by a hallmark inverted CD4:8 ratio at baseline. (100) All these data imply that aging process may be associated with alterations in the immune system, suggesting that genetic determinants of senescence also reside in those polymorphisms for the immune system genes that regulate immune responses. Genes encoding molecules involved in the development of protective immunity are highly polymorphic, and present enormous variation probably resulting from an evolutionary adaptation of the organism facing an ever-evolving pathogen environment. These genes (Table 2), determining acquired and innate immunity, include: HLA genes; genes encoding "atypical" HLA-like molecules (CD1); killer cell immunoglobulin-like receptor genes (KIR); leukocyte Fcγ receptor genes; cytokine and cytokine receptor genes; Toll-like receptor gene family; TNF-receptor associated factors, MBL2. Several studies have focused on the role of HLA and cytokine gene polymorphisms in human longevity. The diversity of these genes might influence successful aging and longevity by modulating an individual's response to life-threatening disorders.

Table 2. Genes of innate and acquired immunity, associated with aging

Acquired immunity genes	
HLA alleles	Effect
DRB1*11, DRB1*07 DRB1*13	Increased in elderly
DRB1*15 DRB1*0101, *1201,*1401	
DQB1*0503; DQA1*0101,*05	
DRB*0403, *1302	Decreased in centenarians
Cytokine genes	
IL-2 (-330 T/C)	Increased (T-low) marginally increased in centenarians
IL-6 (-174 C/G)	Controversial effect: Increased (C-low) in Italian male centenarians; Decreased (G/G-high) in Irish octogenarians and nonagenarians; Increased G allele in Finish elderly survivors; no association
IFN-G (+874 T/A)	Increased (T/T-high) in female Italian centenarians
TNF-A (-308 G/A)	Controversial: Decreased (A-high) in Danish centenarians; no association
IL-10 (-1082G/A,-819C/T,-592C/A)	Increased (-1082G,-819C,-592C) in elderly
Innate Immunity Genes	
TLR 4 (+896A/G)	Associated with age-related diseases. Higher frequency of G allele in centenarians
COX (-765G/C), LOX (-1708G/A)	Associated with age-related diseases. Lower frequency of pro-inflammatory alleles in centenarians
CCR5Delta32	Associated with age-related diseases - atherosclerosis and Alzheimer's disease.
NK Receptor Genes	Controversial data
MBL-2 (cdn 52 (C/T; cdn 54 (G/A; cdn (57 G/A; -619 C/G; -290 G/C; -66 C/T)	Deficient haplotypes are associated with infections

HLA and Longevity

Due to the central role of HLA molecules in the development of protective immunity and significant polymorphism of HLA genes, many studies have addressed the possible impact of these genes on human longevity. Most of the data available so far demonstrated a possible role of HLA class II specificities in human longevity but definitive evidence has remained elusive. In several populations, the DR11 specificity was found to be positively associated with longevity (101, 102, 103). Additionally, in centenarians from the French population, a positive association was found with DR7 and DR13 (103). These specificities have been previously shown to be associated with different diseases: a protective role for infectious diseases (DR13, DR11) or autoimmune diseases (DR11). Additionally centenarians from Sardinia were characterized with increased frequency of HLA-DRB1*15. An increased frequency of several HLA class II alleles: DRB1*0101, 1201, *1401, DQB1*0503, DQA1*0101, *05 was found in Japanese centenarians (107) Studies addressing other genes within the HLA complex are quite limited, and the available data were obtained using serological techniques, which are earlier, pre-molecular and less accurate techniques. In elderly Italians, increased frequencies of B7 and Cw6 were found (105). Association of the HLA-B locus with longevity was also found for Greeks (increased B16 and decreased B15 in elderly) (106), and in elderly Dutch women (decreased B40) (102). These heterogeneous results in different populations suggest that HLA/longevity associations are population-specific, and are likely affected by the population-specific genetic and environmental factors, and hence are difficult to interpret. The MHC-restriction of T cell responses against pathogens confers a positive benefit of HLA heterozygosity. Several investigations demonstrate a positive association of HLA heterozygosity with longevity, but in other studies a similar association was not found (103, 110).

A comparatively small number of investigations have explored possible associations of HLA haplotypes rather than single alleles with longevity, although there is a markedly greater impact of haplotype analysis compared to individual alleles in the genetic predisposition of the HLA-associated diseases. Rea and Middleton (108) found an increased frequency of the serologically-defined haplotype A1-B8-C7-DR3 in centenarian males. However, this observation was not confirmed by later studies (109) Further, other studies found a decreased frequency of the HLA-B8-DR3 haplotype in centenarian females. The possible mechanisms responsible for the different associations of the indicated haplotype in centenarians of both sexes are not clarified yet although it is likely to be related to the influence of the haplotype on immune reactivity. Individuals possessing this haplotype are predominantly characterized by type 2 immune responses. It could be speculated that the HLA-B8-DR3 haplotype is related to a shift of the immune response from type 1 to type 2, which is one of the hallmarks of immune alterations in senescence. A study in the Bulgarian population showed significantly increased frequencies of DRB1*11 and DRB*16 – related haplotypes: A*0101-B*5101-DRB1*1101 and A*0201-B*1801-DRB1*1601 in elderly individuals compared to young controls. It is interesting to note that DRB1*11 and DRB1*16-related haplotypes were found to be protective for different autoimmune diseases in the Bulgarian population.

Cytokine Genes and Longevity

Although the data are limited and controversial, it has been hypothesized that longevity could be associated with cytokine gene polymorphism correlating with different levels of cytokine expression and thereby modulating immune responses in disease (111, 112).

Because of the essential role of cytokines in immune responses, the regulation of cytokine gene expression and their polymorphic nature, the genetic variations of these loci with functional significance could be appropriate immunogenetic candidate markers implicated in the mechanism of successful aging and longevity.

Pro-Inflammatory Cytokine Genes

Genetic variations correlating with elevated levels of pro-inflammatory cytokines have been negatively associated with ageing (113). Several studies showed that cytokine polymorphisms related to different levels of secretion were associated with longevity. Age-related decline in IL-2 production has been observed (114) and studies showed that this reduction in aged subjects is associated with effects on intracellular activation of nuclear transcription pathways (115, 116). Recent studies in Italian (117) and Irish (118) elderly people did not show a statistically significant association of the IL-2 -330 polymorphism with longevity. However, a T allele associated with an IL-2 low-producer genotype was suggested to be marginally associated with longevity, such that a genetic background favoring increased IL-2 production might be detrimental for longevity. Despite the large number of studies on the possible role of IL-6 gene polymorphisms in different diseases, associations still remain controversial (119, 120, 121, 122). It has been hypothesized that the capacity to produce low levels of IL-6 appears to beneficial for longevity (123, 124, 125, 126). Most studies focused on the IL-6 -174 C/G polymorphism and susceptibility to common causes of morbidity and mortality among the elderly, such as type 2 diabetes, cardiovascular diseases, and dementia. The IL-6-174 C/G polymorphism is reported to be predictive for longevity (127). Data on centenarians and elderly individuals from Italy showed an increased frequency of C alleles, associated with low IL-6 expression in male centenarians which seemed to be gender-specific (128). It has also been shown that the proportion of IL-6 high producers (GG genotypes) is increased in individuals affected by age-related diseases with inflammatory pathogenesis – diabetes, atherosclerosis, osteoporosis, and neurodegenerative diseases. Similar negative associations of IL-6 -174 GG with longevity have been observed in the Irish population (118, 115). However data in other populations such as the Finnish (128), Bulgarian (130) and Sardinian showed that IL-6 polymorphism does not affect life expectancy, suggesting that the effect of this polymorphism on longevity might be population-specific and dependent on gene – environment interactions (131, 132).

Data on IFN-γ functional gene polymorphisms and aging are also controversial. While studies in Italian centenarians showed an increased frequency of +874 T/T in female centenarians, investigations among Bulgarian elderly did not show significant differences in IFN-γ (+874) allele distribution compared to young controls 133). Although the polymorphism TNF-A -308 G/A associated with different gene expression is one of the most widely investigated in different diseases, no correlation of this SNP and longevity was found in centenarians in several studies in the Finnish and Italian populations (129, 133) or in elderly Bulgarians (130). However, other studies showed a decreased frequency of the A allele, associated with high production, among centenarians. Additionally it has beeen reported that an anti-inflammatory genotype TNFA GG (low)/ IL-10 GG (high) has a positive role in longevity. It might be due to the fact that TNF-A and IL-10 have complex and opposing roles, and an autoregulatory loop appears to exist (134).

Anti-Inflammatory Cytokine Genes

Considering the important role of IL-10 in limiting inflammatory responses (135), many studies focused on the relevance of polymorphisms in the regulatory region of this gene and their associations with longevity. The IL-10 -1082 A/G polymorphism has been reported to be a male-specific marker for longevity (139). The -1082GG genotype, associated with high IL-10 production, was argued to confer an anti-inflammatory status (136). Studies in Bulgarians demonstrated significant differences for two IL-10 haplotypes: one of them (-1082A,-819T,-592A), possibly associated with low level expression was decreased in the elderly, while the other (-1082G,-819C,-592C) associated with high levels of cytokine gene expression, was significantly more frequent among healthy elderly compared to young controls. This effect was more pronounced in GCC-homozygous individuals as indicated by the analysis of IL-10 genotypes. However, studies in two other populations – Irish nonagenarians (118) and Finnish nonagenarians (129) did not show any association with longevity. A possible explanation for the negative results in the Irish and Finnish studies could be the younger age of the old subjects investigated in comparison with the Italian study. Interestingly, the IL-10 -1082 GG genotype is much less frequent in patients affected by Alzheimer's disease (133). Data on the gene polymorphisms in TGF-B1 are more limited. Analysis of these three SNPs +915 G→C, -509 C→T and -800 G→A showed that the +915 C allele and GC genotype are present at significantly lower frequencies in the elderly. Additionally, decreased frequency of the extended haplotype G -800/C -509/C 869/C 915 and elevated levels of TGF-β1 were observed in elderly people, but no correlation with investigated genotypes in the TGF-B1 gene was found (137). Similarly, no associations of TGF-B1 codons 10 and 25 genotypes with longevity were observed in Bulgarians (130). It has been hypothesized that genetically determined cytokine profiles of TGF-β1 could be involved in mechanisms leading to successful ageing, but more data are needed to confirm these results.

Nonetheless, in general, data on functional cytokine gene polymorphisms are concordant with the hypothesis that longevity is related to anti-inflammatory genotype profiles. Additionally, the pro-inflammatory cytokine profile was correlated with decreased human life span. However, in elderly with different ethnic backgrounds, investigations provide contradictory results on associations with cytokine gene polymorphism. The majority of data were derived from investigations of single polymorphisms in single cytokine genes. The analysis of extended haplotypes which include several polymorphisms in the cytokine genes, as well as haplotypes which consist of SNPs in different cytokine genes, will be required in order to determine the precise immunogenetic basis of longevity. Epigenetic studies on cytokine and chemokine gene expression in elderly people with different immunogenetic profiles will further contribute to better understanding the aging process.

Innate Immunity Genes and Aging

Several genes such as Toll-like receptor genes, Cycloxygenases (COX)/Lipoxygenases (LOX), CCR5, NK receptor genes, MBL2 have been assessed as a possible biomarkers associated with aging.

Toll Like Receptors

TLRs recognize pathogen-associated molecular patterns and have an important role as a component of the innate immune system. One of the members of this family, TLR4, recognizes lipopolysaccharide of Gram-negative bacteria, and initiates innate immunity by activating inflammatory cells via the NF-kB pathway via inducing the expression of a variety of cytokines and other molecules (138, 139). TLR4 expression is involved in human atherosclerotic lesions and the production of inflammatory mediators that stimulate expression of adhesion molecules on endothelial cells, proliferation of smooth muscle cells, activation of immune cells, stimulation of the acute phase responses and matrix break down. A SNP, +896A/G (ASP299GLY), has been found in the TLR4 gene. The +896G allele has been shown to attenuate receptor signalling and to represent a minor risk for developing carotid atherosclerosis. Furthermore, people with this mutant genotype (+896G) have been claimed to display lower levels of some pro-inflammatory cytokines, acute phase reactants and soluble adhesion molecules. Studies of Caruso et al. showed that the +896G TLR4 polymorphism is present at a significantly lower frequency in patients affected by AMI with respect to controls, whereas centenarians have a higher frequency (140). Additionally, TLR4 +896G carriers were shown to produce lower levels of IL-6 andTNF-α and higher levels of IL-10 and therefore to have a lower proinflammatory status.

Cycloxygenases (COX)/Lipoxygenases (LOX)

COX-1 and COX-2 are the key enzymes in the conversion of arachidonic acid to the precursors of the bioactive lipid mediators, prostaglandin, thromboxane and prostacyclin. COXs play a key role in pathophysiological processes of inflammatory diseases and are the main targets for non-steroidal anti-inflammatory drugs. COX-2 is largely expressed in macrophages that infiltrate atherosclerotic plaques. LOX are enzymes that catalyse the stereospecific insertion of molecular oxygen into various positions in arachidonic acid. 5-LOX is the initial key enzyme of the leukotriene pathway. LOX can be induced by pro-inflammatory cytokines and its expression in endothelial cells is relatively low in the basal condition, but can be induced by proinflammatory cytokines. Recent studies have shown that -765GC and -1708GA SNPs in the promoter region of the COX-2 gene and 5-LOX genes, are associated with a significantly lower promoter activity and reduced risk of severe atherosclerosis (141, 142). Additionally, plasma levels of the acute phase protein C-reactive protein are significantly influenced by -765G/C genotype (143). In the Italian population, the frequencies of these proinflammatory alleles were significantly lower in centenarians.

CCR5

The CC chemokine receptor 5 (CCR5) is a member of the CC-chemokine receptor family. CCR5 regulates trafficking and effector functions of memory/effector Th1 cells, macrophages, NK cells, and immature dendritic cells. CCR5 and its ligands are important molecules in viral pathogenesis. Recent evidence has also demonstrated a role for CCR5 in a variety of human diseases, ranging from infectious and inflammatory diseases to cancer. The CCR5Delta32 deletion has been associated with two age-related diseases - atherosclerosis and Alzheimer's disease (144).

NK Receptor Genes

Natural killer (NK) cells play a pivotal role in the innate immune response. During the ageing process, variations occur in NK cell number and function. NK cells mediate their immune function through the recognition and lysis of abnormal cells that either lack the expression, or express inadequate amounts, of HLAclass I molecules (145). The ability of NK cells to discriminate between normal and HLA class I-deficient cells is due to the expression of HLA class I-specific inhibitory receptors (146). Subsequent NK cell-mediated lysis of HLA class I-deficient cells arises from the expression of HLA class I-specific activating receptors by NK cell clonal populations (147). NK cells express two structurally distinct classes of receptor: the C-type lectin-like heterodimeric receptors (148) and receptors belonging to the immunoglobulin superfamily (Ig-SF) (149, 150). Whilst members of the CD94/NKG2 lectin-like receptor family are encoded by a relatively conserved set of genes, many of the NK cell receptors belonging to the Ig-SF display considerable genetic variation, in particular, the killer cell immunoglobulin-like receptors (KIRs). KIR genes are highly polymorphic and this polymorphism has been studied extensively in different populations. Many studies documented a role for KIR gene polymorphism in different diseases, such as infectious diseases, cancer and autoimmunity. Studies in the Irish population (151) did not show significant association of KIR with longevity. However, before applying Bonferroni`s correction, a significant association was observed for the KIR2DS3 and KIR2DL5 genes in the healthy elderly, suggesting that these KIR genes may play a role in successful ageing. To highlight possible gender-specific markers of longevity, KIR genotype and gene frequencies were analysed with respect to gender. KIR2DS2 and KIR2DL2 genes displayed an increased prevalence in aged females relative to young female controls. This suggests that certain combinations of KIR genes may exert subtle gender-dependent effects during the ageing process. Studies in the Bulgarian population also showed that the decreased frequency of the activatory KIR2DS5 and A1B10 haplotypes were associated with a higher CMV antibody level among elderly individuals (unpublished data). However, considering the limited data at present, further investigations are required in order to evaluate the role of KIR and KIR/ligand gene systems in healthy aging, longevity and age associated diseases.

MBL-2

Mannose-binding lectin is a serum protein, a member of the collectin family (152). The protein in the plasma forms a multimeric complex that recognizes mannose- and N-acetylglucosamine-rich oligosaccharides, expressed with high-density in a wide range of bacteria, viruses, fungi and parasites. Upon binding, MBL interacts with mannose-associated serine proteases (MASAP-1,-2) and activates the complement system, leading to opsonization, phagocytosis or direct killing (153, 154). The MBL2 gene, located on chromosome 10 at q11.2-q21, consists of 4 exons and has been shown to be highly polymorphic (155). MBL serum levels are highly variable and are genetically determined. Three independent SNPs: cdn 52 (C/T; Arg/Cys, allele D); cdn 54 (G/A; Gly>Asp, allele B); cdn (57 G/A; Gly>Glu, allele C) disrupt the collagenous structure of the protein and dramatically reduce serum MBL concentrations (156). Any of these mutations (B,C, or D) is referred to as O, while the wild type is referred to as A. In addition to exon 1 SNPs, three regulatory variants in the promoter and in the 5`UTR regions at positions: -619 (C/G, allele L/H), -290 (G/C; allele Y/X) and -66 (C/T; allele P/Q) also influence final serum MBL concentration. Combinations of these 6 SNPs result in widespread haplotypes, determining different serum MBL levels (157, 187) deficiency (haplotypes LYPB, LYQC, HYPD); low level (haplotype LXPA); intermediate level (haplotype LYPA) and high level (haplotypes HYPA and LYQA).

MBL allele and haplotype distribution is quite diverse in different populations and MBL deficiency is one of the most common immune deficiencies, the clinical consequences of which have been extensively studied over the last few years. Although many individuals with low MBL levels are asymptotic, clinical symptoms become apparent in the presence of additional immune defects. Genetically-determined MBL deficiency has been associated with an increase susceptibility to many infections in the case of compromised adaptive immunity – early childhood (159), inherited and acquired immune deficiencies (160), following chemotherapy (161), or following HSCT (162). Furthermore, MBL insufficiency is thought to influence some autoimmune diseases, like SLE (163) and rheumatoid arthritis (164). Preliminary studies in the Bulgarian elderly individuals showed that MBL2-deficient haplotypes are associated with a higher level of CMV antibodies and therefore MBL2 might be another candidate biomarker to be studied in relation to aging (unpublished data).

Diagnostics, Nutrition and Diets

Obviously, nutrition plays an important role in metabolic disease prevention because usually it is in the etiology of the diseases except the monogenic forms. Metabolic balance is influenced by the presence and proportion of essential nutrients and abundance of nonessential components in the diet. To support these approaches new strategies are emerging from genomics and technologies of gene expression to evaluate the efficacy and the safety of specific diets designed to chronically influence metabolism, prevent and reverse metabolic imbalances (165). A problem in assessment is the lack of adequate diagnostics of long-term chronic metabolic imbalance, as biomarkers of damage are not necessarily present until the disease is well established and it may not be possible to reverse chronic diseases by simply restoring normal metabolic balance. The main goal of prevention, including by diet, is to restore optimal metabolism before damage has occurred. Clearly, we need to be able to detect the metabolic imbalance itself by metabolic assessment in any pathways that could lead to disease. Except the rare monogenic inborn errors of metabolism, most common metabolic diseases present with complex traits and single biomarkers are of low diagnostic and prognostic value. A classic example is the chronic imbalance of endogenous cholesterol metabolism participating in the pathogenesis of atherosclerosis. The routine measurement of total cholesterol over decades and its correlation with atherosclerosis and age-related cardiovascular diseases (166) is a good lesson and provides a rationale for new strategies. The U.S. implemented this strategy as public policy by establishing a very ambitious countrywide project, the National Cholesterol Education Program. Reducing cholesterol became a public goal. A number of different population-based studies demonstrated that the relative risk for cardiovascular damage predicted by single biomarkers like total cholesterol, lipoprotein A, homocystein etc. is much lower than the complex prognostic value of high sensitive C-reactive protein values combined with the ratio of total cholesterol to HDL-cholesterol, for example (167). Key elements of these new strategies are to define biomarkers from quantitative metabolite profiles, to use them for population recommendations as well as for individual diets and to prevent disease. It became important to reexamine the definition of toxicity in the context of nutrients i.e. associated not simply with acutely damaging molecules, but with molecules and foods that perturb metabolic regulation. As the changes in metabolic biomarkers caused by foods are small and the metabolic alterations cannot be detected by a single biomarker, modern diagnostics must turn to the complex strategy of applying genomics and biochemistry. Also, the dose-effect relationships and their detection are very important because essential nutrients are by definition necessary up to certain levels; otherwise metabolism is altered in a net destructive direction.

Conclusion

Great advances in our knowledge of the genes involved in ageing are promised by the human genome project and similar projects in other species. The challenge is to test if the candidate longevity genes that have emerged from studies with model organisms exhibit genetic variation for life span in human populations. Future investigations are likely to involve large-scale case-control studies, in which large numbers of genes, corresponding to entire gene functional modules, will be assessed for all possible sequence variation and associated with detailed phenotypic information on each individual over extended periods of time. In addition to information about gene sequences, large amounts of data will emerge from techniques that can compare patterns of the activity of genes in old versus young tissues or those with and without age-related diseases. This should eventually unravel the genetic factors that contribute to each particular aging phenotype. But this avalanche of data will require careful interpretation. A major challenge in evaluating the large numbers of genes that are likely to be picked up by these techniques will be to distinguish which of the many differences are involved in the ageing process, and which are a consequence of it.

References

[1]   Martin GM, Oshima J, Gray MD, and Poot M. What geriatricians should know about the Werner syndrome. *J Am Geriatr Soc.* 1999;47:1136-44.

[2]   Fossel M. Human aging and progeria. *J Pediatr Endocrinol Metab.* 2000;13 Suppl 6:1477-81.

[3]   Herskind AM, McGue M, Holm NV, Sørensen TI, Harvald B, and Vaupel JW. The heritability of human longevity: a population-based study of 2872 Danish twin pairs born 1870-1900. *Human Genetics,* 1996;97:319-23.

[4]   Mitchell BD, Hsueh WC, King TM, et al. Heritability of life span in the Old Order Amish. *Am J Med Genet.* 2001;102:346-52.

[5]   N.Gavrilova, and L. Gavrilov, Data resources for biodemographic studies in familial clustering of human longevity, *Demographic research,* 1999,1, 4, 1-48).

[6]   McGue M, Vaupel JW, Holm N, and Harvald B. Longevity is moderately heritable in a sample of Danish twins born 1870̄1880. *J Gerontol.* 1993; 48: B237-B244.

[7]   Herskind AM, McGue M, Holm NV, Sorensen TI, Harvald B, and Vaupel JW. The heritability of human longevity: a population-based study of 2872 Danish twin pairs born 1870̄1900. *Hum Genet.* 1996; 97: 319-323.

[8]   Yashin AI, and Iachine IA. Genetic analysis of durations, Correlated frailty model applied to survival Danish Twins. *Genet Epidemiol.* 1995; 12: 529-538.

[9]   Perls TT, Wilmoth J, Levenson R, et al. Life-long sustained mortality advantage of siblings of centenarians. *Proc Natl Acad Sci U S A,* 2002;99:8442-7.

[10]   Haseman, J. K., and Elston, R. C. (). The investigation of linkage between a quantitative trait and a marker locus. *Behavior Genetics,*1972; 2, 3–19.

[11]   Kruglyak, L., Dali, M. J., Reeve-Daly, M. P., and Lander, E., S. (1996). Parametric and nonparametric linkage analysis: A unified multipoint approach. *American Journal of Human Genetics,* 1996; 58, 1347–1363.

[12]   Kirkwood TB, and Rose MR. Evolution of senescence: late survival sacrificed for reproduction. *Philos Trans R Soc Lond B Biol Sci.* 1991 332:15-24.

[13]   Hekimi S, and Guarente L. Genetics and the specificity of the aging process. *Science,* 2003;299:1351-4.

[14]   Miller RA. Extending life: scientific prospects and political obstacles. Milbank Q 2002;80:155-74.

[15]   Lin K, Dorman JB, Rodan A, and Kenyon C. daf-16: An HNF-3/forkhead family member that can function to double the life-span of Caenorhabditis elegans *Science,* 1997;278:1319-22.

[16]   Arantes-Oliveira N, Berman JR, and Kenyon C. Healthy animals with extreme longevity. *Science,* 2003;302:611.

[17]   Bartke A, Chandrashekar V, Dominici F, et al. Insulin-like growth factor 1 (IGF-1) and aging: controversies and new insights. *Biogerontology,* 2003;4:1-8.

[18]   Hsu AL, Murphy CT, Kenyon C. Regulation of aging and age-related disease by DAF-16 and heat-shock factor. *Science,* 2003;300:1142-5.

[19]   Kapahi P, Boulton ME, and Kirkwood TB. Positive correlation between mammalian life span and cellular resistance to stress. *Free Radic Biol Med.* 1999;26:495-500.

[20]   Williamson TL, Corson LB, Huang L, et al. Toxicity of ALS-linked SOD1 mutants. *Science,* 2000;288:399.

[21]   Masoro EJ. Caloric restriction and aging: an update. *Exp Gerontol.* 2000;35:299-305.

[22] Sohal RS, and Weindruch R. Oxidative stress, caloric restriction, and aging. *Science,* 1996;273:59-63.

[23] Mair W, Goymer P, Pletcher SD, and Partridge L. Demography of dietary restriction and death in Drosophila. *Science,* 2003;301:1731-3.

[24] Fornieri C, Taparelli F, Quaglino D, Jr., et al. The effect of caloric restriction on the aortic tissue of aging rats. *Connect Tissue Res.* 1999;40:131-43.

[25] Turturro A, Blank K, Murasko D, and Hart R. Mechanisms of caloric restriction affecting aging and disease. *Ann N Y Acad Sci.* 1994;719:159-70.

[26] Roth GS, Ingram DK and Lane MA. Caloric restriction in primates and relevance to humans. *Ann N Y Acad Sci.* 2001;928:305-15.

[27] Howitz KT, Bitterman KJ, Cohen HY, et al. Small molecule activators of sirtuins extend Saccharomyces cerevisiae lifespan. *Nature,* 2003;425:191-6.

[28] Anderson RM, Latorre-Esteves M, Neves AR, et al. Yeast life-span extension by calorie restriction is independent of NAD fluctuation. *Science,* 2003;302:2124-6.

[29] Tissenbaum HA and Guarente L. Increased dosage of a sir-2 gene extends lifespan in Caenorhabditis elegans. *Nature,* 2001;410:227-30

[30] Vaziri H, Dessain SK, Ng Eaton E, et al. hSIR2(SIRT1) functions as an NAD-dependent p53 deacetylase. *Cell,* 2001;107:149-59.

[31] Tatar M, Bartke A, and Antebi A. The endocrine regulation of aging by insulin-like signals. *Science,* 2003;299:1346-51.

[32] Longo VD, and Fabrizio P. Regulation of longevity and stress resistance: a molecular strategy conserved from yeast to humans? *Cell Mol Life Sci.* 2002;59:903-8.

[33] Kenyon C, Chang J, Gensch E, Rudner A, and Tabtiang R. A C. elegans mutant that lives twice as long as wild type *Nature,* 1993;366:461-4.

[34] Kimura KD, Tissenbaum HA, Liu Y, and Ruvkun G. daf-2, an insulin receptor-like gene that regulates longevity and diapause in Caenorhabditis elegans *Science,* 1997;277:942-6.

[35] Garigan D, Hsu AL, Fraser AG, Kamath RS, Ahringer J, and Kenyon C. Genetic analysis of tissue aging in Caenorhabditis elegans: a role for heat-shock factor and bacterial proliferation. *Genetics,* 2002;161:1101-12.

[36] Walker GA, and Lithgow GJ. Lifespan extension in C. elegans by a molecular chaperone dependent upon insulin-like signals. *Aging Cell,* 2003;2:131-9.

[37] Tatar M, Kopelman A, Epstein D, Tu MP, Yin CM, and Garofalo RS. A mutant Drosophila insulin receptor homolog that extends life-span and impairs neuroendocrine function. *Science,* 2001;292:107-10.

[38] Holzenberger M, Dupont J, Ducos B, et al. IGF-1 receptor regulates lifespan and resistance to oxidative stress in mice. *Nature,* 2003;421:182-7.

[39] Bluher M, Kahn BB and Kahn CR. Extended longevity in mice lacking the insulin receptor in adipose tissue. *Science,* 2003;299:572-4.

[40] Atanasova I, N Aslanova, P Gencova, D Koev, G Iankova,S Levi and A Mihailova. Age associated changes in glucocorticoid receptor regulation in healthy people, endokrinnie mehanismi starenia I vozrastnoi patologii /Russ/, 1988, 10,50-55.

[41] Vizev K., I. Atanasova and N.Aslanova. Age related changes in glucocorticoid hormone receptor binding parameters and plasma cortisol levels in macrobiots, *Revue de la societe anthropologique de Yugoslavie*, 36, 2001,131-136.

[42] Orbezova M, I Atanasova, B Milcheva, R Shigarminova, N Aslanova, and S Zacharieva. Adipose tissue hormones in females with different morphotype obesity, Endocrinologia /Bulg/, 2004, 9 (4), 214-224.

[43] Orbezova M, I Atanasova, B Milcheva, R Shigarminova, N Aslanova, V Todorov, and S Zacharieva. Carbohydrate and lipid abnormalities in females with different morphotype obesity , Endocrine diseases /Bulg/, 2005, 4, 123-30.

[44] Bonafe M, Barbieri M, Marchegiani F, et al. Polymorphic variants of insulin-like growth factor I (IGF-I) receptor and phosphoinositide 3-kinase genes affect IGF-I plasma levels and human longevity: cues for an evolutionarily conserved mechanism of life span control. *J Clin Endocrinol Metab.* 2003;88:3299-304.

[45] Goldstein BJ, Bittner-Kowalczyk A, White MF, and Harbeck M. Tyrosine dephosphorylation and deactivation of insulin receptor substrat-1 by protein-tyrosine phosphatase 1B. *J Biol Chem.* 275:4283– 4289, 2000.

[46] Seely BL, Staubs PA, Reichart DR, Bernhanu P, Milarski KL, Saltiel AR, Kusari J, and Olefsky JM. Proteine tyrosine phosphatase 1B interacts with the activated insulin receptor. *Diabetes*, 45:1379 –1385, 1996.

[47] Elchebly M, Payette P, Michaliszyn E, Cromlish W, Collins S, Loy AL,Normandin D, Cheng A, Himms-Hagen J, Chang CC, Ramachandran C,Gresser MJ, Tremblay ML, and Kennedy BP. Increased insulin sensitivity and obesity resistance in mice lacking the protein tyrosine phopsphatase-1B gene. *Science*, 283:1544 –1548, 1999.

[48] Klaman LD, Boss O, Peroni OD, Kim JK, Martin JL, Zabolotny JN, Moghal ,N, Lubkin M, Kim YB, Sharpe AH, Stricker-Krongrad A, Shulman GI, Neel BG, and Kahn BB. Increased energy expenditure decreased adiposity and tissue-specific insulin sensitivity in protein tyrosine phosphatase 1Bdeficient mice. *Mol Cell Biol.* 20:5479 – 5489, 2000.

[49] Gray MD, Shen JC, Kamath-Loeb AS, et al. The Werner syndrome protein is a DNA helicase. *Nat Genet.* 1997;17:100-3.

[50] Huang S, Li B, Gray MD, Oshima J, Mian IS, and Campisi J. The premature ageing syndrome protein, WRN, is a 3'-->5' exonuclease. *Nat Genet.* 1998;20:114-6.

[51] Schulz VP, Zakian VA, Ogburn CE, et al. Accelerated loss of telomeric repeats may not explain accelerated replicative decline of Werner syndrome cells. *Hum Genet.* 1996;97:750-4.

[52] Oshima J, Campisi J, Tannock TC, and Martin GM. Regulation of c-fos expression in senescing Werner syndrome fibroblasts differs from that observed in senescing fibroblasts from normal donors. J Cell Physiol 1995;162:277-83

[53] Yu CE, Oshima J, Fu YH, et al. Positional cloning of the Werner's syndrome gene. *Science* 1996;272:258-62.

[54] Epstein CJ, Martin, G.M., Schultz, A.L., and Motulsky, A.G. Werner's syndrome: a review of its symptomatology, natural history, pathologic features, genetics and relationships to the natural aging process. *Medicine*, 1966;45:172-221.

[55] Goto M. Hierarchical deterioration of body systems in Werner's syndrome: implications for normal ageing. *Mech Ageing Dev.* 1997;98:239-54.

[56] Eriksson M, Brown WT, Gordon LB, et al. Recurrent de novo point mutations in lamin A cause Hutchinson-Gilford progeria syndrome. *Nature,* 2003;423:293-8.

[57] Brown WT. Hutchinson-Gilford progeria syndrome. In: Hisama F, Weissman SM, Martin GM, editors. Chromosomal instability and aging. Basinc science and clinical implications. New York: Marcel Dekker, Inc.; 2003. p. 245-262.

[58] Hirschhorn JN and Daly MJ. Genome-wide association studies for common diseases and complex traits. *Nature reviews,* 2005;6:95–108.

[59] International HapMap Consortium, A haplotype map of the human genome. *Nature,* 2005;437:1299–1320.

[60] Pe'er I, de Bakker PI, Maller J, Yelensky R, Altshuler D, and Daly MJ. Evaluating and improving power in whole-genome association studies using fixed marker sets. *Nature genetics,* 2006;38:663–667.

[61] Almasy L and Blangero J. Multipoint quantitative-trait linkage analysis in general pedigrees. *American journal of human genetics,* 1998;62:1198–1211.

[62] Kathiresan S, A K Manning, S Demissie, R B D'Agostino, A Surti, C Guiducci, L Gianniny, N P Burtt, O Melander, M Orho-Melander, D K Arnett, G M Peloso,[4] Jose M Ordovas, L A and Cupples, A genome-wide association study for blood lipid phenotypes in the Framingham Heart Study, *BMC Med Genet.* 2007; 8(Suppl 1).

[63] Saxena R, Voight BF, Lyssenko V, Burtt NP, de Bakker PI, Chen H, Roix JJ, Kathiresan S, Hirschhorn JN, Daly MJ, et al. Genome-wide association analysis identifies loci for type 2 diabetes and triglyceride levels. *Science* (New York, NY). 2007;316:1331–1336.

[64] Poulsen P, Kyvik KO, Vaag A, and Beck-Nielsen H. Heritability of type II (non-insulin-dependent) diabetes mellitus and abnormal glucose tolerance – a population-based twin study. *Diabetologia,* 1999;42:139–145.

[65] Meigs JB, Cupples LA and Wilson PWF. Parental transmission of type 2 diabetes mellitus: the Framingham Offspring Study. *Diabetes,* 2000;49:2201–2207.

[66] Hirschhorn J and Altshuler D. The inherited basis of diabetes mellitus: implications for the genetic analysis of complex traits. *Annu Rev Genomics Hum Genet.* 2003;4:257–291.

[67] Risch N and Merikangas K. The future of genetic studies of complex human diseases. *Science,* 1996;273:1516–1517.

[68] Altshuler D, Hirschhorn JN, Klannemark M, Lindgren CM, Vohl MC, Nemesh J, Lane CR, Schaffner SF, Bolk S, Brewer C, Tuomi T, Gaudet D, Hudson TJ, Daly M, Groop L, and Lander ES. The common PPARgamma Pro12Ala polymorphism is associated with decreased risk of type 2 diabetes. *Nat Genet.* 2000;26:76–80.

[69] Gloyn AL, Weedon MN, Owen KR, Turner MJ, Knight BA, Hitman G, Walker M, Levy JC, Sampson M, Halford S, McCarthy MI, Hattersley AT, F and rayling TM. Large-scale association studies of variants in genes encoding the pancreatic b-cell KATP channel subunits Kir6.2 (KCNJ11) and SUR1 (ABCC8) confirm that the KCNJ11 E23K variant is associated with type 2 diabetes. *Diabetes,* 2003;52:568–572.

[70] Florez JC, Burtt N, de Bakker PIW, Almgren P, Tuomi T, Holmkvist J, Gaudet D, Hudson TJ, Schaffner SF, Daly MJ, Hirschhorn JN, Groop L, and Altshuler D. Haplotype structure and genotype-phenotype correlations of the sulfonylurea receptor and the islet ATP-sensitive potassium channel gene region. *Diabetes*, 2004;53:1360–1368.

[71] Barroso I, Luan J, Middelberg RPS, Harding A-H, Franks PW, Jakes RW, Clayton D, Schafer AJ, O'Rahilly S, and Wareham NJ. Candidate gene association study in type 2 diabetes indicates a role for genes involved in β-cell function as well as insulin action. *PLoS Biology,* 2003;1:41–55.

[72] Grant SF, Thorleifsson G, Reynisdottir I, Benediktsson R, Manolescu A, Sainz J, Helgason A, Stefansson H, Emilsson V, Helgadottir A, Styrkarsdottir U, Magnusson KP, Walters GB, Palsdottir E, Jonsdottir T, Gudmundsdottir T, Gylfason A, Saemundsdottir J, Wilensky RL, Reilly MP, Rader DJ, Bagger Y, Christiansen C, Gudnason V, Sigurdsson G, Thorsteinsdottir U, Gulcher JR, Kong A, and Stefansson K. Variant of transcription factor 7-like 2 (TCF7L2) gene confers risk of type 2 diabetes. *Nat Genet.* 2006;38:320–323.

[73] Florez JC, Jablonski KA, Bayley N, Pollin TI, de Bakker PIW, Shuldiner AR, Knowler WC, Nathan DM, Altshuler D, and Group tDPPR. TCF7L2 polymorphisms and progression to diabetes in the Diabetes Prevention Program. *N Engl J Med.* 2006;355:241–250.

[74] Beysen D, Raes J, Leroy BP, Lucassen A, Yates JRW, Clayton-Smith J, Ilyina H, Brooks SS, Christin-Maitre S, Fellous M, Fryns JP, Kim JR, Lapunzina P, Lemyre E, Meire F, Messiaen LM, Oley C, Splitt M, Thomson J, Peer YVd, Veitia RA, De Paepe A, and De Baere E. Deletions involving long-range conserved nongenic sequences upstream and downstream of FOXL2 as a novel disease-causing mechanism in blepharophimosis syndrome. *Am J Hum Genet.* 2005;77:205–218.

[75] Drake JA, Bird C, Nemesh J, Thomas DJ, Newton-Cheh C, Reymond A, Excoffier L, Attar H, Antonarakis SE, Dermitzakis ET, Hirschhorn JN. Conserved noncoding sequences are selectively constrained and not mutation cold spots. 2006;38:223–227.

[76] Risch N and Merikangas K. The future of genetic studies of complex human diseases. *Science,* 1996;273:1516–1517.

[77] J B Meigs, A K Manning, C S Fox, J C Florez, C Liu, L A Cupples, and J Dupuis, Genome-wide association with diabetes-related traits in the Framingham Heart Study, *BMC Med Genet.* 2007; 8(Suppl 1): S16.

[78] Grant SF, Thorleifsson G, Reynisdottir I, Benediktsson R, Manolescu A, Sainz J, Helgason A, Stefansson H, Emilsson V, Helgadottir A, Styrkarsdottir U, Magnusson KP, Walters GB, Palsdottir E, Jonsdottir T, Gudmundsdottir T, Gylfason A, Saemundsdottir J, Wilensky RL, Reilly MP, Rader DJ, Bagger Y, Christiansen C, Gudnason V, Sigurdsson G, Thorsteinsdottir U, Gulcher JR, Kong A, and Stefansson K. Variant of transcription factor 7-like 2 (TCF7L2) gene confers risk of type 2 diabetes. *Nat Genet.* 2006;38:320–323.

[79] Groves CJ, Zeggini E, Minton J, Frayling TM, Weedon MN, Rayner NW, Hitman GA, Walker M, Wiltshire S, Hattersley AT, and McCarthy MI. Association analysis of 6,736 U.K. subjects provides replication and confirms TCF7L2 as a type 2 diabetes

susceptibility gene with a substantial effect on individual risk. *Diabetes*, 2006;55:2640–2644.

[80] Zhang C, Qi L, Hunter DJ, Meigs JB, Manson JE, van Dam RM, and Hu FB. Variant of Transcription Factor 7-Like 2 (TCF7L2) Gene and the Risk of Type 2 Diabetes in Large Cohorts of U.S. Women and Men. *Diabetes*, 2006;55:2645–2648.

[81] Scott LJ, Bonnycastle LL, Willer CJ, Sprau AG, Jackson AU, Narisu N, Duren WL, Chines PS, Stringham HM, Erdos MR, Valle TT, Tuomilehto J, Bergman RN, Mohlke KL, Collins FS, and Boehnke M. Association of transcription factor 7-like 2 (TCF7L2) variants with type 2 diabetes in a Finnish sample. *Diabetes*, 2006;55:2649–2653

[82] Damcott CM, Pollin TI, Reinhart LJ, Ott SH, Shen H, Silver KD, Mitchell BD, and Shuldiner AR. Polymorphisms in the transcription factor 7-like 2 (TCF7L2) gene are associated with type 2 diabetes in the Amish: Replication and evidence for a role in both insulin secretion and insulin resistance. *Diabetes*, 2006;55:2654–2659.

[83] Saxena, R.;Gianniny, L.;Burtt, NP.;Lyssenko, V.;Guiducci, C.;Sjögren, M.;Florez, JC.;Almgren, P.;Isomaa, B.;Orho-Melander, M.;Lindblad, U.;Daly, MJ.;Tuomi, T.;Hirschhorn, JN.;Groop, L.; and Altshuler, D. Common SNPs in TCF7L2 are reproducibly associated with type 2 diabetes and reduce the insulin response to glucose in non-diabetic individuals. *Diabetes*, 2006, 55 (10), 2890-5.

[84] Cauchi S, Meyre D, Dina C, Choquet H, Samson C, Gallina S, Balkau B, Charpentier G, Pattou F, Stetsyuk V, Scharfmann R, Staels B, Fruhbeck G, and Froguel P. Transcription factor TCF7L2 genetic study in the French population: expression in human beta-cells and adipose tissue and strong association with type 2 diabetes. *Diabetes*, 2006;55:2903–2908.

[85] van Vliet-Ostaptchouk JV, Shiri-Sverdlov R, Zhernakova A, Strengman E, van Haeften TW, Hofker MH, and Wijmenga C. Association of variants of transcription factor 7-like 2 (TCF7L2) with susceptibility to type 2 diabetes in the Dutch Breda cohort. *Diabetologia*, 2007, 50 (1), 59-62.

[86] Field SF, Howson JM, Smyth DJ, Walker NM, Dunger DB, and Todd JA. Analysis of the type 2 diabetes gene, TCF7L2, in 13,795 type 1 diabetes cases and control subjects. *Diabetologia*, 2007, 50 (1), 212-213.

[87] Humphries, SE.;Gable, D.;Cooper, JA.;Ireland, H.;Stephens, JW.;Hurel, SJ.;Li, KW.;Palmen, J.;Miller, MA.;Cappuccio, FP.;Elkeles, R.;Godsland, I.;Miller, GJ.; and Talmud, PJ. Common variants in the TCF7L2 gene and predisposition to type 2 diabetes in UK European Whites, Indian Asians and Afro-Caribbean men and women. *J Mol Med.* 2006, 84 (12), 1005-14.

[88] Price JA, Brewer CS, Howard TD, Fossey SC, Rich SS, Freedman BI, Weurth JP, and Bowden DW: Construction of a physical map of chromosome 20q12–13.1 and linkage disequilibrium analysis in diabetic nephropathy patients (Abstract). *Am J Hum Genet.* 58 (Suppl.):A241, 1997.

[89] J L Bento, N D Palmer,2 J C Mychaleckyj, L A Lange, C D Langefeld, SS Rich, B I Freedman, and D W Bowden1, Association of Protein Tyrosine Phosphatase 1B GenePolymorphisms With Type 2 Diabetes, *Diabetes*,2004,53, 3007-3012.

[90] Love-Gregory L, Sherva R, Lingwei S, Wasson J, Schappe T, Doria A, Rao DC, Hunt SC, Klein S, Neuman RJ, Permutt MA, and Abumrad NA. Variants in the CD36 gene

associate with the metabolic syndrome and high-density lipoprotein cholesterol. *Human Molecular Genetics,* 2008, 17(11), 1695-1704.

[91] W S Browner, A.Kahn, A Reiner, J Oshima, R Cowthon, W-C Hsueh, and S Cummings, The genetics of human longevity, *Am J Med.* 2004, 117/11/ 851-60

[92] Cohen, HJ, Pieper, CF, Harris, T., et al. The association of plasma IL-6 levels with functional disability in community-dwelling elderly. *J Gerontol A Biol Sci Med Sci.* 1997;52:M201-8.

[93] Chamorro A. Role of inflammation in stroke and atherothrombosis. *Cerebrovasc Dis.* 2004;17 Suppl 3:1-5.

[94] Dandona, P, Aljada, A and Bandyopadhyay A. Inflammation: the link between insulin resistance, obesity and diabetes. *Trends Immunol.* 2004; 25:4-7.

[95] Franceschi, C, Bonafe, M, Valensin, S., et al. Inflamm-aging. An evolutionary perspective on immunosenescence. *Ann N Y Acad Sci.* 2000;908:244-54.

[96] Cavallone, L, Bonafe, M, Olivieri, F., et al. The role of IL-1 gene cluster in longevity: a study in Italian population. *Mech Ageing Dev.* 2003; 124:533-8.

[97] Amadori, A, Zamarchi, R, De Silvestro, G., et al. Genetic control of the CD4/CD8 T-cell ratio in humans. *Nat Med.* 1995; 1:1279-83.

[98] Clementi, M, Forabosco, P, Amadori, A., et al. CD4 and CD8 T lymphocyte inheritance. Evidence for major autosomal recessive genes. *Hum Genet.* 1999; 105:337-42.

[99] Lagaay, AM, D'Amaro, J, Ligthart, GJ., et al. Longevity and heredity in humans. Association with the human leucocyte antigen phenotype. *Ann N Y Acad Sci.* 1991; 621:78-89.

[100] Ferguson, F.G. Immune parameters in a longitudinal study in a very old population of Swedish people: a comparison between survivors and non-survivors. *J. Gerontol.,* 1995,.50A (6), B378–B382.

[101] Soto-Vega E, Richaud-Patin Y, and Llorente L. Human leukocyte antigen class I, class II, and tumor necrosis factor-alpha polymorphisms in a healthy elder Mexican Mestizo population. *Immun Ageing,* 2005;32:13.

[102] Henon N, and Schachter F. Genetics of longevity. *C R Seances Soc Biol Fil.* 1997; 191:553-62.

[103] Ivanova R, Henon N, Lepage V et al. HLA-DR alleles display sex-dependent effects on survival and discriminate between individual and familial longevity. *Hum Mol Genet.* 1998 ;7:187-94.

[104] Akisaka M, and Suzuki M. Okinawa Longevity Study. Molecular genetic analysis of HLA genes in the very old] Nippon Ronen Igakkai Zasshi. 1998; 35:294-8.

[105] Ricci G, Colombo C, Ghiazza B et al. Association between longevity and allelic forms of human leukocyte antigens (HLA): population study of aged Italian human subjects. *Arch Immunol Ther Exp* (Warsz). 1998; 46: 31-4

[106] Papasteriades C, Boki K, Pappa H, et al. HLA phenotypes in healthy aged subjects. *Gerontology,* 1997; 43: 176-81

[107] Takata, H, Suzuki, M, Ishii, T., et al. Influence of major histocompatibility complex region genes on human longevity among Okinawan-Japanese centenarians and nonagenarians. *Lancet,* 1987; 2:824-6.

[108] Rea IM, and Middleton D. Is the phenotypic combination A1B8Cw7DR3 a marker for male longevity? *J Am Geriatr Soc.* 1994; 42:978-83.

[109] Ross O, Curran M, and Rea I. HLA haplotypes and TNF polymorphism do not associate with longevity in Irish. *Mechanisms of Aging and Development*, 2003; 124:563-7.

[110] Caruso, C, Candore, G, Colonna, Romano, G., et al. HLA, aging, and longevity: a critical reappraisal. *Hum Immunol.* 2000; 61:942-9

[111] Ershler WB and Keller ET. Age-associated increased interleukin-6 gene expression, late-life diseases, and frailty. *Annu Rev Med.* 2000;51:245-70.

[112] Volpato, S., Gyralink, J, Ferrucci, L., et al. Cardiovascular disease, interleukin-6, and risk of mortality in older women: the women's health and aging study. *Circulation,* 2001; 103:947-953.

[113] Bruunsgaard H, Pedersen M and Pedersen BK. Aging and proinflammatory cytokines. *Curr Opin Hematol.* 2001;8:131-6.

[114] Bhojak, TJ, DeKosky, ST, Ganguli, M., et al. Genetic polymorphisms in the cathespin D and interleukin-6 genes and the risk of Alzheimer's disease. *Neurosci Lett.* 2000;288:21-4.

[115] Rea IM, Stewart M, Campbell P, Alexander HD, Crockard AD, and Morris TC. 1996. Changes in lymphocyte subsets, interleukin 2, and soluble interleukin 2 receptor in old and very old age. *Gerontology,* . 42, 69–78.

[116] Pawelec G, Barnett Y, Forsey R, Frasca D, Globerson A, McLeod J, Caruso C, Franceschi C, Fulop T, Gupta S, Mariani E, Mocchegiani E, and Solana R. 2002. T cells and aging Front. *Bioscience*,7, 1056–1183 .

[117] Shoskes, DA, Albakri, Q, Thomas, K., et al. 2002. Cytokine polymorphisms in men withchronic prostatitis/chronic pelvic pain syndrome: association with diagnosis and treatment response. *J Urol.* 168, 331-5.

[118] Ross OA, Curran MD, Meenagh A, Williams F, Barnett YA, Middleton D and Rea IM. 2003. Study of age-association with cytokine gene polymorphisms in an aged Irish population. *Mech Ageing Dev.* 124, 199–206.

[119] Terry CF, Loukaci V and Green FR. 2000. Cooperative influence of genetic polymorphisms on interleukin 6 transcriptional regulation. *J Biol Chem.* 275, 18138-44.

[120] Nauck M, Winkelmann BR, Hoffmann M., et al. 2002. The interleukin-6 G(-174)C promoter polymorphism in the LURIC cohort: no association with plasma interleukin-6, coronary artery disease, and myocardial infarction. *J Mol Med.* 80, 507-13.

[121] Humphries SE, Luong LA, Ogg M., et al. 2001. The interleukin-6 -174 G/C promoter polymorphism is associated with risk of coronary heart disease and systolic blood pressure in healthy men.*Eur Heart J.* 22, 2243-52.

[122] Rauramaa R, Vaisanen SB, Luong LA., et al. 2000. Stromelysin-1 and interleukin-6 gene promoter polymorphisms are determinants of asymptomatic carotid artery atherosclerosis. *Arterioscler Thromb Vasc Biol.* 20, 2657-62.

[123] Franceschi C, Olivieri F, Marchegiani F, Cardelli M, Cavallone L, Capri M, Salvioli S, Valensin S, De Benedictis G, Di Iorio A, Caruso C, Paolisso G, and Monti D. 2005. Genes involved in immune response/inflammation, IGF1/insulin pathway and response

to oxidative stress play a major role in the genetics of human longevity: The lesson of centenarians. *Mech Ageing Dev.* 126, 351–361.

[124] Wright N, de Lera TL, Garcia-Moruja C, Lillo R, Garcia-Sanchez F, Caruz A, and Teixido J. 2003. Transforming growth factorbeta1 down-regulates expression of chemokine stromal cell-derived factor-1: Functional consequences in cell migration and adhesion. *Blood*, 102, 1978–1984.

[125] Harris TB, Ferrucci L, Tracy RP., et al. 1999. Associations of elevated interleukin-6 and C-reactive protein levels with mortality in the elderly. *Am J Med.* 106, 506-512.

[126] Christiansen L, Bathum L, Andersen-Ranberg K, Jeune B, and Christensen K. 2004. Modest implication of interleukin-6 promoter polymorphisms in longevity. *Mech Ageing Dev.* 2004; 125, 391–395.

[127] Salvioli S., Olivieri F., Marchegiani F., Cardelli M., Santoro A., Bellavista E., Mishto M., Invidia L., Capri M., Valensin S., Sevini F., Cevenini E., Celani L., Lescai F., Gonos E., Caruso C., Paolisso G., De Benedictis G., Monti D., and Franceschi C., 2006. Genes, ageing and longevity in humans: Problems, advantages and perspectives. *Free Radical Research*, 40, 1303-1323.

[128] Bonafe M, Olivieri F, Cavallone L., et al. 2001. A gender--dependent genetic predisposition to produce high levels of IL-6 is detrimental for longevity. *Eur J Immunol.* 31, 2357-2361.

[129] Wang, XY, Hurme, M, Jylha, M., et al. 2001. Lack of association between human longevity and polymorphisms of IL-1 cluster, IL-6, IL-10 and TNF-alpha genes in Finnish nonagenarians. *Mech Ageing Dev.* 123, 29-38.

[130] Naumova, E, Mihaylova, A, Ivanova, M., et al. 2004. Immunological markers contributing to sucsessful aging in Bulgarians. *Exp Gerontol.* 39, 637-44.

[131] Pes GM, Lio D, Carru C, Deiana L, Baggio G, Franceschi C, Ferrucci L, Oliveri F, Scola L, Crivello A, Candore G, Colonna-Romano G, and Caruso C. 2004. Association between longevity and cytokine gene polymorphisms. A study in Sardinian

[132] Caruso C, Solfrizzi V, D'Introno A, Colacicco AM, Capurso SA, Semeraro C, Capurso A, and Panza F. 2004. Interleukin 6-174 G/C promoter gene polymorphism in centenarians: No evidence of association with human longevity or interaction with apolipoprotein E alleles. *Exp Gerontol.* 39, 1109–1114.

[133] Lio, D, Scola, L, Crivello, A., et al. 2003. Inflammation, genetics, and longevity: further studies on the protective effects in men of IL-10 -1082 promoter SNP and its interaction with TNF-alpha -308 promoter SNP. *J Med Genet.* 40, 296-299

[134] Candore G, Lio D, Colonna Romano G, and Caruso C. 2002. Pathogenesis of autoimmune diseases associated with 8.1ancestral haplotype: Effect of multiple gene interactions. *Autoimmun Rev.* 1, 29–35.

[135] Moore, KW, de Waal Malefyt, R, Coffman, R.L., et al. 2001. Interleukin-10 and the interleukin-10 receptor. *Annu Rev Immunol.* 19, 683-765.

[136] Lio, D, Scola, L, Crivello, A., et al. 2002. Allele frequencies of +874T-->A single nucleotide polymorphism at the first intron of interferon-gamma gene in a group of Italian centenarians. *Exp Gerontol.* 37, 315-9.

[137] Lio D, Scola L, Crivello A, et al. Gender-specific association between -1082 IL-10 promoter polymorphism and longevity. *Genes Immun.* 2002; 3:30-3.

[138] Arroyo-Espliguero, R., Avanzas, P., Jeffery, S., and Kaski, J.C., 2004. CD14 and toll-like receptor 4: a link between infection and acute coronary events? *Heart*, 90, 983–988.

[139] Schroder, N.W., and Schumann, R.R., 2005. Single nucleotide polymorphisms of Toll-like receptors and susceptibility to infectious disease. *Lancet Infect. Dis.* 5, 156–164.

[140] Balistreri, C.R., Candore, G., Colonna-Romano, G., Lio, D., Caruso, M.,Hoffmann, E., Franceschi, C., and Caruso, C., 2004. Role of Toll-like receptor 4 in acute myocardial infarction and longevity. *JAMA*, 292, 2339–2340.

[141] Cipollone, F., and Fazia, M.L., 2006. COX-2 and atherosclerosis. *J. Cardiovasc.Pharmacol.* 47S1, S26–S36.

[142] Dwyer, J.H., Allayee, H., Dwyer, K.M., Fan, J., Wu, H., Mar, R., Lusis, A.J., and Mehrabian, M., 2004. Arachidonate 5-lipoxygenase promoter genotype,dietary arachidonic acid, and atherosclerosis. *N. Engl. J. Med.* 350, 29–37.

[143] Papafili, A., Hill, M.R., Brull, D.J., McAnulty, R.J., Marshall, R.P., Humphries, S.E., and Laurent, G.J., 2002. Common promoter variant in cyclooxygenase-2 represses gene expression: evidence of role in acute-phase inflammatory response. *Arterioscler. Thromb. Vasc. Biol.* 22, 1631–1636.

[144] Balistreri CR, Caruso C, Grimaldi MP, Listì F, Vasto S, Orlando V, Campagna AM, Lio D, and Candore G. CCR5 receptor: biologic and genetic implications in age-related diseases. *Ann N Y Acad Sci.* 2007 ,1100:162-72.

[145] Ljunggren, H.G. and Karre, K., 1990. In search of the 'missing self': MHC molecules and NK cell recognition. *Immunol. Today,* 11, 237–244.

[146] Malaguarnera, L., Ferlito, L., Imbesi, R.M., Gulizia, G.S., Di Mauro, S.,Maugeri, D., Malaguarnera, M., and Messina, A., 2001. Immunosenescence: a review. *Arch. Gerontol. Geriatr.* 32, 1–14.

[147] Radaev, S. and Sun, P.D., 2003. Structure and function of natural killer cell surface receptors. *Annu. Rev. Biophys. Biomol. Struct.* 32, 93–114.

[148] Biassoni, R., Cantoni, C., Falco, M., Pende, D., Millo, R., Moretta, L.,Bottino, C., and Moretta, A., 2000. Human natural killer cell activating receptors. *Mol. Immunol.* 37, 1015–1024.

[149] Carretero, M., Cantoni, C., Bellon, T., Bottino, C., Biassoni, R., Rodriguez, A., Perez-Villar, J.J., Moretta, L., Moretta, A., and Lopez-Botet, M., 1997.The CD94 and NKG2-A C-type lectins covalently assemble to form a natural killer cell inhibitory receptor for HLA class I molecules. *Eur.J. Immunol.* 27(2), 563–567.

[150] Fanger, N.A., Borges, L. and Cosman, D., 1999. The leukocyte immunoglobulin-like receptors (LIRs); a new family of immune regulators. *J. Leukoc. Biol.* 66, 231–236.

[151] Lynn D. Maxwell, Owen A. Ross, Martin D. Curran, I. Maeve Rea, and Derek Middleton, 2004, Investigation of KIR diversity in immunosenecence and longevity within the Irish population. *Experimental Gerontology*, 39, 1223-1232.

[152] MW Turner. Mannose-binding lectin: the pluripotent molecule of the innate immune system. *Immunol Today,* 1996;17(11):532-40.

[153] Petersen SV TS, Jensen L, Steffensen R, Jensenius JC. An assay for the mannan-binding lectin pathway of complement activation. J Immunol Methods. 2001;257(1-2):107-16.

[154] Wallis R DK. Molecular determinants of oligomer formation and complement fixation inmannose-binding proteins. *J Biol Chem.* 1999;274(6):3580-9.

[155] Sastry K HG, Day L, Deignan E, Bruns G, Morton CC, and Ezekowitz RA. The human mannose-binding protein gene. Exon structure reveals its evolutionary relationship to a human pulmonary surfactant gene and localization to chromosome 10. *J Exp Med.* 1989;170(4):1175-89.

[156] Lipscombe RJ SM, Hill AV, Lau YL, Levinsky RJ, Summerfield JA, and Turner MW. High frequencies in African and non-African populations of independent mutations in the mannose binding protein gene. *Hum Mol Genet.* 1992;1(9):709-15.

[157] Madsen HO GP, Thiel S, Kurtzhals JA, Lamm LU, Ryder LP, and Svejgaard A. Interplay between promoter and structural gene variants control basal serum levelof mannan-binding protein. *J Immunol.* 1995;155(6):3013-20.

[158] Madsen HO SM, Hogh B, Svejgaard A, and Garred P. Different molecular events result in low protein levels of mannan-binding lectin in populations from southeast Africa and South *America. J Immunol.* 1998;161(6):3169-75.

[159] Cedzynski M SJ, Swierzko AS, Bak-Romaniszyn L, Banasik M, Zeman K, and Kilpatrick DC. Mannan-binding lectin insufficiency in children with recurrent infections of the respiratory system. *Clin Exp Immunol.* 2004;136(2):304-11.

[160] Boniotto M CS, Pirulli D, Scarlatti G, Spanò A, Vatta L, Zezlina S, Tovo PA, Palomba E, and Amoroso A. Polymorphisms in the MBL2 promoter correlated with risk of HIV-1 vertical transmission and AIDS progression. *Genes Immun.* 2000;1(5):346-8.

[161] Mølle I SR, Thiel S, and Peterslund NA. Chemotherapy-related infections in patients with multiple myeloma: associations with mannan-binding lectin genotypes. *Eur J Haematol.* 2006;77(1):19-26.

[162] Granell M U-IA, Suarez B, Rovira M, Fernández-Avilés F, Martínez C, Ortega M, Uriburu C, Gaya A, Roncero JM, Navarro A, Carreras E, Mensa J, Vives J, Rozman C, Montserrat E, and Lozano F. Mannan-binding lectin pathway deficiencies and invasive fungal infections following allogeneic stem cell transplantation. *Exp Hematol.* 2006;34(10):1435-41.

[163] Lee YH WT, Momot T, Schmidt RE, Kaufman KM, Harley JB, and Sestak AL. The mannose-binding lectin gene polymorphisms and systemic lupus erythematosus: two case-control studies and a meta-analysis. *Arthritis Rheum.* 2005;52(12):3966-74.

[164] Graudal NA HC, and Madsen HO Mannan binding lectin in rheumatoid arthritis. A longitudinal study. *J Rheumatol.* 1998;25:629-35.

[165] Ravussin, E. & Bouchard, C. (2000). Human genomics and obesity:finding appropriate drug targets. *Eur. J. Pharmacol.* 410: 131–145.

[166] Watkins, S. M., Hammock, B. D., Newman, J. W. & German, J. B.(2001) Individual metabolism should guide agriculture toward foods for improved health and nutrition. *Am. J. Clin. Nutr.* 74: 283–286.

[167] Castro E, Edland SD, Lee L, et al. Polymorphisms at the Werner locus: II. 1074Leu/Phe, 1367Cys/Arg, longevity, and atherosclerosis. *Am J Med Genet.* 2000;95:374-80.

[168] Ridker PM, Evaluating novel cardiovascular risk factors: can we better predict heart attacks?, *Ann Intern Med.* 1999, 130, 933-937.

In: Handbook on Longevity: Genetics, Diet and Disease ISBN 978-1-60741-075-1
Editors: Jennifer V. Bentely and Mary Ann Keller © 2009 Nova Science Publishers, Inc.

Chapter XIV

Effects of Chewing Ability on Longevity

Toshihiro Ansai[1]*, Yutaka Takata[2] and Tadamichi Takehara[1]
[1]Division of Community Oral Health Science, Kyushu Dental College
[2]Division of General Internal Medicine, Kyushu Dental College

Abstract

The oral cavity in humans has a variety of functions, such as eating, swallowing, and speaking, as well as chewing, which is one of its most important roles. Although the association of chronic periodontitis with systemic health has become an important issue, few studies have been conducted regarding the association between chewing ability and systemic health status. Recently, we conducted a population-based prospective study to determine the association between chewing ability and longevity in 697 (277 males, 420 females) community-dwelling elderly subjects in Japan, and herein present some of those results. Chewing ability was assessed based on the number of types of food each subject reported able to chew in answers to a questionnaire, which showed that individuals with higher chewing ability lived longer, after adjusting for various confounding factors (multivariate hazard ratio: 2.6; 95% confidence interval: 1.2-5.5). When the associations between causes of death and chewing ability were further analyzed, subjects reporting the lowest numbers of chewable foods were associated with a higher risk of mortality from cardiovascular disease (CVD) as compared with those able to chew all the types of food surveyed (multivariate hazard ratio: 5.1; 95% confidence interval: 1.1-23.8). On the other hand, there was no significant association between chewing ability and other causes of death including cancer. Our results indicate that maintenance of chewing ability in

---

* Correspondence to: Toshihiro Ansai, DDS, Ph.D.,
Division of Community Oral Health Science, Department of Health Promotion,
Kyushu Dental College, 2-6-1 Manazuru, Kokurakita-ku, Kitakyushu 803-8580, Japan
Tel: +81-93-582-1131 (ext. 2102)
Fax: +81-93-591-7736
E-mail: ansai@kyu-dent.ac.jp

elderly individuals contributes to longevity. In addition, we discuss the significance of masticatory function in light of nutrition status.

Key words: masticatory; chewing; nutrient; longevity; systemic health.

Introduction

The oral cavity has various roles and functions, as demonstrated in Figure 1, among which chewing ability is thought to be one of the most important, in addition to eating, swallowing, and speaking. Masticatory function is considered to have an influence on various functions related to systemic health including brain activity. However, epidemiological studies of the associations of oral functions including masticatory function, with systemic health tend to be disregarded. Although a number of studies have focussed on the associations between chronic periodontitis and systemic health in elderly subjects, reports of the effects of chewing ability on systemic health are limited, and findings are scarce. In addition, those associations have been mainly discussed in regard to the inflammatory pathway, whereas epidemiological studies of nutritional status are few.

- Chewing
- Swallowing
- Speech
- Breathing
- Sense of taste
- Sense of touch
- Thermoesthesia
- Support for saliva functions
- Forming expressions

Ansai, et al.

Figure 1. Roles of the oral cavity.

Recently, we performed a cohort study of community-dwelling elderly subjects in regard to the association between oral functions, including masticatory function, and systemic health condition. In this chapter, we present results of data regarding the association of dental status, reflected by a lower level of chewing ability, and mortality. In addition, we discuss the influence of decreased chewing ability on systemic health from the viewpoint of nutritional status and also show the significance of chewing ability in light of prevention against impaired systemic functions.

Factors Associated with Masticatory Function

Number of teeth (or missing teeth), occlusion, salivary flow rate, periodontal disease (including gingival swelling and mobility of teeth), psychological aspects, and quality of life (QOL) are known to be associated with chewing ability. However, we should note that even in individuals with several teeth in the mouth, enough chewing ability is not necessarily obtained. Whether the occlusal status in the mouth is adequate is important. For example, occlusal status with no occluding pairs of teeth in the jaws, in which the upper and lower teeth do not contact each other, results in a lack of masticatory ability. According to the work of Österberg et al. [1], chewing ability significantly correlated to the Eichner Index, in which Class A denotes dental support in all four quadrants. Class B denotes contact in one to three zones or in the frontal region only, and Class C denotes an absence of tooth contact. Maximal bite force is reduced to half in cases of Class B in the Eichner Index and a third in cases with occlusion only in the frontal region, while it is reduced to one fourth in Class C, as compared with an occlusal status of dental support in all quadrants. Thus, the existence of occluding pairs of teeth in the upper and lower jaws as well as number of teeth is necessary for better chewing ability. Although patients who have teeth extracted because of severe periodontitis and other teeth left untreated are often observed in a clinical situations, it is important to understand that such situations can lead to a reduction in chewing ability. In an investigation of the association between maximal bite force and salivary flow, Yeh et al. [2] reported that subjects with higher levels of bite force had higher unstimulated and stimulated salivary flows as compared with those with lower levels of bite force. These findings suggest that a daily habit of chewing well, from a younger age if possible, is a key for higher masticatory function.

Method of Masticatory Function Evaluation

Various terms are used to refer to masticatory function, including masticatory efficiency, masticatory ability, and masticatory performance [3]. Herein, we use the phrase masticatory function to cover the meaning of those terms. The most frequently used method of determining masticatory functionis the sieve method, which peanuts or agar bits are chewed, and the size and rates evaluated. This method involves drying, filtering, and weighing the materials, and is slow and complicated, thus it is not considered useful for epidemiological studies. Recently, a new method of measuring glucose content resolved by chewing gummy jelly as a test specimen has been developed, and reported to be simple and easy to use in the field such in epidemiological study [4]. On the other hand, in epidemiological studies performed to date, questionnaire methods based on self-evaluation have been often used. While self-assessed and dentist-assessed chewing ability tends to be weakly correlated [5], perceived chewing ability is considered to be likely to have a greater impact on food choice [6]. Among those, Yamamoto's chart, in which subjects are asked about their ability to chew foods in order to form an evaluation chart of masticatory function, is the most popular in Japan, and was also used in the present study. As the other method to assess perceived chewing ability, the questionnaire in the oral health component of the National Diet and Nutrition survey id often used [7].

Effects of Masticatory Function on Nutrition Status

To date, there are few reports of the association between masticatory function and nutrition status based on population-based epidemiological studies. In an epidemiological study using a community-dwelling population aged 70 -years old (512 subjects) in Niigata Prefecture, Japan, relationships between chewing ability and total calorie intake, nutrients and food were investigated [8]. They found that the mean total calorie intake for males was 1706 kcal (SD = 350.8), while it was 1474 kcal (SD = 252.3) for females. Variables that significantly affected low chewing ability were gender, number of teeth present, presence of swelling and pain in the gums, presence of mobile teeth, degree of saliva flow, and low QOL. In males, total calorie intake and vegetable and fruit intake were found to be significantly lower in the poor chewing category than in the good category, when chewing ability was divided into two categories: able to chew all foods was considered (good), and not being able to chew any of the foods was considered (poor), while there was no such significant association in females.

In people aged 65 years and older studied in the United Kingdom, 881 free-living and 275 institutionalized subjects underwent a dental exam and were interviewed about their ability to eat 16 kinds of key foods. They were asked which foods they could eat easily, with some difficulty, and not at all [9]. There were mor edentate subjects who stated that they had eating difficulties than the dentate subjects, and perceived chewing ability increased with increasing numbers of natural teeth and pairs of opposing posterior teeth. Among people with teeth, the number of natural teeth affected the ease with which apples, raw carrots, nuts, toast, tomatoes, crisps, and oranges could be eaten. Also, the number of posterior occluding pairs of natural teeth showed similar relationships with the ease of eating certain foods to the number of natural teeth. For example, difficulty eating or not being able to eat apples had a significant relationship with the number of posterior occluding pairs. Similar trends were reported for hard-to-chew foods, such as raw carrots, nuts, and well-done steak. These associations remained valid after statistical adjustment for age, gender, social class, denture wearing status, and region.

Findings from the British National Diet and Nutrition Survey of adults aged 65 and over showed that intake levels of non-starch polysaccharides, protein, calcium, non-heme irons, niacin, and vitamin C were significantly lower in edentate subjects [10]. Plasma ascorbate (vitamin C) levels showed significant differences between dentate and edentate individuals, and the levels were also significantly related to numbers of teeth and posterior occluding pairs, even after controlling for confounding factors. On the other hand, plasma retinol (analyte indicating plasma level of vitamin A) was significantly lower in the edentate individuals, but was not significantly related to the numbers of teeth or posterior occluding pairs in dentate subjects.

Denture- wearing and its relationship to diet and nutritional status have also been studied. Using a representative sample of the adult population in the United States, differences in the intake of specific nutritious food items, dietary fiber, and levels of blood analyte were analyzed between subjects wearing complete upper and lower dentures and those who had all of their natural teeth. Multivariate analysis results indicated that intake of some nutrient-rich foods, such as carrots and tossed salads, as well as levels of beta carotene, folate, and vitamin C in serum were significantly lower in the denture -wearers [11].

Association between Masticatory Function and Systemic Health Condition

As described above, significant reductions in ingested nutrients including fiber, and antioxidants such as vitamin C and vitamin E, were observed in elderly individuals with lower chewing ability. Dietary fiber is an important component of the diet and is particularly associated with gastro-intestinal disease. A Japanese epidemiological study found that elderly individuals with lower chewing ability, irrespective of denture wearing, had a significantly higher risk of gastrointestinal disease, which supports the association between masticatory function and nutrients [12].

It has been speculated that higher intakes of fruits and vegetables, cruciferous vegetables, and antioxidant nutrients can decrease the risks of all-cause, cancer, and cardiovascular disease (CVD) mortality. However, whether particular antioxidants, such as ascorbic acid (vitamin C), alpha-tocopherol (vitamin E), and beta-carotene, may underlie these associations remains to be determined, though higher intakes of fruits and vegetables have been associated with a lower risk of disease mortality [13].

Association between Masticatory Function and Longevity Based on Results of Community-Based Cohort Study

There are few studies of the association between chewing ability and longevity. Among recent reports, Nakanishi et al. [14] studied 1405 community-dwelling people aged 65 and older and noted that self-assessed chewing disability may be associated with a greater risk of mortality. A 9-year follow-up program was completed by 1245 of those subjects, which showed that self-assessed masticatory disability remained a significant predictor of mortality, after controlling for potential predictors of mortality [hazard ratio (HR) = 1.63, 95% CI = 1.30- 2.03]. However, as that survey only included questions regarding demographics, health status, and psychosocial variables, adjustment for variables commonly associated with chronic diseases including metabolic syndrome, such as results of laboratory blood examinations, smoking status, and medical history, were not included in the statistical analyses.

In order to address the above-mentioned issues, we conducted a large population-based survey, and analyzed the association between masticatory function and longevity using prospective cohort study [15]. The subjects were 697 individuals born in 1917 (80 years old) and residing in Fukuoka Prefecture, Kyushu, in southern Japan. All 80-year-old individuals residing in 9 districts, including 3 cities, 4 towns, 1 village, and 1 ward, were invited to participate in the survey, of whom 697 applied. Of those, 672 completed physical, laboratory blood, and oral examinations, including a questionnaire regarding life style, and oral and systemic health at the beginning of the investigation and then followed up during 4 years. The subjects took part in face-to-face interviews, and answered all of the questions. Assessment of masticatory function was based on the following question regarding the number of types of food: "Can you chew any of the following 15 types of food?", according to a chart based on Yamamoto's chewing assessment. The response was a simple dichotomous variable (yes/no) for each type. The 15 different types of food were divided into 4 groups, ranging from very hard-to-chew to easy-to-chew. Briefly, 3 foods were very hard to chew (hard rice crackers, peanuts, and yellow pickled radish), 6 foods were moderately hard to chew (French bread, beefsteak, octopus in vinegar, pickled shallots, dried scallop, and dried cuttlefish), 3 foods were slightly hard to chew (konnyaku, a tubular roll of boiled fish paste, and squid sashimi), and 3 foods were easy to chew (boiled rice, tuna sashimi, and grilled eel) (Figure 2). In our analysis, masticatory function was categorized as follows: group A was composed of individuals who could eat all 15 foods, group B could eat 5-14 foods, and group C could eat 0-4 foods. As for subjects who died, we recorded the date and cause of death according to resident registration cards and official death certificates, which were available in the register of the Public Health Center of each district included in the study. Deaths were classified by trained physicians according to the International Classification of Disease (ICD), tenth revision (ICD-10). During the 4-year follow-up period, 108 participants (58 men, 50 women) died.

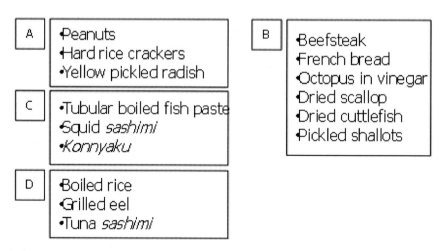

Ansai, et al.

Figure 2. Surveyed food types (n = 15). A: very hard-to-chew, B: moderately hard-to-chew, C: slightly hard-to-chew, D: easy-to-chew.

When general characteristics in individuals aged 80 years old who did or did not survive during 4-year follow-up were compared, individuals who died during the 4-year follow-up period were more likely to be male, and had lower serum total cholesterol and albumin concentrations than those who remained alive. Body mass index was higher in the survivors. Furthermore, smokers were more likely to die during the follow-up period, while alcohol consumption did not differ between individuals who survived and those who did not, nor did serum glucose concentrations, systolic blood pressure, and diastolic blood pressure. Also, the percentage of subjects with a medical history of CVD, cancer, or pneumonia did not differ between individuals who died and those who survived. There were no significant differences in the numbers of teeth, missing teeth, and chewable foods between individuals who survived and those who did not. In addition, the prevalence of edentulous subjects and subjects with severe periodontal disease did not differ between the groups. In Cox proportional hazards analyses, factors showing a statistically significant relationship with mortality were gender, smoking status, physical health status, body mass index, serum total cholesterol, and serum albumin.

The association between masticatory function and longevity was analyzed using multivariate Cox analysis, after adjustment for potential confounding factors, including gender, cigarette smoking status (never, past, current), blood pressure, and laboratory serum data [15]. Those results showed that individuals able to chew the lowest number of chewable foods were associated with a higher risk of all-cause mortality than those with the ability to chew all 15 types of food surveyed [HR = 2.6, 95% confidence interval (95% CI) = 1.2-5.5] (Figure 3). In addition, physical health status (poor), smoking status (current), and serum albumin (continuous) were also significantly associated with mortality (HR = 2.31, 95% CI = 1.21-4.39; HR = 2.63, 95% CI = 1.47-4.70; HR = 0.27, 95% CI = 0.14-0.53, respectively). Furthermore, we analyzed multivariate-adjusted hazard ratios according to the differences in the 4 types of chewable foods, i.e., from easy to very hard-to-chew, and found that reduced chewing ability of the easy-to-chew foods increased the risk of all-cause mortality (HR for 0-1 vs 3 = 2.7, 95% CI = 1.20-5.87) (Figure 3). Also, a reduction in ability to chew slightly hard-to-chew foods tended to be associated with a risk of mortality (HR for 0-1 vs 3 = 1.8, 95% CI = 0.93-3.42, P = 0.08).

Results of additional follow-up examinations of the same subjects conducted 1 year later (i.e., 5 years from the baseline) were also analyzed. During the 5-year follow-up period, a total of 157 subjects died. With additional year, a stronger association between chewing ability and all-cause mortality was found. Those with the lowest number of chewable foods were associated with a higher risk of all-cause mortality than those with the ability to chew all of the 15 types of food surveyed (HR = 3.6, 95% CI = 1.5-8.5). We also found that subjects with more intact teeth had a significantly decreased risk of all-cause mortality. The odds ratios for all-cause mortality were 2.1-fold (95% CI = 1.1-4.1) and 2.1-fold (95% CI = 1.1-4.0) greater for subjects with 1 to 9 and edentate subjects, respectively, as compared to subjects with 20 or more teeth (unpublished data).

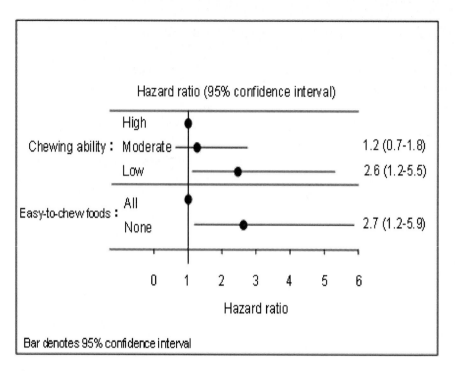

Ansai, et al.

Figure 3. Effects of chewing ability on mortality risk in 80-year-old subjects.

Next, we analyzed whether masticatory function is associated with causes of death [16]. As described above, during the 4-year follow-up period, 108 participants died, of whom 27 died from CVD (8 heart failures, 5 myocardial infarctions, 5 strokes, 4 aortic aneurysms, 3 ischemic heart diseases, 1 sick sinus syndrome, 1 hypertensive heart disease), 27 from cancer (6 lung, 3 pancreatic, 3 hepatic, 2 colon, 2 gastric, 2 uterine, 2 urinary system cancers, 7 cancers of other organs), 22 from pneumonia, and the others from other causes. As shown in Figure 4, Group C, which consisted of participants able to chew the lowest number of chewable foods, and group B had a 5.1-fold (95% CI = 1.1-23.8) and 2.1-fold (95% CI = 0.7-6.4), respectively, higher risk of CVD mortality, than group A, which consisted of participants able to chew all 15 foods and who had the greatest number of teeth. On the other hand, smoking was 2.1-fold higher risk of CVD mortality, though it did not reach statistical significance. These findings remained significant even after adjusting for various potential confounders, including gender, cigarette smoking status, serum laboratory data, body mass index, and blood pressure, which suggest that poor masticatory function is an independent risk factor for CVD mortality, at least in this group of subjects. On the other hand, no significant associations between masticatory function and other causes of death, such as cancer, pneumonia, were found, whereas the effect of smoking status on mortality due to cancer was found to be significant.

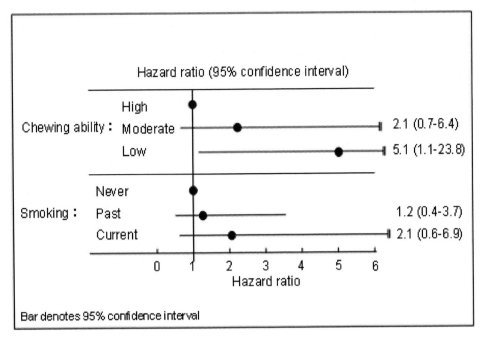

Ansai, et al.

Figure 4. Effects of chewing ability on CVD mortality risk in 80-year-old subjects.

Relationship between Masticatory Function and Systemic Health Condition

Based upon the results described above, a hypothetical flow chart showing the association between masticatory function and systemic health, or longevity, is presented in Figure 5. Reduction of masticatory function is thought to be mainly attributed to missing teeth, for which the most frequent cause is severe periodontitis. Missing teeth and consequently mal-dentition status lead to poor masticatory function. It is possible that two biological pathways are linked to a reduction in masticatory function; an infection and inflammation pathway, and a nutritional pathway, as suggested by Janket et al. [17]. Some studies have reported that periodontal disease might contribute to generation of inflammatory mediators [18, 19]. In a meta-analysis of 5 cohort studies, an increased relative risk of CVD due to periodontal disease was reported, whereas well-conducted epidemiological studies reported null results [20]. Thus, these issues remain controversial, presumably due to differences in assessment of periodontal disease, or confounders for socioeconomic and behavioral risk factors for CVD. However, we consider that periodontitis is associated with past infection and the burden of past inflammation, which leads to missing teeth and impaired masticatory function.

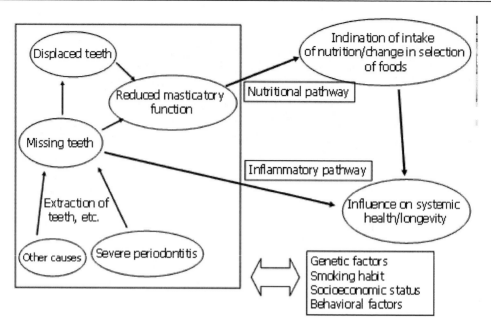

Ansai, et al.

Figure 5. Relationship between masticatory function and systemic health.

Evidence supporting the latter pathway is limited at present. A hypothetical argument has been proposed, which states that poor masticatory function is a limiting factor for adequate intake of beneficial nutrients and selection of food items. For example, intake of foods that prevent CVD, including fiber, antioxidants, and fruit and vegetables, should be considered. Furthermore, another researcher reported that edentulism encourages intake of high levels of fat and carbohydrates. Also, Joshipura and colleagues [21] observed that edentulous subjects in a cohort of 49,501 men had significantly lower intake levels of vegetables, fiber, and carotenoids, and higher intake levels of cholesterol and saturated fat than subjects with 25 or more teeth. Thus, it is possible that oral health including masticatory function, affects the risk of CVD via nutrition intake, at least indirectly.

Association between Masticatory Function and Prevention of Impaired Systemic Function

In 2006, the Japanese Ministry of Health, Labour and Welfare started a system of disease prevention and nursing care for elderly individuals, in which 3 pillars for health promotion were presented; improvement of physical fitness, improvement of nutrition, and improvement of oral function. We previously investigated the association between chewing self-assessment and performance of activities of daily living (ADL) in 80-year-old subjects using a cross-sectional study [22], in which the numbers and the types of foods that the subjects could chew were used as indicators of chewing ability. We found that the number of chewable foods was linked to independent function, based on results of multiple regression analysis (β

= 0.223, P < 0.001), after adjustment for gender. Furthermore, logistic regression analysis showed that functional dependency was 7.5 times more prevalent in individuals capable of chewing 4 foods or fewer and 3.3 times more prevalent in those able to chew 5 to 9, as compared to those who could chew all 15 items. We also found an association between high-level functional capacity and chewing ability in another study of those 80-year-old subjects [23]. For determining high-level functional capacity, the Tokyo Metropolitan Institute of Gerontology Index of Competence (TMIG index) was used, which consists of instrumental self-maintenance, intellectual activity, and social roles. Using multiple regression and logistic analyses adjusted for various confounding factors, high-level functional capacity, including intellectual activity and social roles, was found to be more associated with the ability to chew hard foods than easily chewable foods.

It is important to note that an association between cognitive function and chewing ability was observed. Onozuka et al. [24] evaluated brain activation associated with chewing in intact humans (n = 17, 20 - 31 years old) using functional magnetic resonance imaging (fMRI). In all subjects, chewing resulted in a bilateral increase in blood oxygenation level-dependent (BOLD) signals in the senosorimotor cortex, supplementary motor area, insula, thalamus, and cerebellum, which suggested that chewing causes regional increases in brain neuronal activities that are related to biting force. They also assessed the effect of aging on brain regional activity using fMRI. Interestingly, in aged subjects, gum-chewing resulted in an increased BOLD signals in the right prefrontal area, which were 4 times greater than those seen in young subjects [25]. These findings suggest that chewing stimulates neuronal activity within a network between the right prefrontal cortex and hippocampus, which might be useful for maintaining cognitive function. Interesting findings from our epidemiological study have also been presented. Cognitive function was evaluated using a Mini-Mental State Examination (MMSE), a standardized test that is widely used in epidemiological studies. A full score on the MMSE is 30, while cognitive impairment is defined as a score of less than 24. Multiple regression analysis of the same 80-year-old community-dwelling subjects showed a significant association between chewing ability at baseline and MMSE score 5 years later, even after adjusting for confounders (unpublished data).

Using the same subjects, we also found a significant association between a decrease in chewing ability and deterioration in physical fitness [26]. Chewing ability was related positively with physical fitness measurements of hand grip strength, leg extensor strength, isokinetic leg extensor power, stepping rate, and one-leg standing time. In addition, using logistic regression analysis, several physical fitness measurements of isokinetic leg extensor power and one-leg standing time, were significantly associated with chewing ability, even after adjustment for potential confounders. Another epidemiological study of approximately 750 individuals aged 70 and 80 years old found the similar associations between physical fitness and masticatory function [27]. In that study, Eichner index was used as a measurement of occlusal condition. In multiple regression models, the Eichner index showed significant independent effects for leg extensor power (Class A, p = 0.031), stepping rate (Class A, p = 0.044), and one-leg standing time (Class A, p = 0.022; Class B, p = 0.021)., indicating that dental occlusal condition is associated with lower extremity dynamic strength, agility, and balance function in the elderly individuals. Along with our results, these findings suggest that chewing ability in elderly individuals with adequate occlusal status may be an independent predictor of physical fitness.

Based on the association of individual general health with chewing ability described above, a mal-circulation cycle of impaired masticatory function is proposed, as shown in Figure 6. Reduction of masticatory ability is linked to undesirable eating -habits caused by an inability to chew well, which limits eating pleasure and healthy diet choice, thus influencing nutrition. These individuals tend to choose softer and more easily chewed foods that are lower in fiber and nutriential density, resulting in marked changes in the dietary intake of some key nutrients, such as non-starch polysaccharides [28]. A reduction in masticatory function is linking to a lack of appetite and malnutrition as well as eating and swallowing dysfunctions. A Japanese research group investigated that the effects of professional oral health care on improvement of oral functions including masticatory function, and found that professional treatment resulted in an increased level of serum albumin, which reflected an improvement in nutritional status in impaired elderly individuals in a nursing home [29]. In addition, oral cleaning and oral function practices were associated with an improved sense of taste in those subjects [29]. When an impaired elderly individual develops a better sense of taste and eats a greater variety of foods as a result, physical capacity and willingness can be improved, with improvements in QOL expected. To lower the number of impaired elderly individuals with lower ADL, promotion of oral functions including chewing ability, as well as improvements in physical fitness and nutritional status, and prevention of anxiety and depression, are indispensable for self-support and QOL. We propose masticatory function as an indicator for the degree of assistance needed by elderly individuals.

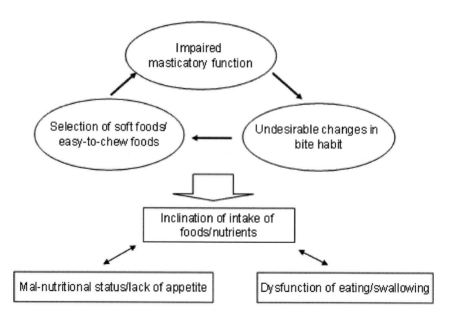

Ansai, et al.

Figure 6. Mal-circulation cycle of impaired masticatory function.

Conclusion

In this chapter, the association between masticatory function and systemic health was discussd in light of nutritional status. Based on recent findings, we concluded that maintaining masticatory function can lead to prevention of general health impairment and promote eating/feeding support in the elderly individuals. Accumulated epidemiological evidence suggests a close relationship between masticatory function and systemic health condition, ADL, physical fitness, and QOL. Masticatory function is one of the important roles of oral function. Oral health promotion can greatly contribute to encourage independence in elderly individuals and prevent a bedridden situation.

References

[1]   Österberg, T., Tsuga, K., Rothenberg, E., et al. (2002). Masticatory ability in 80-year-old subjects and its relation to intake of energy, nutrients and food items. *Gerodontology*, 19:95-101.

[2]   Yeh, C.-K., Johnson, D., Dodds, M., et al. (2000). Association of salivary flow rates with maximal bite force. *J Dent Res.* 79:1560-1565.

[3]   Boretti G, Bickel M, Geering AH. (1995). A review of masticatory ability and efficiency. *J Prothet Dent.* 74: 400-403.

[4]   Okiyama,, S., Ikebe, K. & Nokubi, T. (2003). Association between masticatory performance and maximal occlusal force in young men. *J Oral Rehabil.* 30:278-282.

[5]   Feine, J.S., & Lund, J.P. (2006). Measuring chewing ability in randomized controlled trials with edentulous populations wearing implant protheses. *J Oral Rehabil* 33:301-308.

[6]   Bradbury, J., Thomason, J.M., Jepson, N.J.A., Walls, A.W.G., Mulvaney, C.E., Allen, P.F., Moynihan, P.J. (2008). Percieved chewing ability and intake of fruit and vegetables. *J Dent Res.* 87:720-725.

[7]   Steel, J.G., Sheiham, A., Marcenes, W., & Walls A.W.G. (1998). National diet and nutrition survey: people aged 65 years and over. Vol. 2: Report of the oral health survey, London: The Stationery Office (HMSO).

[8]   Kanmori, H., Yoshihara, A., Ando, Y., & Miyazaki, H. (2003). The effect of chewing ability on the dietary intake of healthy elderly people. *J Dent Health* (in Japanese), 53:13-22.

[9]   Sheiham, A., Steele, J., Marcenes, W., et al. (1999). The impact of oral health on stated ability to eat certain foods; Findings from the national diet and nutrition survey of older people in Great Britain. *Gerodontology,* 16:11-20.

[10]   Sheiham, A., Steele, J., Marcenes, W. et al. (2001). The relationship among dental status, nutrient intake, and nutritional status in older people. *J Dent Res.* 80:408-413.

[11]   Nowjack-Raymer, R.E. & Sheiham, A. (2003). Association of edentulism and diet and nutrition in US adults. *J Dent Re.s* 82:123-126.

[12] Ikebe, K., Sajima, H., Namba, H., Ono, T., Yamamoto, M. et al. (1999). Oral and general health in the independent elderly Part 2: relarion between mastication and general disease. *Jpn J Gerodontol* (in Japanese) 14:131-138.

[13] Genkinger, J.M., Platz, E.A., Hoffman, S.C., Comstock, G.W., & Helzlsouer, K.J. (2004). Fruit, vegetable, and antioxidant intake and all-cause, cancer, and cardiovascular disease mortality in a community-dwelling population in Washington County, Maryland. *Am J Epidemiol.* 160:1223-1233.

[14] Nakanishi, N., Fukuda, H., Takatorige, T., & Tatara, K. (2005). Relationship between self-assessed masticatory disability and 9-year mortality in a cohort of community-residing elderly people. *J Am Geriatr Soc.* 53:54-58.

[15] Ansai, T., Takata, Y., Soh, I., et al. (2007). Relationship between chewing ability and 4-year mortality in a cohort of 80-year-old Japanese people. *Oral Dis.* 13:214-219.

[16] Ansai, T., Takata, Y., Soh, I., et al. (2008). Association of chewing ability with cardiovascular disease and cancer mortality in 80-year-old Japanese population. *Eur J Cardiovasc Prev Rehabil* 15:104-106.

[17] Janket, S.J., Qvarnström, M., Meurman, J.H., Baird, A.E., Nuutinen, P., Jones, J.A. (2004). Asymptotic dental score and prevalent coronary heart disease. *Circulation* 109:1095-1100.

[18] Beck, J., Garcia, R., Heiss, G., et al. (1996). Periodontal disease and cardiovascular disease. *J Periodontol.* 67:1123-1137.

[19] Wu, T., Trevisan, M., Genco, R.J. et al. (2000). Examination of the relation between periodontal health status and cardiovascular risk factors: serum total and high density lipoprotein cholesterol, C-reactive protein, and plasma fibrinogen. *Am J Epidemiol.* 151:273-282.

[20] Danesh, J. (1999). Coronary heart disease, Helicobacter pylori, denta; disease, Chlamydia pneumoniae, and cytomegalovirus: meta-analyses of prospective studies. *Am Heart J.* 138:S434-S437.

[21] Joshipura, K.J, Willett, W.C, & Douglass, C.W. (1996). The impact of edentulousness on food and nutrient intake. *JADA* 127:459-467.

[22] Takata, Y., Ansai, T., Awano, S., Sonoki, K., Fukuhara, M., Wakisaka, M., & Takehara, T. (2004). Activities of daily living and chewing ability in an 80-year-old population. *Oral Dis* 10:365-368.

[23] Takata, Y., Ansai, T., Soh, I., Akifusa, S., Sonoki, K., Fujisawa, K., et al. Relationship between chewing ability and high-level functional capacity in an 80-year-old population in Japan. *Gerodontol* 25: 147-154, 2008.

[24] Onozuka, M., Fujita, M., Watanabe, K., Hirano, Y., Niwa, M., Nishiyama, K., & Saito, S. (2002). Maping brain region activity during chewing: a functional magnetic resonance imaging study. *J Dent Res* 81:743-746.

[25] Onozuka, M., Fujita, M., Watanabe, K., Hirano, Y., Niwa, M., Nishiyama, K., & Saito S. (2003). Age-related changes in brain regional activity during chewing: a functional magnetic resonance imaging study. *J Dent Res.* 82:657-660.

[26] Takata, Y., Ansai, T., Awano, S., Hamasaki, T., Yoshitake, Y., Kimura, Y., Sonoki, K., Wakisaka, M., Fukuhara, M., & Takehara, T. (2004). Relationship of physical fitness to chewing in an 80-year-old population. *Oral Dis* 10:44-49.

[27] Yamaga, T,. Yoshihara, A., Ando, Y., Yoshitake, Y., Kimura, Y,. Shimada, M., Nishimuta, M., & Miyazaki, H. (2002). Relationship between dental occlusion and physical fitness in an eldely population. *J Gerontol:Madical Sciences* 57:M616-M620.

[28] Walls, A.W.G. (1999). Oral health and nutrition (Editorial). *Age Ageing* 28:419-420.

[29] Kikutani, T., Yoneyama, T., Teshima, T., et al. (2005). Effect of oral function and eating support on nutritional improvement of the elderly. *Jpn J Gerodontol* (in Japanese) 21:208-213.

In: Handbook on Longevity: Genetics, Diet and Disease   ISBN 978-1-60741-075-1
Editors: Jennifer V. Bentely and Mary Ann Keller   © 2009 Nova Science Publishers, Inc.

Chapter XV

Research on Aging and Longevity in the Parthenogenetic Marbled Crayfish, with Special Emphasis on Stochastic Developmental Variation, Allocation of Metabolic Resources, Regeneration, and Social Stress

Günter Vogt
Department of Zoology, University of Heidelberg, Heidelberg, Germany
E-mail: vogt@zoo.uni-heidelberg.de

Abstract

This article presents first results on aging and longevity in the marbled crayfish, an isogenic invertebrate with indeterminate growth. The marbled crayfish is the only known parthenogenetic species of more than 10.000 decapod crustaceans and has a maximal life span of roughly 3.5 years. Its main advantages, aside from genetically identical offspring and lifelong growth, are the alternation of growth and reproduction phases, a high regeneration capacity and easy handling in the laboratory. In a group of seven genetically identical batch-mates life span varied from 437 to 910 days although the sibs were communally reared and fed ad libitum with the same pellet food. In the same group there was no clear-cut relationship between longevity and growth or reproduction frequency. However, the specimen with the lowest life span showed fast growth, early onset of reproduction, and short time intervals between reproduction cycles. Damages like loss of appendages were repaired and did not negatively affect longevity. Social stress, in contrast, shortened life expectancy. The biological peculiarities of the marbled crayfish and the data obtained so far argue for a more intense use of this animal in research on aging and longevity.

Introduction

The ultimate goal of aging research is the understanding of the parameters and mechanisms that determine senescence and longevity in order to increase the life span, and particularly the healthy span, in humans. This aim is achieved by two approaches, the direct study of human aging and age related diseases, and biogerontological experiments with laboratory animals.

The most common animal models for research on aging and longevity are the mouse *Mus musculus*, the rat *Rattus norvegicus*, the nematode *Caenorhabditis elegans*, and the fruit fly *Drosophila melanogaster* [e.g. Conn, 2006; Braeckman & Vanfleteren, 2007; Bartke, 2008; Johnson, 2008; Kennedy, 2008; Lepperdinger et al., 2008]. These models served to investigate fundamental aspects of gerontology such as the genetics of aging and longevity [e.g. Braekman & Vanfleteren, 2007; Kuningas et al., 2008], the association of telomere length with aging [e.g. Jiang et al., 2007; Baird, 2008], the relationship of aging and diseases including cancer [e.g. Anisimov, 2007; Serrano & Blasco, 2007; Enns et al., 2008; Salminen et al., 2008], the influence of environmental factors on longevity [e.g. Braendle et al., 2008; Mangel, 2008], the effects of caloric restriction on life span [e.g. Houthoofd & Vanfleteren, 2006; Smith et al., 2008], the relationship of cellular dysfunction and aging [e.g. Brys et al., 2007; Passos et al., 2007a], or the extension of life span by drugs [e.g. Kitani, 2007; Evason et al., 2008].

Aside from these commonly used laboratory models further species were tested for their suitability to investigate special aspects of aging and longevity. For instance, the fish *Nothobranchius furzeri*, which has the shortest life span documented for a vertebrate of just three months, was suggested as a useful model for comparative genomics of aging [Valdesalici & Cellerino, 2003; Terzibasi et al., 2007]. The zebra fish *Danio rerio*, a common laboratory model in development and genetics, was propagated to be used for investigation of the molecular biology of aging with the help of transgenic lineages [Gerhard & Cheng, 2002; Kishi, 2004]. The honey bee *Apis mellifera* is of interest because of its unique diversity in life span, which varies from a few weeks to more than two years, depending on the social environment. Therefore, this species is expected to provide insight into regulatory pathways that can shape the time-course of aging by delaying, halting or even reversing processes of senescence [Münch et al., 2008]. Bdelloid rotifers, tardigrades and soil nematodes are of interest for research on longevity because they can extend their life spans for months or even years by anhydrobiosis, which is cryptobiosis by dessication. Interestingly, they can either ignore, partially count, or fully register the time spent in the anhydrobiotic state, depending on species [Ricci & Pagani, 1997]. For instance, in the rotifer *Adineta ricciae* [Ricci & Covino, 2005] and the tardigrade *Milnesium tradigradum* [Hengherr et al., 2008] the time spent dry was completely ignored. In the nematode *Panagrolaimus rigidus*, in contrast, long-term anhydrobiosis resulted in a partial reset of the internal clock whereas short-term anhydrobiosis was fully registered [Ricci & Pagani, 1997].

In this article, I present first data on aging and longevity in the marbled crayfish, a recently introduced laboratory model in development, epigenetics, and evolutionary biology [Vogt, 2008a]. Although rather well investigated, the marbled crayfish or Marmorkrebs (Figure 1A) has no scientific name as yet. It is genetically very similar to *Procambarus alleni*

(Faxon, 1884) and *Procambarus fallax* (Hagen, 1870) (Astacida, Cambaridae) [Scholtz et al., 2003; Keith Crandall, personal communication]. Both species look alike and coexist in some tropical sloughs of South Florida. The marbled crayfish appeared in the German aquarium trade in the mid-1990ies and has been used as an experimental animal approximately since the year 2000 [Tolley & Vogt, 2002; Scholtz et al., 2003; Vogt et al., 2004; Seitz et al., 2005]. This all-female crayfish is unique because it is the first of more than 10.000 decapod crustaceans that was shown to produce high amounts of genetically identical offspring by apomictic thelytoky [Martin et al., 2007; Vogt et al., 2008].

Life Cycle and Biology of the Marbled Crayfish

The life cycle of the marbled crayfish can be subdivided into embryonic, juvenile, adolescent, and adult phases [Vogt et al., 2004; Vogt, 2008a]. The embryonic period is completed within the eggs (Figure 1B), which are carried on the maternal pleopods. It lasts approximately 17 to 28 days, depending on female and environmental conditions. The juvenile phase includes seven to eight stages, which are characterized by a spotted pigmentation pattern (Figure 1C). The following seven to ten adolescent stages become increasingly marmorated and have clearly visible external female characters. First reproduction usually occurs at an age of five to six months and a total length of roughly 4 cm. The adult phase (Figure 1A) includes several alternating molting and reproduction cycles.

Marbled crayfish thrive best at temperatures of 18-25 °C. Maximum growth is obtained at 25 °C and maximum survival at 20 °C. They can stand temperatures below 8 °C and above 30 °C for many weeks but mortality increases under such conditions and reproduction stops [Seitz et al., 2005]. Marbled crayfish eat almost everything. In the laboratory, all life stages can be fed with a single pellet food as a sole food source (e.g. TetraWafer Mix, Tetra, Melle, Germany). Marbled crayfish can be cultured either individually or communally in all kinds of containers. The embryos and juvenile stages 1 to 4 can even be raised in micro-plates [Vogt, 2007, 2008a, b; Vogt et al., 2004, 2008].

Under favorable conditions marbled crayfish have a generation time (egg to spawning) of roughly six months. They can grow to a total length (see Figure 1A) of almost 9 cm but mostly remain smaller. The biggest Marmorkrebs, which I ever had in my laboratory, had a total length of 8.8 cm and a weight of 23.5 g. The maximal age so far recorded in my laboratory population is 1325 days (specimen still alive). Marbled crayfish can reproduce all year round with minimal intervals of 10 weeks between spawnings and have clutch sizes of 50 to 500 eggs, depending on size of the female. The viability of the eggs is often higher than 80%. The eggs and the first two lecithotrophic juvenile stages are permanently carried under the mother's abdomen. Stage 3 juveniles, and sometimes also stage 4 and stage 5 juveniles, also adhere to the maternal pleopods for resting but leave them regularly for feeding. The entire brooding period (embryonic development plus post-embryonic brood care) lasts between 35 and 55 days, depending on female and environmental conditions [Vogt & Tolley, 2004; Vogt et al., 2004; Seitz et al., 2005; Alwes & Scholtz, 2006; Vogt, 2008a, b].

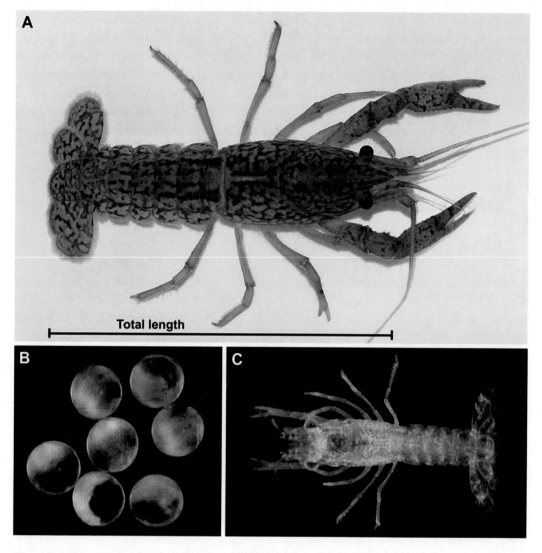

Figure 1. Life stages of the parthenogenetic marbled crayfish. A: Adult female showing eponymous marbled coloration. Horizontal bar indicates total length (tip of rostrum to end of telson), a common measure of body size in crayfish. B: In vitro cultured eggs including developing embryos. C: Juvenile with spotted pigmentation.

The marbled crayfish shares some characteristics with the well established gerontological model organisms but has several special features that qualify for use as an additional experimental animal on aging and longevity. In common with other models are easy culture, high fertility, rather short generation time, breeding at any time of the year, easy accessibility of all life stages, high tolerance to physical manipulation, and adaptability to a wide spectrum of experimental conditions [Vogt *et. al.*, 2004; Seitz et al., 2005; Vogt, 2008a, b; Vogt et al., 2008]. The generation time of the marbled crayfish of approximately six months is longer than in *Caenorhabditis elegans*, *Drosophila melanogaster*, *Mus musculus*, and *Rattus norvegicus* but within the range of *Danio rerio*. The same holds for the maximal life span of roughly 3.5 years, which is much longer than in worm and fruit fly, comparable to mouse and rat, but shorter than in zebrafish. Marbled crayfish usually die between 1.5 and 2.5 years. Only few specimens of our laboratory population reached ages exceeding three years (e.g. specimens A1 and B3$_1$, Figure 2B).

Special advantages of the marbled crayfish for research on aging and longevity are genetically identical offspring, direct embryonic development outside the body, indeterminate growth, repeated reproduction, a broad spectrum of social behavior, high regeneration ability, functionally different stem cell systems, and methylation of the DNA [Vogt et. al., 2004; Martin et al., 2007; Vogt, 2008a; Vogt et al., 2008]. The ability to thrive in very simple housing systems on a single pellet food facilitates performance of highly standardized experiments.

Longevity and Developmental Stochasticity

Aging is an inherently stochastic process that is characterized by heterogeneity between cell types and organisms. There is even variation within clonal populations raised in the same environment [e.g. Finch & Kirkwood, 2000; Herndon et al., 2002; Aranda-Anzaldo & Dent, 2003; Kirkwood et al., 2005; Rea et al., 2005; Bahar et al., 2006; Golden et al., 2006; Passos et al., 2007b; Kirkwood, 2008; Vogt et al., 2008]. Stochastic developmental variation is generated by a variety of processes like gene expression, intracellular signaling, spatial distribution of cell organelles, reaction-diffusion-like patterning mechanisms, stem cell activity during organogenesis, and non-linear self-reinforcing circuitries involving behavior, metabolism and neuronal and hormonal control [e.g. Finch & Kirkwood, 2000; Kærn et al., 2005; Maamar et al., 2007; Neildez-Nguyen et al., 2008; Vogt et al., 2008]. In freshwater crayfish, which are characterized by step-wise alteration of the phenotype via molting (see below), time and frequency of molting is a further source of randomness.

In the marbled crayfish, stochastic developmental variation can be produced in all life stages and can cause variation of practically all morphological characters and life history traits including longevity, as revealed by experiments with genetically identical sibs [Vogt et al., 2008]. The life spans of seven communally reared batch-mates, which were exposed to the same environmental and nutritional conditions at any time of their life, varied between 437 and 910 days (Figure 2, specimens B1-B7). Specimens B1 and B3-B6, which had life spans of 437, 610, 571, 910 and 568 days, respectively, died of natural causes during molting. Specimens B2 and B7 were sacrificed at day 626 for measurement of DNA-methylation.

Longevity and Epigenetic Code

It seems reasonable to assume that differences in aging and longevity among genetically identical siblings are based on differences in their epigenetic code. The epigenetic code includes methylation of cytosines, histone modifications, and DNA-binding proteins and can, unlike the genetic code, be erased and rewritten during life-time. Alteration of the epigenetic code can result in activation or silencing of genes and thus affect aging and susceptibility to diseases. Of the various epigenetic markers that regulate expression of the genome, DNA methylation is the best investigated one [e.g. Bennett-Baker et al., 2003; Jaenisch & Bird, 2003; Fraga et al., 2005; Anway et al., 2006; Whitelaw & Whitelaw, 2006; Dolinoy et al., 2007; Schiewek et al., 2007].

The marbled crayfish has methylated DNA in both the juvenile and adult life stages [Vogt et al., 2008], which is in contrast to *Caenorhabditis elegans* that lacks methylated DNA at all [Bird, 2002] and *Drosophila melanogaster* that possesses methylated DNA only through the embryonic stages [Lyko et al., 2006]. Measurement of global 5-methyl cytosine methylation in two communally reared batches of the marbled crayfish revealed variations among batch-mates, tissues and age. In a group of four 188-days old adolescents with total lengths of 3.2-4.2 cm (mean: 3.58 cm) and weights of 0.68-1.71 g (mean: 1.01 g) methylation values were 1.75-1.94% (mean: 1.86%) in the hepatopancreas and 1.96-2.09% (mean: 2.01%) in the abdominal musculature [Vogt et al., 2008]. These values were higher than those of a group of three 626-days old adults of 6.2-7.0 cm (mean: 6.7 cm) and 6.04-10.32 g (mean: 7.99 g), which had methylation ratios of 1.52-1.78% (mean: 1.65%) in the hepatopancreas and 1.77-1.92% (mean: 1.84%) in the abdominal musculature. These data suggest that in the marbled crayfish DNA methylation is reduced with age both in the hepatopancreas, the main metabolic organ of crayfish [Vogt, 2002], and the abdominal musculature. This result is contradictory to findings obtained with human monozygotic twins where the 5-methyl cytosine methylation values increased from 2.5% in 3-year old children to 3.5-4.6% in 50-year old individuals [Fraga et al., 2005]. Interestingly, in this study the youngest twins were similar with respect to their epigenetic code, whereas the oldest twins were clearly distinct.

Longevity and Allocation of Metabolic Resources

The trade-off between investment in maintenance and repair and other activities like growth and reproduction is the mainstay of the disposable soma theory, one of the mainstream theories of aging [Kirkwood, 1977, 2008]. In some species the optimal allocation of the metabolic resources is apparently fixed, whereas in others it seems to be adjusted in response to changes in circumstances [Kirkwood, 2008]. Freshwater crayfish seems to belong to the second type.

The marbled crayfish is characterized by indeterminate growth, i.e. growth that continues throughout the entire life span of an individual. This is in contrast to the most common laboratory models of gerontology like *Mus musculus*, *Rattus norvegicus*, *Caenorhabditis elegans*, and *Drosophila melanogaster*, which display determinate growth, the more or less rapid growth to a mature conclusive size. In animals with indeterminate growth like crustaceans and fish the genetic component is less important for growth and determination of the final size than the environmental conditions, which is in contrast to animals with determinate growth like mammals, birds, reptiles or holometabolous insects [Sebens, 1987; Charnov & Berrigan, 1991].

A further difference between the marbled crayfish and the common aging models with respect to growth is its step-wise increase of body size by molting [Reynolds, 2002; Vogt et al., 2004; Vogt, 2008b; Vogt et al., 2008]. During ecdysis the rigid old exoskeleton is shed and the body is enlarged by uptake of water. The new exoskeleton is then adjusted to this new size and is not significantly changed until the next ecdysis. In the intermolt period the water content of the tissues is reduced and replaced by organic material. This period is also the time of accumulation of reserves, which are mainly deposited in the hepatopancreas to be used for energy consuming processes like tissue repair, regeneration of damaged appendages, molting, or reproduction [Vogt, 1994, 2002; Vogt et al., 2004]. In their lifetime, marbled crayfish molt approximately 20-25 times [Vogt, 2008a].

Marbled crayfish usually alternate between growth and reproduction periods once they have reached sexual maturity. Mostly, there is one or two growth periods interspersed between subsequent reproduction phases. Only occasionally there are more than two growth phases intercalated. Specimen B, for instance, showed a rather typical sequence of growth and reproduction: 1st oviposition – 49 days – molt – 39 days – molt – 62 days – 2nd oviposition – 71 days – molt – 80 days – 3rd oviposition. Specimen A, in contrast, showed a rather extreme pattern: 1st oviposition – 70 days – molt – 50 days – molt – 68 days – molt – 94 days – molt – 149 days – 2nd oviposition – 43 days – molt – 39 days – 3rd oviposition – 31 days – molt – 45 days – 4th oviposition – 55 days – molt – 68 days – 5th oviposition. Specimen A was the mother of specimen A1 (Figure 2), had a total of six reproduction cycles and reached an age of 1040 days and a final total length of 7.8 cm. Specimen B was the mother of specimens B1-B7 (Figure 2), had four reproduction cycles, and reached an age of 620 days and a final total length of 6.3 cm.

In the reproduction period, a relatively high amount of energy and metabolites is required to equip the numerous eggs with yolk [Vogt et al., 1989a, 2004; Reynolds, 2002; Vogt, 2002]. Therefore, and since a certain amount of energy is required for the basic metabolism of the mother, growth stops in this period. Most breeding females even lose some weight because during breeding, and sometimes also during post-embryonic brood care, feeding is either completely suppressed or at least drastically reduced, depending on female. Under laboratory conditions with unlimited access to food, reproduction related temporal growth stop may remain without consequences for the individual concerned. However, in wild crayfish populations with limited food resources the individual decision to either grow or reproduce can have severe consequences, since dominance is positively correlated with body size. Smaller specimens also have a higher risk to be preyed upon by conspecifics or predators [Gherardi, 2002; Reynolds, 2002].

One might hypothesize that extensive allocation of metabolic resources to growth or reproduction may result in shorter life because of inadequate maintenance and tissue repair but our experiment with the communally raised batch-mates B1-B7 suggest that things are not that simple. Marked variation was not only recorded for the life span (437-910 days), but also for final total length (5.8-7.0 cm) and final weight (5.2-10.3 g) (Figure 2). The number of reproduction cycles varied from 1 to 5 and the time point of first egg laying from 157 to 531 days. There was also a broad range of variation with respect to the timing of oviposition: female B1 laid eggs at days 157, 267 and 375, B2 at days 160, 369 and 497, B3 at days 168, 392 and 502, B4 at days 183, 390 and 516, B5 at days 315, 394, 507, 643 and 850, B6 at days 328 and 507, and B7 at day 500 (Figure 2).

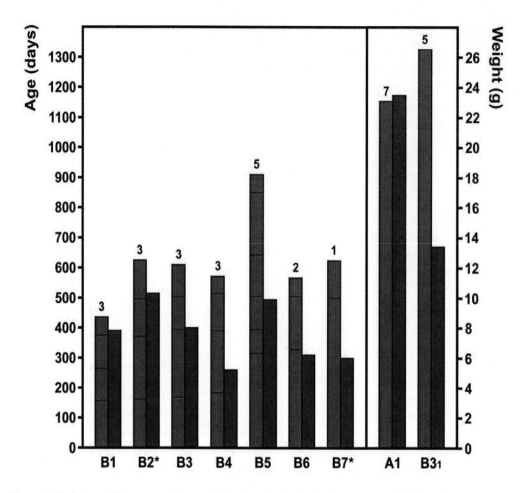

Figure 2. Variation of life span, weight, and reproduction frequency among genetically identical marbled crayfish. Shown are the data for seven communally reared batch-mates (B1-B7) and two individually reared specimens (A1 and B3$_1$) of different laboratory strains (A and B). Life span is indicated by left columns, weight by right columns, the number of reproductive cycles by figures on left columns, and the time points of egg laying by horizontal bars in left columns. Specimens B1-B7 were housed in a 60 x 30 x 30 cm aquarium filled at a water level of 15 cm and equipped with a layer of fine gravel and three stones to provide shelter and to enable breathing of atmospheric air. Temperature fluctuated between 18.0°C and 23.5°C throughout the experimental period. The crayfish were fed daily ad libitum with TetraMin Wafer Mix pellets. Water was completely changed once a week. Specimens A1 and B3$_1$ were communally reared in similar aquaria for 301 and 182 days, respectively, and then held individually in 30 x 20 x 15 cm aquaria filled at a water level of 6 cm. Water and feeding conditions were the same as for specimens B1-B7. Crayfish B3$_1$ is a progeny of female B3 and was heavily damaged during early adolescence. Specimens indicated by asterisks (B2 and B7) were sacrificed for analysis of DNA-methylation. The other crayfish died of natural causes. Specimen B3$_1$ was still alive at the end of the experimental period.

Our results suggest that, under the conditions of our experiment, longevity, growth, and reproduction were not narrowly correlated (Figure 2). There are examples like the pair B1 and B6, which seem to corroborate shortening of life expectancy by fast growth and intense reproduction. Female B1, the specimen with the shortest life span of 437 days only, showed the fastest growth during the juvenile, adolescent and early adult phases (final weight 7.8 g) and the highest number of reproduction cycles in this period of time. Specimen B6 grew slower (final weight 6.3 g) and reproduced less frequently (2 reproductive cycles) but lived longer (568 days). But there are also contradictory examples in our data set, for instance the pair B2 and B4. Specimen B2 lived longer than B4 (626 days versus 571 days) although it had grown to a considerably larger final size (7.4 g versus 5.2 g) and had reproduced as often as B4 (3 reproductive cycles).

Longevity and Social Environment

Longevity is influenced not only by the genes or developmental randomness but also by the environment [Kirkwood & Austad, 2000; Braendle et al., 2008; Kirkwood, 2008; Mangel, 2008]. The environmental component is apparently predominant in taxa with indeterminate growth such as freshwater crayfish [Sebens, 1987]. As a poikilothermic animal the marbled crayfish is particularly sensitive to water temperature [Seitz et al., 2005] but was also shown to respond to other environmental factors such as pollutants [Vogt, 2007]. Lower water temperature reduces the metabolism and may have life span extending effects similar to caloric restriction (see below) but this hypothesis was not yet tested by us. However, Seitz et al. [2005] have shown that mortality in the marbled crayfish was lower at 20 °C compared to 25 °C, which is the optimal temperature for growth.

Environmental stress is not only caused by suboptimal water parameters, inadequate food or pollutants but also by social stress. Freshwater crayfish display a variety of social behaviors including a broad spectrum of agonistic interactions, which are used to establish and maintain dominance hierarchies when living in groups. Usually, the largest specimen is the most dominant one [Gherardi, 2002; Lundberg, 2004]. In the marbled crayfish, aggressiveness among group members is not as pronounced as in other crayfish species because there are no males, which are usually bigger and more aggressive than the females. Nevertheless, when adult marbled crayfish meet in the free arena of an aquarium they often show agonistic behaviors. The intensity of such interactions increases if food or hiding possibilities are limited [Vogt et al., 2008]. Agonistic interactions are expected to cause stress and may therefore affect individual life span.

At present, we have not much data on this topic but our three oldest specimens (A, A1, B3$_1$) have in common that they were reared individually for most of their lifetime. For instance, specimen A1, the biggest and most fertile crayfish of my laboratory population with a final total length of 8.8 cm and more than 800 offspring, was reared in a group of 5 batch-mates until its first oviposition at day 301. Thereafter, it was kept individually until the end of life at day 1154 (Figure 2). Specimen B3$_1$, the oldest specimen of my laboratory population (1325 days, still alive), was communally reared in a group of ten until day 182, and then housed individually (Figure 2). These three individually reared females were kept under the same water conditions and fed ad libitum with the same pellet food as the communally reared specimens B1-B7 but lived considerably longer, suggesting that social stress may reduce life expectancy.

Longevity and Dietary Restriction

Dietary or caloric restriction, the significant reduction of food intake in the absence of malnutrition, has been shown to increase life span in mice, rats, hamsters, dogs, fish, and some invertebrates. It apparently extends life by slowing of the aging processes but the underlying mechanisms are not known as yet [Masoro, 2005; Houthoofd & Vanfleteren, 2006; Mathers, 2006; Shanley & Kirkwood, 2006; Mangel, 2008; Smith et al., 2008]. There is evidence that dietary restriction causes increased resistance against environmental stressors but no decrease of the metabolic rate [Houthoofd & Vanfleteren, 2006]. We have not yet performed experiments on caloric restriction in the marbled crayfish but highly standardized experiments on this topic are easily feasible because marbled crayfish can be fed with a single pellet food throughout all life stages. Pellets enable a much better control of the caloric intake than other food sources and their biochemical composition can be changed as desired.

Dietary restriction is experimentally accomplished either by reducing the amount of food consumed daily or by imposing intermittent fasting regimens. The marbled crayfish is well adapted to temporal fasting periods because feeding is regularly suppressed in the days before and after ecdysis and also during breeding, as described above. Therefore, comparison of dietary restriction and longevity in the marbled crayfish and species lacking regular periods of fasting may provide new insight into this topical field of aging research.

Longevity and Functional Senescence

Functional senescence is the intrinsic age-related decline in functional status with death as its ultimate consequence [Grotewiel et al., 2005]. It can be measured at the organismic, organ, or cellular level. Organismic indicators of functional senescence are, for instance, reduced motor activity, reproduction and heart rate, declined ability to respond to stress, restricted function of the immune system, and increased risk of age-associated diseases. Cellular indicators are the decline of metabolic processes, oxidative damage, loss of the ability to divide, DNA damage, shortening of the telomeres, alteration of the epigenome, or changes in quantity and structure of the cell organelles [Fraga et al., 2005; Grotewiel et al., 2005; Jiang et al., 2007; Passos et al., 2007a; Serrano & Blasco, 2007; Rossi et al., 2008]. Functional senescence is not only a valuable approach to measure the decline of particular functions across age but is also promising to identify key organs that fail with age and cause death [Kishi, 2004; Grotewiel et al., 2005].

There is apparently a considerable difference in functional senescence between animals with determinate and indeterminate growth. Animals with determinate growth like insects and mammals usually show a decline of function with increasing age [Kishi, 2004; Grotewiel et al., 2005; Rossi et al., 2008]. For instance, in rodents cellular function is increasingly impaired by oxidative damage, and in *Drosophila melanogaster* production of offspring is gradually reduced. Egg-laying in the fly reaches a maximum at day 4 of adulthood and is minimal at around 50 days of age [Grotewiel et al., 2005]. In contrast, animals with indeterminate growth like some fish and decapod crustaceans seem to show very slow or negligible functional senescence [Klapper et al., 1998a, b; Kishi, 2004].

In the marbled crayfish, there is apparently no age-related decrease in reproduction. The reproductive success rather increases with the size of a female, which is roughly correlated with age. For instance, specimen A1, which had a life span of 1154 days (Figure 2), produced 421 juveniles in its seventh and last reproduction period at around 1100 days of age. This batch comprised more than half of the total juvenile production of this female. There was also no marked age-related reduction in motor or feeding activity, suggesting that marbled crayfish show no or only little functional senescence at the organismic level. The same seems to hold for the tissue and organ level because microscopic analyses of the hepatopancreas and ovaries in juveniles, adolescents, and adults revealed no evidence for age-related alterations [Vogt et al., 2004; Vogt, 2007]. The organs of freshwater crayfish and their relatives are well investigated, both under normal and pathological conditions [e.g. Johnson, 1980; Vogt, 1987, 1990, 1992, 1994, 1999, 2002; Vogt et al., 1989a, b; Harrison & Humes, 1992; Lightner & Redman, 1998; Vogt & Štrus, 1998; Edgerton et al., 2002], providing a good data base for more detailed future investigations into this topic.

Age-related decline is at least partly caused by an imbalance between cell loss and cell renewal by stem cells. Therefore, one focus of future research on aging should be on functioning and dysfunctioning of stem cells [Rossi et al., 2008]. Particularly promising results can be expected from the stem cells of species with indeterminate growth because these remain functional until death. Such material is ideally suited to investigate the molecular mechanisms that keep stem cells working even in advanced age. The marbled crayfish harbors a variety of stem cell systems with different activity patterns, which may be well suited for research in this direction. Some types of stem cells are continuously active over long periods of time, for instance during embryonic development or limb regeneration, but others are cyclically active for short periods of time only, for instance after ecdysis or feeding [Vogt, 2008a].

Molt-related stem cells are probably located in all tissues and organs of the marbled crayfish and serve for growth and repair. For instance, in the heart we have found numerous small satellite cells distributed along the muscular fiber network. In the noble crayfish *Astacus astacus* these heart myogenic stem cells were shown to be quiescent during intermolt but were activated after ecdysis for a short period of time to enlarge the heart [Martynova, 1993]. In its lifetime, the marbled crayfish passes through 20-25 molting cycles [Vogt, 2008a; Vogt et al., 2008], and accordingly, the molt-related stem cells are activated and silenced 20-25 times as well. However, it is not yet known whether an individual stem cell divides only once or several times during a molt-related growth pulse.

Another cyclically active stem cell system independent from the molting cycle is provided by the E-cells of the hepatopancreas. The hepatopancreas is the central organ of metabolism in crayfish and other decapods and includes functions like absorption and metabolism of nutrients, storage of reserves, synthesis of digestive enzymes, and detoxification of xenobiotics [e.g. Vogt et al., 1989a, b; Vogt & Quinitio, 1994; Vogt, 1994, 2002; James et al., 1995; Möhrlen et al., 2001]. The E-cells divide in the final phase of each feeding cycle to replace regularly discharged epithelial cells [Vogt, 1994, 2002, 2007]. The E-cell system is particularly interesting because its cells are not homogeneously distributed across the organ but concentrated at the blindly ending tips of the numerous hepatopancreas tubules, propagating their descendants in one direction only. This particular division pattern results in the establishment of a distinct age gradient along the hepatopancreas tubules, resembling the situation in the crypts of Lieberkühn of the small intestine of mammals (Bach et al., 2000), or even more, the terminal meristems of plants. E-cells are apparently multipotent as they give rise to three mature cell types with different functions [Vogt, 1994, 2002]. They are thought to undergo more than 1.000 division pulses in their life-time, resembling closely the stem cells in the small intestine of mouse [Bach et al., 2000]. The hepatopancreas of crayfish has a high cellular turnover and seems to be completely renewed after approximately two weeks, as demonstrated by means of radioactive labeling [Davis & Burnett, 1964].

Further interesting stem cells are located in the brain of crayfish. In the red swamp crayfish *Procambarus clarkii*, a species closely related to the marbled crayfish [Scholtz et al., 2003], neurogenic stem cells were shown to reside in a special area of the brain, the neurogenic niche [Sullivan et al., 2007]. From there, they migrate to their site of destination and give rise to new neurons, resembling closely the situation in higher vertebrates. These and the other stem cell systems of the marbled crayfish offer promising material to investigate the molecular mechanisms that govern activation, maintenance, and silencing of adult stem cells. By comparison with mammalian stem cells they are expected to contribute to the understanding of loss of activity during aging.

One of the molecular mechanisms that lead to the decline of tissue and organ integrity during aging is telomere shortening in their stem cells [Jiang et al., 2007; Baird, 2008; Rossi et al., 2008]. The telomeres form the ends of the chromosomes and are shortened with each round of cell division. For instance, in the human pancreas telomere erosion occurs at an average rate of 36 bp per year [Ishii et al., 2006]. The initial length of the telomeres can vary and is a heritable trait [Kappei & Londono-Vallejo, 2008]. Since premature aging symptoms and age-related diseases are often associated with short telomeres, telomere length is regarded as an indicator of life expectancy [Klapper et al., 1998a; Jiang et al., 2007; Baird, 2008; Rossi et al., 2008].

Loss of the replicative capacity of cells by telomere shortening can be counteracted by activation of telomerase, a reverse transcriptase, which adds new repeats to the ends of the chromosomes. In the adults of animals with determinate growth including humans, most somatic tissues lack telomerase activity, whereas it is expressed in embryonic tissues, stem cells and tumor cells [Jiang et al., 2007; Rossi et al., 2008]. Animals with indeterminate growth, in contrast, express telomerase also in the tissues and organs of the adults, as was shown for rainbow trout *Oncorhynchus mykiss* and the American lobster *Homarus americanus* [Klapper et al., 1998a, b]. Continuous telomerase expression is thought to be the primary route for maintaining long term cell proliferation capacity and may therefore be responsible for the slow or negligible functional senescence of animals with indeterminate growth.

The marbled crayfish has not yet been investigated with respect to chromosomes, telomeres and telomerase but data obtained with its relatives suggest that research in this direction is promising. Crayfish have generally high numbers of chromosomes, and thus, plenty of telomeres to investigate. For instance, the con-generic *Procambarus clarkii* has a chromosome number (n) of 100 [Lécher et al., 1995]. Telomere structure and telomerase activity were analyzed in detail in the American lobster *Homarus americanus* [Klapper et al.,

1998b]. Telomerase activity was measured in all organs investigated and was still high in specimens of advanced age. It was highest in the hepatopancreas, which is presumably the organ with the fastest cellular turnover in decapod crustaceans.

Longevity and Diseases and Regeneration

It is trivial, that diseases can reduce the mean life span of a population and also considerably influence individual life expectancy. Interestingly, age-related diseases have not been recorded as yet in the marbled crayfish, other freshwater crayfish, or decapod crustaceans in general, although a broad spectrum of infectious, nutritional, or environmental diseases is known in this taxon [e.g. Stewart, 1984; Lightner & Hedrick, 1987; Lightner & Redman, 1998; Vogt, 1999; Edgerton et al., 2002; Vogt, 2008c]. Likewise, age-related cancer, and cancer in general, is virtually absent in crayfish and other decapods [Vogt, 2008c], although some species like lobsters can grow almost as old as humans. This scarcity of age-related diseases and tumors is probably due to the preservation of stem cell function throughout life, possession of sophisticated detoxification systems for carcinogens [James et al., 1995], and specific properties of the proPO immune system in these crustaceans. The proPO system is an arthropod-specific immune response, which is based on the activation of prophenoloxidase. It eliminates pathogens and damaged tissue areas by encapsulation and melanization [Cerenius & Söderhäll, 2004].

In contrast to crayfish, approximately 30% of the laboratory rodents have tumors at the end of their 2-3 year life span [Chandra & Frith, 1992; Anisimov et al., 2001; Rangarajan & Weinberg, 2003]. In humans and mammalian laboratory models of aging, age-related cancer is at least partly caused by the same mechanisms that ensure longevity, e.g. maintenance of the genomic stability and replicative integrity via telomere length preservation by telomerase [e.g. Hahn, 2001; Shay et al., 2001; Anisimov, 2007; Serrano & Blasco, 2007; Rossi et al., 2008]. Comparison of the marbled crayfish and the mouse, which have similar maximal body sizes and life spans but strikingly different tumor incidences, may contribute to the understanding of the causes of age-related cancer. The absence or low rate of age-associated cancer as observed in the marbled crayfish and its relatives [Vogt, 2008c] is apparently not a general feature of animals with indeterminate growth because in zebrafish age-related tumors are quite common [Rangarajan & Weinberg, 2003].

The marbled crayfish also appears very suitable to investigate the repair and regeneration of organs in detail, which is another topical aspect of aging and longevity. Like other crayfish, the marbled crayfish can autotomize and regenerate its limbs from the first juvenile stage to death. Autotomy of limbs is a natural reflex and occurs at a pre-formed fracture plane in the basis-ischium segment [Hopkins, 1993; Mykles, 2001; Vogt, 2002]. Regeneration of an autotomized limb is initiated by formation of a blastema, which is made up of mitotically active epidermis cells and immigrant cells [Hopkins, 1993]. The regenerative blastema produces different types of tissue like musculature, connective tissue, epidermis, and nervous tissue.

Our experiments revealed that damages are repaired in the marbled crayfish and do not necessarily shorten life expectancy. For instance, specimen $B3_1$, which had lost 3 of 8 walking legs and one of the two chelae in the adolescent period, recovered fully in an individual housing system throughout the next two molting cycles and reached the highest age (1325 days, still alive) ever recorded in my population. However, growth and frequency of reproduction were lower than in undamaged specimen A1 (Figure 2), although both were reared under very similar environmental and nutritional conditions, suggesting that regeneration of limbs requires a considerable proportion of the metabolic resources at cost of growth and reproduction.

Conclusion

First experiments with isogenic marbled crayfish revealed that longevity is considerably influenced by several non-genetic factors. One of them is developmental stochasticity, which was found to cause a remarkably broad range of life spans even among identically reared batch-mates. These life span differences are probably based on variations of the epigenetic code, as may be concluded from first DNA methylation data. Another life span modifying parameter is social stress that obviously reduced life expectancy in the marbled crayfish. Damages like loss of appendages had no adverse effects on longevity, at least when the regenerating specimens were isolated from conspecifics and other predators. However, growth and reproduction frequency was lower in damaged than in undamaged specimens. Due to the small sample size of our experiment we could not establish a clear relationship between longevity and growth and reproduction in normal crayfish but the strict temporal separation of growth and reproduction periods make the marbled crayfish particularly suitable to investigate this topic in depth. And first investigations into functional senescence indicate that marbled crayfish remain vital until death, which occurred during ecdysis in most of our specimens. Although the results of this study have to be regarded as preliminary they provide a first data base and may encourage future research on aging and longevity with the marbled crayfish.

References

Alwes, F. & Scholtz, G. (2006). Stages and other aspects of the embryology of the parthenogenetic Marmorkrebs (Decapoda, Reptantia, Astacida). *Dev. Genes Evol. 216*, 169-184.

Anisimov, V. N. (2007). Biology of aging and cancer. *Cancer Contr. 14*, 23-31.

Anisimov, V. N., Zabezhinski, M. A., Rossolini, G., Zaia, A., Piantanelli, A., Basso, A. & Piantanelli, L. (2001). Long-live euthymic BALB/c-nu mice. II: Spontaneous tumors and other pathologies. *Mech. Ageing Dev. 122,* 477-489.

Anway, M. D., Leathers, C. & Skinner, M. K. (2006). Endocrine disruptor vinclozolin induced epigenetic transgenerational adult-onset disease. *Endocrinology 147*, 5515-5523.

Aranda-Anzaldo, A. & Dent, M. A .R. (2003). Developmental noise, ageing and cancer. *Mech. Ageing Dev. 124*, 711-720.

Bach, S. P., Renehan, A. G. & Potten, C. S. (2000). Stem cells: the intestinal stem cell as a paradigm. *Carcinogenesis 21*, 469-476.

Bahar, R., Hartmann, C. H., Rodriguez, K. A., Denny, A. D., Busuttil, R. A., Dollé, M. E. T., Calde, R. B., Chisholm, G. B., Pollock, B. H., Klein, C. A. & Vijg, J. (2006). Increased cell-to-cell variation in gene expression in ageing mouse heart. *Nature 441*, 1011-1014.

Baird, D. M. (2008). Telomeres II. *Exp. Gerontol. 43*, 15-19.

Bartke, A. (2008). New findings in gene knockout, mutant and transgenic mice. *Exp. Gerontol. 43*, 11-14.

Bennett-Baker, P. E., Wilkowski, J. & Burke, D. T. (2003). Age-associated activation of epigenetically repressed genes in the mouse. *Genetics 165*, 2055-2062.

Bird, A. (2002). DNA methylation patterns and epigenetic memory. *Genes Dev. 16*, 6-21.

Braekman, B. P. & Vanfleteren, J. R. (2007). Genetic control of longevity in *C. elegans*. *Exp. Gerontol. 42*, 76-80.

Braendle, C., Milloz, J. & Félix, M. A. (2008). Mechanisms and evolution of environmental responses in *Caenorhabditis elegans*. *Curr. Top. Dev. Biol. 80*, 171-207.

Brys, K., Vanfleteren, J. R. & Braeckman, B. P. (2007). Testing the rate-of-living/oxidative damage theory of aging in the nematode model *Caenorhabditis elegans*. *Exp. Gerontol. 42, Sp. Iss.*, 845-851.

Cerenius, L. & Söderhäll, K. (2004). The prophenoloxidase-activating system in invertebrates. *Immunol. Rev. 198*, 116-126.

Chandra, M. & Frith, C. H. (1992). Spontaneous neoplasms in aged CD-1 mice. *Toxicol. Lett. 61*, 67-74.

Charnov, E. L. & Berrigan, D. (1991). Evolution of life history parameters in animals with indeterminate growth, particularly fish. *Evol. Ecol. 5*, 63-68.

Conn, P. M. (2006). *Handbook of models for human aging*. New York: Academic Press.

Davis, L. E. & Burnett, A. L. (1964). A study of growth and cell differentiation in the hepatopancreas of the crayfish. *Dev. Biol. 10*, 122-153.

Dolinoy, D. C., Weidman, J. R. & Jirtle, R. L. (2007). Epigenetic gene regulation: linking early developmental environment to adult disease. *Reprod. Toxicol. 23*, 297-307.

Edgerton, B. F., Evans, L. H., Stephens, F. J. & Overstreet, R. M. (2002). Synopsis of freshwater crayfish diseases and commensal organisms. *Aquaculture 206*, 57-135.

Enns, L. C., Wiley, J. C. & Ladiges, W. C. (2008). Clinical relevance of transgenic mouse models for aging research. *Crit. Rev. Eukaryot. Gene Expr. 18*, 81-91.

Evason, K., Collins, J. J., Huang, C., Hughes, S. & Kornfeld, K. (2008). Valproic acid extends *Caenorhabditis elegans* lifespan. *Ageing Cell 7*, 305-317.

Finch, C. E. & Kirkwood, T. B. L. (2000). *Chance, development and aging*. New York: Oxford University Press.

Fraga, M. F., Ballestar, E., Paz, M. F., Ropero, S., Setien, F., Ballestar, M. L., Heine-Suñer, D., Cigudosa, J. C., Urioste, M., Benitez, J., Boix-Chornet, M., Sanchez-Aguilera, A., Ling, C., Carlsson, E., Poulsen, P., Vaag, A., Stephan, Z., Spector, T. D., Wu, Y.-Z.,

Plass, C. & Esteller, M. (2005). Epigenetic differences arise during the lifetime of monozygotic twins. *PNAS 102*, 10604-10609.

Gerhard, G. S. & Cheng, K. C. (2002). A call to fins! Zebrafish as a gerontological model. *Aging Cell 1*, 104-111.

Gherardi, F. (2002). Behaviour. In D. M. Holdich (Ed.), *Biology of freshwater crayfish* (pp. 258-290). Oxford: Blackwell.

Golden, T. R., Hubbard, A. & Melov, S. (2006). Microarray analysis of variation in individual aging *C. elegans*: Approaches and challenges. *Exp. Gerontol. 41*, 1040-1045.

Grotewiel, M. S., Martin, I., Blandari, P. & Cook-Wiens, E. (2005). Functional senescence in *Drosophila melanogaster. Ageing Res. Rev. 4*, 372-397.

Hahn, W. C. (2001). Telomerase and cancer: where and when? *Clin. Cancer Res. 7*, 2953-2954.

Harrison, F. W. & Humes, A. G. (Eds.) (1992). *Microscopic anatomy of invertebrates, vol. 10: Decapod Crustacea*. New York: Wiley-Liss.

Hengherr, S., Brümmer, F. & Schill, R. O. (2008). Anhydrobiosis in tardigrades and its effects on longevity traits. *J. Zool. 275*, 216-220.

Herndon, L. A., Schmeissner, P. J., Dudaronek, J. M., Brown, P. A., Listner, K. M., Sakano, Y., Paupard, M. C., Hall, D. H. & Driscoll, M. (2002). Stochastic and genetic factors influence tissue-specific decline in ageing *C. elegans. Nature 419*, 808-814.

Hopkins, P. M. (1993). Regeneration of walking legs in the fiddler crab, *Uca pugilator. Amer. Zool. 33*, 348-356.

Houthoofd, K. & Vanfleteren, J. R. (2006). The longevity effect of dietary restriction in *Caenorhabditis elegans. Exp. Gerontol. 41*, 1026-1031.

Ishii, A., Nakamura, K., Kishimoto, H., Honma, N., Aida, J., Sawabe, M., Arai, T., Fujiwara, M., Takeuchi, F., Kato, M., Oshimura, M., Izumiyama, N. & Takubo, K. (2006). Telomere shortening with aging in the human pancreas. *Exp. Gerontol. 41*, 882-886.

Jaenisch, R. & Bird, A. (2003). Epigenetic regulation of gene expression: how the genome integrates intrinsic and environmental signals. *Nat. Genet. Suppl. 33*, 245-254.

James, M. O., Altman, A. H., Li, C.-L. J. & Schell, J. D. Jr. (1995). Biotransformation, hepatopancreas DNA binding and pharmacokinetics of benzo[*a*]pyrene after oral and parenteral administration to the American lobster, *Homarus americanus. Chem.-Biol. Interact. 95*, 141-160.

Jiang, H., Ju, Z. & Rudolph, K. L. (2007). Telomere shortening and ageing. *Z. Gerontol. Geriat. 40*, 314-324.

Johnson, P. T. (1980). *Histology of the blue crab, Callinectes sapidus*. New York: Praeger.

Johnson, T. E. (2008). *Caenorhabditis elegans* 2007: The premier model for the study of aging. *Exp. Gerontol. 43*, 1-4.

Kærn, M., Elston, T. C., Blake, W. J. & Collins, J. J. (2005). Stochasticity in gene expression: from theories to phenotype. *Nat. Rev. Genet. 6*, 451-464.

Kappei, D. & Londono-Vallejo, J. A. (2008). Telomere length inheritance and aging. *Mech. Ageing Dev. 129*, 17-26.

Kennedy, B. K. (2008). The genetics of ageing: insight from genome-wide approaches in invertebrate model organisms. *J. Int. Med. 263*, 142-152.

Kirkwood, T. B. L. (1977). Evolution of ageing. *Nature 270*, 301-304.

Kirkwood, T. B. L. (2008). Understanding ageing from an evolutionary perspective. *J. Intern. Med. 263*, 117-127.

Kirkwood, T. B. L. & Austad, S. N. (2000). Why do we age? *Nature 408*, 233-238.

Kirkwood, T. B. L., Feder, M., Finch, C. E., Franceschi, C., Globerson, A., Klingenberg, C. P., LaMarco, K., Omholt, S. & Westendorp, R. G. J. (2005). What accounts for the wide variation in life span of genetically identical organisms reared in a constant environment? *Mech. Ageing Dev. 126*, 439-443.

Kishi, S. (2004). Functional aging and gradual senescence in zebrafish. *Ann. N. Y. Acad. Sci. 1019*, 521-526.

Kitani, K. (2007). Pharmacological interventions in aging and age-associated disorders. *Geriat. Gerontol. Int. 7*, 97-103.

Klapper, W., Heidorn, K., Kühne, K., Parwaresh, R. & Krupp, G. (1998a). Telomerase activity in 'immortal' fish. *FEBS Letters 434*, 409-412.

Klapper, W., Kühne, K., Singh, K. K., Heidorn, K., Parwaresh, R. &, Krupp, G. (1998b). Longevity of lobsters is linked to ubiquitous telomerase expression. *FEBS Letters 439*, 143-146.

Kuningas, M., Mooijaart, S. P., Van Heemst, D., Zwaan, B. J., Slagboom, P. E. & Westendorp, R. G. J. (2008). Genes encoding longevity: from model organisms to humans. *Aging Cell 7*, 270-280.

Lécher, P., Defaye, D. & Nöel, P. (1995). Chromosomes and nuclear DNA of Crustacea. *Invertebr. Reprod. Dev. 27*, 85-114.

Lepperdinger, G., Berger, P., Breitenbach, M., Frohlich, K.-U., Grillari, J., Grubeck-Loebenstein, B., Madeo, F., Minois, N., Zwerschke, W. & Jansen-Durr, P. (2008). The use of genetically engineered model systems for research on human aging. *Front. Biosci. 13*, 7022-7031.

Lightner, D. V. & Hedrick, R. P. (1987). Embryonal carcinoma of developing embryos of grass shrimp *Palaemon orientis* (Crustacea, Decapoda). *Dis. Aquat. Org. 3*, 101-106.

Lightner, D. V. & Redman, R. M. (1998). Shrimp diseases and current diagnostic methods. *Aquaculture 164*, 201-220.

Lundberg, U. (2004). Behavioural elements of the noble crayfish, *Astacus astacus* (Linnaeus, 1758). *Crustaceana 77*, 137-162.

Lyko, F., Beisel, C., Marhold, J. & Paro, R. (2006). Epigenetic regulation in *Drosophila*. *Curr. Top. Microbiol. Immunol. 310*, 23-44.

Maamar, H., Raj, A. & Dubnau, D. (2007). Noise in gene expression determines cell fate in *Bacillus subtilis*. *Science 317*, 526-529.

Mangel, M. (2008). Environment, damage and senescence: modelling the life-history consequences of variable stress and caloric intake. *Funct. Ecol. 22*, 422-430.

Martin, P., Kohlmann, K. & Scholtz, G. (2007). The parthenogenetic Marmorkrebs (marbled crayfish) produces genetically uniform offspring. *Naturwissenschaften 94*, 843-846.

Martynova, M. G. (1993). Satellite cells in the crayfish heart muscle function as stem cells and are characterized by molt-dependent behaviour. *Zool. Anz. 230*, 181-190.

Masoro, E. J. (2005). Overview of caloric restriction and ageing. *Mech. Ageing Dev. 126*, 913-922.

Mathers, J. C. (2006). Nutritional modulation of ageing: Genomic and epigenetic approaches. *Mech. Ageing Dev. 127*, 584-589.

Möhrlen, F., Baus, S., Gruber, A., Rackwitz, H.-R., Schnölzer, M., Vogt, G. & Zwilling, R. (2001). Activation of pro-astacin. Immunological and model peptide studies on the processing of immature astacin, a zinc-endopeptidase from the crayfish *Astacus astacus*. *Eur. J. Biochem. 268*, 2540-2546.

Münch, D., Amdam, G. V. & Wolschin, F. (2008). Ageing in a eusocial insect: molecular and physiological characteristics of life span plasticity in the honey bee. *Funct. Ecol. 22*, 407-421.

Mykles, D. L. (2001). Interactions between limb regeneration and molting in decapod crustaceans. *Amer. Zool. 41*, 399-406.

Neildez-Nguyen, T. M. A., Parisot, A., Vignal, C., Rameau, P., Stockholm, D., Picot, J., Allo, V., Le Bec, C., Laplace, C. & Paldi, A. (2008). Epigenetic gene expression noise and phenotypic diversification of clonal cell populations. *Differentiation 76*, 33-40.

Passos, J. F., von Zglinicki, T. & Kirkwood, T. B. L. (2007a). Mitochondria and ageing: winning and losing in the numbers game. *BioEssays 29*, 908-917.

Passos, J. F., Saretzki, G., Ahmed, S., Nelson, G., Richter, T., Peters, H., Wappler, I., Birket, M. J., Harold, G., Schaeuble, K., Birch-Machin, M. A., Kirkwood, T. B. L. & von Zglinicki, T. (2007b). Mitochondrial dysfunction accounts for the stochastic hetero-geneity in telomere-dependent senescence. *PLoS Biol. 5*, e110.

Rangarajan, A. & Weinberg, R. A. (2003). Comparative biology of mouse versus human cells: modelling human cancer in mice. *Nat. Rev. Cancer 3*, 952-959.

Rea, S. L., Wu, D., Cypser, J. R., Vaupel, J. W. & Johnson, T. E. (2005). A stress-sensitive reporter predicts longevity in isogenic populations of *Caenorhabditis elegans*. *Nat. Genet. 37*, 894-898.

Reynolds, J. D. (2002). Growth and reproduction. In D. M. Holdich (Ed.), *Biology of freshwater crayfish* (pp. 152-191). Oxford: Blackwell.

Ricci, C. & Covino, C. (2005). Anhydrobiosis of *Adineta ricciae*: costs and benefits. *Hydrobiology 546*, 307-314.

Ricci, C. & Pagani, M. (1997). Desiccation of *Panagrolaimus rigidus* (Nematoda): survival, reproduction and the influence on the internal clock. *Hydrobiology 347*, 1-13.

Rossi, D. J., Jamieson, C. H. M. & Weissman, I. L. (2008). Stem cells and the pathways to aging and cancer. *Cell 132*, 681-696.

Salminen, A., Huuskonen, J., Ojala, J., Kauppinen, A., Kaarniranta, K. & Suuronen, T. (2008). Activation of innate immunity system during aging: NF-κB signaling is the molecular culprit of inflamm-aging. *Ageing Res. Rev. 7*, 83-105.

Schiewek, R., Wirtz, M., Thiemann, M., Plitt, K., Vogt, G. & Schmitz O. J. (2007). Determination of the DNA methylation level of the marbled crayfish: an increase in sample throughput by an optimised sample preparation. *J. Chromatogr. B 850*, 548-552.

Scholtz, G., Braband, A., Tolley, L., Reimann, A., Mittmann, B., Lukhaup, C., Steuerwald, F. & Vogt, G. (2003). Parthenogenesis in an outsider crayfish. *Nature 421*, 806.

Sebens, K. P. (1987). The ecology of indeterminate growth in animals. *Ann. Rev. Ecol. Syst. 18*, 371-407.

Seitz, R., Vilpoux, K., Hopp, U., Harzsch, S. & Maier, G. (2005). Ontogeny of the Marmorkrebs (marbled crayfish): a parthenogenetic crayfish with unknown origin and phylogenetic position. *J. Exp. Zool. A 303*, 393-405.

Serrano, M. & Blasco, M. A. (2007). Cancer and ageing: convergent and divergent mechanisms. *Nat. Rev. Mol. Cell Biol. 8*, 715-722.

Shanley, D. P. & Kirkwood, T. B. L. (2006). Caloric restriction does not enhance longevity in all species and is unlikely to do so in humans. *Biogerontology 7*, 165-168.

Shay, J. W., Zou, Y., Hiyama, E. & Wright, W. E. (2001). Telomerase and cancer. *Hum. Mol. Genet. 10*, 677-685.

Smith, E. D., Kaeberlein, T. L., Lydum, B. T., Sager, J., Welton, K. L., Kennedy, B. K. & Kaeberlein, M. (2008). Age- and calorie-independent life span extension from dietary restriction by bacterial deprivation in *Caenorhabditis elegans*. *BMC Dev. Biol. 8*, 49.

Stewart, J. E. (1984). Lobster diseases. *Helgoland Mar. Res. 37*, 243-254.

Sullivan, J. M., Benton, J. L., Sandeman, D. C. & Beltz, B. S. (2007). Adult neurogenesis: a common strategy across diverse species. *J. Comp. Neurol. 500*, 574-584.

Terzibasi, E., Valenzano, D. R. & Cellerino, A. (2007). The short-lived fish *Nothobranchius furzeri* as a new model system for aging studies. *Exp. Gerontol. 42*, 81-89.

Tolley, L. & Vogt, G. (2002). Reproduction of the marble crayfish, a presumptive partheno-genic decapod. *8th Colloquium Crustacea Decapoda Mediterranea, Corfu, Greece, Sept. 2-6, 2002. Abstracts*, 97.

Valdesalici, S. & Cellerino, A. (2003). Extremely short lifespan in the annual fish *Nothobranchius furzeri*. *Proc. R. Soc. Lond. B (Suppl.) 270*, S189-S191.

Vogt, G. (1987). Monitoring of environmental pollutants such as pesticides in prawn aqua-culture by histological diagnosis. *Aquaculture 67*, 157-164.

Vogt, G. (1990). Pathology of midgut gland-cells of *Penaeus monodon* postlarvae after *Leucaena leucocephala* feeding. *Dis. Aquat. Org. 9*, 45-61.

Vogt, G. (1992). Transformation of anterior midgut and hepatopancreas cells by *Monodon Baculovirus* (MBV) in *Penaeus monodon* postlarvae. *Aquaculture 107*, 239-248.

Vogt, G. (1994). Life-cycle and functional cytology of the hepatopancreatic cells of *Astacus astacus* (Crustacea, Decapoda). *Zoomorphology 114*, 83-101.

Vogt, G. (1999). Diseases of European freshwater crayfish, with particular emphasis on interspecific transmission of pathogens. In F. Gherardi & D. M. Holdich (Eds.), *Crayfish in Europe as alien species* (pp. 87-103). Crustacean Issues 11. Rotterdam: Balkema.

Vogt, G. (2002). Functional anatomy. In D. M. Holdich (Ed.), *Biology of freshwater crayfish* (pp. 53-151). Oxford: Blackwell.

Vogt, G. (2007). Exposure of the eggs to 17α-methyl testosterone reduced hatching success and growth and elicited teratogenic effects in postembryonic life stages of crayfish. *Aquat. Toxicol. 85*, 291-296.

Vogt, G. (2008a). The marbled crayfish: a new model organism for research on development, epigenetics, and evolutionary biology. *J. Zool. 276*, 1-13.

Vogt, G. (2008b). Investigation of hatching and early post-embryonic life of freshwater crayfish by *in vitro* culture, behavioral analysis, and light and electron microscopy. *J. Morphol. 269*, 790-811.

Vogt, G. (2008c). How to minimize formation and growth of tumours: potential benefits of decapod crustaceans for cancer research. *Int. J. Cancer 123*, 2727-2734.

Vogt, G. & Quinitio, E. T. (1994). Accumulation and excretion of metal granules in the prawn, *Penaeus monodon,* exposed to water-borne copper, lead, iron and calcium. *Aquat. Toxicol. 28*, 223-241.

Vogt, G. & Štrus, J. (1998). Diseases of the shrimp *Palaemon elegans* (Crustacea, Decapoda) in the Bay of Piran, Adriatic Sea. *J. Nat. Hist. 32*, 1795-1806.

Vogt, G. & Tolley, L. (2004). Brood care in freshwater crayfish and relationship with the offspring´s sensory deficiencies. *J. Morphol. 262*, 566-582.

Vogt, G., Quinitio, E. T. & Pascual, F. P. (1989a). Interaction of the midgut gland and the ovary in vitellogenesis and consequences for the breeding success: a comparison of unablated and ablated spawners of *Penaeus monodon*. In N. de Pauw, E. Jaspers, H. Ackefors & N. Wilkins (Eds.), *Aquaculture: a biotechnology in progress* (pp. 581-592). Bredene: European Aquaculture Society.

Vogt, G., Stöcker, W., Storch, V. & Zwilling, R. (1989b). Biosynthesis of *Astacus* protease, a digestive enzyme from crayfish. *Histochemistry 9,* 373-381.

Vogt, G., Tolley, L. & Scholtz, G. (2004). Life stages and reproductive components of the Marmorkrebs (marbled crayfish), the first parthenogenetic decapod crustacean. *J. Morphol. 261*, 286-311.

Vogt, G., Huber, M., Thiemann, M., van den Boogaart, G., Schmitz, O. J. & Schubart, C. D. (2008). Production of different phenotypes from the same genotype in the same environment by developmental variation. *J. Exp. Biol. 211*, 510-523.

Whitelaw, N. C. & Whitelaw, E. (2006). How lifetimes shape epigenotype within and across generations. *Hum. Molec. Genet. 15, Rev. Iss. 2*, R131-137.

In: Handbook on Longevity: Genetics, Diet and Disease   ISBN 978-1-60741-075-1
Editors: Jennifer V. Bentely and Mary Ann Keller   © 2009 Nova Science Publishers, Inc.

Chapter XVI

Genetic Background for Longevity in Livestock Species: A Review

Joaquim Casellas
Genètica i Millora Animal, IRTA-Lleida, 25198 Lleida, Spain

Introduction

Longevity is a trait of major interest in livestock with important implications on both economic and animal welfare grounds. The relevance of longevity within the animal production framework was highlighted during the twentieth century with a plethora of studies focusing on environmental sources of variation. Although the specific molecular mechanisms involved in the longevity of domestic species remains unclear, recent studies have provided plenty of evidence of genetic determinism for aging-related traits in livestock. Indeed, longevity must be viewed as the final expression of a dynamic system governed by intrinsic (e.g. immunology, reproduction, and growth) and extrinsic determinants (e.g. temperature, food, and predators), in which every intrinsic determinant (and some extrinsic determinants, such as resistance to cold temperatures) is virtually modulated by genes. As the influence of genes is inextricably intertwined with longevity, it is virtually impossible to consider the broad determinants of longevity without a basic understanding of the underlying genetics.

Although longevity is not a conceptually new trait in livestock production, several advances relating to genetic background and genetic mechanisms have been achieved during the last few decades. The earliest investigations focused on non-additive genetic effects (i.e. inbreeding depression and crossbreeding/heterosis) that have a non-negligible impact on livestock longevity. Nevertheless, the recent development of specific analytical models has allowed a straightforward characterization of additive genetic sources of variation with moderate to low heritabilities in all species, and an increasing number of quantitative trait loci and candidate genes that influence the aging process. These models have resulted in systematic international genetic evaluations for cow longevity in dairy cattle and in some local breeding programs in other species and breeds. This has produced the first evidence of genetic progress due to selection programs. Future research into livestock longevity will focus on new technological platforms such as massive single nucleotide polymorphism genotyping and gene expression microarray in order to provide a more detailed characterization of the aging process in our domestic breeds. Within this context, the genetics of longevity in livestock species encompasses not only estimations of preliminary additive and non-additive genetic effects, but also national/international breeding programs and the latest technologies for addressing the genetic mechanisms that determine livestock lifespan.

Longevity under Farm Management

Longevity is straightforwardly defined as "length of life", a biological event that starts at birth (or at early stages of gestation) and finishes at death. This process can be viewed as a genetically determined and environmentally modulated phenomenon, although the respective contributions of the two components vary greatly across species and even across individuals within a given species. This huge variability is highlighted in Table 1, where a wide range of species-specific longevity values are reported. For example, potential life expectancy is around 10 years for the majority of domestic mammals (carnivores, ruminants and pigs), with it being slightly shorter for birds (e.g. chickens, ducks and pigeons) and clearly longer for equine species (horses and donkeys; Table 1). Note that these are average values and that maximum longevities may be much greater, ranging from 18 years (in the case of rabbits) to 62 years (in that of horses; Carey and Judge, 2000).

Although this chapter focuses on genetics, environmental influences can also play a key role in the longevity of domestic livestock. A substantial percentage of individuals does not die of natural causes on the farm but is culled due to insufficient performance. Note that these human-induced deaths do not invalidate the usefulness of longevity studies relating to domestic livestock, although they may require a more specific description of the longevity process. In such cases, longevity must be viewed as the length of "productive" life, where the term "productive" implies a second criterion modulating animal longevity: the productive life span during the period in which the animal is alive and reaches or surpasses a minimal, and often arbitrary, level of performance which is measured in terms of growth, milk yield, progeny, or other factors. This is an additional source of variability in longevity studies and requires additional efforts to appropriately model lifespan data for different livestock species. These data must be treated with a certain degree of caution, principally in the case of breeds reared under more intensive production systems. Dairy and beef cattle provide very representative examples of this phenomenon. The average longevity of the former is dramatically reduced in milk-producing systems (~3 years; Caraviello et al., 2004b), whereas beef cattle longevities tend to be similar to their biological potentials (Tarrés et al., 2004). The productive lives of dairy cows are greatly reduced by extraordinary milk yields and high energy demands that, on average, cannot be maintained for more than a couple of lactations. Other intensive production systems show similar trends, as observed in the case of pigs (~3 years; Yazdi et al., 2000a) and rabbits (~1.5 years; Sánchez et al., 2004). In contrast, non-intensive beef production systems are associated with rather natural conditions that allow an almost complete expression of potential longevity. As suggested in Table 1, environmental modulation of longevity could have a huge impact on final performance. Specific statistical approaches are therefore required to appropriately correct for environmental sources of variation and to precisely estimate genetic effects. In this way, it will be possible to avoid bias due to farm management practices or artificial reductions in animal lifespan.

Table 1. Potential longevity (adapted from Carey and Judge (2000)) and expected longevity under standard farm management of domestic species (years)

Species	Potential longevity		Expected longevity under standard farm management (reference)	
	Expected	Maximum		
Cat	10 - 12	34		
Chicken	7 - 8	30		
Cow	9 - 12	20	~3 ~9	(dairy; Caraviello et al., 2004b) (beef; Tarrés et al., 2004)
Dog	10 - 12	30		
Donkey	18 - 20	47		
Duck	10	20		
Goat	12	21		
Horse	20 - 25	62		
Pig	10	27	~3	(Yazdi et al., 2000a)
Pigeon	10	35		
Rabbit	6 - 8	18	~1.5	(Sánchez et al., 2004)
Sheep	12	24	~6	(El-Saied et al., 2005)

Additive Polygenic Background

The first evidence of selective breeding in pigeons, dogs and cattle was reported by Darwin (1859). This human-related influence on the genetics of domestic livestock persisted during the late 19th century and throughout the 20th century, with a plethora of animal breeding initiatives, which mainly focused on the additive genetic component (Fisher, 1918; Henderson, 1973). Within this context, current breeding schemes are based on the availability of reliable additive genetic variance components and breeding value estimates. This is a key point for livestock longevity because of the peculiarities of failure time data (i.e. censoring, non-Gaussian patterns; Ducrocq et al., 1988a) and the availability of proper methods to model longevity. Indeed, the controversy over the application of survival analysis techniques (Cox, 1972; Ducrocq et al., 1988a,b) and linear/threshold mixed models (VanRaden & Klaaskate, 1993; Guo et al., 2001; Caraviello et al., 2004a) has reached its maximum expression with regard to heritability and estimations of additive breeding value for the length of productive life (Serenius & Stalder, 2006).

Survival analysis relies on the proportional hazard model first described by Sir. D. R. Cox (Cox, 1972) and based on the modeling of a flexible (non-)parametric baseline hazard function that properly accounts for a wide range of departures from data normality (Casellas et al., 2006). Given its ability to properly account for censored data and time-dependent effects, survival analysis is considered theoretically superior for the analysis of longevity data (Ducrocq et al., 1988a; Caraviello et al., 2004a), although the greater computational demands (Ducrocq et al., 2000) and the complexity of constructing multi-trait models (Damgaard & Korsgaard, 2006; Tarrés et al., 2006) have limited its implementation in favor of more conventional threshold/linear mixed model approaches. Length of productive life has been analyzed using linear mixed models that also account for censored records within a Bayesian framework through a data augmentation step (Guo et al., 2001). On the other hand, stayability - recorded as a binary trait indicating whether an animal has reached some fixed age - is typically modeled using mixed threshold models (Boettcher et al., 1999; López-Serrano et al., 2000). Estimates obtained under this heterogeneity of analytical approaches are not totally comparable, but provide us with a complex scenario in which the magnitude of the additive genetic background for livestock longevity can be roughly characterized.

The heritability estimates presented in the literature indicate that it is possible to select for livestock longevity; however, the magnitude of heritability estimates varies greatly according to different definitions of the longevity traits in question, the analytical models applied, and the populations studied (Serenius & Stalder, 2006). In dairy cattle, 21 of the 37 references shown in Table 2 (57%) obtained heritability estimates that were equal to or lower than 0.10. Almost null estimates were also obtained, although they were inferred under linear mixed models and with a discrete characterization of longevity (Dematawewa & Berger, 1998). It should be noted that proportional hazard models typically provide higher heritabilities than linear or threshold mixed models (Serenius & Stalder, 2006). The remaining 16 articles reported a wide range of values, with a maximum estimate of 0.22 (Neerhof et al., 2000), although provision was also made for estimates of lower than 0.10. These values suggested two main relationships: a) longevity must be additively influenced by genes, and b) the additive polygenic effect has a moderate to low impact on longevity. More specifically, this genetic effect could be split into two different contributions. Firstly, longevity in dairy cows could, theoretically, be regulated by genes that have a direct influence on animal lifespan and aging, as previously demonstrated in mice and humans (Osiewacz, 1997; de Magalhães et al., 2005; Casellas & Medrano, 2008). Alternatively, the genetic variability in some culling factors (e.g. cow fertility, milk production or composition, and udder health; Weigel et al., 2003; Hadley et al., 2006) could be accumulated in the infinitesimal genetic effect of longevity when these systematic effects are not completely accounted for by the analytical model (see below). Whatever the case, this does not invalidate the use of additive genetic background for dairy cattle longevity but rather suggests that specific and indirect genes could act together.

Table 2. Estimated heritabilities for longevity in dairy cattle populations

Breed	Country	Model[1]	Heritability	Reference
Ayrshire	Canada	PHM, C	0.09^2	Sewalem et al., 2006
Braunvieh	Switzerland	PHM, C	$0.06^2, 0.18^3$	Vukasinovic et al., 2001
Crossbred	Australia	LMM, D	0.01 to 0.09	Madgwick & Goddard, 1989
Danish BW[4]	Denmark	PHM, C	$0.06^2, 0.22^3$	Neerhof et al., 2000
Dutch BW	The Netherlands	PHM, C	$0.04^2, 0.11^3$	Vollema et al., 2000
Dutch RW[4]	The Netherlands	PHM, C	$0.04^2, 0.10^3$	Vollema et al., 2000
Guernsey	USA	LMM, C	0.12	Cruickshank et al., 2002
Holstein	Canada	LMM, C	0.08	Jairath et al., 1994
Holstein	Canada	LMM, D	0.04 to 0.05	Boettcher et al., 1999
Holstein	Canada	TMM, D	0.07	Boettcher et al., 1999
Holstein	Canada	PHM, C	0.05 to 0.07^2 0.09 to 0.12^3	Boettcher et al., 1999
Holstein	Canada	PHM, C	0.08 to 0.09^2 0.15 to 0.20^3	Dürr et al., 1999
Holstein	Canada	PHM, C	0.14^2	Sewalem et al., 2005
Holstein	Czech Republic	PHM, C	$0.03^1, 0.04^3$	Páchová et al., 2005
Holstein	Germany	PHM, C	0.11 to 0.12^2 0.17 to 0.18^3	Buenger et al., 2001
Holstein	Spain	PHM, C	0.02 to 0.03^2 0.05 to 0.07^3	Chirinos et al., 2007
Holstein	Spain	TMM, D	0.11	González-Recio & Alenda, 2007
Holstein	Switzerland	PHM, C	$0.07^2, 0.18^3$	Vukasinovic et al., 2001
Holstein	The Netherlands	LMM, D	0.01 to 0.12	Vollema & Groen, 1996
Holstein	The Netherlands	LMM, C	0.03 to 0.14	Vollema & Groen, 1996
Holstein	The Netherlands	LMM, C	0.07 to 0.08	Vollema & Groen, 1998
Holstein	The Netherlands	PHM, C	0.02	Vollema & Groen, 1998
Holstein	USA	LMM, D	0.02 to 0.05	Hudson & Van Vleck, 1981
Holstein	USA	PHM, C	0.09^2	Ducrocq et al., 1988b
Holstein	USA	LMM, C	0.03	Boldman et al., 1992
Holstein	USA	LMM, D	0.01 to 0.04	Short & Lawloar, 1992
Holstein	USA	LMM, D	0.03 to 0.09	VanRaden & Klaaskate, 1993
Holstein	USA	LMM, D	0.002 to 0.01	Dematawewa & Berger, 1998
Holstein	USA	PHM, C	0.06 to 0.13^2	Caraviello et al., 2004b
Holstein	USA	LMM, C	0.08 to 0.10	Tsuruta et al., 2005
Holstein	Canada	LMM, D	0.01 to 0.06	Van Doormaal et al., 1985

Table 2 (Continued).

Breed	Country	Model[1]	Heritability	Reference
Jersey	Canada	PHM, C	0.10^2	Sewalem et al., 2005
Jersey	USA	LMM, C	0.07	Caraviello et al., 2004a
Jersey	USA	PHM, C	$0.05^2, 0.18^3$	Caraviello et al., 2004a
Simmental	Switzerland	PHM, C	$0.06^2, 0.20^3$	Vukasinovic et al., 2001
Swedish RW	Sweden	PHM, C	$0.06^2, 0.10^3$	Röxtrom and Strandberg, 2002
Swedish RW	Sweden	PHM, C	0.14 to 0.18^3	Roxtröm et al., 2003

[1]PHM: proportional hazard model; LMM: linear mixed model; TMM: threshold mixed model; C: continuous trait (time interval); D: discrete trait (dead or alive at a given age).
[2] Heritability on the log-transformed scale.
[3] Heritability on the observed scale.
[4] BW: Black and White; RW: Red and White.

As indicated in the previous section, beef cattle commonly demonstrate greater longevities than dairy cattle (Caraviello et al., 2004b; Tarrés et al., 2004). This could be one of the main reasons for the slightly higher heritabilities reported in Table 3. Note that some evidence of heritabilities increasing with age has been reported by VanRaden & Klaaskate (1993), Vega (1999) and Martínez et al. (2005), while the formula proposed by Tarrés et al. (2005) relied on this peculiarity of longevity data. Moreover, beef breeds are typically associated with smaller selection intensities than dairy breeds (e.g. Holstein; Mc Parland et al., 2006), which should lead to smaller losses of genetic variability and produce higher heritabilities. Table 3 shows a wide range of estimates fluctuating from 0 (Vega, 1999) to 0.68 (Snelling et al., 1995). Even so, the majority of estimates fell between 0.10 and 0.20. Within the substantial heterogeneity of heritability estimates, it is important to note that analyses performed on a discrete characterization of cow longevity (i.e. stayability at a given age) provided the highest values. Analyses of longevity defined on a continuous scale provided estimates of between 0.03 (Roughsedge et al., 2005) and 0.16 (Tanida et al., 1988). The only two analyses performed using proportional hazards models reported a small range of heritabilities of between 0.09 and 0.11 for Chianina cattle (Forabosco et al., 2006b) and of between 0.11 and 0.14 for a crossbred population (Rogers et al., 2004). The reported superiority of survival analyses techniques (Ducrocq et al., 1988a; Caraviello et al., 2004a) suggests that, although slightly greater than in dairy breeds, the genetic background of longevity in beef cows should be considered modest. Nevertheless, these estimates could be used support genetic selection programs for cow longevity, as reported below.

In 2003, genomic causes of sheep longevity caused considerable controversy and were discussed worldwide by scientists and non-scientists alike due to the premature death of Dolly (Wilmut et al., 1997), the first cloned mammal. Nevertheless, the genetic backgrounds for the longevity of the remaining 1,000 million sheep and rams in the world remain unclear. Very few studies have been conducted (Table 4), with reported heritabilities ranging from 0 (Brash et al., 1994) to 0.33 (Vatankhah & Zamani, 2007). Nevertheless, these heritabilities were generally low and suggested a pattern similar to those observed for dairy cattle. These estimates contrast with the moderate heritabilities reported for lamb survival in recent studies. Although early survival cannot be compared with adult longevity, it is important to note that Southey et al. (2001, 2003) obtained heritabilities ranging from 0.13 to 0.21 in a 50% Columbia, 25% Hampshire and 25% Suffolk composite population. These findings were further corroborated in more specific competing risk analyses in which values ranged from 0.08 to 0.16 (Southey et al., 2004). These values are not exempt from controversy given that small heritabilities for lamb survival have also been reported (0.027; Casellas et al., 2007).

Table 3. Estimated heritabilities for longevity in beef cattle populations

Breed	Country	Model[1]	Heritability	Reference
Angus	Canada	LMM, D	0.23 to 0.24	Rasali et al_2005
Angus	USA	LMM, D	0.02 to 0.68	Snelling et al., 1995
Angus	USA	LMM, C	0.05	Tanida et al., 1988
Angus	USA	TMM, D	0.14 to 0.15	Doyle et al., 2000
Angus	United Kingdom	LMM, C	0.13	Roughsedge et al., 2005
Canchim	Brazil	TMM, D	0.07 to 0.08	Nieto et al., 2007
Chianina	Italy	LMM, D	0.03 to 0.05	Forabosco et al., 2006
Chianina	Italy	LMM, C	0.08	Forabosco et al., 2006
Chianina	Italy	PHM, C	0.09 to 0.11[2]	Forabosco et al., 2006
Crossbred	South Africa	TMM, D	0.03 to 0.11	van der Westhuizen et al., 2001
Crossbred	USA	PHM, C	0.11 to 0.14[2]	Rogers et al., 2004
Crossbred	USA	TMM, D	0 to 0.28	Vega, 1999
Hereford	USA	LMM, C	0.16	Tanida et al., 1988
Hereford	USA	LMM, D	0.07	Mwansa et al., 2002
Hereford	USA	LMM, C	0.05 to 0.15	Martínez et al., 2004
Hereford	USA	LMM, D	0.09 to 0.35	Martínez et al., 2005
Hereford	USA	TMM, D	0.09 to 0.30	Martínez et al., 2005
Limousine	United Kingdom	LMM, C	0.08	Roughsedge et al., 2005
Nellore	Brazil	TMM, D	0.12 to 0.18	Silva et al., 2003
Nellore	Brazil	TMM, D	0.22 to 0.24	Silva et al., 2006
Nellore	Brazil	TMM, D	0.22 to 0.28	Van Melis et al., 2007
Simmental	United Kingdom	LMM, C	0.03	Roughsedge et al., 2005
South Devon	United Kingdom	LMM, C	0.10	Roughsedge et al., 2005

[1]PHM: proportional hazard model; LMM: linear mixed model; TMM: threshold mixed model; C: continuous trait (time interval); D: discrete trait (dead or alive at a given age).

[2] Heritability on the log-transformed scale.

[3] Heritability on the observed scale.

Table 4. Estimated heritabilities for longevity in sheep populations

Breed	Country	Model[1]	Heritability	Reference
Churra	Spain	LMM, C	0.02 to 0.06	El-Saied et al., 2005
Dorset	Australia	LMM, C	0.00 to 0.03	Brash et al., 1994
Lori-Bakhtiari	Iran	LMM, C	0.33	Vatankhah & Zamani, 2007
Scottish Blackface	United Kingdom	LMM, C	0.08	Conington et al., 2001

[1]LMM: linear mixed model; C: continuous trait (time interval).

Table 5. Estimated heritabilities for longevity in swine populations

Breed	Country	Model[1]	Heritability	Reference
Duroc	Spain	PHM, C	0.07[2]	Fernàndez de Sevilla et al., 2008
Landrace	Finland	LMM, C	0.05	Serenius & Stalder, 2004
Landrace	Finland	PHM, C	0.16 to 0.17[2]	Serenius & Stalder, 2004
Landrace	Germany	TMM, D	0.07 to 0.11	López-Serrano et al., 2000
Landrace	Sweden	PHM, C	0.05 to 0.12[2] 0.11 to 0.27[3]	Yazdi et al., 2000b
Landrace	USA	LMM, C	0.23 to 0.25	Guo et al., 2001
Large White	Finland	LMM, C	0.10	Serenius & Stalder, 2004
Large White	Finland	PHM, C	0.17 to 0.19[2]	Serenius & Stalder, 2004
Large White	Germany	TMM, D	0.08 to 0.10	López-Serrano et al., 2000
Yorkshire	Sweden	PHM, C	0.09 to 0.13[2] 0.21 to 0.31[3]	Yazdi et al., 2000a

[1]PHM: proportional hazard model; LMM: linear mixed model; TMM: threshold mixed model; C: continuous trait (time interval); D: discrete trait (dead or alive at a given age).
[2] Heritability on the log-transformed scale.

Sow longevity is an important factor in the pig industry, although selection for this trait is not commonly practiced. There is relatively little scientific literature concerning the additive genetic background for sow longevity, with a moderate range of heritabilities (Table 5). In addition to differences due to longevity trait definitions, estimates also vary according to the analytical method used and the formula applied for heritability. Estimates of sow longevity heritabilities based on survival analysis have ranged from 0.05 (Serenius & Stalder, 2004) to 0.31 (Yazdi et al., 2000a) and from 0.05 (Serenius & Stalder, 2004) to 0.25 (Guo et al., 2001) in linear and threshold model analyses, respectively. Moreover, Guo et al. (2001) suggested that heritability estimates tend to decrease with increasing censoring rates, even when a linear mixed model is applied. As Serenius & Stalder (2006) concluded, the heritability estimates presented in the literature indicate that sufficient genetic variation is present in most swine populations for sow longevity to be improved through direct selection. As observed in sheep populations, heritabilities for the early survival of piglets is a controversial subject, as observed values ranged from 0.03 (Casellas et al., 2004; Cecchinato et al., 2008) to 0.18 (Mesa et al., 2006).

Heritabilities for longevity in other domestic species are shown in Table 6. Ricard & Fournet-Hanocq (1997) reported a moderate estimate in jumping horses, whereas controversial heritabilities were reported for both laying hens (Ducrocq et al., 2000; Ellen et al., 2008) and rabbits (Piles et al., 2006a; Sánchez et al., 2004, 2006). Even so, these values were within the range previously reported for other species of livestock, which suggests that breeding programs for livestock longevity could be carried out.

Table 6. Estimated heritabilities for longevity in other domestic species

Species	Country	Model[1]	Heritability	Reference
Jumping horse	France	PHM, C	0.18^2	Ricard & Fournet-Hanocq, 1997
Laying hen	France	PHM, C	0.17 to 0.49^2	Ducrocq et al., 2000
Laying hen	The Netherlands	LMM, C	0.02 to 0.10	Ellen et al., 2008
Rabbit	Spain	PHM, C	0.05^2	Sánchez et al., 2004
Rabbit	Spain	PHM, C	0.19 to 0.31	Piles et al., 2006a
Rabbit	Spain	PHM, C	0.10^2	Sánchez et al., 2006

[1]PHM: proportional hazard model; LMM: linear mixed model; C: continuous trait (time interval).
[2] Heritability on the log-transformed scale.

Non-Additive Polygenic Background

Historically, farmers have been interested in two main sources of non-additive genetic effects in livestock: heterosis and inbreeding. The two phenomena have opposite effects on livestock performance and were systematically taken into account in breeding and crossbreeding programs in the last century. Nevertheless, a more general point of view can be assessed in mixed models through the inclusion of random dominance effects (see Hoeschele & VanRaden [1991] for additional details) in which the magnitude of the effect can be expressed as a percentage of the total phenotypic variance. Relevant dominance variance relating to stayability and the length of productive variance has been reported for Landrace, Large White and crossbred sows (3% to 12%; Serenius et al., 2006). Similar values were reported by Van Tassell et al. (2000; 5.7%) for Holstein cows, whereas Fuerst & Sölkner (1994) obtained the greatest values for dominance variance, accounting for between 19% and 35% of phenotypic variance, in purebred Simmental, crossbred Simmental, and Braunvieh crossed with Brown Swiss cows. These estimates highlight the relevant contribution of non-additive genetic sources of variation to livestock longevity.

Heterosis, also known as hybrid vigor, is defined as the deviation from the mean of reciprocal F_1 crosses from the mean of the two parent breeds. In cattle, heterosis increases cow longevity, with crossbred animals exhibiting lower mortality rates than purebreds (Bailey, 1991). More specifically, Rohrer et al. (1988) reported a significant average increase of 829.2 days in the productive longevity (28.4%) of first-generation crosses between Angus, Brahman, Hereford, Holstein and Jersey cattle breeds. Núñez-Dominguez et al. (1991) observed an increase ranging from 15.2% to 16.8% (from 0.99 to 1.36 years; with differences due to culling policies) in a complete diallel cross involving three beef cattle breeds: Angus, Hereford and Shorthorn. Similar percentage increases in cow longevity due to heterosis were reported by Spelbring et al. (1977) for Angus × Milking Shorthorn cows (16.5%; 0.56 years), Sharma et al. (2000; 15.0% to 18.0%) for Friesian × Sahiwal cows, and Heins et al. (2006) for crossbreds of Holstein with Normande, Montbeliarde and Scandinavian Red dairy cows. These estimates suggest a moderate influence of heterosis on cow survival, with expected increases for full heterosis of around 15-20%, although higher values cannot be discarded.

The effect of heterosis on the longevity of rabbit has been recently analyzed within the context of proportional hazard models (Piles et al., 2006b). This analysis was performed on three selected lines and their reciprocal crosses, with almost null and positive effects on longevity, according to the lines involved. Significant estimates reported 1.28 ($P<0.10$) and 1.42 ($P<0.05$) times higher death risks associated with parental lines than reciprocal crosses. Although these values could not be transformed into percentages, they were similar to estimates for between-line differences of direct and maternal genetic effects relating to rabbit doe longevity.

On the other hand, inbreeding occurs when related animals are mated and this is quantified by a coefficient which measures the probability of the two alleles at any autosomal locus in an individual being identical by descent (i.e. descending from the same allele carried by a particular ancestor; Wright, 1922). In theory, inbreeding reduces genetic variability and increases homozygosis for recessive deleterious alleles. The effect of inbreeding in livestock has only been addressed in dairy cattle and sows, but available information suggests that longevity decreases with inbreeding (Thompson et al., 2000a,b; Van Tassell et al., 2000; Caraviello et al., 2003; Sewalem et al., 2006). Despite slight discrepancies between papers, a reduction of approximately 5 days of productive life for each 1% increase in inbreeding was reported by Fuest & Sölkner (1994) and Smith et al. (1998). This estimate implies a reduction of around half a lactation for a 25% inbred cow.

A recent study addressed the effect of inbreeding depression on Landrace sow longevity, accounting for heterogeneous effects across founder-specific partial inbreeding (Casellas et al., 2008b). Analyses were performed on a population of more than 4,000 sows in which inbreeding was generated from 35 founders. A substantial degree of heterogeneity between founder-specific inbreeding depression effects was revealed, with negative and neutral effects on sow longevity. For the most penalizing founder, risk of death respectively increased 1.078 and 2.138 times for 1% and 10% of inbred descendants (Casellas et al., 2008b). This study confirmed the overall average negative effect of inbreeding on longevity traits, although suggested that relevant differences would exist, with these depending on the deleterious genetic load of each founder. Although further studies are required, these results could facilitate more accurate management of inbreeding and inbreeding depression in livestock.

Quantitative Trait Loci and Candidate Genes

With the molecular revolution in full swing and, in particular, the development of gene markers covering all livestock chromosomes, several quantitative trait loci (QTL) and candidate genes for influencing the aging process of domestic animals have been reported during the last decade (Tables 7 and 8). Note that there are a huge number of lethal and disease-related loci with obvious effects on livestock longevity (OMIA, 2008), but this section concentrates on genes or QTL that influence longevity under standard physiological and productive conditions. Within this context, reliable data are scarce and this poses a challenge when compiling lists of such genetic polymorphisms. The majority of studies has addressed this phenomenon in dairy cattle.

Although several genomic regions have been significantly associated with productive longevity or neonatal survival, these results are not exempt from controversy. The genetic mechanism involved in this phenotypic change cannot be easily characterized. Both direct influences on the aging process and indirect effects through factors affecting livestock survival would be involved, with the final inference being highly dependent on the model applied. We could take locus bone morphogenetic protein 1B receptor (BMP1BR) in sheep as an example, where a mutation in the intracellular kinase domain gives rise to the Booroola phenotype. Lambs with mutant alleles are born with lighter weights (Southey et al., 2002) and consequently suffer a greater risk of death during the neonatal period (Southey et al., 2002; Casellas et al., 2007). Could this locus be considered a genetic regulator of lamb survival? Direct effects on lamb survival obviously cannot be discarded, although the most plausible mechanism would seem to be linked to impaired survivability due to lighter birth weight. Within this context, the BMP1BR locus could be viewed as an indirect genetic regulator of lamb survival. This would be a plausible assumption for several of the QTL and candidate genes reported in Tables 7 and 8, respectively. However, readers must be cautious in interpreting the associations summarized in these tables because they are simply a collection of genetic components potentially involved in the direct or indirect regulation of livestock survival and longevity.

As shown in Table 7, several of the QTL distributed in six chromosomes were associated with productive longevity in dairy cattle. These results suggest a joint contribution of multiple genomic regions in the genetic regulation of longevity, which was previously suggested by the statistically relevant detection of additive and dominant polygenic effects on longevity (see sections above). In a similar way, several candidate genes have been reported to have significant associations with productive longevity and neonatal survival in cattle, as well as in other livestock species, such as sheep, chicken and pigs (Table 8). Many of the QTL of candidate genes are only of minor interest, as they have been the subject of one report but lack additional confirmations. Nevertheless, the assimilation of the results obtained in experimental species (de Magalhães et al., 2005) and the molecular and gene-mapping revolutions now underway will lead to an explosion of knowledge in this area in the years ahead. To fully exploit the genetic variation that does occur, breeders and researchers need to be continually on the lookout for unusually long-lived animals and must save them and their progeny whenever possible.

Table 7. Quantitative trait loci detected for length of productive life

Species	Chromosome	QTL location (cM)	Reference
Cattle	2	60 to 75	Kuhn et al. (2003)
Cattle	4	28	Heyden et al. (1999)
Cattle	7	77 to 83	Ashwell et al. (2004)
Cattle	16	1 to 39	Zhang et al. (1998)
Cattle	18	30 to 50	Muncine et al. (2006)
Cattle	18	77	Kuhn et al. (2003)
Cattle	21	66	Heyden et al. (1999)
Chicken	10	62 to 82	Rabie et al. (2005)

Table 8. Candidate genes with significant effects on longevity and survival

Gene	Species	Trait	Reference
α_{S1}-casein	Cattle	Productive life	Prinzenberg et al. (2005)
β3-adrenergic receptor	Sheep	Neonatal survival	Forrest et al. (2003, 2006, 2007)
β-hydroxylase	Pig	Neonatal survival	Casellas et al. (2008a)
Bone morphogenetic protein 1B receptor	Sheep	Neonatal survival	Southey et al. (2002)
Fibroblast growth factor 2	Cattle	Productive life	Wang et al. (2008)
Calpastatin	Cattle	Productive life	García et al. (2006)
Mammalian follicle stimulating hormone	Pig	Neonatal survival	Li et al. (2008)
MX1	Chicken	Neonatal survival	Livant et al. (2007)
POU class 1 homebox 1	Cattle	Productive life	Huang et al. (2008)
Protease inhibitor	Cattle	Productive life	Khatib et al. (2005)
Uterine milk proteins	Cattle	Productive life	Khatib et al. (2007)
Microsatellites (BMS2519, BM103 and 513)	Cattle	Productive life	Ashwell & Van Tassell (1999)
Multiple single nucleotide polymorphisms	Chicken	Neonatal survival	Long et al. (2007)

Breeding Programs and the Generation of Long-Lived Lines

After their initial domestication, for centuries, livestock were unconsciously selected (Darwin, 1959) for productive traits of interest, which would no doubt have also included longevity (Zohary et al., 1998). Indeed, long lived individuals would have been present in a greater number of breeding seasons and would therefore have contributed more offspring to the next generation. This mechanism was the basis of the empirical methods of selection applied by individual farmers which eventually led to the huge number of livestock breeds currently available. When selection became a scientifically based technique, which progressed with the knowledge of the biological and genetic processes involved, the development of breeding plans focused on direct productive traits such as milk yield, litter size and growth penalized fitness traits (e.g. fertility, stayability). Longevity was omitted for decades and the breeds with the shortest longevities (and the highest production levels) were favored (Table 1), although some of the results obtained are rather controversial (Theilgaard et al., 2006). This phenomenon was characterized by Everett et al. (1976) in USA dairy cattle, where Ayrshire, Guernsey and Holstein cows showed a significant negative trend for stayability from 1965 onwards, which was phenotypically corroborated by Nieuwhof et al. (1989).

Interest in livestock longevity in dairy cattle has increased in recent years, and national genetic evaluations were implemented in France (Ducrocq, 1999), Austria and Germany (Pasman & Reinhardt, 1999), The Netherlands (De Jong et al., 1999) and Italy (Schneider & Miglior, 1999) in 1997, 1998, 1999 and 1999, respectively. An international genetic evaluation is currently being performed by the International Bull Evaluation Service (INTERBULL; http://www.interbull.org/framesida-home.htm) for direct longevity of dairy bulls from Australia, Belgium, Canada, Denmark, Finland, France, Germany, Hungary, Ireland, Israel, Italy, New Zealand, Spain, Sweden, Switzerland, The Netherlands, The United Kingdom and The United States of America. This initiative includes the Red Dairy Cattle, Brown Swiss, Guernsey, Jersey, Holstein and Simmental breeds. The service will contribute very interesting data about genetic trends in dairy cow longevity over the next few years, although initial estimates have not detected any significant changes in average breeding value associated with longevity (Ducrocq, 2005). A breeding scheme including longevity as a selection objective has also been proposed for the Chianina beef cattle breed (Forabosco et al., 2006a).

Possibly the most interesting initiative within the framework of livestock longevity is the recent generation of a long-lived rabbit line (Sánchez et al., 2008). This line was founded by selecting females from commercial farms that had extremely productive lives (measured in terms of the number of parturitions) but whose prolificacy was near of above average for the Spanish commercial rabbit population. Founder females were subject to very high intensity selection: 25 to 38 parturitions at an average of 8.7 live-born rabbits per parturition (see Sánchez et al. (2008) for a detailed description of the foundation process). As seen in the exhaustive study performed by Sánchez et al. (2008), this long-lived line was as productive as other commercial lines with an average increase in mean productive life across farms of 31.63 days. Note that this value is approximately half of the average interval between parturitions for this species. The longer productive life of this new rabbit line could be partially understood as an indication of the success of the selection procedure during foundation. This result must be viewed as the first successful selection experiment for productive longevity in domestic livestock.

Conclusion

Our current knowledge of genetic background for livestock longevity has been outlined in this chapter, in which relevant evidence of additive and non-additive genetic mechanisms has been discussed. Although the genetics of longevity remains a relatively novel research field in domestic species, recent studies have provided very appealing results and substantial efforts are currently being made to genetically improve our livestock, particularly in the case of dairy cattle. Moreover, the molecular and statistical revolutions currently underway will lead to an explosion of knowledge in this area in the years ahead. Further efforts will focus on detecting specific genes linked with long-lived variants and also on generating long-lived lines, following on from the work pioneered by Sánchez et al. (2008).

This kind of research is particularly relevant in the context of current production systems and its relevance will increase in the coming years. There has been an underlying philosophical change in production strategies. Livestock had to be more and more productive the 20th century, almost to their biological limit in several species. This led to a drastic and rather unnatural reduction of the productive lives. Recently, several studies have shown that longevity must be considered in selection programs (Forabosco et al., 2006) and that economic productivity could increase with greater longevity, albeit at the expense of a reduction in other classical production parameters. Note that the economic relevance of livestock longevity on our farms is high (Jalvingh et al., 1992), given its close relation with culling costs. Furthermore, society's concern for the well-being of domestic animals has increased in recent years (Camm & Bowles, 2000), with animal welfare and short longevities becoming increasingly important issues. Further studies are needed into livestock production systems and breeding programs in order to better understand and manage the genetic mechanisms involved in animal longevity and generate, or genetically improve, current breeds and thereby extend the productive life of our livestock without substantial losses of economic efficiency.

References

Ashwell MS; Heyen DW; Sonstegard TS; Van Tassell CP; Da Y; VanRaden PM; Ron M; Weller JI, Lewin HA. Detection of quantitative trait loci affecting milk production, health, and reproductive traits in Holstein cattle. *Journal of Dairy Science*, 2004, 87, 468-475.

Ashwell, MS; Van Tassell, CP. Detection of putative loci affecting milk, health, and type traits in a US Holstein population using 70 microsatellite markers in a genome scan. *Journal of Dairy Science*, 1999, 82, 2497-2502.

Bailey, CM. Life span of beef-type Bos Taurus and Bos indicus × Bos Taurus females in a dry, temperate climate. *Journal of Animal Science*, 1991, 69, 2379-2386.

Boettcher, PJ; Jairath, LK; Dekkers, JCM. Comparison of methods for genetic evaluation of sires for survival of their daughters in the first three lactations. *Journal of Dairy Science*, 1999, 82, 1034-1044.

Boldman, KG; Freeman, AE; Harris, BL. Prediction of sire transmitting abilities for herd life transmitting abilities for linear type traits. *Journal of Dairy Science*, 1992, 75, 552-563.

Borg, RC. 2007. Phenotypic and genetic evaluation of fitness characteristics in sheep under a range environment. Ph.D. Thesis. Virgina Polytechnic Institute and State University, Blacksburg, VI, USA.

Brash, LD; Fogarty, NM; Gilmour, AR. Reproductive performance and genetic parameters for Australian Dorset sheep. *Australian Journal of Agricultural Research*, 1994, 45, 427-441.

Buenger, A; Ducrocq, V; Swalve, HH. Analysis of survival in dairy cows with supplementary data on type scores and housing systems from a regions of Northwest Germany. *Journal of Dairy Science*, 2001, 1531-1541.

Camm, T; Bowles, D. Animal welfare and the reaty of Rome – legal analysis of the protocol on animal welfare and welfare standards in the European Union. *Journal of Environmental Law*, 2000, 12, 197-205.

Caraviello, DZ; Weigel, KA; Gianola, D. Analysis of the relationship between type traits, inbreeding, and functional survival in Jersey cattle using a Weibull proportional hazards model. *Journal of Dairy Science*, 2003, 86, 2984-2989.

Caraviello, DZ; Weigel, KA; Gianola, D. Comparison between a Weibull proportional hazards model and a linear model for predicting the genetic merit of US Jersey sires for daughter longevity. *Journal of Dairy Science*, 2004a, 87, 1469-1476.

Caraviello, DZ; Weigel, KA; Gianola, D. Prediction of longevity breeding values for US Holstein sires using survival analysis methodology. *Journal of Dairy Science*, 2004b, 87, 3518-3525.

Carey, JR; Judge, DS. Longevity records: life spans of mammals, birds, amphibians, reptiles and fish. Odense: Odense University Press; 2000.

Casellas, J; Caja, G; Such, X; Piedrafita, J. Survival analysis from birth to slaughter of Ripollesa lambs under semi-intensive management. *Journal of Animal Science*, 2007, 85, 512-517.

Casellas, J; Medrano, JF. Lack of Socs2 expression reduces lifespan in high-growth mice. *Age*, 2008, 30, 245-249.

Casellas, J; Noguera, JL; Varona, L; Sánchez, A; Arqué, M; Piedrafita, J. Viability of Iberian × Meishan F_2 newborn pigs. II. Survival analysis up to weaning. *Journal of Animal Science*, 2004, 82, 1925-1930.

Casellas, J; Tarrés, J; Piedrafita, J; Varona, L. Parametric bootstrap for testing model fitting in the proportional hazards framework: An application to the survival analysis of Bruna dels Pirineus beef calves. *Journal of Animal Science*, 2006, 84, 2609-2616.

Casellas, J; Tomás, A; Sánchez, A; Alves, E; Noguera, JL; Piedrafita, J. Using haplotype probabilities in categorical survival analysis: a case study with three candidate genes in an Iberia × Meishan F$_2$ population of newborn pigs. *Journal of Animal Breeding and Genetics*, 2008a, 125, 5-12.

Casellas, J; Varona, V; Ibáñez-Escriche, N; Noguera, JL. Analysis of founder-specific inbreeding depression on Landrace sow longevity. *Journal of Animal Science*, 2008b, 86 (E-suppl. 2), 209.

Cecchinato, A; Bonfatti, V; Gallo, L; Carnier, P. Survival analysis of pre-weaning piglet survival in a dry-cured ham-producing crossbred line. *Journal of Animal Science*, 2008,, 86, 2486-2495.

Chirinos, Z; Carabaño, MJ; Hernández, D; Genetic evaluation of length of productive life in Spanish Holstein-Friesian population. Model validation and genetic parameters estimation. *Livestock Science*, 2007, 106, 120-131.

Conington, J; Bishop, SC; Grundy, B; Waterhouse, A; Simm, G. Multi-trait selection indexes for sustainable UK hill sheep production. *Animal Science*, 2001, 73, 413-423.

Cox, DR. Regression models and life tables (with discussion). *Journal of the Royal Statistical Society Series B*, 1972, 34, 187-220.

Cruickshank, J; Weigel, KA; Dentine, MR; Kirkpatrick, BW. Indirect prediction of herd life in Guernsey Dairy Cattle. *Journal of Dairy Science*, 2002, 85, 1307-1313.

Damgaard, LH; Korsgaard, IR. A bivariate quantitative genetic model for a linear Gaussian trait and a survival trait. *Genetics, Selection, Evolution*, 2006, 38, 45-64.

Darwin, CR. On the Origin of Species by Means of Natural Selection, or the Preservation of Favoured Races in the Struggle for life. 1st edition. London: John Murray; 1959.

De Jong, G; Vollema, AR; Van der Beek, S; Harbers, A. Breeding value for functional longevity in the Netherlands. *Interbull Bulletin*, 1999, 21, 68-72.

de Magalhães, JP; Cabral, JAS; de Magalhães, D. The influence of genes on the aging process of mice: a statistical assessment of the genetics of aging. *Genetics*, 2005, 169, 265-274.

Dematawewa, CMB; Berger, PJ. Genetic and phenotypic parameters for 305-day yield, fertility, and survival in Holsteins. *Journal of Dairy Science*, 1998, 81, 2700-2709.

Doyle, SP; Golden, BL; Green, RD; Brinks, JS. Additive genetic parameter estimates for heifer pregnancy and subsequent reproduction in Angus females. *Journal of Animal Science*, 2000, 78, 2091-2098.

Ducrocq, V; Extension of survival analysis to discrete measures of longevity. *Interbull Bulletin*, 1999, 21, 41-47.

Ducrocq, V; An improved model for the French genetic evaluation of dairy bulls on length of productive life of their daughters. *Animal Science*, 2005, 80, 249-255.

Ducrocq, V; Besbes, B; Protais, M. Genetic improvement of laying hens viability using survival analysis. *Genetics, Selection, Evolution*m, 2000, 32, 23-40.

Ducrocq, V; Quaas, RL; Pollak, EJ; Casellas, G. Length of productive life of dairy cows. 1. Justification of a Weibull model. *Journal of Dairy Science*, 1988a, 71, 3061-3070.

Ducrocq, V; Quaas, RL; Pollak, EJ; Casellas, G. Length of productive life of dairy cows. 2. Variance component estimation and sire evaluation. *Journal of Dairy Science*, 1988b, 71, 3071-3079.

Dürr, JW; Monardes, HG; Cue, RI. Genetic aspects of herd life in Quebec Holsteins using Weibull models. *Journal of Dairy Science*, 1999, 82, 2503-2513.

Ellen, ED; Visscher, J; van Arendonk, JAM; Bijma, P. Survival of laying hens: genetic parameters for direct and associative effects in three purebred layer lines. *Poultry Science*, 2008, 87, 233-239.

El-Saied, UM; De La Fuente, LF; Carriedo, JA; San Primitivo, F. Genetic and phenotypic parameter estimates of total and partial lifetime traits for dairy ewes. *Journal of Dairy Science*, 2005, 88, 3265-3272.

Everett, RM; Keown, JF; Clapp, EE. Production and stayability trends in dairy cattle. *Journal of Dairy Cattle*, 1976, 59, 1532-1539.

Fernàndez de Sevilla, X; Fàbrega, E; Tibau, J; Casellas J. Effect of leg conformation on survivability of Duroc, Landrace, and Large White sows. *Journal of Animal Science*, 2008, 86, 2392-2400.

Fisher, RA. The correlation between relatives on the supposition of Mendelian inheritance. *Transactions of the Royal Society of Edinburgh*, 1918, 52, 399-433.

Forabosco, F; Boettcher, P; Bozzi, R; Filippini, F; Bijma, P. Genetic selection strategies to improve longevity in Chianina beef cattle. *Italian Journal of Animal Science*, 2006a, 5, 117-127.

Forabosco, F; Bozzi, R; Filippini, F; Boettcher, P; Van Arendonk, JAM; Bijma, P. Linear model vs. survival analysis for genetic evaluation of sires for longevity in Chianina beef cattle. *Livestock Science*, 2006b, 101, 191-198.

Forrest, RH; Hickford, JGH; Frampton, CM. Polymorphism at the bovine β3-adrenergic receptor locus (ADRB3) and its association with lamb mortality. *Journal of Animal Science*, 2007, 85, 2801-2806.

Forrest, RH; Hickford, JGH; Hogan, A; Frampton, C. Polymorphism at the ovine β3-adrenergic receptor locus: associations with birth weight, growth rate, carcass composition and cold survival. *Animal Genetics*, 2003, 34, 19-25.

Forrest, RH; Hickford, JGH; Wynyard, J; Merrick, N; Hogan, A; Frampton, C. Polymorphism at the β3-adrenergic receptor (ADRB3) locus of Merino sheep and its association with lamb mortality. *Animal Genetics*, 2006, 37, 465-468.

Fuerst, C; Sölkner, J. 1994. Additive and nonadditive genetic variances for milk yield, fertility, and lifetime performances traits of dairy cattle. *Journal of Dairy Science*, 1994, 77, 1114-1125.

Garcia, MD; Michal, JJ; Gaskins, CT; Reeves, JJ; Ott, TL; Liu, Y; Jiang, Z. Significant association of the calpastatin gene with fertility and longevity in dairy cattle. *Animal Genetics*, 2006, 37, 304-305.

González-Recio, O; Alenda, R. Genetic relationship of discrete-time survival with fertility and production in dairy cattle using bivariate models. *Genetics, Selection, Evolution*, 2007, 39, 391-404.

Guo, S-F; Gianola, D; Rekaya, R; Short, T. Bayesian analysis of lifetime performance and prolificacy in Landrace sows using a linear mixed model with censoring. *Livestock Production Science*, 2001, 72, 243-252.

Hadley, GL; Wolf, CA; Harsh, SB. Dairy cattle culling patterns, explanations, and implications. *Journal of Dairy Science*, 2006, 89, 2286-2296.

Heins, BJ; Hansen, LB; Seykora, AJ. Fertility and survival of pure Holstein versus crossbreds of Holstein with Normande, Montbeliarde, and Scandinavian Red. *Journal of Dairy Science*, 2006, 89, 4944-4951.

Henderson, CR. Sire evaluation and genetic trends. In: *Proceedings of the Animal Breeding and Genetics Symposium in Honor of Jay L. Lush*, Champaign, ASAS and ADSA; 1973; 10-41.

Heyden DW; Weller JI; Ron M; Band M; Beever JE; Feldmesser E; Da Y; Wiggans GR; VanRaden PM; Lewin HA. A genome scan for QTL influencing milk production and health traits in dairy cattle. *Physiological Genomics*, 1999, 1, 165-175.

Hoeschele, I; VanRaden, PM. Rapid inversion of dominance relationship matrices for noninbred populations by including sire by dam subclass effects. *Journal of Dairy Science*, 1991, 74, 557-569.

Huang, W; Maltecca, C; Khatib, H. A praline-to-histidine mutation in POUF1F1 is associated with production traits in dairy cattle. *Journal of Animal Breeding and Genetics*, 2008, (in press).

Hudson, GFS; Van Vleck, LD. Relationship between production and stayability in Holstein cattle. *Journal of Dairy Science*, 1981, 64, 2246-2250.

Jairath, LK; Hayes, JF; Cue, RI. Multitrait resticted maximum likelihood estimates of genetic and phenotypic parameters of lifetime performance traits for Canadian Holsteins. *Journal of Dairy Science*, 1994, 77, 303-312.

Jalving, AW; Dijkhuizen, AA; van Arendonk, JAM; Brascamp, EM. An economic comparison of management strategies on reproduction and replacement in sow herds using a dynamic probabilistic model. *Livestock Production Science*, 1992, 32, 331-350.

Khatib, H; Heifetz, E; Dekkers, JC. Association of the protease inkibitor gene with production traits in Holstein dairy cattle. *Journal of Dairy Science*, 2005, 88, 1208-1213.

Khatib, H; Schutzkus, V; Chang, YM; Rosa, GJM. Pattern of expression of the uterine milk protein gene and its association with productive life in dairy cattle. *Journal of Dairy Science*, 2007, 90, 2427-2433.

Kuhn CH; Bennewitz J; Reinsch N; Xu N; Thomsen H; Looft C; Brockmann GA; Schwerin M; Weimann C; Hiendleder S; Erhardt G; Medjugor R. Quantitative trait loci mapping of functional traits in the German Holstein cattle population. *Journal of Dairy Cattle*, 2003, 86, 360-368.

Li, FE; Mei, SQ; Deng, CY; Jiang, SW; Zuo, B; Zheng, R; Li, JL; Xu, DQ; Lei, MG; Xiong, YZ. Association of a microsatellite flanking FSHB gene with reproductive traits and reproductive tract components in pig. *Czech Journal of Animal Science*, 2008, 53, 139-144.

Livant, EJ; Avedaño, S; McLeod, S; Ye, X; Lamont, SJ; Dekkers, JCM; Ewald, SJ. MX1 exon 13 polymorphisms in broiled breeder chickens and associations with commercial traits. *Animal Genetics*, 2007, 38, 177-190.

Long, N; Gianola, D; Rosa, GJM; Weigel, KA; Avedaño, S. Machine learning classification procedure for selecting SNPs in genomic selection: application to early mortality in broilers. *Journal of Animal Breeding and Genetics*, 2007, 124, 377-389.

López-Serrano, M; Reinsch, N; Looft, H; Kalm, E. Genetic correlations of growth, backfat thickness and exterior with stayability in large white and landrace sows. *Livestock Production Science*, 2000, 64, 121-131.

Madgwick, PA; Goodard, ME. Genetic and phenotypic parameters of longevity in Australian dairy cattle. *Journal of Dairy Science*, 1989, 72, 2624-2632.

Martinez, GE; Koch, RM; Cundiff, LV; Gregory, KE; Kachman, SD; Van Vleck, LD. Genetic parameters for stayability, stayability at calving, and stayability at weaning to specific ages for Hereford cows. *Journal of Animal Science*, 2005, 83, 2033-2042.

Martinez, GE; Koch, RM; Cundiff, LV; Gregory, KE; Van Vleck, LD. Genetic parameters for six measures of length of productive life and three measures of lifetime production by 6 yr after first calving for Hereford cows. *Journal of Animal Science*, 2004, 82, 1912-1918.

Mc Parland, S; Kearney, JF; Rath, M; Berry, DP. Inbreeding and pedigree analysis of Irish dairy and beef cattle populations. *Journal of Animal Science*, 2006, 85, 322-331.

Mesa, H; Safransky, TJ; Cammack, KM; Weaber, RL; Lamberson, WR. Genetic and phenotypic relationships of farrowing and weaning survival to birth and placental weights in pigs. *Journal of Animal Science*, 2006, 84, 32-40.

Muncine SA; Cassady JP; Ashwell MS. Refinement of quantitative trait loci on bovine chromosome 18 afecting health and reproduction in US Holsteins. *Animal Genetics*, 2006, 3, 273-275.

Mwansa, PB; Crews Jr., DH; Wilton, JW; Kemp, RA. Multiple trait selection for maternal productivity in beef cattle. *Journal of Animal Breeding and Genetics*, 2002, 119, 391-399.

Neerhof, HJ; Madsen, P; Ducrocq, VP; Vollema, AR; Jensen, A; Korsgaard, IR. Relationships between mastitis and functional longevity in Danish Black and White dairy cattle estimated using survival analysis. *Journal of Dairy Science*, 2000, 83, 1064-1071.

Nieto, LM; Campos de Silva, LO; Marcondes, CR; Rosa, AN; Martins, EN; Torres Jr, RAA. Heredabilidade da habilidade de parmanência no rebanho em fêmeas de bovines da raça Canchim. *Pesquisa Agropecuaria Brasileira*, 2007, 42, 1407-1411.

Nieuwhof, GJ; Norman, HD; Dickinson, FN. Phenotypic trends in herdlife of dairy cows in the United States. *Journal of Dairy Science*, 1989, 72, 726-736.

Núñez-Dominguez, R; Cundiff, LV; Dickerson, GE; Gregory, KE; Koch, RM. Heterosis for survival and dentition in Hereford, Angus, Shorthorn, and crossbred cows. *Journal of Animal Science*, 1991, 69, 1885-1898.

OMIA, Online Mendelian Inheritance in Animal. Reprogen, Faculty of Veterinary Science and Australian National Genomic Information Service, University of Sydney. 2008. Available at http://omia.angis.org.au/.

Osiewacz, HD. Genetic regulation of aging. *Journal of Molecular Medicine*, 1997, 75, 715-727.

Páchová, E; Zavadilová, L; Sölkner, J. Genetic evaluation of the length of productive life in Holstein cattle in the Czech Republic. *Czech Journal of Animal Science*, 2005, 50, 493-398.

Pasman, E; Reinhardt, F. Genetic evaluation for length of productive life of Holstein cattle in Germany. *Interbull Bulletin*, 1999, 21, 55-59.

Piles, M; Garreau, H; Rafel, O; Larzul, C; Ramon, J; Ducrocq, V. Survival analysis in two lines of rabbits selected for reproductive traits. *Journal of Animal Science*, 2006a, 84, 1658-1665.

Piles, M; Sánchez, JP; Orengo, J; Rafel, O; Ramon, J; Baselga, M. Crossbreeding parameter estimation for functional longevity in rabbits using survival analysis methodology. *Journal of Animal Science*, 2006b, 84, 58-62.

Prinzenberg, EM; Brandt, H; Bennewitz, J; Kalm, E; Erhardt, G. Allele frequencies for SNPs in the α_{S1}-casein gene (CSN1S1) 5' flanking region in the European cattle and association with economic traits in German Holstein. *Livestock Production Science*, 2005, 98, 155-160.

Rabie, TS; Crooijmans, RP; Bovenhuis, H; Vereijken, AL; Veenendaal, T; van der Poel, JJ; Van Arendonk, JA; Pakdel, A; Groenen, MA. Genetic mapping of quantitative trait loci affecting susceptibility in chicken to develop pulmonary hypertension syndrome. *Animal Genetics*, 2005, 36, 468-476.

Rasali, DP; Crow, GH; Shrestha, JNB; Kennedy, AD; Brûlé-Babel, A. Genetic association between cows' stayability to three years of age and juvenile growth traits in Canadian Angus herds. *Canadian Journal of Animal Science*, 2005, 85, 139-143.

Ricard, A; Fournet-Hanocq, F. Analysis of factors affecting length of competitive life of jumping horses. *Genetics, Selection, Evolution*, 1997, 29, 251-267.

Rogers, PL; Gaskins, CT; Johnson, KA; MacNeil, MD. Evaluating longevity of composite beef females using survival analysis techniques. *Journal of Animal Science*, 2004, 82, 860-866.

Rohrer, GA; Baker, JF; Long, CR; Cartwright, TC. Productive longevity of firt-cross cows produced in a five-breed diallel: II. Heterosis and general combining ability. *Journal of Animal Science*, 1988, 66, 2836-2841.

Roughsedge, T; Amer, PR; Thompson, R; Simm, G. Genetic parameters for a maternal breeding goal in beef production. *Journal of Animal Science*, 2005, 83, 2319-2329.

Roxström, A; Ducrocq, V; Strandberg, E. Survival analysis of longevity in dairy cattle on a lactation basis. *Genetics, Selection, Evolution*, 2003, 35, 305-318.

Roxtröm, A; Strandberg, E. Genetic analysis of functional, fertility-, mastitis-, and production-determined length of productive life in Swedish dairy cattle. *Livestock Production Science*, 2002, 74, 125-135.

Sánchez, JP; Baselga, M; Ducrocq, M. Genetic and environmental correlations between longevity and litter size in rabbits. *Journal of Animal Breeding and Genetics*, 2006, 123, 180-185.

Sánchez, JP; Baselga, M; Peiró, R; Silvestre, MA. Analysis of factors influencing longevity of rabbit does. *Livestock Production Science*, 2004, 90, 227-234.

Sánchez, JP; Theilgaard, P; Mínguez, C; BAselga, M. Constitution and evaluation of a long-lived productive rabbit line. *Journal of Animal Science*, 2008, 86, 515-525.

Schneider, MP; Miglior, F. A proposal for genetic evaluation for functional herd life in Italian Holstein. In: *Proc. 50th EAAP Meeting*. Zurich: EAAP; 1999; 11-15.

Serenius, T; Stalder, KJ. Genetics of length of productive life and lifetime prolificacy in the Finnish Landrace and Large White pig populations. *Journal of Animal Science*, 2004, 82, 3111-3117.

Serenius, T; Stalder, KJ. Selection for sow longevity. *Journal of Animal Science*, 2006, 84 (E. Suppl.), E166-E171.

Serenius, T; Stalder, KJ; Puonti, M. Impact of dominance effects on sow longevity. *Journal of Animal Breeding and Genetics*, 2006, 123, 355-361.

Sewalem, A; Kistemaker, GJ; Ducrocq, V; Van Doormaal, BJ. Genetic analysis of herd life in Canadian dairy cattle on a lactation basis using a Weibull proportional hazards model. *Journal of Dairy Science*, 2005, 88, 368-375.

Sewalem, A; Kistemaker, GJ; Miglior, F; Van Doormaal, BJ. Analysis of inbreeding and its relationship with functional longevity in Canadian dairy cattle. *Journal of Dairy Science*, 2006, 89, 2210-2216.

Sharma, BS; Prabhakaran, VT; Pirchner, F. Gene action and heterosis in lifetime traits of Friesian × Sahiwal crosses. *Journal of Animal Breeding and Genetics*, 2000, 117, 319-330.

Short, TH; Lawlor, TJ. Genetic parameters of conformation traits, milk yield, and hed life in Holstein. *Journal of Dairy Science*, 1992, 75, 1987-1988.

Silva, JAV; Eler, JP; Ferraz, JBS; Golden, BL; Oliveira, HN. Heritability estimate for stayability in Nelore cows. *Livestock Production Science*, 2003, 79, 97-101.

Silva, JAV; Formigoni, IB; Eler, JP; Ferraz, JBS. Genetic relationship among stayability, scrotal circumference and post-weaning weight in Nellore cattle. *Livestock Science*, 2006, 99, 51-59.

Smith, LA; Cassell, BG; Pearson, RE. The effects of inbreeding on the lifetime performance of dairy cattle. *Journal of Dairy Science*, 1998, 81, 2729-2737.

Snelling, WM; Golden, BL; Bourdon, RM. Within-herd genetic analyses of stayability of beef females. *Journal of Animal Science*, 1995, 73, 993-1001.

Southey, BR; Rodriguez-Zas, SL; Leymaster, KA. Survival analysis of lamb mortality in a terminal sire composite population. *Journal of Animal Science*, 2001, 79, 2298-2306.

Southey, BR; Rodriguez-Zas, SL; Leymaster, KA. Discrete time survival analysis of lamb mortality in a terminal sire composite population. *Journal of Animal Science*, 2003, 81, 1399-1405.

Southey, BR; Rodriguez-Zas, SL; Leymaster, KA. Competing risks analysis of lamb mortality in a terminal sire composite population. *Journal of Animal Science*, 2004, 82, 2892-2899.

Southey, BR; Thomas, DL; Gottfredson, RG; Zelinsky, RD. Ewe productivity of Booroola Merino-Rambouillet crossed sheep during early stages of the introgression of the Fec[B] allele into a Rambouillet population. *Livestock Production Science*, 2002, 75, 33-44.

Spelbring, MC; Martin, TG; Drewry, KJ. Maternal productivity of crossbred Angus × Milking Shorthorn cows. II. Cow reproduction and longevity. *Journal of Animal Science*, 1971, 45, 976-982.

Tanida, H; Hohenboken, WDDeNise, SK. Genetic aspects of longevity in angus and Hereford cows. *Journal of Animal Science*, 1988, 66, 640-647.

Tarrés, J; Piedrafita, J; Ducrocq, V. Validation of an approximate approach to compute genetic correlations between longevity and linear traits. *Genetics, Selection, Evolution*, 2006, 38, 65-83.

Tarrés, J; Puig, P; Ducrocq, V; Piedrafita, J. Factors influencing length of productive life and replacement rates in the Bruna dels Pirineus beef breed. *Animal Science*, 2004, 78, 13-22.

Theilgaard, P; Sánchez, JP; Pascual, JJ; Friggens, NC; Baselga, M. Effect of body fatness and selection for prolificaciy on survival of rabbit does assessed using a cryopreserved control population. *Livestock Science*, 2006, 103, 65-73.

Thompson, JR; Everett, RW; Hammerschmidt, NL. Effects of inbreeding on production and survival in Holsteins. *Journal of Dairy Science*, 2000a, 83, 1856-1864.

Thompson, JR; Everett, RW; Wolfe, CW. Effects of inbreeding on production and survival in Jerseys. *Journal of Dairy Science*, 2000b, 83, 2131-2138.

Tsuruta, S; Misztal, I; Lawlor, TJ. Changing definition of productive life in US Holsteins: Effect on genetic correlations. *Journal of Dairy Science*, 2005, 88, 1156-1165.

van der Westhuizen, RR; Schoeman, SJ; Jordaan, GF; van Wyk, JB. Heritability estimates derived from threshold analyses for reproduction and stayability traits in a beef cattle herd. *South African Journal of Animal Science*, 2001, 31, 25-32.

Van Doormaal, BJ; Schaeffer, LR; Kennedy, BW. Estimation of genetic parameters for stayability in Canadian Holsteins. *Journal of Dairy Science*, 1985, 68, 1763-1769.

Van Melis, MH; Eler, JP; Oliveira, HN; Rosa, GJM; Silva, JAV; Ferraz, JBS; Pereira, E. Study of stayability in Nellore cows using a threshold model. *Journal of Animal Science*, 2007, 85, 1780-1786.

VanRaden, PM; Klaaskate, EJK. Genetic evaluation of length of productive life including predicted longevity of live cows. *Journal of Dairy Science*, 1993, 76, 2758-2764.

Van Tassell, CP; Misztal, I; Varona, L. Method R estimates of additive genetic, dominance genetic, and permanent environmental fraction of variance for yield and health traits of Holstein. *Journal of Dairy Science*, 2000, 83, 1873-1877.

Vatankhah, M; Zamani, F. Phenotypic and genetic characteristics of longevity in Lori-Bakhtiari sheep. *Biotechnology in Animal Husbandry*, 2007, 23, 323-329.

Vega, VE. Herdlife, stayability and lifetime production in beef cattle. Ph.D. dissertation, University of Nebraska, Lincoln, 1999.

Vollema, AR; Groen, AF. Genetic parameters of longevity traits of an upgrading population of dairy cattle. *Journal of Dairy Science*, 1996, 79, 2261-2267.

Vollema, AR; Groen, AF. A comparison of breeding value predictors for longevity using a linear model and survival analysis. *Journal of Dairy Science*, 1998, 81, 3315-3320.

Vollema, AR; Van Der Beek, S; Harbers, AGF; De Jong, G. Genetic evaluation for longevity of Dutch dairy bulls. *Journal of Dairy Science*, 2000, 83, 2629-2639.

Vukasinovic, N; Moll, J; Casanova, L. Implementation of a routine genetic evaluation for longevity based on survival analysis techniques in dairy cattle populations in Switzerland. *Journal of Dairy Science*, 2001, 84, 2073-2080.

Wang, X; Maltecca, C; Tal-Stein, R; Lipkin, E; Khatib, H. Association of bovine fibroblast growth factor 2 (FGF2) gene with milk fat and productivelife: an example of the ability of the candidate pathway strategy to identify quantitative trait genes. *Journal of Dairy Science*, 2008, 91, 2475-2480.

Weigel, KA; Palmer, RW; Caraviello, DZ. Investigation of factors affecting voluntary and involuntary culling in expanding dairy herds in Wisconsin using survival analysis. *Journal of Dairy Science*, 2003, 86:1482-1486.

Wilmut, I; Schnieke, AE; McWhir, J; Kind, AJ; Campbell, KH. Viable offspring derived from fetal and adult mammalian cells. *Nature*, 1997, 385, 810-813.

Wright, S. Coefficients of inbreeding and relationship. *The American Naturalist*, 1922, 56, 330-338.

Yazdi, MH; Lundheim, N; Rydmer, L; Ringmar-Cederberg, E; Johansson, K. Survival of Swedish Landrace and Yorkshire sows in relation to osteochondrosis: a genetic study. *Animal Science*, 2000a, 71, 1-9.

Yazdi, MH; Rydhmer, L; Ringmar-Cederberg, E; Lundeheim, N; Johansson, K. Genetic study of longevity in Swedish Landrace sows. *Livestock Production Science*, 2000b, 63, 255-264.

Zhang, Q; Boichard, D; Hoeschele, I; Ernst, C; Eggen, A; Murkve, B; Pfister-Genskow, M; Witte, LA; Grignola, FE; Uimari, P; Thaller, G; Bish, J. Mapping quantitative trait loci for milk production and health of dairy cattle in a large outbreed pedigree. *Genetics*, 1998, 149, 1959-1973.

Zohary, D; Tchernov, E; Kolska Horwitz, L. The role of unconscious selection in the domestication of sheep and goats. *Journal of Zoology*, 1998, 245, 129-135.

In: Handbook on Longevity: Genetics, Diet and Disease   ISBN: 978-1-60741-075-1
Editors: Jennifer V. Bentely and Mary Ann Keller   ©2009 Nova Science Publishers, Inc.

Chapter XVII

Genetic and Environmental Factors Affecting Inflammatory Responses to Infection

C.C. Blackwell, S.M. Moscovis, S.T. Hall, J. Stuart,
C.J. Ashhurst-Smith, J. Roberts-Thomson,
D. Yarnold and R.J. Scott

University of Newcastle, Newcastle, NSW, Australia
John Hunter Hospital, New Lambton, NSW, Australia

Introduction

The incidence of notifiable infectious diseases is higher in Indigenous Australians compared with the non-Indigenous population (Table 1), and there are higher incidences of heart and kidney diseases for which infection and inflammation are thought to play important roles in their pathogenesis [Australian Bureau of Statistics, 2001]. These discrepancies in health have been attributed mainly to poor socioeconomic conditions in which many Indigenous families live. New evidence is emerging that indicates there are significant genetic differences which might contribute to susceptibility to or severity of infections. The objective of this review is to examine these differences in relation to classical risk factors to determine potential interactions between genetic background and environmental conditions that contribute to susceptibility to these diseases.

For at least 40,000 years, epidemic infections considered to be major selective pressures for many genetic characteristics associated with immunity and infection were absent among Indigenous Australians. Until the late 18th century, because of its geographic isolation, the population was not regularly exposed to new infectious agents such as those which spread through Europe and Asia. In addition to its geographic isolation, Australia had other factors that reduced the likelihood of acute epidemic diseases. Indigenous Australians were nomadic and often relocated once food sources were depleted. This did not allow large amounts of human waste to accumulate and become a significant reservoir of infection. The low population density, scattered tribal groups, and the limited rate of travel reduced swift spread of any diseases with short incubation periods. If an individual or group became infected, the epidemic would most likely be restricted and not transmitted to another group. Except for the north of the country, there was little exposure to invasion or to "foreign trade routes" such as those between Europe and Asia along which epidemics traveled. The lack of domesticated animals in Indigenous tribes might also have been a contributing factor. Animals, like humans, require large populations to maintain epidemics. The development of agriculture and herding provided opportunities for transfer of pathogens from domesticated animals to humans. In addition, there is evidence that many of the most common epidemic viral and bacterial diseases are derived from those that affect domesticated animals: measles and tuberculosis from cattle; influenza from pigs and poultry; whooping cough from pigs and dogs [Diamond, 1997].

Table 1. Notifications of selected diseases[1] to the National Notifiable Diseases Surveillance System (NNDSS) by Indigenous status[2] 2001 [Australian Bureau of Statistics, 2005]

Disease	Crude rate per 100,000 population		Rate ratio[3]
	Indigenous	Non-Indigenous	
Routine childhood immunisation			
Measles	1.1	0.4	2.8
Mumps	4.6	0.6	7.7
Rubella	2.7	0.6	4.5
Pertussis	353.6	59.1	6.0
Haemophilus influenzae type b	1.1	0.1	11.0
Hepatitis B (incident)	11.0	1.2	9.2
Pneumococcal disease (invasive)	39.0	8.7	4.5
No routine immunisation			
Meningococcal infection	20.1	3.1	6.5
Chlamydial infection	1213.3	66.5	18.2
Hepatitis A	18.6	2.4	7.8
Hepatitis C (incident)	36.5	3.9	9.4
Salmonellosis	238.1	29.0	8.2
Shigellosis	71.4	1.6	44.6
Ross River virus infection	79.7	10.8	7.4
Syphilis	225.2	5.4	41.7
Donovanosis	8.0	<0.1	..
Gonococcal infection	1059.2	15.4	68.8
Leprosy	1.1	<0.1	..
Tuberculosis	9.8	1.0	9.8

[1]Disease have been categorised into those where routine immunisation was or was not provided
[2]Data from South Australia, Western Australia and the Northern Territory are combined. Except for pneumococcal disease (invasive) where data are from metropolitan New South Wales, Victoria, South Australia, Western Australia, Tasmania, and the Northern Territory.
[3]Rate ratio is equal to the rate of Indigenous notifications divided by the rate of non-Indigenous notifications.

Initial studies of DNA samples from a remote Indigenous Australian community indicate that their cytokine gene polymorphisms differ significantly from those of non-Indigenous, mainly European/Caucasian Australians [Moscovis et al., 2004a,b;2006; Titmarsh et al., 2008]. The arrival of Europeans introduced not only epidemic diseases characteristic of agrarian societies but also the conditions for their survival and spread. In addition to new microorganisms, Europeans also introduced changes in diet that included tobacco use and alcohol consumption.

Immune and Inflammatory Responses

The increased susceptibility of Aboriginal Australians to infection does not appear to be an inherent problem in regards to the development of an immune response. Earlier studies reported that Indigenous Australian children have higher levels of serum IgG at birth than non-Indigenous children, and the decline in these levels is not as dramatic as in non-Indigenous children [Stuart, 1978]. Despite what appear to be powerful immunoglobulin responses, Indigenous children have high incidences of perinatal mortality due to infection and higher incidences of respiratory and ear infections, bacterial meningitis, and Sudden Infant Death Syndrome (SIDS) for which infection has been suggested to be an important trigger [Alessandri et al., 1994; Allesandri et al., 2001; Currie and Brewster, 2001; Blackwell et al., 2004; 2005]. As noted for other Indigenous groups, there might also be less efficient responses to polysaccharide antigens such as the capsules of pneumococci and meningococci. For example the vaccine for *Haemophilus influenzae* type b (Hib) induces significantly lower levels of antibodies to the capsular polyribotolphosphate (PRP) antigen in Indigenous infants [Guthridge et al., 2000].

We investigated the hypothesis that among Indigenous Australians, the distribution of single nucleotide polymorphisms (SNP) for the inflammatory cytokines might reflect combinations that result in extremes of inflammatory responses: 1) low levels of pro-inflammatory responses and high levels of anti-inflammatory responses such as those suggested by Westendorp et al. [1997] to contribute to susceptibility to meningococcal infection; 2) high levels of pro-inflammatory responses and low levels of anti-inflammatory responses contributing to severity of disease (*e.g.* tissue / organ damage) or fatal outcome of infection. For example, there is a higher incidence of hospitalization for infections such as pertussis among very young infants prior to the initiation of childhood immunizations. The more remote the Indigenous community in which the child lives, the greater the risk of hospitalization. This pattern is not observed among non-Indigenous infants [Kolos et al., 2007].

To explore the hypothesis, we examined the distribution of cytokine gene polymorphisms for both pro-inflammatory and anti-inflammatory cytokines. The population was a community in Central Australia living in relative isolation and unlikely to have much admixture of Caucasian genes. The pro-inflammatory factors assessed included interleukin-1β (IL-1β), interleukin-6 (IL-6), interleukin-8 (IL-8), tumour necrosis factor-α (TNF-α), and interferon-γ (INF-γ). Anti-inflammatory factors included interleukin-10 (IL-10), interleukin-4 (IL-4) and IL-1 receptor antagonist (IL-1Ra).

There were highly significant differences in the distributions of these genotypes between Indigenous Australians and non-Indigenous Australians who are mainly of European origin (Table 2). Aboriginal Australians have an increased proportion of alleles associated with increased production of pro-inflammatory cytokines: *IL1B* -511T; *IL6* -174G; and *IFNG* +874T and decreased production of anti-inflammatory cytokines: *IL10* -1082A; *IL10* -592A; and *IL1RN* +2018C. The IL-8 polymorphism among Indigenous Australians was also significantly different from that of non-Indigenous Australians; however, the effect of this SNP on levels of IL-8 responses differs in the various systems used to assess its role in pathogenesis in different conditions (see below).

Table 2. Distribution of cytokine gene polymorphisms in Aboriginal Australians and Caucasians [Moscovis et al., 2004a,b;2006; submitted for publication; Titmarsh et al., 2008.%

SNP / Reference	Genotype	Aboriginal Australian	Caucasian
IL1B C-511T	CC	4	50
	CT	23	41
	TT	73	9
IL1RN T+2018C	TT	44	59
	TC	47	27
	CC	8	14
IL6 G-174C	CC	1	17
	GC	11	41
	GG	88	42
IFNG T+874A	AA	12	37
	TA	49	47
	TT	39	16
TNF G-308A	GG	99	68
	GA	1	29
	AA	0	3
IL8 A-251T	AA	3	20
	AT	31	52
	TT	66	28
IL4 C-589T	CC	56	78
	CT	39	19
	TT	5	3
IL10 G-1082A [6]	GG	(0	31
	GA	15	38
	AA	85	31
IL10 C-592A	CC	44	59
	CA	41	36
	AA	15	6

The levels of cytokine responses associated with some of the polymorphisms have been characterized (e.g., IL-10). For others, there have been varying reports of responses associated with different genotypes. Differences in populations tested, methods of assessment and various factors such as polymorphisms in IL-10, environmental pollutants, body mass index and asymptomatic viral infection and chronic infections need to be considered in assessment of inflammatory responses. Few studies have considered these confounding factors, much less the possible interactions among them. The following sections examine interactions between genetic and environmental factors that could contribute to susceptibility to or severity of infections and conditions for which infections are suggested to be triggers.

Infection and Inflammation

Bacteria can cause disease in two general ways. They can invade areas of the body that are normally sterile (meningitis or septicaemia) or they can remain on mucosal surfaces and produce powerful toxins that result in disease (cholera, food poisoning or toxic shock syndrome due to toxins of *Staphylococcus aureus*). The primary reaction to all infectious agents or their products in the non-immune host is the inflammatory response, and cytokine production plays a major role in these innate host defenses. The model of a strong initial pro-inflammatory reaction leading to protection from infection has been previously proposed [Netea et al., 2003]. An initially weak cytokine response results in defective bacterial clearance, leading to proliferation of the pathogen and excessive stimulation of the pro-inflammatory cytokine response by large quantities of bacterial antigens. By preventing bacterial proliferation through a strong pro-inflammatory response in the early stages of infection, the severely unbalanced inflammatory response does not occur. If these responses are too low, the host is at greater risk of invasive infection [Westendorp et al., 1997]. If these responses are too high, there is danger of tissue damage or death due to these normally "protective" inflammatory mediators that have profound effects on physiological homeostasis. There is, however, a second and very important need to balance inflammatory responses as there appears to be a trade off between fertility and survival to reach the age of reproduction [Van Bodegom et al., 2007]

Invasive Diseases Controlled by Antibodies to the Pathogen

Meningococcal disease is used as an example of this type of infection. Among Indigenous Australians, the incidence of invasive meningococcal disease (IMD), meningitis and/or septicaemia, can be up to 6 times that observed for non-Indigenous populations (Table 1). Regardless of age, in the non-immune host lacking specific antibody protection, inflammatory responses are a major defense against IMD. These responses are mediated mostly by cytokines. A few key cytokines appear to orchestrate the host's inflammatory responses to meningococcal disease. These include the pro-inflammatory cytokines: TNF-α,

IL-1, IL-6 and IL-8. Anti-inflammatory cytokines that are of interest in meningococcal disease include IL-10 and IL-1ra.

TNF-a

TNF-α is produced by a variety of cell sources including macrophages and monocytes, T cells, mast cells and polymorphonuclear leukocytes (PMNs). It causes macrophage activation, stimulating the superoxide pathway and the nitric oxide pathways which produce reactive oxygen and nitrogen species respectively, both of which have bactericidal activity. PMN stimulation causes enhanced phagocytosis, production of superoxides, and induction of degranulation [Vassalli, 1992]. First degree relatives of individuals who died of meningococcal disease had genotypes associated with low levels of TNF-α [Westendorp et al., 1997]. The predominant genotype for the *TNF* G-308A SNP among Aboriginal Australians (GG) was that associated with low responses of the cytokine (Table 2). This could be an important risk factor among Aboriginal populations if the observations of Westendorp et al. [1997] apply to non-Caucasian groups.

IL-1β

IL-1β is produced by monocytes and macrophages, endothelial cells, and granulocytes [Dinarello, 1996]. Examples of IL-1β activity influencing the immune responses are: increased PMN activity; enhancement of blood brain barrier permeability for leukocytes and plasma; induction of the coagulant response in blood; increased proliferation of B cells and $CD4^+$ T cells; production of nitric oxide and prostaglandin [Dahmer et al., 2005; Hackett et al., 2001; van Furth et al., 1996]. Patients who were homozygous for either the common or rare allele at position –511 on the IL-1β gene had increased odds ratios for death compared to heterozygous individuals. The homozygous genotype for the IL1B C-511T SNP that is rare in Europeans (TT) is found in 73% of Aboriginal subjects we tested [Moscovis et al., 2004b]. One explanation for this is the phenomenon of heterosis, in which there is an increased response observed for heterozygote carrier of a SNP compared to either type of homozygous SNP carriers; for example, the advantage conferred by being heterozygous for the MBL2 genotype compared to having a homozygous genotype [Helleman et al., 2007] .

IL-6

IL-6 is produced by fibroblasts, endothelial cells, monocytes, macrophages, keratinocytes, mast cells, fat cells and T cell lines. Its production is stimulated by endotoxin, IL-1, and TNF-α alone or in conjunction with IFN-γ [Snick, 1990]. It is involved in induction of acute phase proteins, increased platelet formation, and increased proliferation and differentiation of B and T cells [Hackett et al., 2001; Snick, 1990]. In a northern European population [Balding et al., 2003], severity and fatality of meningococcal infection was associated with the GG genotype of *IL6* G-174C SNP. This genotype has been linked with high responses of this cytokine and the wildtype allele is also predominant in other Indigenous populations [Moscovis et al., 2006; Vozarova et al., 2003].

IL-8

IL-8 is produced predominantly by macrophages and is a potent chemo-attractant for neutrophils (Hacking et al., 2004). Production of IL-8 is stimulated by endotoxin and the cytokines TNF-α and IL-1, but not IL-6 [DeForge et al., 1992]. It is produced by meningeal cells in response to meningococcal infection [Christodoulides et al., 200]. Meningoccal infections elicit strong neutrophil responses in the cerebrospinal fluid; in contrast, lymphocytes are the predominant cell type in viral meningitis (VM). In a Greek population, genotype distributions between patients with IMD differed significantly from patients with viral meningitis (VM) ($p < 0.0001$). A significant difference was observed between AA and TT genotype distributions between the two groups ($p < 0.0001$) and for the AA genotype and T allele carriage ($p < 0.0001$). Allele distribution between patients with VM and healthy controls was significantly different ($p = 0.0004$); the A allele was associated with increased risk of viral meningitis (OR 2.242, CI 1.438-3.496) [Titmarsh et al., submitted for publication]. This observation was of particular interest in that Aboriginal Australians have predominantly the T allele.

There are conflicting reports of phenotypes associated with different genotypes of this *IL8* SNP. There is functional evidence that the A allele of the *IL8* -251 SNP is associated with higher levels of IL-8 [Jiang et al., 2006; Ohyauchi et al., 2005; Taguchi et al., 2005]. In an Indian population, the TT allele was associated with higher IL-8 responses to live tuberculosis organisms and culture filtrates from the bacteria [Selvaraj et al., 2006]. Assuming that the A allele is associated with higher levels of the chemo-attractant, an individual with one or both alleles might have more IL-8 -sensitive cells recruited to sites of infection. In the case of meningococcal infection, increased recruitment of leukocytes, in particular neutrophils, to the site of infection would result in strong initial pro-inflammatory responses enhancing destruction of the bacteria. Among patients with IMD, the AA genotype was found for only 12.2 % compared with VM patients (43.3%). This should subsequently result in a more effective response against the pathogen early in the infection. This scenario would be consistent with improved outcome. Factors associated with adverse outcome (limb amputation/death) in children with invasive meningococcal disease were a leukocyte count less than 5000/mm³, an absolute neutrophil count less than 3000/mm³ and a CSF leukocyte count less than 10/mm³ [Malley et al., 1996]. Alternatively, if the TT genotype is associated with higher IL-8, excessive responses could contribute to the physiological shock and tissue damage characteristic of severe IMD.

IL-1ra

IL-1ra is an acute phase protein that binds the same receptors as IL-1β and IL-1α. It has an anti-inflammatory role as it does not induce cell activation, thereby, counterbalancing the pro-inflammatory effects of IL-1β and IL-1α [Arend, 2002; Chiche et al., 2001]. The soluble receptor protein is involved in non-functional binding to IL-1β which disables the interaction of IL-1β with functional IL-1 receptors present on the cell surfaces. The IL1RN T+2018C polymorphism results in the decreased expression of the IL1RN gene, which encodes for the IL-1Ra protein. This ultimately leads to increased IL-1β biological activity, and susceptibility to enhanced pro-inflammatory responses. The IL1RN polymorphism is also associated with increased levels of IL-1β secretion [Santilla et al., 1998]; however, the mechanism responsible for this remains unknown.

SNP analysis of the cytokine IL-1β in a northern European population found that the likelihood of survival is increased in IMD patients who possess the C allele at *IL1B* -511, with odds ratio of 2.01 (CI 1.11 to 3.79); however, mortality is increased if in combination with the variant C allele *IL1RN* +2018, OR 0.61, CI 0.38 to 0.993 [Read et al., 2003]. The CC genotype was found in only 8% of the Indigenous Australian population examined [Moscovis et al., 2004b].

IL-10

IL-10 is produced mainly by monocytes, but it is also produced in T and B cells. IL-10 down-regulates the pro-inflammatory cytokines TNF-α, IL-1 (both α and β), IL-6, and IL-8. It is a strong suppressor of the immune response by inhibiting leukocyte migration and chemokine production via down regulation of chemo-attractant proteins and intracellular adhesion molecules. It down-regulates the T cell response through inhibitory interactions with dendritic cells [Mocellin et al., 2004; van Furth et al., 1996]. IL-10 also inhibits the activation of coagulation and fibrinolysis pathways caused by endotoxin release from meningococci [Pajkrt et al., 1997]. High IL-10 concentrations (≥1,000 pg/ml) in human serum have been associated with fatality in patients with meningococcal septic shock (Lehmann et al., 1995).

The AA genotype for the G-1082A SNP in the promoter sequence is associated with low IL-10 production [Turner et al., 1997]. Peripheral blood mononuclear cells from individuals with the -1082A allele showed significantly lower inducible IL-10 levels compared with individuals with the −1082G allele [Hajeer et al., 1988], and this was independent of the other polymorphisms at positions −819 and −592 [Reich et al., 1999].

Associations between severity of infection and invasive infections have been reported for the genotype associated with high levels of IL-10 responses for meningococcal disease, and community acquired pneumonia and pneumococcal infections [Westendorp et al., 1997; Boehmke et al., 2003]. Polymorphisms associated with low levels of IL-10 have been associated with severity of disease among patients with Epstein Barr Virus (EBV) infection [Helminen et al., 1999]. The AA genotype for the G-1082A SNP associated with low levels of IL-10 responses was predominant among the Indigenous Australian population tested (85%) [Moscovis et al., 2004a].

In an *in vitro* model using human leukocytes, we found that levels of IL-10 were significantly reduced in smokers, both the baseline levels before stimulation with bacterial toxins and the responses to both endotoxin [Blackwell et al., 2002]. The greatest effect of smoking on reduction of IL-10 responses was observed for individuals with the genotype associated with low IL-10 responses [Moscovis et al., 2004a]. This is also the genotype predominant among groups with higher incidences of infection such as Indigenous people in Australia, Native Americans and African Americans.

The higher incidence of IMD among Aboriginal Australians could reflect greater exposure to important risk environmental risk factors such as cigarette smoke or close physical contact indentified in other populations. It might also reflect the higher proportion of genotypes associated with high pro-inflammatory (IL-1 β and IL-6) and low anti-inflammatory (IL-10 and IL1RN) responses.

Tuberculosis (TB)

The incidence of TB is about 10 times higher among Indigenous Australians compared with the non-Indigenous population (Table 1). Several studies have examined associations between SNPs for cytokine genes and susceptibility to TB in different ethnic groups in Europe and north America. The two for which there is most evidence are IFN-γ and IL-8

IFN-γ

IFN-γ plays a key role in control of disease due to *Mycobacterium tuberculosis* [Collins & Kaufmann, 2001]. The TT genotype for the +874 T→A SNP is suggested to be associated with increased production of IFN-γ [Pravica et al., 2000]. Among Caucasians, the TT homozygote for the +874 T→A SNP was significantly lower among patients in Sicily with TB (8.9%) compared with healthy controls (25.8%) [Lio et al., 2002]. In a Spanish population, individuals homozygous for AA had an increased risk of 3.75 for TB; and stimulation of mononuclear cells from individuals with the AA genotype resulted in lower levels of IFN-γ than cells of the non-AA genotype [Lopez-Maderuelo et al., 2003]. Among Indigenous Canadians and American Blacks who are at higher risk of TB, the pattern of SNP distributions is similar to that of the Sicilian patients with TB. There are low proportions of individuals with the TT genotype in their population compared to Caucasian controls [Larcombe et al., 2005] (Table 3). In contrast, the Indigenous Australian group examined had one of the highest proportions of individuals with the TT genotype (Table 3). This indicates that although IFN-γ plays an important role in resistance to TB, it cannot adequately control the infection without the contribution of other critical cytokines.

Table 3. Distribution of the IFNG T+874A genotypes among populations at high risk of tuberculosis compared with those at low risk. %

Group	TT	TA	AA	Ref
Low risk				
Caucasian				
Italy	25.8	42.4	25.8	Lio et al., 2002
Canada	20	53	27	Larcombe et al., 2005
US	22	51	27	Hoffmann et al., 2002
Australia	37	47	16	Table 2
High risk				
US Black	9	52	39	Ma et al., 2003
Aboriginal Canadian	4	20	76	Larcombe et al., 2005
Indigenous Australian	39	49	12	Table 2

IL-8

IL-8 has become a major interest for research on TB world wide. Clinical and pathological levels of IL-8 were elevated in pleural exudate, bronchoalveolar lavage fluid, and cerebrospinal fluid of TB patients. Il-8 concentrations in plasma are higher in patients who die of TB than those who survive [Ma et al., 2003]. There have been varying reports on the effect of the IL-8 A-251T SNP on levels of IL-8 responses. Both T and A alleles have been reported to be associated with high IL-8 responses. Peripheral blood monocytes from patients with TB and uninfected controls from the same population in India were stimulated with culture filtrate antigen (CFA) or live *M. tuberculosis.* Cells from patients or control donors with the TT genotype showed significantly higher IL-8 responses to CFA or the live organisms compared with donors with the AA genotype [Selvaraj et al., 2006]. Both American Caucasian and Black patients with TB were more likely to be homozygous for the AA allele (OR = 3.41, 95% CI 1.52-7.64), and the AA allele was predominant among the Black population (56%) compared with the Caucasian group (14%) [Ma et al., 2003] (Table 4). This might contribute to the higher risk of TB among African American populations compared with Caucasian populations exposed to similar environmental conditions [Stead et al., 1990]; however, the TT genotype was predominant among Indigenous Australians examined (66%) [Titmarsh et al., 2008].

Table 4. Distribution of the IL-8T-251A genotypes among populations at high risk of tuberculosis compared with those at low risk. %

Group	TT	TA	AA	Ref
Low risk				
Caucasian				
US	39.3	46.7	14	Ma et al., 2003
Australian	28	52	20	
High risk				
US Black	13.8	29.9	56.3	Ma et al., 2003
Aboriginal Australian	66	31	3	Titmarsh et al., 2008

For Indigenous Australians, the distribution of genotypes for both IFN-γ and IL-8 differ significantly from the other two high risk groups considered. Among the ethnic groups examined, Aboriginal Australians had the highest proportion of the TT genotype (39%) for IFN-γ compared with the other two high risk groups, African Americans (9%) and Canadian Aboriginals (4%). For the IL-8 genotypes, the proportions for the AA genotype associated with increased risk of disease among American Blacks (63% in the patient group) was the minority genotype among Aboriginal Australians (3%). If the predominant AA genotype is associated with low IL-8 responses this might contribute to the susceptibility noted for this genotype in both Caucasian and Black population in the US. The reported high level responses associated with the TT genotype in the study from India might reflect the model suggested by Ma et al. [2003]. Increased levels of IL-8 attracts an excess of leukocytes to the area of infection. This results in the extensive tissue damage often noted in pulmonary TB. This damage is mediated by free radicals, proteases and elastases released in response to the infection. High IL-8 secretion might also enhance inflammation by delaying the apoptosis of PMN [Ma et al., 2003]. For all three high-risk groups, the predominant genotype for the anti-inflammatory cytokine IL-10 (*IL10* G-1082A) is the AA associated with low levels of IL-10 responses which are further reduced by smoking [Moscovis et al., 2004].

Cigarette Smoke and Susceptibility to Infection

Tobacco smoking was introduced to Australia at the same time as European diseases. Active smoking and exposure of children or adults to cigarette smoke are major factors for respiratory infections, bacterial meningitis and SIDS. The term "passive" smoking implies a lower level of exposure to cigarette smoke among both adults and children exposed to this environmental pollutant. There is evidence, however, that some infants have as much cotinine in their body fluids as active smokers [Daly et al., 2001]. Cotinine is a metabolic breakdown product of nicotine and is readily measurable thereby making it an excellent surrogate for nicotine exposure. Exposure to cigarette smoke could affect susceptibility to infection at two stages, colonization by potentially pathogenic bacteria and enhancement or suppression of inflammatory responses [Blackwell et al., 2004].

Smokers are more frequently colonised by potentially pathogenic bacteria such as meningococci or staphylococci [Blackwell et al., 1992; Musher and Fainstein, 1981]. Buccal epithelial cells (BEC) from smokers bound significantly more *S. aureus, Bordetella pertussis*, and several Gram-negative bacteria [El Ahmer et al., 1999a]. The enhanced binding was not associated with upregulation of cell surface antigens observed with virus-infected cells [El Ahmer et al., 1999b]. Pre-treatment of cells from non-smokers with a water-soluble cigarette smoke extract (CSE) significantly enhanced bacterial binding. The enhancement was observed with CSE dilutions up to 1 in 300. Coating of mucosal surfaces by passive exposure to cigarette smoke in the child's environment might enhance attachment of a variety of bacterial species [El Ahmer et al., 1999a]

In an animal model, nicotine significantly enhanced the lethal effect of bacterial toxins [Sayers et al., 1995]. Studies with human monocytes found that cotinine, enhanced production of some inflammatory mediators. In this model system, it was also demonstrated that a water-soluble cigarette smoke extract enhanced TNF-α responses of RSV infected human monocytes, and it also enhanced nitric oxide production from monocytes exposed to TSST [Raza et al., 1999]. .

Modulation of the inflammatory responses by cigarette smoke had not been considered previously in relation to genotype. There were no significant differences between IL-10 responses to endotoxin observed with cells from non-smokers for the three genotypes of the IL10 G-1082A polymorphism. Smoking had a significant effect on IL-10 responses of two of the three genotypes to endotoxin. This is consistent with our previous study indicting that smokers had lower levels of IL-10 responses to TSST and endotoxin [Blackwell et al., 2002]. Although IL-10 responses to endotoxin were lower from leukocytes of smokers with the GG genotype, the differences were not significant; however, the cells from smokers who were heterozygotes had significantly lower IL-10 responses and leukocytes from donors of the AA genotype had the lowest IL-10 responses [Moscovis et al., 2004a]. These observations help to explain some of the differences reported for cytokine responses associated with genotype.

Infection and Inflammation in Other Conditions

For classical infections the effects of important environmental risk factors such as exposure to cigarette smoke appear to play a important role in disturbing the balance of the inflammatory responses by enhancing susceptibility to virus infections and also enhancing colonisation by potential bacterial pathogens. The powerful pro-inflammatory responses that would be predicted to be protective against invasive bacterial infections might result in excessive or prolonged production of these cytokines if the modulating effect of anti-inflammatory cytokines are lowered as we have shown for IL-10. As smoking is a risk factor for a number of conditions in which infection and inflammation have also been implicated, the remainder of this review will assess five of these which are prevalent among Indigenous Australians: Sudden Infant Death Syndrome (SIDS); ischaemic heart disease; type II diabetes; kidney disease; preterm births and stillbirths.

Sudden Infant Death Syndrome (SIDS)

Despite successful public health campaigns to reduce the risk factors for SIDS, it is still the major cause of death between 1 month to 1 year of age among infants in industrialized countries. SIDS is a diagnosis of exclusion. The original definition was "… the sudden death of any infant or young child which is unexpected by history, and in which a thorough post mortem examination fails to demonstrate an adequate cause of death"[Beckwith, 1970]. The definition was revised in 1989 to "the sudden death of an infant under one year of age which remains unexplained after a thorough case investigation, including performance of a complete autopsy, examination of the death scene, and review of the clinical history" [Rognum, 2001].

Two recent reviews summarised the evidence for inflammatory responses in SIDS [Goldwater, 2004; Vege & Rognum, 2004]. Inflammatory changes particularly in the respiratory tract are common findings in SIDS and probably reflect recent infections which have been noted in the two weeks prior to death for over 40% of SIDS babies [Hoffman et al., 1988; Wilson, 1999]. Perturbation of the clotting system [Goldwater et al., 1990] has been suggested to be responsible for the high proportion of SIDS infants in whom blood remains liquid. This could be associated with increased numbers of mast cells [Howat et al., 1994] and mast cell degranulation products [Holgate et al., 1994] noted for many SIDS infants. Release of heparin might account for liquid blood and release of preformed tumour necrosis factor α (TNF-α) or other vasoactive compounds could contribute to anaphylactic-like responses. Identification of toxins in brain tissue has been proposed as one explanation for the brain oedema noted in many SIDS infants [Goldwater, 2004]. Evidence of immune/inflammatory activation in tissues and secretions of SIDS infants has been reported [Gleeson et al., 1993; Rognum & Vege, 2004].

The most direct evidence for cytokine involvement comes from studies in which half of the SIDS infants investigated had IL-6 concentrations in their CSF equivalent to those found for infants dying from infectious diseases such as meningitis or septicaemia [Vege et al., 1995]. Other cytokines implicated in experimental studies of SIDS include interleukin-1β (IL-1β) which has been shown in animal models to interact with nicotine and interfere with auto-resuscitation in animal models [Froen et al., 2000].

Table 5. Comparison of risk factors among ethnic groups with low (Bangladeshi), moderate (Caucasian) and high (Aboriginal Australian) incidences of SIDS (adapted from Blackwell et al., 2005)

Factor	Caucasian European	Bangladeshi	Aboriginal Australian
SIDS / 1000 live births	2	0.3	6.1
Prone sleeping	+	-	-
IgG levels at birth	+	++	++
Bed Sharing	+	+++	+++
Switch to circadian rhythm (age in weeks)	8-16	12-20	?
Breast feeding	+	+++	+++
Bacterial colonisation	+	?	+++
Genotype high IL-6 responses (%)	38	94	88
Genotype high IL-1β responses (%)	9	56	71
Genotype low IL-10 responses (%)	31	84	83
Mothers who smoke (%)	25	3	75

-, +, ++, +++ = rare to common
? = not known

By definition, invasive bacterial infections are explainable causes of death and, therefore, not involved in SIDS. Although virus infection might be an important co-factor in the series of events leading to death, there is little evidence that SIDS is due to an unrecognised viral disease [An et al., 1993]. Toxigenic bacteria and/or their toxins have been identified in SIDS infants in studies from several different countries [Blackwell et al.,1995;

2005; Zorgani et al., 1999]. Many bacterial species express molecules that act as superantigens and the cytokines they induce, if not moderated, can cause tissue damage or death. They are responsible for the pathology of septic and toxic shock [Bone, 1993]. It has been suggested that SIDS is due to rapid, uncontrolled release of inflammatory mediators in response to infectious agents or their toxins [Blackwell et al., 2005]. Surveys of SIDS infants found little or negligible levels of antibodies to a range of bacterial toxins [Siarakas et al., 1999; Oppenheim et al., 1994]. In the absence of protective anti-toxins, the inflammatory mediators induced by these toxins could produce significant changes in each of the physiological mechanisms proposed to explain these deaths: hypoxia; poor arousal; hypoglycaemia; vascular shock; cardiac arrythmias; hyperthermia; and anaphylaxis [Raza & Blackwell, 1999]

There is now significant evidence that infection and inflammation play a role in inducing the physiological changes leading to SIDS [Blackwell *et al.*, 2005]. There are variations in the incidence of these deaths in different ethnic groups within the same country. For example, before the campaigns to reduce the environmental and infant care practices identified as significant risk factors for SIDS, the lowest incidence published was for Bangladeshi infants living in Britain (0.3/1000 live births) [Balarajan,1989]. One of the highest incidences was that reported for Indigenous Australian infants (6.1/1000 live births [Allesandri et al.,1994]. These differences could not be explained on variations in infant care practices and other factors have been assessed in relation to the incidence of SIDS. These differences could not be explained on the basis of major genetic differences in cytokine gene polymorphisms as those observed for Aboriginal Australians was very similar to those for Bangladeshis [Moscovis et al., 2004a,b; 2006]. The major risk factor that differs between these two groups is the proportion of mothers who smoke [Blackwell et al., 2004; 2005]. At the time the epidemiological studies were carried out, smoking was low among Bangladeshi women in Britain (3%) [Hilder, 1994] compared with Aboriginal Australian mothers (75%) [Eades et al., 1999] (Table 5)

Heart Disease

Ischaemic heart disease (IHD) is a major cause of mortality in the Aboriginal population of Australia [Ring et al., 2002]. Inflammatory responses triggered by chronic infections, e.g., Chlamydia pneumoniae, Helicobacter pylori, cytomegalovirus (CMV), have been implicated in the aetiology of IHD [Vallance et al., 1997; Bhagat et al., 1996]. Our work indicates that inflammatory cytokine gene polymorphisms most commonly found among Indigenous Australians in a remote community might result in strong pro-inflammatory cytokine responses and that smoking might further enhance these responses to infectious agents [Moscovis et al., 2004a,b;2006]. These observations, in the context of a recent report of an unusually high prevalence of H. pylori infection among Aboriginal communities (60% in an urban population and 91% in a remote population) [Windsor et al., 2005], led us to consider the interactions between the genetics of cytokine responses to H. pylori, and some of the risk factors for IHD, e.g., gender and smoking.

Evidence for Chronic Infection as a Risk Factor for IHD

Following brief exposure to endotoxin or certain cytokines, endothelium-dependent relaxation was impaired for several days; impairment was greater than that induced by chronic risk factors. It was suggested that after the acute stage of infection when vasodilator effects are induced, "the residual inability of endothelium to generate nitric oxide and prostanoids in response to agonists would tip the balance of mediators produced in favor of thrombosis and vasospasm" [Bhagat et al., 1996]. Studies on an Aboriginal community in Western Australia found very high plasma concentrations of C reactive protein (CRP), a marker for inflammation, and soluble E-selectin, a marker for vascular endothelium activation [Rowley et al., 2003].

The overall prevalence of infection with *H. pylori* among two Indigenous Australian populations was 76%; and 60% of an urban community had evidence of *H. pylori* infection compared with 91% of a rural community [Windsor et al., 2005]. There is conflicting evidence for associations between chronic infection with *H. pylori* and IHD [Pellicano et al., 2003]. Some studies indicated *H. pylori* is a marker for poor socioeconomic conditions in early life such as overcrowding, low educational level, and unhygienic conditions [Brown, 2000]. Other considerations are that reported associations are due to chance or preferential publication of positive results [Wald et al., 1997; Danesh & Peto, 1998]. Major criticisms include undetected heart disease in controls and qualitative not quantitative tests for antibodies to *H. pylori* [Wald *et al.*, 1997; Danesh & Peto, 1998, Alkout et al., 2000b].

In patients with gastrointestinal disease, levels of IgG antibodies to *H. pylori* correlated with the density of antral colonisation by the bacteria and with the degree of gastritis in the antrum [Kreuning et al., 1994]. Levels of IgG to *H. pylori* were related to severity of gastrointestinal disease [Atherton et al., 1996]. Quantitative assessment of IgG specific for *H. pylori* among patients in a European population was compared among individuals who survived a myocardial infarction (MI) and those who died of IHD. Sera were obtained from 4 groups: 1) men who survived one MI; 2) men matched for age and socioeconomic background to group 1; 3) individuals who died suddenly of IHD; 4) accidental deaths with no evidence of heart disease at autopsy matched for age and sex to group 3. Levels of IgG to *H. pylori* increased with age but were not associated with smoking or socioeconomic groups. There was a correlation between IgG to the bacteria and decreasing socioeconomic levels only among group 1 (P < 0.01). IgG levels were higher for subjects who died suddenly of heart disease (median = 151 ng ml^{-1}) compared with survivors of a first MI (median = 88 ng ml^{-1}) (P = 0.034) and higher for survivors compared with their controls (median = 58 ng ml^{-1}) (P = 0.039) [Alkout et al., 2000b].

Inflammation and Genetics in IHD

Our previous studies on inflammatory responses to *H. pylori* indicated that the host response plays a major role in pathogenesis of peptic ulcer disease and requires as much detailed examination as the virulence factors for the bacteria. Blood group O is associated with peptic ulceration and leukocytes of individuals of blood group O had significantly higher IL-6 and TNF-α responses to the whole bacteria, an outer membrane vesicle (OMV) preparation or a purified adhesin that binds to the O antigen. With all three antigen preparations, there was a dose dependent response of the pro-inflammatory cytokines [Alkout et al., 2000a].

One hypothesis suggested to explain the association between *H. pylori* and IHD is that chronic infection induces inflammatory mediators which increase levels of coagulation factors (*e.g.,* fibrinogen) [Patel et al., 1995]. Ethnic groups other than Aboriginal Australians have higher incidences of IHD compared to Caucasian populations. IHD is more common among South Asians living in Britain and their higher levels of fibrinogen are not associated with common polymorphisms in the fibrinogen gene [Kain et al., 2002]. Sera from South Asians and Europeans in the Newcastle-upon-Tyne Heart Project in Britain were examined quantitatively for IgG to *H. pylori*. After adjustment for confounding factors (age, sex, income, social class, educational level), geometric mean IgG was increased among Asian men with evidence of IHD, but this was not observed among Europeans in the study [Fischbacher et al., 2004]. Cardiovascular disease and deaths among Indigenous Australians between the ages of 25-55 years are 5-10 times that of non-Indigenous groups [Veroni et al., 1994]. While smoking and diabetes which are traditional risk factors for heart disease are more common among Indigenous communities, others such as high cholesterol levels are not [Wang & Hoy, 2003]. In a study of a remote Aboriginal population, it was found that higher CRP concentrations were associated with fibrinogen levels, IgG concentrations and with IgG seropositivity for *H. pylori, C. pneumoniae* or CMV [McDonald et al., 2004].

Increasing intima-media thickness in an Aboriginal population was associated with increased CRP concentrations over a range that suggested infection and inflammation might be important risk factors for cardiovascular disease [McDonald et al., 2004]. Plasma fibrinogen production is mediated mainly by IL-6 from monocytes and macrophages [Akira & Kishimoto, 1992]. In an Italian population, a polymorphism in the IL6 gene (C-174G) was higher among patients with peripheral artery occlusive disease (PAOD). The GG genotype was significantly more common among PAOD patients and the CC genotype more common in the control group [Flex et al., 2002]. The GG genotype is associated with production of higher levels of IL-6 responses [Fishman et al., 1998], and we found that the GG genotype is predominant among the remote Indigenous population we examined. The majority of the European/Caucasian population tested possessed either the GC (41%) or CC (17%) genotypes. The GG genotype was predominant among the Bangladeshi and Indigenous Australian populations. The distribution of the GG genotype differed significantly between the European group (42%) and both Bangladeshis (94%) (χ^2 = 32.39, df = 2, p = 0.00) and Indigenous Australians (88%) (χ^2 = 52.57, df = 2, p = 0.00) [Moscovis et al.,2006].

Smoking, Gender and Cytokine Responses in Relation to Genotype

In the model system tested using human leukocytes [Gordon et al., 1999], the highest median IL-6 responses to endotoxin were observed for smokers with the GG genotype. Higher median levels of IL-6 were not observed among non-smokers for this genotype compared with those with the GC or CC genotypes. For non-smokers, there were no differences between median IL-6 responses among the GG, GC or CC genotypes [Moscovis et al.,2006].

Because of previous reports of significantly higher levels of IL-6 responses in males compared with females [Heesen et al., 2002], we assessed the data by gender. The median IL-6 level for the 60 women tested was 4.9 ng ml^{-1} and that for the 40 men was 8 ng ml^{-1} but the difference was not significant. When the levels were assessed for non-smokers, the differences were significant: women (n = 34), 5.2 ng ml^{-1}; men (n = 24) 8.1 ng ml^{-1} (p = 0.025). The difference for the smokers was not significant: women (n = 25) 4.6 ng ml^{-1}; men (n = 15) 7.85 ng ml^{-1} (p = 0.366). There were not enough subjects to assess the data by both smoking and gender.

The AA genotype is associated with low levels of IL-10 production [Hajeer et al., 1988; Reich et al., 1999] and it was predominant among Aboriginal Australians and Bangladeshis (>80% for both) compared with European/Caucasian subjects (31%) (P = 0.00). The GG genotype was absent in both the Bangladeshi and Aboriginal populations tested [Moscovis et al., 2004a]. Endotoxin induced significantly lower levels of IL-10 from leukocytes from smokers (25.6 ng ml^{-1}, range 1-171.4 ng ml^{-1}) than from non-smokers (57.7 ng ml^{-1}, range 1-1608.0 ng ml^{-1}) (p=0.00). There were no significant differences for IL-10 responses from leukocytes from non-smokers to endotoxin for the three genotypes of the IL-10 (G-1082A) SNP. There were significant differences between smokers and non-smokers for individuals with the GA genotype (p = 0.04) and the AA genotype (p = 0.01). The difference between smokers and non-smokers for the GG genotype was not significant (p = 0.09) [Moscovis et al., 2004a].

Seasonal Variation in IHD and Virus Infection

In winter fatal and non-fatal MI and stroke increase among the elderly [Woodhouse et al., 1994; Stout & Crawford, 1991]. Elderly individuals studied in their homes, sheltered or residential accommodation had increased levels of fibrinogen, plasma viscosity and HDL cholesterol in winter. Institutionalized individuals had greater changes in plasma fibrinogen compared with those in the community. Respiratory tract infections are more common in winter and also more common among institutional residents [Stout & Crawford, 1991]. Interferon-γ (IFN-γ) responses play an important role in dealing with virus infections and virus infections also enhance inflammatory responses to bacteria or their components [Sarawar et al., 1994; Blood-Siegfried et al., 2004]. The distribution of the IFN-γ T+874A polymorphism in the remote Indigenous community we examined varied significantly in comparison with both the Bangladeshi (p=0.02) and European (p=0.00) ethnic groups. Within each ethnic group the majority of individuals (~50%) possessed the heterozygous genotype. The Indigenous Australian population differed from the two other ethnic groups in that 39% of individuals possessed the TT genotype associated with high IFN-γ responses, compared to 16% and 13% for the European and Bangladeshi populations, respectively (Table 2). The interactions between chronic infections such as *H. pylori* and acute viral infections might result in increased levels of IL-6 and subsequent increases in fibrinogen.

The evidence for the role of *H. pylori* in IHD has been mixed. The recent finding that these bacteria are present in over 90% of some Aboriginal communities indicates that it would be worthwhile examining their potential role in the aetiology of IHD. If the genetic and environmental factors common among Aboriginal Australians enhance pro-inflammatory responses (particularly IL-6) to chronic infections, assessment of these interactions could provide insights into the higher incidence of IHD in this group. If there is evidence that *H. pylori* contributes significantly to the aetiology of IHD, programs to prevent and eradicate these infections would be justified and might lead to long term reduction of heart disease in Indigenous Australians. The information to support such public health measures is not available at present [Talley, 2005].

Type 2 Diabetes

It has been proposed that atherosclerosis and type 2 diabetes share a common inflammatory basis [Pradhan et al., 2001] indicated by a growing body of evidence that low grade chronic activation of the inflammatory system associated with development of type 2 diabetes which affects up to 30% of Indigenous Australians over the age of 55. Those living in remote areas (16%) were approximately twice as likely to have type 2 diabetes as those living in non-remote areas (9%) [Australian Bureau of Statistics, 2004]. A major study of the *IL6* gene promoter polymorphisms and type 2 diabetes (>20,000 patients from 8 different countries) found evidence for an association between reduced risk of developing the disease and the GC and CC alleles (OR 0.91, p = 0.037) corresponding to a risk modification of nearly 9% [Huth et al., 2006]. High IL-6 levels and insulin resistance has been reported for the Pima Indians of North America and among Caucasians [Vozarova et al., 2001; Fernandez-Real et al., 2001]. A similar pattern for the *IL6* G-174CSNP is observed among the Indigenous Aboriginal and population examined and among South Asians [Moscovis et al., 2006].

In addition to the IL-6 genotype, obesity (a significant factor for type 2 diabetes) needs to be considered as fat cells produce cytokines. It has been estimated that 25-30% of total circulating concentrations of IL-6 originates from subcutaneous adipose tissue in healthy adults [Mohamed-Ali et al., 1997].

It has been suggested that an insulin-resistant genotype associated with an activated immune system might have been advantageous when life span was short and injury and infectious disease prevalent. Lindsey et al. (2001) found that gamma globulin levels were predictors for type 2 diabetes among Pima Indians, and they proposed the hypothesis that repeated epidemics in Native Americans introduced by Europeans in the fifteenth century led to selection of individuals who were resistant to infections but consequently prone to type 2 diabetes. Our findings of this genotype in Aboriginal Australians and south Asians do not support this hypothesis. The Australian population was isolated from acute epidemic diseases until the late 18th century and the South Asian population exposed to a large number of epidemics. High levels of IgG have been found among Indigenous Australians, both children and adults. Serum concentrations of CRP were significantly correlated with IgG concentrations. Higher CRP levels were associated with IgG antibodies to *H. pylori, C. pneumoniae* and higher titres for CMV. Higher CRP levels were also associated with older age group, females, skin sores, high BMI, waist circumference, blood pressure, glycated haemoglobin and albuminuria. The increased evidence of inflammatory mediators was suggested to result from higher incidences of chronic infection [McDonald et al., 2004]. If this hypothesis is correct, adapting strategies to reduce the chronic infection load (e.g., eradication of *H. pylori* and *C. pneumoniae* and addressing chronic skin infections) and improvement in skin hygiene might help reduce the risks of cardiovascular disease and diabetes.

Low IL-10 levels have been reported among elderly individuals with type 2 diabetes markers and CRP levels. The predominant genotype for Indigenous Australians was that for low IL-10 responses [Moscovis et al., 2004;]. A positive correlation between serum levels of the anti-inflammatory IL-10 and insulin sensitivity has been reported [Straczkowski et al., 2005; Van Exel et al., 2002]. In healthy young adults, the correlation remained significant after adjustment for age, gender, BMI, fasting and postload glucose and insulin, lipids and hs-CRP [Straczkowski et al., 2005].

Identification of individuals at risk for both type 2 diabetes and atherosclerosis at an early stage when risk factor modification might delay or prevent the clinical onset of these diseases is considered to be a major challenge. For Indigenous Australians, there is considerable information on the potential role of chronic infections and obesity; there is an urgent need to assess these factors in relation to the genetic markers for high pro-inflammatory and low anti-inflammatory responses .

Kidney Disease

One of the areas in which the health of Indigenous Australians differs most significantly from that of non-Indigenous populations is kidney disease. The most severe form is end stage renal disease (ESDR) in which dialysis and kidney transplantation are required to maintain life. One of the major questions being asked is, "Are kidney, cardiovascular and infectious diseases related?" [McDonald, 2004]. Among Indigenous people, all stages of kidney disease have been shown to predict cardiovascular morbidity and mortality [Go et al., 2004; Hillege et al., 2001; Janssen et al., 2000]. Infection has been known to play a role in kidney disease, in particular post streptococcal glomerulonephritis, but this is responsible for only a small proportion of ESDR among Indigenous Australians [McDonald & Excell, 2005]. It has been suggested that a series of insults through life, including small kidneys associated with low birth weight, progressing through higher rates of infection and diabetes explains the increased incidence of kidney disease [Hoy et al., 2001].

There is a strong correlation between Chronic Kidney Disease (CKD) and cardiovascular disease (CVD). With increased proteinuria and decreased glomerular flow rate (GFR) the traditional CVD risk factors, such as hypertension and dyslipidaemia, are also increased. In conjunction with traditional factors CKD related changes to many systems increase the individual's CVD risk. These non-traditional risk factors include disruption to: red blood cell production, inflammation, calcium and phosphorus metabolism, infections, oxidative stress, increased levels of homocystine, uraemia, and proteinuria.

Infection and inflammation are thought to be the common thread linking cardiovascular disease, diabetes and kidney disease. In a study of a remote Aboriginal population, it was found that higher CRP concentrations were associated with fibrinogen levels, IgG concentrations and with IgG seropositivity for *H. pylori, C. pneumoniae* or CMV [McDonald et al., 2004]. ESRD is inversely correlated with markers of socioeconomic deprivation in non-Aboriginal communities [Cass et al., 2002]. ESRD is more common in remote Indigenous communities and this is thought to reflect the living conditions associated with social deprivation - overcrowding; higher cigarette consumption, obesity, low birth weight infants. These are factors that have been consistently identified in different countries and cultures [Marmot, 1999]. In addition to the socioeconomic factors and the increased burden of infection in these communities, the influence of inflammatory cytokine genes needs to be considered. Members of the remote community examined in our studies had a higher proportion of the SNP associated with strong pro-inflammatory responses and low anti-inflammatory responses compared with Indigenous people from costal of rural communities [Ashhurst-Smith et al., 2008]. The genotypes were similar to those observed among Indigenous Canadians with ESDR [Larcombe et al., 2005] (Table 6).

Approximately 30-50% of dialysis patients have evidence of markedly activated inflammatory responses and is suggested to be an indicator of poor outcome of ESRD [Yao et al., 2004]. High levels of IL-6 are associated with poor outcome of ESRD [Bologa et al., 1998; Pecoits-Filho et al., 2002; Panichi et al., 2004] and this genotype associated with high IL-6 production is predominant in Aboriginal populations in both Australia and North America. IL-1β is suggested to lead to malnutrition through inducing anorexia and muscle wasting among ESRD patients.

Table 6. Cytokine SNP among Indigenous groups with high incidences of ESRD. %

SNP	Phenotype of response	Australian Caucasian N = 124	Australian Indigenous N =119	Control Canadian N =130	ESRD Canadian Indigenous N = 78
IL1B C-511T	Low	50	4		
	Medium	41	23		
	high	9	73		
IL6 G-174C	Low	17	1	0	4
	Medium	41	11	14	0
	High	42	88	86	96

SNP	Phenotype of response	Australian Caucasian N = 124	Australian Indigenous N =119	Control Canadian N =130	ESRD Canadian Indigenous N = 78
IFNG T+874A	Low	37	12	76	69
	Medium	47	49	20	24
	High	16	39	4	6
TNF G-308A	Low	68	99	93	96
	Medium	29	1	7	4
	High	3	0	0	0
IL8 A-251T	Low	20	3		
	Medium	52	31		
	High	28	66		
IL10 G-1082A	Low	31	85	62	96
	Medium	38	15	32	4
	High	31	0	6	0

Preterm Birth and Stillbirths

Aboriginal women have double the rates of preterm birth and birth of a low birthweight baby compared to non-Aboriginal women (Table 7). The incidence of stillbirths is also higher among Aboriginal (10.8/1000) than non-Aboriginal (4.57/1000) women [Allesandri et al., 2008]. A recent review summarized the effects of inflammatory responses on survival and reproductive function as a trade off between fertility (survival *in utero*) and survival to reach reproductive age [Van Bodegom et al., 2007]. If the hypothesis is correct, powerful pro-inflammatory responses evolved to promote survival to the age of reproduction could contribute to prematurity and low birthweight as a result of chronic or acute infection. Chronic infection which is more common among Aboriginal Australians might be an important factor for low birthweight, preterm births and stillbirths. In a European population, antibodies to *Chlamydia trachomatis* were more prevalent among mothers who and a still birth (33.3%) or preterm delivery (18.8%) [Gencay et al., 2000] and chlamydial infections are 18 times more prevalent among Aboriginal Australians (Table 1). In a study of intrauterine growth retardation (IUGR) in an urban population, non-Caucasians (including Aboriginal) women were more often seropositive for *H. pylori*, and IUGR was more common among women who were seropositive for *H. pylori* (OR 2.4 95% CI1.14-5.08). Both smoking and *H. pylori* infection were independent risk factors for IUGR [Eslick et al., 2002].

Exposure to environmental stressors such as cigarette smoke, has been shown to affect profoundly the outcomes of pregnancy [Horta et al., 1997; Chan *et al.*, 2001; Moshin et al., 2003]; however, little is understood about how cigarette exposure reduces birthweight and affects gestational length. In addition, obesity is associated with higher levels of interleukin-6 (IL-6), and the genotype for high levels of IL-6 was associated with spontaneous preterm birth [Simhan et al., 2003]. This is the genotype predominant among Indigenous Australians [Moscovis et al., 2006] along with the genotype for low IL-10 production [Moscovis et al., 2004a].

Table 7. Comparison of Aboriginal to non-Aboriginal measurable fetal outcomes.
Modified from Laws et al., 2006.

Measurable Outcomes	Aboriginal n (%)	Non- Aboriginal n (%)
Total number of deliveries	9004	248300
Preterm deliveries	(14.3%)	(7.9%)
Low birthweight	(13.2%)	(6.1%)

Infections as a Selective Pressure?

Parasitic infection represents a chronic long-term environmental insult that involves the parasite triggering host reactivity that creates an anti-inflammatory environment primarily through the activation of IL-4, IL-5, IL-10 and IL-13 as well as the immunoglobulin IgE. Together these responses orchestrate the activation of T-helper 2 (Th2) immune response (for review see Maizels et al. 2004). How a decrease in anti-inflammatory control might relate to improved survival is not yet clear; however, similar patterns of SNPs for low levels of TNF, IFN and high levels of IL-4 and IL-6 were observed among Aboriginal Canadians [Larcombe et al., 2005]. Further work in understanding the relationship between microbial pathogens and parasitic infection is required to reconcile these differences. Nevertheless, the cytokine profiles observed in Indigenous populations are best explained by the respective parasitic load or perhaps chronic viral infections to which the populations were exposed compared to that observed in the European population.

Summary

The cytokine profiles observed in the different populations examined should be considered as responses to their respective natural environments. Not only will the host organism, in this case man, be responding to the immediate environment but also the respective pathogens will be doing likewise. The evidence for this divergence is no more striking that when one environment is transposed for another, as in the Indigenous populations in whom within a very short time in terms of evolution their environments were changed from sparsely populated nomadic hunter gatherer populations to increasingly crowded conditions, contact with new diseases of human populations and their domesticated animals, profound changes in diet and the introduction of tobacco and alcohol usage. The effects various risk factors for both infectious diseases and conditions for which infectious triggers are postulated can be explained in relation to their effects on inflammatory responses. Future studies should focus on assessment of these interactions with the goal of developing interventions, both social and medical/biological, to reduce the imbalances in health among Indigenous people.

References

Akira S, Kishimoto T. IL-6 and NF IL-6 in acute phase responses and viral infection. *Immunol Rev* 1992; 127: 25-50

Alessandri LM, Stanley FJ, Waddell, VP, Newnham J. Stillbirths in Western Australia 1980–1983: Influence of Race, Residence and Place of Birth *ANZJOG 2008*; 28: 284-292.

Allesandri LM, Chambers HM, Blair EM, Read AW. Perinatal and postneonatal mortality among Indigenous and non-Indigenous infants born in Western Australia. *Med J Aust* 2001; 175: 185-189.

Alessandri LM, Read AW, Stanley FJ, Burton PR, Dawes VP. Sudden infant death syndrome in aboriginal and non-aboriginal infants. *J Paediatr Child Health* 1994; 30: 234-241.

Alkout AM, Blackwell CC, Weir DM. The inflammatory response to *Helicobacter pylori* in relation to ABO blood group antigens. *J Infect Dis* 2000; 181: 1364-1369.

Alkout AM, Ramsay E, Blackwell CC, Bentley AJ, Elton RA, Weir DM, Busuttil. IgG levels to *Helicobacter pylori* among individuals who died of ischaemic heart disease compared with patients who experienced a first heart attack. *FEMS Immunolo Medi Microbiol* 2000; 29: 271-274.

An SF, Gould S, Keeling JW, Fleming KA. The role of viral infection in SIDS: detection of viral nucleic acid by in situ hybridization. *J Pathol* 1993; 171: 271-278.

Arend W. P.The balance between IL-1 and IL-1Ra in disease. *Cytokine Growth Factor Rev* 2002; 13: 323-340.

Ashhurst-Smith C, Stuart JE, Moscovis SM, Titmarsh CJ, Hall ST, Walker P, Dorrington R, Eisenberg R, Burns C, Scott RJ, Blackwell CC *Alloiococcus otitidis*, gene polymorphisms and otitis media with effusion (OME) in Aboriginal children [Abstract 57]. *In: Program and abstracts of the 2nd Aboriginal Health Research Conference* (Sydney) 29-30 March 2008

Atherton JC, Tham KT, Peek RM, Cover TL, Blaser MJ. Density of *Helicobacter pylori* infection *in vivo* as assessed by quantitative culture and histology. *J Infect Dis* 1996; 174: 552- 56.

Australian Bureau of Statistics. *Diabetes in Australia: a snapshot 2001* 4820.0.55.001 2004.

Australian Bureau of Statistics, in *ABS cat no. 4704.0 AIHW cat no. IHW14.* (ABS, Canberra, 2005).

Balding J, Healy C M, Livingstone W J, White B, Mynett-Johnson L, Cafferkey M, Smith, O P. Genomic polymorphic profiles in an Irish population with meningococcaemia: is it possible to predict severity and outcome of disease? *Genes Immun 2003*; 4: 533-40.

Balarajan R, Raleigh VS, Botting B. Sudden infant death syndrome and post neonatal mortality in immigrants in England and Wales. *BMJ* 1989; 298: 716-20.

Beckwith JB. (Discussion of terminology and definition of the sudden infant death syndrome. In *Sudden Infant Death Syndrome; Proceedings of the Second International Conference on the Causes of Sudden Death in Infants* (A.B. Bergman, J.B. Beckwith and G.C. Ray, eds.), University of Washington Press, 1970: 14-22.

Bhagat K, Collier J, Vallance, P. Endothelial stunning following a brief exposure to endotoxin: a mechanism to link infection to infarction. *Cardiovasc Res* 1996; 32: 822-29

Blackwell CC, Gordon AE, James VS, et al. The role of bacterial toxins in Sudden Infant Death Syndrome (SIDS). *Int J Med Microbiol* 2002; 291: 561-70.

Blackwell CC, Moscovis SM, Gordon AE, et al. Ethnicity, Infection and Sudden Infant Death Syndrome. *FEMS Immunol Med Microbiol* 2004; 42: 53-65.

Blackwell CC, Moscovis SM, Gordon AE, et al. Cytokine responses and sudden infant death syndrome: genetic, developmental, and environmental risk factors *J Leukocyte Biol* 2005; 78: 1242-54.

Blackwell CC, Tzanakaki G, Kremastinou J, Weir DM, Vakalis N, Elton RA, Mentis A. Factors affecting carriage of *Neisseria meningitidis* among Greek military recruits. *Epidemiol Infect* 1992; 108: 441-48.

Blackwell, C.C., Weir, D.M., Busuttil A. Infectious agents, the inflammatory responses of infants and sudden infants death syndrome (SIDS). *Molecular Medicine Today* 1995; 1: 72-78.

Blood-Siegfried J, Nyska A, Geisenhoffer K., Lieder H, Moomaw C, Cobb K, Sheldon B, Coombs W, Germolec D. Alteration in Regulation of Inflammatory Response to Influenza A Virus and Endotoxin In Suckling Rat Pups: A Potential Relationship to Sudden Infant Death Syndrome. *FEMS Immunol Med Microbiol* 2004; 42: 85-93.

Boehmke F, Esnaashari H, Seitzer U, Kothe H, Maass M, Zabel P, Dalhoff K. Pneumococcal septic shock is associated with the interleukin-10-1082 gene promotor polymorphism. *Am J Resp Crit Care Med* 2003; 168: 476-80.

Bologa RM, Levine DM, Parker TS. et al. 1998. Interleukin-6 predicts hypoalbuminemia, hypocholesterolemia, and mortality in hemodialysis patients. *Am J Kidney Dis* 1998; 32: 107-14.

Bone RC. Gram-negative sepsis: a dilemma of modern medicine. *Clin Microbiol Rev* 1993; 6: 57-68.

Brown L. *Helicobacter pylori*: epidemiology and routes of transmission. *Epidemiol Rev.* 2000; 22: 283-297.

Cass A, Cunningham J, Snelling P et al. End-stage renal disease in indigenous Australians: a disease of disadvantage. *Ethn Dis 2002*; 12: 373-78.

Chan A, Keane RJ, Robinson JS. The contribution of maternal smoking to preterm birth, small for gestational age and low birthweight among Aboriginal and non-Aboriginal births in South Australia. *Med J Aust.* 2001; 174: 389-93.

Chiche J-D, Siami S, Dhainaut J-F D Mira J-P. Cytokine polymorphisms and susceptibility to severe infectious diseases. *Sepsis* 2001; 4: 209-15.

Christodoulides M, Makepeace B L, Partridge KA, Kaur D, Fowler M I, Weller RO, Heckels J E. Interaction of *Neisseria meningitidis* with human meningeal cells induces the secretion of a distinct group of chemotactic, Ppoinflammatory, and growth-factor cytokines. *Infect Immun* 2002; 70: 4035-44.

Collins HL & Kaufmann SHE. The many faces of host response to tuberculosis. *Immunol* 2001; 103: 1-9.

Currie BJ, Brewster DR.. Childhood infections in the tropical north of Australia. *J Paediatr Child Health* 2001; 37: 326-30.

Dahmer, M. K., Randolph, A., Vitali, S. and Quasney, M. W.: Genetic polymorphisms in sepsis. *Pediatr Crit Care Med* 2005; 6: S61-73.

Daly JB, Wiggers JH, Considine RJ.(Infant exposure to environmental tobacco smoke: a prevalence study in Australia. *Aust N Z J Pub Health* 2001; 25: 132-7.

Danesh J, Peto, R. Risk factors for coronary heart disease and infection with *Helicobacter pylori*: meta-analysis of 18 studies. *BMJ* 1998; 316,: 1130-2.

DeForge L, Kenney J, Jones M, Warren J, Remick D. Biphasic production of IL-8 in lipopolysaccharide (LPS)-stimulated human whole blood. Separation of LPS- and cytokine-stimulated components using anti-tumor necrosis factor and anti-IL-1 antibodies. *J Immunol* 1992; 148: 2133-41.

Diamond J. *Guns, Germs and Steel*. London: Vintage Random House, 1997.

Dinarello C. Biologic basis for interleukin-1 in disease. *Blood* 1996; 87: 2095-2147.

Eades SJ, Read AW, the Bibbulung Gnarneep Team. (1999) Infant care practices in a metropolitan Aboriginal population. *J Paediatr Child Health* 1999; 5: 541-44.

El Ahmer OR, Essery SD, Saadi AT, Raza MW, Ogilvie MM, Weir DM, Blackwell CC. The effect of cigarette smoke on adherence of respiratory pathogens to buccal epithelial cells. FEMS Immunol Me. *Microbiol 1999a*; 23: 27-36.

El Ahmer OR, Raza MW, Ogilvie MM, Elton RA, Weir DM., Blackwell, C.C. Binding of bacteria to HEp-2 cells infected with influenza A virus. *FEMS Immunol Med. Microbiol.* 1999b; 23: 331-41.

Eslick GD, Yan P, Xia H-X, Murray H, Spurrett B, Talley NJ. Fetal intrauterine growth restrictions with *Helicobacter pylori* infection. *Aliment Pharmacol Ther 2002*; 16: 1677-82.

Fernandez-Real JM, Vayreda M, Richart C, Gutierrez C, Broch M, Vendrell J, Ricart W. Circulating interleukin 6 levels, blood pressure, and insulin sensitivity in apparently healthy men and women. *J Clin Endocrinol Metab* 2001; 86: 1154-59.

Fischbacher CM, Bhopal R, Blackwell CC, Ingram R, Unwin NC, White M, Alberti KGMM. IgG is higher in South Asians than Europeans: Does infection contribute to ethnic variation in cardiovascular disease? *Arterioscler Thromb Vasc Biol* 2003; 2: 703-4.

Fischbacher CM, Blackwell CC, Bhopal R, Ingram R, Unwin NC, White M. Serological evidence of *Helicobacter pylori* infection in UK South Asian and European populations: implications for gastric cancer and coronary heart disease. *J Infect 2004;* 48: 168-74.

Fishman D, Faulds G, Jeffery R, Mohamed-Ali V, Yudkin JS, Humphries S, Woo P. The effect of novel polymorphisms in the interleukin-6 (IL-6) gene on IL-6 transcription and plasma IL-6 levels, and an association with systemic-onset juvenile chronic arthritis. *J Clin Invest* 1998; 102: 1369-76.

Flex A, Gaetani E, Pola R, et al. The -174 G/C polymorphism of the interleukin-6 gene promoter is associated with peripheral artery occlusive disease. *Eur J Endovas Surg* 2002; 24: 264-68.

Froen T F, Aker H, Stray-Pedersen B, Saugstad OD. Adverse effects of nicotine and interleukin-1 beta on autoresuscitation after apnea in piglets: Implications for sudden infant death syndrome. *Pediatrics* 2000; 105: E52

Gencay M, Koskiniemi M, Ammala P, Fellerman V, Narvanen A, Wahlstrom T, Vaheri A, Puolakkainen M. *Chalmydia trachomatis* seropostititivity is associated with both stillbirth and preterm delivery. *APMIS 2000*; 108: 584-88.

Gleeson M, Clancy RL, Cripps AW. Mucosal immune response in a case of sudden infant death syndrome. *Pediatr Res 1993*; 33: 554–56.

Go AS, Chertow GM, Fan D et al. Chronic kidney disease and the risks of death, cardiovascular events and hospitalisation. *N. Engl. J. Med.* 2004; 351: 1296-1305.

Goldwater P. SIDS pathogenesis: pathological findings indicate infection and inflammatory responses are involved. *FEMS Immunol Med Microbiol* 2004; 42: 11-20.

Goldwater PN, Williams V, Bourne AJ, Byard RW. Sudden infant death syndrome: a possible clue to causation. *Med J Austral 1990;* 153: 59-60.

Gordon AE, Al Madani OM, Raza MW, Weir DM, Busuttil A, Blackwell CC (1999) Cortisol levels and control of inflammatory responses to toxic shock syndrome toxin (TSST-1): The prevalence of night time deaths in Sudden Infant Death Syndrome. *FEMS Immunol Med Microbiol 1999;* 25: 199-206.

Guthridge S, McIntyre P, Isaacs C, Hanlon M, Patel M. Differing serologic responses o an *Haemophilus influenzae* type b polysaccharide-*Neisseria meningitidis* outer membrane protein conjugate (PRP-OMPC) vaccine in Australian Aboriginal and Caucasian infants – implications for disease epidemiology. *Vaccine 2000;* 18: 2584-91.

Hackett S J, Thomson AP, Hart CA. Cytokines, chemokines and other effector molecules involved in meningococcal disease. *J Med Microbiol 2001*; 50: 847-59, 2001

Hacking D, Knight JC, Rockett K, Brown H, Frampton J, Kwiatkowski DP, Hull J, Udalova IA. Increased in vivo transcription of an IL-8 haplotype associated with respiratory syncytial virus disease-susceptibility. *Genes Immun 2004*; 5: 274-82.

Hajeer AH, Lazarus M, Turner D, Mageed RA, Vencovsky J, Sinnott P, Hutchinson IV, Ollier WER. IL-10 gene promoter polymorphisms in rheumatoid arthritis. *Scand J Rheumatol* 1988; 27: 142 - 45.

Heesen M, Bloemeke B, Heussen N, Kunz D. Can the interleukin-6 response to endotoxin be predicted? Studies of the influence of a promoter polymorphism of the interleukin-6 gene, gender, the desity of the endotoxin receptor CD14 and inflammatory cytokines. *Crit Care Med 2002;* 30: 664-669.

Helminen M, Lahdenpohja N, Hurme M. Polymorphism of the interleukin-10 gene is associated with susceptibility to Epstein-Barr virus infection. *J Infect Dis 1999;* 180: 496 - 99.

Helleman D, Larrson A, Madsen O et al. Heterozogosity of mannos-binding lectin (MBL2) genotypes predicts advantage (heterosis in relation to fatal outcome in intensive care patients. *Hum Mol Genet* 2007; 24: 3071-80.

Hilder AS. Ethnic differences in the sudden infant death syndrome: what can we learn from immigrants to the UK. *Early Hum Devel 1994;* 38: 143-49.

Hillege HL, Hanssen WM, Bak AA et al. 2001. Microalbuminuria is common, also in a nondiabetic, nonhypertensive population, and an independent indicator of cardiovascular risk factors and cardiovascular morbidity. *J Intern Med 2001*; 249: 519-26

Hoffman HJ, Damus, K, Hillman L, and Krongrad E . Risk factors for SIDS: results of the ntional Institute of Child Health and Human Development SIDS Cooperative Epidemiological Study. *Ann NY Acad Sci 1988*; 533: 13-30.

Holgate ST, Walters C, Walls AF, Lawrence S, Shell DJ, Variend S, Fleming PJ, Berry PJ, Gilbert RE, Robinson C. The anaphylaxis hypothesis of sudden infant death syndrome

(SIDS): mast cell degranulation in cot death revealed by elevated concentrations of tryptase in serum. *Clin Exp Allergy 1994*; 24: 115-123.

Horta BL, Victora CG, Menezes AM, Halpern R, Barros FC. Low birthweight, preterm births and intrauterine growth retardation in relation to maternal smoking. *Paediatr Perinat Epidemiol*. 1997; 11:140-51.

Howat WJ, Moore IE, Judd M, Roche WR. Pulmonary immunopathology of sudden infant death syndrome. *Lancet 1994;* 343:1390-1392.

Hoy W, Wang Z, van Buynder P *et al*. 2001. The natural history of renal disease: Part 1. Changes in albuminuria and glomerular filtration rate over time in a community-based cohort of Australian Aborigines with high rates of renal disease. *Kidney Int 2001;* 60: 243-48.

Huth C, Heid IM, Vollmert C et al. IL gene promoter polymorphisms and type 2 diabetes. Joint analysis of individual participants' data from 21 studies. *Diabetes 2006*; 55: 2915-21.

Janssen WM, Hillege H, Pinto-Sietsma SJ et al. Low levels of urinary albumin excretion are associated with cardiovascular risk factors in the general population. *Clin Chem Lab Med 2000;* 38:1107-10.

Jiang ZD, DuPont HL, Garey K et al. A common polymorphism in the interleukin 8 gene promoter is associated with *Clostridium difficile* diarrhea. *Am J Gastroenterol 2006;* 101: 1112-6, 2006

Kain K, Blaxill JM, Catto AJ, Grant PJ, Carter AM. Increased firbrinogen levels among South Asians versus whites in the United Kingdom are not explained by common polymorphisms. *Am. J. Epidemiol. 2002;* 156: 174-179.

Kolos V, Menzies R, McIntyre P. Higher pertussis hospitalization rates in indigenous Australian infants, and delayed vaccination. *Vaccine 2007;* 25:588-90.

Kreuning J, Lindeman J, Biemond I, Lamers CB. Relation between IgG and IgA antibody titres against Helicobacter pylori in serum and severity of astritis in asymptomatic subjects. *J Clin Pathol 1994*; 47: 227-31.

Larcombe L, Rempel JD, Dembinski I, Tinckam K, Rigatto C, Nickerson P. Differential cytokine genotype frequencies among Canadian Aboriginal and Caucasian populations. *Genes Immun 2005*; 5: 140-144.

Laws P, Grayson N, Sullivan EA. Australia's Mothers and Babies 2004. In: Unit ANPS, ed.: *Australian Institute of Health and Welfare 2006.*

Lehmann A K, Halstensen A, Sornes S, Rokke O, Waage A. High levels of interleukin 10 in serum are associated with fatality in meningococcal disease. *Infect Immun 1995;* 63: 2109-12.

Lio D, Marino V, Serauto A, et al. (2002) Genotype frequencies of the +874T→A single nucleotide polymorphism in the first intron of the interferon-γ gene in a sample of Sicilian patients affected by tuberculosis. *Eur J Immunogenet 2002*; 29: 371-4.

Lindsey R S, Krakoff J, Hanson RL, Bennett PH, Knowler WC. Gamma globulin levels predict type 2 diabetes in the Pima Indian population. *Diabetes 2001;* 50: 1598-1603.

Lopez-Maderuelo D, Arnalich F, Serantes R et al. 2003. Interferon-γ and interleukin-10 gene polymorphisms in pulmonary tuberculosis. *Am J Resp Crit Care Med 2003*; 163: 970-5.

Ma X, Reich RA, Wright JA, Toker HR, Teeter LD, Musser JM, Graviss EA. Association between interleukin-8 gene alleles and human susceptibility to tuberculosis disease. *J Infect Dis 2003*; 188: 349-55.

Maizels RM, Balic A, Gomez-Excobar N, Nair M, Taylor MD, Allen JE. Helminth parasites – masters of regulation. *Immunological Rev. 2004*; 201:89-116.

Malley R, Huskins WC, Kuppermann N. Multivariable predictive models for adverse outcome of invasive meningococcal disease in children, *J Pediatrics 1996*; 129: 702-10.

Marmot M. Epidemiology of socioeconomic status and health: are determinants within countries the same as between countries? *Ann NY Acad Sci 1999;* 896: 16-29.

McDonald SP, Excell L. ANZDATA Registry Report. Adelaide, Australia and New Zealand *Dialysis and Transplant Registry; 2005.*

McDonald S, Maguire G, Duartes N, Wang XL, Hoy W C-reactive protein, cardiovascular risks, and renal disease in a remote Australian Aboriginal community. *Clin Sci 2004;* 106: 121-8.

Mocellin, S, Marincola F, Riccardo Rossi C, Nitti D, Lise, M.: The multifaceted relationship between IL-10 and adaptive immunity: putting together the pieces of a puzzle. *Cytokine Growth Factor Rev 2004;* 15: 61-76.

Mohamed-Ali V, Goodrick S, Rawesh A et al. Subcutaneous adipose tissue releases interleukin-6 but not tumor necrosis factor-alpha in vivo. *J Clin Endocrinol Metab 1997;* 82: 4196-4200.

Mohsin M, Wong F, Bauman A, Bai J. Maternal and neonatal factors influencing premature birth and low birth weight in Australia. *J Biosoc Sci 2003*; 35:161-74.

Moscovis SM, Gordon AE, Al Madani OM, et al. Interluekin-10 and Sudden Infant Death Syndrome. *FEMS Immunol Med Microbiol 2004a*; 42: 130-8.

Moscovis SM, Gordon AE, Al Madani OM et al. Interleukin-1β and Sudden Infant Death Syndrome. *FEMS Immunol. Med. Microbiol. 2004b*; 42, 139-45.

Moscovis SM, Gordon AE, Al Madani OM et al. IL6 G-174C associated with sudden infant death syndrome in a Caucasian Australian cohort. *Hum Immunol 2006*; 67:819-25.

Musher DM, Fainstein V. Adherence of *Staphylococcus aureus* to pharyngeal cells from normal carriers and patients with viral infections. In: J. Jeljaswiecz, ed. *Staphylococci and staphylococcal infections*. New York: Gustav Fischer Verlag, 1981: 1011-16.

Netea MG, van der Meer JWM, van Deuren M, Kullberg B. Proinflammatory cytokines and sepsis syndrome: not enough, or too much of a good thing? *Trends Immunol. 2003;* 24: 254-8.

Ohyauchi M, Imatani A, Yonechi M et al .The polymorphism interleukin 8 -251 A/T influences the susceptibility of Helicobacter pylori related gastric diseases in the Japanese population *Gut 2005*; 54: 330-5.

Oppenheim BA, Barclay RG et al. Antibodies to endotoxin core in sudden infant death syndrome. *Arch Dis Child 1994*; 70: 95-8.

Pajkrt D, van der Poll T, Levi M et al. Interleukin-10 Inhibits Activation of Coagulation and Fibrinolysis During Human Endotoxemia. *Blood 1997;* 89: 2701-2705.

Panichi V, Maggiore U, Taccola D et al. Interleukin-6 is a strong predictor of total and cardiovascular mortality than C-reactive protein in haemodialysis patients. *Nephrol Dial Transpl 2004*; 19: 1154-60.

Patel P, Mendall MA, Carrington D et al. Association of *Helicobacter pylori* and *Chlamydia pneumoniae* infection with coronary heart disease and cardiovascular risk factors. *BMJ 1995*; 311: 711-4.

Pecoits-Filho R, Barahy B, Lindholm B, Helmburger O, Stenvinkel Pl. 2002. Interleukin-6 and its receptor is an independent predictor of mortality in patients starting dialysis treatment. *Nephrol Dial Transpl. 2002*; 17: 1684-6

Pellicano R, Fagoonee S, Rizzetto M, Ponzetto A. *Helicobacter pylori* and coronary heart disease: which directions for future studies ? *Crit Rev Microbiol 2003;* 29: 351-9.

Pradhan AD, Manson JE, Rifai N, Buring JE, Ridker PM. C-reactive protein, interleukin 6, and risk of developing type 2 diabetes mellitus. *JAMA 2001*; 286: 327-34.

Pravica V, Perrey C, Stevens A, Lee JH and Hutchinson IV. A single nucleotide polymorphism in the first intron of the human IFN-gamma gene: absolute correlation with a polymorphic CA microsatellite marker of high IFN-gamma production. *Hum Immunol 2000;* 61: 863-6

Raza MW, Blackwell CC. Sudden infant death syndrome: virus infections and cytokines *FEMS Immunol Med Microbiol 1999*; 25: 85-96

Raza MW, Essery SD, Elton RA, Weir DM, Busuttil A, Blackwell CC. Exposure to cigarette smoke, a major risk factor for Sudden Infant Death Syndrome: effects of cigarette smoke on inflammatory responses to viral infection and toxic shock syndrome toxin-1. *FEMS Immunol Med Microbiol 1999*; 25, 145-54.

Read RC, Camp NJ, di Giovine FS et al. (2000) An interleukin-1 genotype is associated with fatal outcome of meningococcal disease. *J Infect Dis 2000*; 182, 1557-60.

Reich K, Westphal G, Schulz T et al. Combined analysis of polymorphisms of the TNF-α and IL-10 promoter regions and polymorphic xenobiotic metabolizing enzymes in psoriasis. *J Invest Dermatol 1999*; 113: 214-20.

Ring IT, Brown N.I Indigenous health: chronically inadequate responses to damning statistics. *Med J Aust 2002*; 177: 629-631.

Rognum TO. Definition and pathologic features. In: Byard RW and Krouse HF eds. *Sudden Infant Death Syndrome: Problems, Progress and Possibilities*. London: Arnold, 2001: 4-30.

Rowley K, Walker KZ, Cohen J et al. Inflammation and vascular endothelial activation in an Aboriginal population: relationships to coronary disease risk factors and nutritional markers. *Med J Aust 2003;* 178: 495-500

Santilla S, Savinainen K, Hurme M. Presence of the IL-1RA allele 2 (IL1RN*2) is associated with enhanced IL-1[beta] production in vitro. *Scand J Immunol 1998*; 47: 195-8.

Sarawar SR, Blackman MA, Doherty PD. (1994) Superantigen shock in mice with inapparent viral infection. *J. Infect Dis 1994*; 170: 1189-94.

Sayers NM, Drucker DB, Telford DR, Morris JA. (1995) Effects of nicotine on bacterial toxins associated with cot death. *Arch Dis Child 1995*; 73: 549-51.

Selvaraj P, Prabhu Anand S, Haeahar MS, Chandra G, Banurekha B, Narayanau PR. Promoter polymorphism of IL-8 gene and IL-8 production in pulmonary tuberculosis. *Curr Sci 2006;* 90: 952-4.

Siarakas S, Brown AJ, Murrell WG. Immunological evidence for a bacterial toxin aetiology in sudden infant death syndrome *FEMS Immunol Med Microbiol 1999*; 25: 37-50.

Simhan HN, Krohn MA, Roberts JM, Zeeve A, Caritis SN. Interleukin-6 promotor -174 polymorphism and spontaneous preterm birth. *Am J Obstet Gynecol 2003*; 189:915-918.

Snick J V. Interleukin-6: An Overview. *Ann Rev Immunol 1990;* 8: 253-78.

Stead WW, Senner JW, Reddick WT, Lofgren JP. Racial differences in susceptibility to infection by *Mycobacterium tuberculosis*. *N Engl J Med 1990;* 322: 422-7.

Stout RW, Crawford V. Seasonal variation in fibrinogen concentrations among elderly people. *Lancet 1991;* 338: 9-13.

Straczkowski M, Kowalska I, Nikolajuk A, Krukowska A, Gorska M. Plasma interleukin-10 concentration is positively related to insulin sensitivity in young healthy individuals. *Diabetes Care 2005*; 28: 2036-37.

Stuart J. The development of serum immunoglobulins G, A and M in Australian Aboriginal infants. *Med J Austral 1978*; 1 (suppl): 4-5.

Taguchi A, Ohmiya N, Shirai K, et al. Interleukin-8 promoter polymorphism increases the risk of atrophic gastritis and gastric cancer in Japan. *Cancer Epidemiol Biomarkers Prev 2005*; 14: 2487-93.

Talley NJ. *Helicobacter pylori* infection in Indigenous Australians: a serious health issue? *Med J Austral 2005*; 182: 205-206.

Titmarsh CJ, Moscovis SM, Hall ST, Tzanakaki G, Kremastinou J, Scott RJ, Blackwell CC. *Cytokine gene polymorphisms among Greek patients with meningococcal disease* (submitted for publication).

Titmarsh C J, Moscovis SM, Hall ST, Scott RJ, Blackwell CC. Interleukin-8 gene polymorphisms in Aboriginal Australians: basis for investigation of significant infections. (Abstract 58) *In: Program and Abstracts of the 2nd Aboriginal Health Research Conference (Sydney)* 29-30 March 2008

Turner DM, Williams DM, Sankaran D, Lazarus M, Sinnott PJ, Hutchinson IV. An investigation of polymorphism in the interleukin-10 gene promoter. *Eur J Immunogenet 1997;* 24: 1-8.

Vallance P, Collier J, Bhagat. Infection, inflammation, and infarction: does acute endothelial dysfunction provide a link? *Lancet 1997*; 349: 1391-2.

Van Bodegom D, May L, Meij HJ, Westendorp RGJ. Regulation of human life histories: the role of the inflammatory host response. *Ann. N.Y. Acad. Sci 2007*; 1100: 84-97.

Van Exel E, Gussekloo J, de Craen AJM, Frolich M, Mootsma-van der Wiel A, Westendorp RGJ. Low production capacity of interleukin-10 associates with the metabolic syndrome and type 2 diabetes. *Diabetes 2002*; 51: 1088-92.

van Furth A M, Roord JJ, van Furth R. Roles of proinflammatory and anti-inflammatory cytokines in pathophysiology of bacterial meningitis and effect of adjunctive therapy. *Infect Immun 1996*; 64: 4883-90.

Vassalli, P. The Pathophysiology of Tumor Necrosis Factors *Ann Rev Immunol 1992*; 10: 411-52.

Vege Å , Rognum TO. Sudden infant death syndrome, infection and nflammatory response. *FEMS Immunol Med Microbiol 2004*; 42: 3-10.

Vege Å, Rognum TO, Ånestad G. IL-6 cerebrospinal fluid levels are related to laryngeal IgA and epithelial HLA-DR response in sudden infant death syndrome. *Pediatr Res 1999*; 45: 803-9.

Veroni M, Gracey M, Rouse I. Patterns of mortality in Western Australian Aboriginals, 1983-1989. *Int J epidemiol 1994*; 23: 73-81.

Vozarova B, Fernandez-Real J-M, Knowler WC et al. The interleukin-6 (-174) G/C promoter polymorphism is associated with type-2 diabetes mellitus in native Americans and Caucasians. *Hum Genet 2003*; 112: 409-13.

Vozarova B, Weyer C, Lindsay RS, Pratley RE, Bogardus C, Tataranni PA. High white blood cell count is associated with a worsening of insulin sensitivity and predicts the development of type 2 diabetes. *Diabetes. 2002*; 51: 455-61.

Wald NJ, Law MR, Morris JK, Bagnall, AM. *Helicobacter pylori* infection and mortality from ischaemic heart disease: negative results from a large prospective study. *BMJ 1997;* 315: 1199-1201.

Wang Z, Hoy WE. Hypertension, dyslipidaemia, body mass index, diabetes and smoking status in Aboriginal Australians in a remote community. *Ethnicity & Disease 2003;* 13: 324-330.

Westendorp RGJ, Langemans JAM, Huizinga TW, Elouali AH, Verweij CL, Boomsma DI, Vandenbrouke JP Genetic influence on cytokine production and fatal meningococcal disease. *Lancet 1997*; 349: 170-3.

Wilson CE. Sudden infant syndrome and Canadian Aboriginals: bacteria and infections. *FEMS Immunol Med Microbiol 1999*; 25: 221-6.

Windsor HM, Abioye-Kuteyi EA, Leber JM et al. (2005) Prevalence of *Helicobacter pylori* in Indigenous Western Australians: comparison between urban and remote rural populations. *Med J Aust 2005*; 182: 210-13.

Woodhouse PR, Khaw KT, Plummer M, Foley A, Meade TW. Seasonal fariations of plasma fibrinogen and factor VII activity in the elderly: winter infection and death from cardiovascular disease. *Lancet 1994*; 343: 435-9.

Yao Q, Lindholm B, Stenvinkel P. 2004. Inflammation as a cause of malnutrition, atherosclerotic cardiovascular disease, and poor outcome in hemodialysis patients. *Hemodialy Int 2004*; 8: 118-29.

Zorgani AA, Al Madani OM, Essery, SD et al. (1999) Detection of pyrogenic toxins of *Staphylococcus aureus* in cases of Sudden Infant Death Syndrome (SIDS). *FEMS Immunol Med Microbiol 1999*; 25: 103-8.

In: Handbook on Longevity: Genetics, Diet and Disease   ISBN: 978-1-60741-075-1
Editors: Jennifer V. Bentely and Mary Ann Keller   ©2009 Nova Science Publishers, Inc.

Chapter XVIII

Mammalian Cell Sporulation – A Possible Link to Disease and Aging

Yonnie Wu[1], Kyle Heim[2] and Erick Vasquez[3]

[1]Clemson University Genomics Institute
[2]Department of Biochemistry and Genetics,
[3]Department of Chemical and Biomolecular Engineering,
Clemson University, SC

Abstract

This chapter reviews the physiochemical properties of mammalian spores and straw cells, which develop in vitro from the transformation of normal mammalian cells exposed to desiccative conditions. We hypothesize that this transformation is directly linked with aging and aging related diseases. Unlike many of the current damage related aging theories involving damage to DNA and protein molecules (leading to improper gene expression and protein function), this transformation is an active process at the cellular level. The metamorphosis of a normal cell into a mammalian spore is an inherited survival mechanism that can cause the loss of the body's most basic life-sustaining unit, the cell.

Mammalian spores are extremely prevalent. It is estimated that a typical person currently possesses billions of spores in their blood; the amount of spores may fluctuate in a day, perhaps influenced by physiological conditions such as diet and exercise that affect the overall sporulation stress. These mammalian spores form long extensive and extremely hydrophilic filamentous network that could contribute to blood viscosity. Blood cholesterol level may be increased from sporulation of billions of cells per day.

The metamorphosis of a mammalian spore from a normal mammalian cell is marked by a variety of distinct physical changes. First, the nuclei is broken into many pieces and reassembled within a tiny tube shaped structure. Second, tubular walls are constructed. Finally, upon the reintroduction of water, mammalian spores revert to normal mammalian cells and begin to divide. The early steps of this transformation resemble the development of apoptotic bodies. However, instead of destroying itself, the cell enters a robust spore-like cell survival phase, allowing it to remain viable under severe external conditions. Mammalian spores construct a strong cell wall using sulfated-glucose polymers and glycosylated acidic proteins, allowing it to withstand harsh treatment such as UV-C radiation.

A direct inverse relationship is displayed between the number of mammalian spores present in the blood of 9 domestic animals and these animals' average lifespan. The number of mammalian spores present in the heart and lung tissues, as well as excreted in the urine, also increases with the age of the mammal. This increased production of mammalian spores may play a role in disrupting normal cell and organ function. The large number of mammalian spores produced by a variety of tissues makes this transformation appear to be a natural physiological process embedded within a cell's environmental response machinery. The universal nature of mammalian spores and their mobility within the bloodstream allow them to affect many parts of the body. The mobile character of these cells displays a potential link to longevity and the development of aging-related diseases, including the metastasis of various cancers.

Water is the most essential component for cell survival. Throughout evolution organisms have developed many novel adaptations for particular environmental deficiencies and conditions. The formation of spores may be an early form of environmental adaptation for single celled organisms. However, in multicellular organisms the mammalian spore survival mechanism may not be beneficial because the organism loses necessary functional cells. Inhibiting mammalian spore biogenesis would prevent the depletion of normal healthy cells, as well as the spread of potentially harmful cells, and therefore improve mammalian longevity. Intervention of sporulation using membrane interacting molecules is discussed. Exogenous phosphotidylcholines (DOPC) significantly promote dehydration-induced sporulation while other phospholipids (DOPG, DOPE, DOPA, and DOPS) are ineffective.

Introduction

Multicellular organisms composed of same life-supporting molecules (DNA, protein, lipid etc) can all have very different lifespan. Most mammals typically live for a few years while some plants (bristlecone pine and creosote bush) can live for a few hundred years, or longer. This diversity suggests that an organism's lifespan is genetically programmed and environmentally developed. The aging process in mammals is thought to be associated with harmful modifications to DNA and protein molecules, which result in an accumulation of damage to the organism. We hypothesize that another active mechanism embedded within the cellular machinery also plays an important role in the aging process of an organism by involving an individual cell's desire to survive by transforming into a dormant spore [1].

This theory involves a "programmed cell survival" process that may profoundly contribute to human aging. Over millions of years of evolutionary time, living creatures from primitive cells to multi-cellular organisms have been subjected to frequent episodes of dehydration related stress. Bacteria and fungi produce spores to survive through a drought. Mammalian cells evolving from bacteria may have retained this mechanism to transform into spores for survival when faced with dehydration occurring naturally *in vivo*.

However, this "cell survival" mechanism is undesirable in multicellular organisms since the transformation removes functional cells, vital for sustaining life. Over time the loss of cells gradually pushes the body into disintegrative stages and may produce chronic diseases such as osteoporosis, cardiovascular disease, Alzheimer's, cancer, etc. These diseases often take many years to develop and appear to be age related.

Mammalian Spores

The structure of a mammalian spore is composed of three major parts: a tubular center (i) with typically two to three filaments (ii) protruding out with numerous microscopic hairs (iii) on the surface of these filaments (Figure 1).

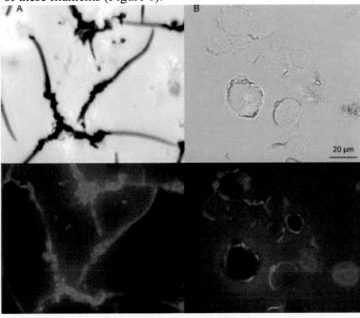

Figure 1. Human colon cancer (CACO2) mammalian spores induced from dehydration of cell culture *in vitro* (A) mammalian spores in bright field (up) and fluorescent (MT-Red, bottom). Untransformed cells when dried whose cellular contents are pushed to the edge and often in a fragmented section displaying relatively less contrast compared to mammalian spores.

Production *in Vitro*

Subjecting normal mammalian cells (Figure 2A) to dehydration (air dry) *in vitro* produces spore-like cells. Cells first begin to develop short thin spiked branches (Figure 2B). These tiny branches then elongate to develop long thin filaments (C). As these filaments develop from surrounding cells, they begin to connect and form an elaborate filamentous network that is independent of any specific cell type (E). The wall of the spore is 200 nm thick (F). The appearance of the sporulation resembles the initial phases of apoptosis with membrane blebbing (G). However, as the sporulation continues to the later stages it begins to differ from the formation of apoptotic bodies in several areas: (1) mammalian spores develop an extended tubular structure instead of the disintegrated sections of apoptotic bodies; (2) the filamentous extensions and network are extremely hydrophilic and unable to be seen in water (G) and only present themselves once the water has evaporated (H); (3) chromatin is compacted within the tubes and produces an intense green fluorescent emission only within the tubes in which it is present, not within the remaining cellular debris isolated away from the tubes (C); (4) in addition to the filaments and tubular center, many microscopic hairs also protrude from the filamentous extensions (D). When examined under a scanning electron microscope using scattering background electrons, mammalian spores in solution displayed an interconnected network during growth (E). Upon completion of a successful sporulation the plasma matrix is finally dispensed and separated from the tube. The tubes are then sealed off with a patch at the intersection between two corresponding tubes, which connect to form the filamentous network. These patches are easily observed due to their lighter color relative to the rest of the tube [2].

Similar to bacterial spores, mammalian spores revive after a period of dormancy. When these spores were taken from rabbit serum stored at 4°C and -20°C for over two years and incubated, new filaments began to grow within the first 24 hours. There is a 5-day layover period between the time of incubation and the production of new generations of regular cells from mammalian spores. Due to the large number of newly formed mammalian spores, the mammalian spores incubated from the 2-year old rabbit serum were almost certainly the result of residual mammalian spores containing only the tubular center. This rapid rate of formation of new mammalian spores suggests that these cells may not only be the product of normal cells, but also the product of the previously formed mammalian spores as well. When mammalian spores with a coordinated growth period were incubated at 22°C and 37°C in 10% medium (DEME, ATCC) the filament elongation rate was 0.6 μm/hr for floating mammalian spores (not attached to the plate) and 1.1 μm/hr for those mammalian spores attached to the bottom of the plate. Tubular centers attached to the bottom of the plate displayed a growth rate of 3.8 μm^3 /hr over a five day period. Normal spherical cells began to appear within the 4-well chambers two ~ four weeks after synchronized spores lacking any filamentous extensions began incubation [1, 2].

Are Mammalian Spores Artifacts from Dehydration?

The initial questions that arise while investigating the development and transformation of these cells are: "Are these structures simply artifacts of dehydration?" Even more specifically, do these structures appear to be dead cell polymerization or medium precipitation? Or does a physical process that does not involve a living organism form these spore-like mammalian spores? These are the same questions we have asked ourselves over the last two years. Table 1 summarizes physical and chemical examinations in an attempt to distinguish a complex biological process from dehydration related phenomena.

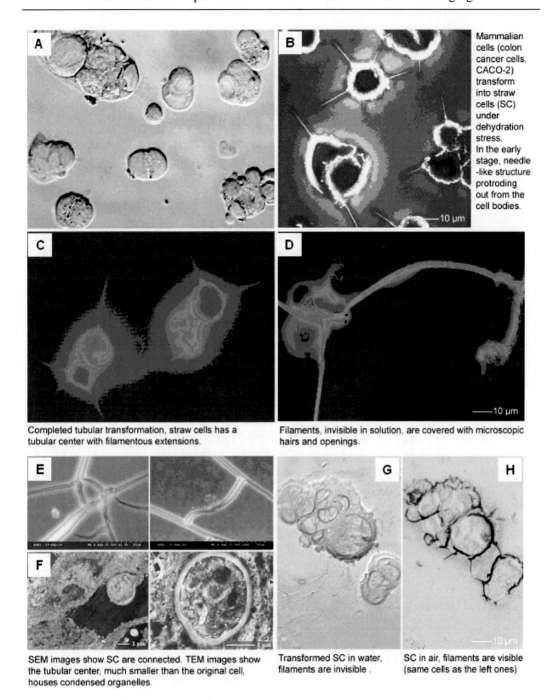

Mammalian cells (colon cancer cells, CACO-2) transform into straw cells (SC) under dehydration stress. In the early stage, needle-like structure protroding out from the cell bodies.

Completed tubular transformation, straw cells has a tubular center with filamentous extensions.

Filaments, invisible in solution, are covered with microscopic hairs and openings.

SEM images show SC are connected. TEM images show the tubular center, much smaller than the original cell, houses condensed organelles.

Transformed SC in water, filaments are invisible.

SC in air, filaments are visible (same cells as the left ones)

Figure 2. Confocal, SEM and TEM images of mammalian spores produced by dehydration of CACO2 cells *in vitro.*

The sporulation process appears to be sensitive to physiochemical conditions. Physically, conditions such as volume to area ratio, speed of drying, and the presences of compounds that alter osmosis all affect the transformation process. Sensitivity to changes in osmotic pressure suggests that the potential sensor(s) that triggers the transformation may be membrane bound on the cell surface because the separation of the plasma membrane from the cytoplasm occurs when water is extracted outward by changes in osmotic pressure across the membrane.

Free energy, mainly in the form of the elastic energy, is needed to account for the remarkable transformation from a spherical-to-tubular shape. A spontaneous life-less physical process appears to contradict the laws of thermodynamics.

Chemically, incubation of cells with 0.2% sodium azide (preventing the cells from using oxygen) halts the production of mammalian spores. No filaments extrude from the tubular bodies at the edge of the drying cells. Incubation with 3.5% paraformaldehyde (fixes cells in PBS at pH 7.4 for 10-15 min at room temperature) also prevents the formation of mammalian spores. These treatments suggest strongly that the transformation involves active enzymatic processes in the cellular metabolism.

Addition of trichloroacetic acid (0.4%) denatures protein also prevented mammalian spore formation. Using an acid or a base to adjust the pH of the medium to extremes, also affects the transformation, but not completely. A few mammalian spores survived a pH below 4 or above 12. Apoptosis inhibitors and organic solvents (5% methanol or ethanol, 0.2% DMSO) are ineffective in inhibiting sporulation. Metabolically, C-14 labeled glucose was measured in greater quantities in the dehydrating culture than in the control culture, suggesting that transforming cells consume energy and that sporulation is a metabolically active process [2].

Control conditions, using medium-free cells in PBS produced no mammalian spores. Dehydration of saline, medium, lipid vesicles, polysaccharide, or dead cells, were all found to produce nothing resembling the tubular structure of mammalian spores. The dried substances formed under these conditions were either tree-shaped salt crystal, round or rod shaped dots, or pieces of cell debris. Since "artifacts" supposedly produced either by dead cell polymerization or medium precipitation have not yet been characterized by anyone, and whose physical entity is unknown, we can only speculate as to how these "artifacts" might react to added chemicals. We used N/A in place for such an event. Based on the evidence collected in table 1, it appears extremely unlikely that such a complex and highly organized structure is the result of medium precipitation or dead cell polymerization.

Mammalian Spores Found in Tissues and Blood

Mammalian spores were found in all tissue fluid from the animals investigated [2], as well as within the blood of humans and domestic animals[1]. These cells can be counted two different ways: (1) using a Hemacytometer while counting the number of dark dots around 1μm within a defined volume of solution without any distortion to the blood samples or (2) count the tubular mammalian spores from 1μl of a dried blood droplet on a glass slide directly. The numbers derived from both methods (in solution vs. in air) are in good agreement with each other, suggesting that no artifacts were introduced in the counting process and that straw (or spore) blood cell counts (SBCs) reflect their blood content.

Table 1. Characterization of mammalian spores by physical and chemical treatment during dehydration induced sporulation in CACO2 cells.

Treatment Physical	Observation (SC in 4 well)	Note effect during drying	Artifacts spontaneous	Metabolism programmed
Sonication/vortex	no SC	cells are damaged prior to drying	N/A*	Pro
Volum e/area ratio	afect	change local osmostic pressure	Con	Pro
Transformation time	> 4hr	extension can grow over time	Con	Pro
Sugar (1%), NaCl(1%)	no SC	change osmostic pressure	N/A	Pro
PEG (1%)	no SC	change osmostic pressure	N/A	Pro
Elastic energy modeling	Energy	required to maintain the tubes	Con	Pro
Structural				
Light microscopy	structural	hairs, openings, extensions	Con	Pro
SEM	structural	tubes, connection	Con	Pro
TEM	structural	cells, cell walls, organelles	Con	Pro
Protein analysis	Yes	flament contains proteins	N/A	Pro
Polysaccharides analysis	Yes	flament contains proteins	N/A	Pro
Chemical**				
Sodium azide (0.2%)	no SC	inhibits oxygen usage	Con	Pro
Paraform aldehyde (3.5%)	no SC	cross-linking of proteins in fixation	N/A	Pro
TCA (0.4%)	no SC	denatures proteins	Con	Pro
Fomic acide (0.1%)	reduce	pH < 2.0	N/A	Pro
Diethylamine (0.1%)	reduce	pH > 10	N/A	Pro
Extreme pH	reduce	pH from 2 ~ 12 with HCl or NaOH	N/A	Pro
p38 MPAK inhibitor	reduce	binds to MAPK protein kinase	Con	Pro
Membrane interacting***	afect	incorporate into the lipid bilayer	Con	Pro
Apoptosis inhibitor	no effect	inhibits Caspases	N/A	N/A
Ethanol (0.5%)	no effect	decrease hydrophilicity	N/A	N/A
DMSO (0.1%)	no effect	solvent	N/A	N/A

Treatment	Observation	Note	Artifacts	Metabolism
Physical	(SC in 4 well)	effect during drying	spontaneous	programmed
Energy consumption				
C-14 Glucose labeling	increase	more than regular growth	Con	Pro
Medium-free in PBS	no SC	cells are intact	Con	Pro
Cell-free control				
Growth medium	no SC	form salt crystals	Con	Pro
Lipids (200ppm)	no SC	form round dots	Con	Pro
PBS	no SC	form salt crystals	Con	Pro

Physical conditions are defined in the method section. Chemicals were added to the growth medium prior to dehydration.

* N/A = effect unknown,

** compound added to the medium,

*** more in Table 3

We were able to consistently and reproducibly purify several grams of isolated mammalian spore filaments from cell cultures. Protein and carbohydrate compositions from these isolated filaments were then analyzed spectrometrically in order to determine the unique chemical properties of mammalian spores.

The filament purification technique utilizes the hydrophilic properties of these cells while using filtration, differential centrifugation, acid and base (strong and mild) catalyzed hydrolysis, and LC chromatography. Based upon our robust purification techniques, it is unlikely that "random artifacts" could be consistently isolated in large enough quantities to be detected in the analytical assays performed throughout this investigation.

The evidence collected thus far suggests that tubular mammalian spores are newly discovered biological phenomena that develop from normal mammalian cells into dormant spore-like structures. These spore-like structures differ slightly from traditional bacterial and fungal spores, but maintain the ability to germinate, grow, and stay dormant while resisting harsh environmental conditions.

At least five different types of mammalian spores can be grouped according to their size and morphology in humans, mice, cows and pigs. These types include: large mammalian spores from epithelial cells, small mammalian spores with short extensions from lymphocytes, hairy mammalian spores covered with many microscopic hairs, smooth mammalian spores, and mammalian spores stacked with nodules on the surface from lung tissue. The straw blood cells with the greatest number of filaments were those isolated from chickens, dogs, rats, and cattle, while those isolated from humans, mice, and rabbits possessed the fewest filamentous extensions [1].

Upon the reintroduction of water *in vitro* these tubular cells use their extensive filaments to rapidly absorb the surrounding water, functioning similar to a straw (hence the name straw cell). Once the growth medium becomes fully hydrated, several of the mammalian spores revert to regular sphere shaped cells and begin to propagate. During this process of reversion to normal cells and propagation, these cells undergo periods of detachment and reattachment to the base of the incubation chambers.

When the straw blood cell count (or spore blood cell count, SBC) of nine domestic animals (mouse, rat, rabbit, chicken, dog, sheep, pig, cow, and horse) were plotted against the animal's average lifespan, a direct inverse correlation was discovered. According to this graph, an animal's average lifespan is inversely correlated to the number of mammalian spores present within that animal's blood stream. The coefficient of correlation for this relationship is $R^2 = 0.7$ (Figure 3). Based upon this inverse relationship between the length an animal lives and its SBC, it appears that SBC may be an indicator of an animal's inherent stress level. This inverse relationship also suggests that the production of mammalian spores within the body may eventually disrupt normal cellular and organ function. Also, using fresh bovine tissue and human urine samples, we discovered that the number of mammalian spores increases with the age of the animal, as well as the level of polysaccharides (a component of the mammalian spore's cell wall) within the urine. We speculate that this increased level of mammalian spores within the body collectively lead to the loss of normal healthy cells while disrupting cellular and organ function and may also significantly contribute to the aging process.

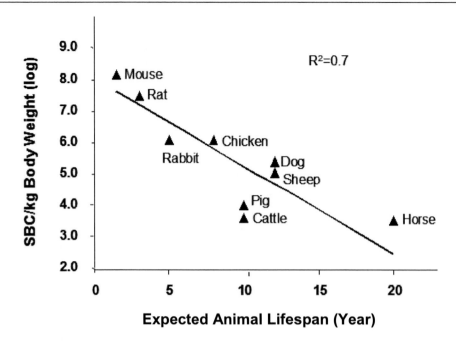

Figure 3. The relationship between SBC and expected animal lifespan [1].

Mammalian spores within the blood can typically be isolated from the matrix using basic differential centrifugation and filtration techniques, depending on the extent and magnitude of the filamentous extensions. The hydrophilic nature of the extended filaments prevents spores from precipitating at 10,000 rpm (9,530 x g), while bare spores (without filamentous extension) do precipitate at 10,000 rpm.

The prevalence of mammalian spores within the blood was determined for 9 mammals and a bird by estimating the percentage of the dry blood weight that is made up of mammalian spores. Mice contained the highest percentage of mammalian spores by dry weight with 10.4% and pigs having the lowest percentage with 0.6%. The mean weight for all ten animals was 4%. Humans and mice contained the highest raw SBC with approximately 45 million/ml of blood, with an average SBC for all ten animals and humans of 10 million/ml of blood.

The largest quantity of mammalian spores within human blood appears to be those originating from lymphocytes (T and/or B cells) containing distinctive short filamentous extensions. These characteristic mammalian spores of lymphocyte origin make up ~40% of the 45million mammalian spores/ml within the blood. The number of mammalian spores characteristic of lymphocytes also appears to be in good agreement with the ~50billion lymphocytes that die each day through apoptosis. Counting that the half-life of filaments are ~20hr within the bloodstream, we estimate that ~100 billion of all cells are converted into mammalian spores every day. This sporulation occurs naturally in both fresh and postmortem tissues [2].

Chemical Composition

Grams of mammalian spore filaments were harvested from cell cultures and purified to homogeneity. They were then analyzed to determine the chemical composition, as well as the protein and carbohydrate content using FTIR and mass spectrometry. Partial hydrolysis was also performed to help dissect the complex into monomers, allowing for easier identification. Chemical analysis reveals that the filaments are primarily composed of sulfated glucose polysaccharides containing little protein [2]. The protein sequences are currently being investigated.

Mammalian spore physiological properties are summarized in Figure 4. Like our single celled microbial ancestor, mammalian cells also transform from vegetative cells into dormant spores. Unlike the lipid bilayer of the plasma membrane composed of phospholipids, the spore surface is made of sulfated polysaccharide, which makes the spores hydrophilic and mobile in polar aqueous biofluid.

Contribution to Blood Cholesterol Level

High blood cholesterol is a risk factor for coronary heart disease [3, 4]. Mammalian spores may contribute to blood cholesterol levels significantly. The estimated 100 billion regular cells that undergo sporulation each day most likely shed their membrane lipid components into the bloodstream, increasing free lipid concentrations in circulation. The amount of cholesterol contributed to this membrane shedding is estimated from an individual cell's cholesterol contribution. The cell cholesterol content is measured from a known amount of cells before and after dehydration-induced sporulation. Cells were extracted and the total lipids were then profiled for individual lipid species by counting ions in positive and negative ion mode of ESI-mass spectrometry [5]. Data presented are from four experiments, each with a duplicate cell population of 100,000. The MS and MS/MS scan of cholesterol ions (369.35, M-H_2O+H^+) were identical between cell and standard samples. The linear standard curve was constructed by adding known amounts of cholesterol to cell cultures so the ionization was in the same background for the sample and standard, from which the cholesterol ion counts from 100,000 cells was converted to µg. The analysis revealed that an individual cell, on average, contains 0.01ng cholesterol. For 100 billion cells, it contributes to ~15% of blood cholesterol at 200mg/dL.

This estimation agrees with calculations made using data from literature [6, 7]: if one mammalian cell weighs an average of 4~8 (ng), of which 10% is protein and 1.8% of this protein is sterol [7], then there are ~0.3 mg of cholesterol/ml of blood when a cell is resolved in blood through sporulation, or 15% of the cholesterol at 200mg/dL blood. This 15% contributed by mammalian spores is less than dietary cholesterol, which accounts for 1/3 of total cholesterol in circulation [3]. It is has long been observed that the relative amount of lipid species remains stable, while the absolute amount may fluctuate in the ESI. Using a normalized ion count against the total ion count appears to be reproducible when profiling is in the linear responses range.

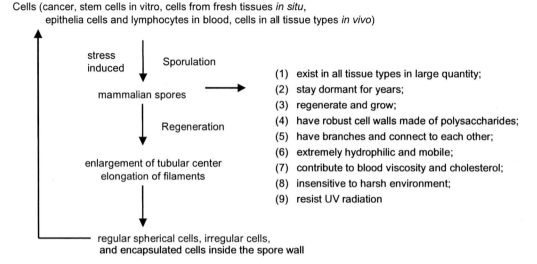

Figure 4. Physiological pathways of mammalian spores.

Contribution to Blood Viscosity

Mammalian spores floating freely within the bloodstream may contribute to blood viscosity through their connected network of hydrophilic filaments with hairy extensions (hyphae). Viscosity intrinsically determines an individual's blood pressure. We purified straw cells from fresh human blood samples using a filtration method [1] and measured their viscosity using methods described in literature [8]. The results indicated that mammalian spores contribute to 10% of overall blood viscosity.

Two types of different spores were discovered depending on the ethnic group from which samples were taken. Caucasian samples contained spores with hairy extensions and Oriental samples contained smooth extensions (Fig1B and C, [1]). While straw cells contribute to 10% of overall viscosity, straw cells with hairy extensions could contribute more to the overall viscosity compared to those with smooth extensions. The cause of death by heart disease for Americans is almost twice that of Chinese (39% versus 21%, [9, 10]). Differences in blood viscosity associated with hairy spores and hyphae that are physically more resistant to flow may be another contributing factor to heart disease by reducing blood flow.

Perhaps differences between the diets of the western and far-east cultures (meat-rich and carbohydrate-rich, respectively) are not as responsible for heart disease as once thought. These hereditary structures of the spores/hyphae could be causing a 10% difference in the blood viscosity between various ethnic groups. Increased surface area of the hairy spores causes extra-drag in solution and adds resistance to blood flow. Viscosity measurements of the control serum (albumin solution at 100 mg/ml) were used to determine residual viscosity from remaining protein molecules associated with straw cell preparation.

Signaling Pathway

The ability of such a wide variety of cell and tissue types to undergo a sporulation process suggests that these cells may have a water activity sensor(s) to specifically interpret the water status of the surrounding environment. The depletion of water from the local environment activates these sensors, which in turn produces a signal cascade that propagates through the cytoplasm and into the nucleus. Upon reaching the nucleus, the signal tells the cell to prepare for a drastic transformation process, which includes nuclei fragmentation and the synthesis of a protective cell wall (Figure. 5). Drosophila *melanogaster* use specific hygrosensation sensors to identify slight variations in humidity. These sensors use the receptors wtrw and nan for detecting moist and dry air, respectively [11]. One may be able to use these hygrosensation sensors as a basis to determine potential membrane interacting inhibitors that may interfere with the water activity sensors present on the cell surface. The discovery of a successful inhibitor would help identify and grant insight into the structure and function of these sensors.

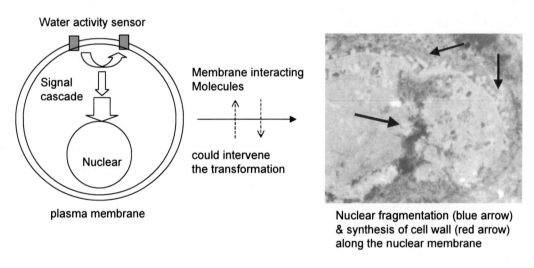

Nuclear fragmentation (blue arrow)
& synthesis of cell wall (red arrow)
along the nuclear membrane

Figure. 5. Mechanism of sporulation. There may be water activity sensors on the cell surface that survey the hydration status of the environment. Once triggered, they send signals to the nucleus and mobilize the cell to go through drastic changes that result in a fragmented nucleus (blue arrow) and synthesis of cell wall materials (red arrow). The fragmented nucleus resides in the center of the fortified tubular structure with filamentous branches.

Despite the similar physical characteristics and morphology in the early stages of transformation, it appears that the formation of apoptotic bodies and mammalian spores are ultimately governed by separate mechanisms based on studies using apoptosis inhibitors and a sporulation inhibitor in both CACO2 cells and in mice. Although the pathways of sporulation and apoptosis eventually diverge, these processes may share a similar signaling pathway in the early stages. However, it is not surprising that the two pathways deviate from each other in the late stages because the apoptotic pathway destroys the cell, while sporulation produces a viable organism.

The P38 MAPK inhibitor interferes with environmental response machinery by interrupting P38 kinase activity, which is activated by receptors located on the outer membrane surface as a reaction to external stress [12]. The SBC in mice was reduced by up to 30% by injecting 1mg/kg body weight/day of a pyridinyl imidazole, which inhibits an inducible P38 MAPK [1]. The P38 MAP kinases are a family of serine/threonine protein kinases which are essential for specific cellular responses to environmental stress signals [12]. The resulting reduction in SBC suggests that the protein kinase cascade, mediated through IL-1, TNF, IL-18 to MEKK1, 3, NIK, to MKK3, 6, is significant in the external stress response associated with a sporulation.

Aging Theory

Water is the most essential component for life. The ability for organisms to possess a means to utilize water and overcome dire circumstances in which such a fundamental resource becomes scarce is necessary for survival. *Bdelloid rotifers* (aquatic microinvertebrates) adapt to desiccation by contracting into a compact shape and staying dormant until conditions improve [13, 14]; nematodes accumulate trehalose, a non-reducing sugar, to protect membranes and proteins from desiccation [15]; plants express late embryogenesis abundant (LEA) proteins in maturing seeds and pollen in response to desiccation [16]. The adaptability of organisms in response to dehydration through a state of suspended metabolism is essential for long-term survival [14]. Mammalian sporulation that forms a dormant spore may simply be the product of selective evolution driven by the need for water. Mammalian spores withstand long periods of time without water and form an extensive network that searches for new sources of water. The sporulation process may be a conserved mechanism in mammalian and animal cells.

Steady production of mammalian spores within the body as people age, may be linked to the decreased amount of water present in the tissues of older people or the waning desire to drink water as one grows older [17, 18]. As one sleeps the body is less active and the metabolism slows down, resulting in reduced circulation and flow of water to the brain. A publication recently discovered that nerve cells attempted to divide before they died in mice with Alzheimer's disease [19]. A wide variety of life threatening human diseases such as Alzheimer's, tumor metastasis, pulmonary obstruction, and cardiovascular thrombosis are often associated with older individuals. These diseases may share a common mechanism associated with the aging process, inherited through our critical dependence upon water and selective evolution.

Mammalian spores occur naturally and are produced at an almost constant rate per body weight in all the humans and animals we tested. The direct correlation between an animal's SBC and its average expected lifespan, suggests a simple connection between the number of normal healthy cells that undergo the sporulation process and the amount of cells needed to sustain life (Figure 3). Aging begins at birth and continues steadily throughout an individuals life [20]. Assuming that the loss of functional cells dominates the aging (a very large assumption due to the variety of other factors that contribute to the aging process), then the aging rate per year from the current average human lifespan of 75 years that lost 3.2×10^{15} cells (Figure 6) can be expressed as:

$$K_a = 3.2 \times 10^{15}/75 = 43 \times 10^{12} \text{ (cell/year)} \tag{1}$$

Over 75 years, an individual has lost ~70% of his/her total functional cells (4.5×10^{15}). An individual's life expectancy can then be projected by:

$$L_e = C_t / K_a \tag{2}$$

Where C_t is the total number of functional cells and K_a is an aging rate, a function of cell loss, likely resulting from overall stress on the body, including dehydration, radiation, DNA damage, oxidative stress, etc. People who do not live to the average age of 75 years due to age-related diseases, their K_a is higher than 43 (trillion cells/year). An accelerated local sporulation rate may have resulted in a specific age-related disease, which, subsequently may have further advanced sporulation and lead to a shortened life.

There are two ways to increase L_e: one is by increasing the total number of cells within the body; the second is by decreasing K_a. If one is able to decrease sporulation by 50% through medicinal applications that specifically inhibit the sporulation machinery, the resulting $K_{a50} = \frac{1}{2} K_a$, producing a life expectancy which doubles that of the uninhibited K_a. Even more, if K_{a10} equals one tenth of K_a, then L_e multiplies by 10.

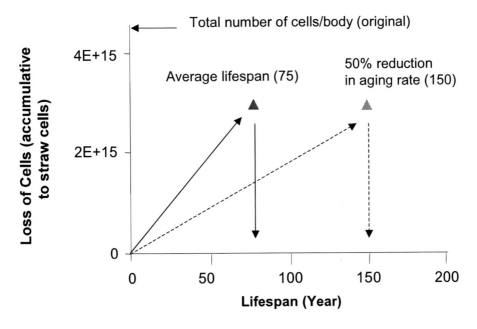

Figure 6. Current Human lifespan versus hypothetical lifespan with reduced aging rate assuming death is only associated with the loss of cells through sporulation. Daily loss of ~ 100 billion cells to spores could accumulate to 3,200 trillion cells at age 75.

If one is able to prevent all cells from being lost through sporulation, K_a becomes infinitesimally small, and then equation (2) calls for an infinite value of L_e. The potential lifespan reaches a point of eternity, or singularity as introduced by Ray Kurzweil in 2005 [21]. If no cells are lost and all cells present are healthy and functioning properly, then an individual will not approach the critical threshold of cells required to sustain life and therefore will not die according to this model.

Age–Related Diseases

Targeting age-related tumorgenesis using apoptosis promoters is an active route of treatment [22-26]. It appears that physical and chemical stress not only induces apoptosis but also produces viable mammalian spores. Mammalian spores and apoptotic bodies may be the co-products of the same upstream stress responding pathway. It is hypothesized that vast numbers of free circulating mammalian cancer spores in the blood are capable of regenerating back into actively growing tumor cells at new locations, under the proper conditions. This ability to transport within the bloodstream and reproduce under proper conditions is a possible mechanism for metastasis, the establishment of new sites in the body for tumorgenesis. The potential for normal mammalian spores to colonize and grow into tumors may be very small, depending upon the availability of nutrients, DNA mutations, and interactions with the host immune system. The mammalian spore's robust cell wall [2] may allow them to tolerate the harsh conditions provided by radiation and chemotherapy, which enables mammalian spores to remain viable even after the original cancer cells die off (i.e. remission in cancer patients). Cancerous mammalian spores would then able to propagate when growth conditions improve *in vivo*.

The hydrophilic nature of mammalian spores allows them to flow freely within the blood circulatory system. *In vitro*, mammalian spores originating from both normal cells and cancer cells germinate and grow back into vegetative cells within a few days to a few weeks. In general, after the remission of the original cancer, the recurrence of tumors in cancer patients frequently occurs within 2~3 years after initial treatments [27, 28].

Aging-related cancer occurrence remains a leading cause of morbidity and mortality in humans, mainly due to the propensity of primary tumors to metastasize to various regions of the body [29]. Metastasis after the removal of a primary tumor can be difficult to identify, creating uncertainty in patients with regards to possible cancer recurrence. This difficulty of identifying metastasized tumors is especially a problem in breast cancer patients; exemplified by the fact that recurrence can take place even after decades of apparent disease-free survival. The mechanisms underlying tumor dormancy in breast cancer remain poorly understood [29]. Mammalian spores have only recently become a subject of investigation in 2007 for potential involvement in tumorgenesis.

Intervention

Noninfectious diseases, such as chronic age-related cardiovascular diseases and cancers, can take 10 - 20 years to develop. These age-related diseases lack therapeutic targets for chemical intervention, and currently no treatments are 100% effective. Natural lipid mixtures have been used as therapeutic agents for treating aging-related diseases. For example, fish oil and omega-type fatty acids have been used to treat high blood pressure [30-32]. These lipid mixtures have even been used in treating some cancers and have shown activity in mouse models to reduce prostate tumor size [33, 34]. In our screening program of natural compounds that inhibit sporulation, we found methanol extracts in yellow fish eggs (Croaker) contain diverse lipid species with a relatively high quantity of lysophospholipids, as well as unsaturated fatty acids, which exert potent anti-sporulation activity *in vitro* (Table 2).

Eggs may be important in protecting fish against unwanted sporulation. Lysophospholipids and fatty acids can also serve as detergents to protect from invading microorganisms. Although the normal concentrations of lysophospholipids in membranes are relatively low compared to phospholipids (<1:100), at least 37 lysophospholipids have been identified in the fish egg methanol extraction.

Inhibition of sporulation was carried out using pure chemicals (Table 3) to exam if anti-sporulation activities can be reproduced in a chemically defined system. We have discovered that molecules which can be readily incorporated into the plasma membrane, or become a native component of the lipid bilayer of a cell's membrane system have various anti-sporulation activities. Listed in Table 3, are examples of the chemicals tested, some have no influence, some promote, and others inhibit sporulation. The structure of these lipids with respect to their anti-sporulation activities and interactions with the membrane bilayer may provide insight into the mechanism of sporulation.

Interestingly, a major lipid component of the plasma membrane, Phosphatidylcholine (PC) is involved in promoting dehydration-induced sporulation when perturbed. PC carries a positive net charge at physiological pH, and dramatically promotes sporulation at concentrations as low as 0.2 ppm during exogenous addition to cell culture (Table 3). PC increases sporulation by ~2-10-fold compared to controls and other membrane-building glycerophospholipids with connected synthetic pathways (Figure 7). The length of the aliphatic chain and degree of unsaturation of the phospholipids appears to play a role in the level of activity. PC 36:4 promotes sporulation less than PC 36:2, while PC 24:0 has essentially no activity.

Available PC 36:2 (the most abundant PC species) was increased by 5%, compared to the total PC present within the cellular membrane, enhanced sporulation by 7-fold, as estimated by positive ESI-MS. This dramatic increase in straw cell transformation suggests an association of PC 36:2 and PC 36:4 with the sporulation machinery, perhaps by ionic interactions between positively charged PC and the anionic proteins on the membrane surface. PC may also provide fuel for the energy required during sporulation. The surface of the plasma membrane is slightly anionic containing more negative lipids (PI, PS, PG, PE and PA) than positive ones (PC, PE and Sphingolipids) when estimated by ESI-MS in both positive ion and negative ion mode for both positive and negative lipids, respectively.

**Table 2. Screening of fish egg (Croaker) methanol extract for
anti-sporulation compounds**

HPLC RT (min)	Lipid	Chain	MW (Dalton)	Charge (M)
32.0	LPC	14:0	468.30	+1
		18:3	518.33	+1
		20:5	542.31	+1
		22:6	568.33	+1
		22:5	570.35	+1
	LP E	20:5	500.28	+1
		22:5	526.32	-1
	LPA	20:6	453.24	-1
	LPI	16:3	555.27	-1
		20:4	619.32	-1
		22:6	643.29	-1
38.9	LPA	16:1p	373.21	-H_2O-H
		16:0	391.21	-H_2O-H
		16:2	405.22	-1
	PA	40:4	751.44	-1
	LPG	14:0	405.22	-1
	LPE	18:3p a/o 18:4e	440.32	-H_2O-H
	LPI	24:5	655.47	-1
	FA	18:3	277.22	-1
		18:0	283.24	-1
		20:5	301.21	-1
		22:6	327.22	-1
		24:4	359.22	-1
	LPC	16:0	496.33	+1
		18:1	522.35	+1
	LPG	18:2	507.44	-1
		20:3	533.44	-1
	PE	36:0	748.54	-1
		38:1	774.55	-1
	LPI	20:0	609.50	-1
		22:2	633.49	-1
		24:3	659.52	-1
	FA	14:0	227.20	-1
		16:4	253.20	-1
		18:2	279.23	-1
		20:4	303.23	-1
		22:5	329.24	-1
		24:6	355.27	-1

Retention times are fractions collected from a linear acetonitrile gradient at 2% B/min of 1min/ml flow rate on a C18 reverse-phase column – lysophospholipids and free fatty acids are the major component identified from these fractions by ESI mass spectrometry at positive and negative ion mode.

Lipids with a similar chain length and unsaturation but different head group (DOPE, DOPG, and DOPS) are mostly ineffective. DOPE, however, is slightly inhibitory of sporulation at 20 ppm, although PE can give rise to PC via two independent pathways (Figure 7). DOPG slightly promotes straw cell formation while carrying negative charge. PA 36:0 displayed inhibitory activity, but at 20 ppm it becomes cytotoxic to cells. Sphingosine is also inhibitory but becomes cytotoxic as well (Table 3). Lysophospholipids and fatty acids also contain small amounts of inhibitory activity. The concentration of these lysolipids within the membrane in their native state is low [35].

Table 3. Effect of lipid and membrane-interacting small molecules on dehydration induced sporulation in production of mammalian spores

	Membrane interacting molecule (lipids and small molecules)	Mass (Dalton)	Activity (qualitative)	Amount (ppm)
Ineffective	Cholesterol	386.7	same as control	67
	n-octyl-ß-D-Glucopyranoside	294.4	same as control	67
	Phosphatidylglycerol	246.05	same as control	67
	Tetraoleoyl cardiolipin	1501.97	same as control	67
	Sphingomyelin	731.09	same as control	67
	DOPG	774.52	slightly promotional	20
	PG 36:4	770.49	slightly promotional	20
	DOPS	792.57	same as control	2 and 20
	DOPE	748.07	slightly inhibitory	2 and 20
	PE 36:4	735.98	slightly inhibitory	2 and 20
	PC 24:0	621.8	slightly promotional	22
Promotional	PC 36:4	781.56	2-fold of control	2
	PC 36:4	781.56	10-fold of control	20

Abbreviations: DOPG,   L-α-dioleoylphosphatidylglycerol;   DOPE,   L-α-dioleoylphos-
phatidylethanolamine; PE 36:4, 1,2-dilinolenoyl-sn-glycero-3-phosphoethanolamine; PC 36:4, 1,2-
dilinoleoyl-sn-glecero-3-phosphocholine; DOPC, 1,2-dioleoyl-sn-glecero-3-phosphocholine ;PA
36:0, L-α phosphotidic acid; ANTs, 8-aminonaphthalene-1,3,6-trisulfonic acid. * With respect to
total PC species.

A dose of 2 ppm, equivalent to 200 mg/day for a 75kg person, is in the range of applicable potency and indicates a reasonable selectivity for specific molecules. Understanding the process and mechanisms involved in sporulation could assist in identifying and developing lipids with more potent inhibitory activity. Toxicity of lipids may not be as large of a concern as synthetic compounds because lipids naturally exist within the cell. These glycerophospholipids provide insight and opportunities to continue our investigation of this newly discovered biological phenomenon.

PC, Cell Death and Sporulation

Phosphatidylcholine (PC) constitutes a major portion of cellular phospholipids (30 ~ 40%) and displays unique molecular properties in different cell types and tissues. PC contains a comprehensive system of phospholipases, acyltransferases and other metabolism related enzymes which allow it to function as the origin for a variety of unique signaling mediators with diverse physical properties and great sensitivity to changes in the physical environment.

PC homeostasis lies within the balance of the CDP–choline (Figure 7) and phosphatidylethanolamine methylation (PEM) pathways. Disruption of these pathways, both by inhibition of the CDP-choline pathway or over expression of the HPEM pathway in hepatocytes, disturbs PC homeostasis and may retard cell growth or even lead to cell death. Current evidence reveals that apoptosis and necrosis may have certain common mediators and often occur simultaneously throughout the process of cell death [36, 37] Apoptosis can be activated by simply reducing PC synthesis. This link between apoptosis and PC synthesis was first suggested through the inactivation of CT within a cell line containing modified temperature-sensitive CT, in which inactivated CT lead to a 50% decrease in PC followed by retarded cell growth and eventually apoptosis. [38].

The process of sporulation resembles that of necrosis more than apoptosis. During necrosis cell death is accompanied by the rupture of membranes and the release of subcellular components into the immediate vicinity, while in the event of apoptosis the cellular membrane integrity is retained. Reduced PC triggers either apoptosis or necrosis, while increased PC promotes sporulation, and all three events lead to the loss of functional cells. The use of PC to minimize both cell death and sporulation may be a difficult task due to its opposite effect on both transformations. Molecules such as farnesol, geranylgeraniol, and chelerythrine that induce cell death, and thought to inhibit CPT activity and PC synthesis [40, 41], could be tested at sub-μmole range to identify if sporulation could be inhibited while not inducing apoptosis. Farnesol at 8 ppm has some inhibitory activity on dehydration-induced sporulation in CACO2 cells but does not block PC-promoted sporulation.

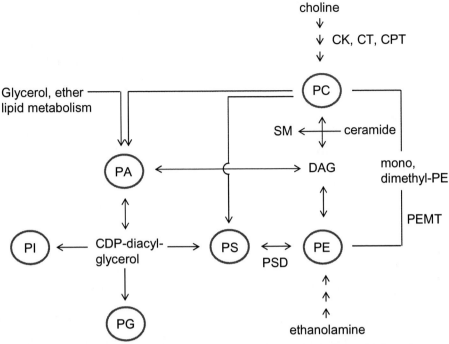

Abbreviations: CK, choline kinase; CT, CTP-phosphocholinecytidyltransferase; CPT, cholinephosphotransferase; DAG, diacylglycerol; PC phosphatidylcholine; PE, phosphatidylethanolamine; PEMT, phosphatidylethanolanie-*N*-methyl-transferase; PS, phosphatidylserine;PSD, phosphatidylserine decarboxylase; PA, 1,2-diacyl-sn-glycerol-3-phosphate; PG, phosphatidylglycerol; PI, phosphatidylinositol; SM, sphingomyelin.

Figure 7. Pathways for the synthesis of Glycerophospholipids.

In fungus *Aspergillus niger* farnesol blocks the yeast-to-filamentous growth transition by acting as an inhibitor of conidiation [42], a process of fungal spore formation. Conidiation is usually induced by exposure of hyphae to air, the mechanism of which is not well understood [43], but reminiscent of mammalian sporulation induced by air-dehydration. The initial signal may involve PC in the outer-leaflet of the lipid bilayer. However, PC may eventually move toward the inner-leaflet as the outer lipid bilayer begins to collapse due to the removal of proton rich water, diminishing the ionic interaction between the water and lipid molecules. Cationic PC may interact with anoic membrane proteins such as G-proteins, thus triggering the signal cascade. In many filamentous fungi a G-protein coupled signaling pathway, including protein kinase A, plays a crucial role in asexual spore formation [43].

Conclusion

Mammalian straw cells found with spore-like structures could very likely be mammalian spores. Extensive experiments analyzing a variety of elements of the straw cell's biology indicate that these cells are not artifacts rising from dead cell polymerization or medium precipitation. Inherited from and analogous to bacterial spores, their biological roles may be to survive harsh environmental conditions. These spores are abundant in the blood and tissues of all 8 mammals observed, including humans. Sporulation releases cholesterol into the blood stream, increases blood viscosity, and reduces the number of functional cells. Sporulation may play an important role in the process of aging and the development of aging-related diseases. The concentration of phosphotidylcholines within the cell appears to regulate both cell death and cell survival by inducing apoptosis when the concentration is reduced and promoting sporulation when increased. Gaining a better understanding of mammalian sporulation may grant a novel perspective, as well as potential treatments, of aging and aging-related diseases.

References

[1]   Wu, Y., Henry, D. C., Heim, K., Tomkins, J. P. and Kuan, C. Y. (2008) Straw blood cell count, growth, inhibition and comparison to apoptotic bodies. *BMC cell biology*, 9:26.

[2]   Wu, Y., Laughlin, R. C., Henry, D. C., Krueger, D. E., Hudson, J. S., Kuan, C. Y., He, J., Reppert, J. and Tomkins, J. P. (2007) Naturally occurring and stress induced tubular structures from mammalian cells, a survival mechanism. *BMC Cell Biology,* 8, 36.

[3]   McNamara, D. J. (2000) Dietary cholesterol and atherosclerosis. *Biochimica et Biophysica Acta*, 1529, 310-320.

[4]   No_authors_listed (1984) The Lipid Research Clinics Coronary Primary Prevention Trial results. I. Reduction in incidence of coronary heart disease. *JAMA*, 251, 351-364.

[5]   Milne, S., Ivanova, P., Forrester, J. and Brown, H. A. (2006) Lipidomics: An analysis of cellular lipids by ESI-MS. *Methods*, 39, 92–103.

[6]   Chabanel, A., Flamm, M., Sung, K. L. P., Lee, M. M., Schachter, D. and Chien, S. (1983) Influence of cholesterol content on red cell membrane viscoelasticity and fluidity. *Biophys. J.* 44, 171-176.

[7]   Limanek, J. S., Chin, J. and Chang, T. Y. (1978) Mammalian cell mutant requiring cholesterol and unsaturated fatty acid for growth. *PNAS,* 75, 5452-5456.

[8]   Sehyun Shin, Yunhee Ku, Myung-Su Park and Jang-Soo Suh (2004) Measurement of red cell deformability and whole blood viscosity using laser-diffraction slit rheometer. *Korea-Australia Rheology Journal,* 16, 85-90.

[9]   (2002) Leading Causes of Death in the United States. *National Vital Statistics Report,* 50.

[10]   Jiang He, Dongfeng Gu, Xigui Wu, Kristi Reynolds, Xiufang Duan, Chonghua Yao, Jialiang Wang, Chung-Shiuan Chen, Jing Chen, Rachel P. Wildman, Michael J. Klag and Paul K. Whelton (2005) Major Causes of Death among Men and Women in China. *New England J. of Medicine,* 353.

[11]   Liu, L., Li, Y., Wang, R., Yin, C., Dong, Q., Hing, H., Kim, C. and Welsh, M. J. (2007) Drosophila hygrosensation requires the TRP channels water witch and nanchung. *Nature,* 450, 294-298.

[12] Kumar, S., Boehm, J. and Lee, J. C. (2003) P38 MAP kinases: key signaling molecules as therapeutic targets for inflammatory diseases. *Nature Reviews*, 2, 717-726.

[13] Dickson, M. R. and Mercer, E. H. (1967) Fine structural changes accompanying desiccation in Philodina roseola (Rotifera). *J. Microscopie*, 6, 331-348.

[14] Ricci, C. and Caprioli, M. (2005) Anhydrobiosis in bdelloid species, populations and individuals. *Integr. Comp. Biol.* 45, 759-763.

[15] Browne, J., Tunnacliffe, A. and Burnell, A. (2002) Plant desiccation gene found in a nematode. *Nature,* 416, 38-38.

[16] Delseny, M., Bies-Etheve, N., Carles, C., Hull, G., Vicient, C., Raynal, M., Grellet, F. and Aspart, L. (2001) Late Embryogenesis Abundant (LEA) protein gene regulation during Arabidopsis seed maturation. *Journal of Plant Physiology*, 158, 419-427.

[17] Ellis, K. J. (2000) Human Body Composition: In Vivo Methods. *Physiol. Rev.* 80, 649-680.

[18] Tuuri, G., Keenan, M. J., West, K. M., Delany, J. P. and Mark, J. (2005) Body water indices as markers of aging in male masters swimmers. *J. Sports Science and Medicine,* 4, 406-414.

[19] Yang, Y., Varvel, N. H., Lamb, B. T. and Herrup, K. (2006) Ectopic cell cycle events link human Alzheimer's disease and APP transgenic mouse models. *J. Neuroscience*, 26, 775-784.

[20] Gavrilov, L. A. and Gavrilova, N. S. (2006) *The Handbook of the Biology of Aging.* Academic Press.

[21] Kurzweil, R. (2005) The Singularity is Near: When Humans Transcend Biology. Viking.

[22] Bian, X., Giordano, T. D., Lin, H. J., Solomon, G., Castle, V. P. and Opipari, A. W. (2004) Chemotherapy-induced Apoptosis of S-type Neuroblastoma Cells Requires Caspase-9 and Is Augmented by CD95/Fas Stimulation. *The Journal of Biological Chemistry,* 279, 4663–4669.

[23] Hwang, J. T., Ha, J. and Park, O. J. (2005) Combination of 5-fluorouracil and genistein induces apoptosis synergistically in chemo-resistant cancer cells through the modulation of AMPK and COX-2 signaling pathways. *Biochem Biophys Res Commun.* 332, 433–440.

[24] Reed, J. C. (2002) Apoptosis-based therapies. Nat. Rev. Drug Discov. 1, 111–121.

[25] Reed, J. C. and Pellecchia, M. (2005) Apoptosis-based therapies for hematologic malignancies. *Blood,* 106, 408-418.

[26] Somasundaram, S., Edmund, N. A., Moore, D. T., Small, G. W., Shi, Y. Y. and Orlowski, R. Z. (2002) Dietary Curcumin Inhibits Chemotherapy-induced Apoptosis in Models of Human Breast Cancer. *Cancer Research,* 62, 3868–3875.

[27] Greco, C., Castiglioni, S., Fodor, A., De Cobelli, O., Longaretti, N., Rocco, B., Vavassori, A. and Orecchia, R. (2007) Benefit on biochemical control of adjuvant radiation therapy in patients with pathologically involved seminal vesicles after radical prostatectomy. *Tumori,* 93, 445-451.

[28] Klass, C. M. and Shin, D. M. (2007) Current status and future perspectives of chemoprevention in head and neck cancer. *Curr Cancer Drug Targets*, 7, 623-632.

[29] Allan, A. L., Vantyghem, S. A., Tuck, A. B. and Chambers, A. F. (2006-2007) Tumor dormancy and cancer stem cells: implications for the biology and treatment of breast cancer metastasis. *Breast Dis.* 26, 87-98.

[30] Daviglus, M. L., Stamler, J., Orencia, A. J. and al., e. (1997) Fish consumption and the 30-year risk of fatal myocardial infarction. *New England J. Medicine*, 336, 1046-1053.

[31] Mozaffarian, D., Lemaitre, R. N., Kuller, L. H., Burke, G. L., Tracy, R. P. and Siscovick, D. S. (2003) Cardiac benefits of fish consumption may depend on the type of fish meal consumed: the Cardiovascular Health Study. *Circulation,* 107, 1372-1377.

[32] Sun, Q., Ma, J., Campos, H., Rexrode, K. M., Albert, C. M., Mozaffarian, D. and Hu, F. B. (2008) Blood concentrations of individual long-chain n-3 fatty acids and risk of nonfatal myocardial infarction. *Am J Clin Nutr.* 88, 216-223.

[33] McEntee, M. F., Ziegler, C., Reel, D., Tomer, K., Shoieb, A., Ray, M., Li, X., Neilsen, N., Lih, F., O'Rourke, D. and Whelan, J. (2008) Dietary n-3 polyunsaturated fatty acids enhance hormone ablation therapy in androgen-dependent prostate cancer. *Am J Pathol.* 173, 229-241.

[34] Wallstrom, P., Bjartell, A., Gullberg, B., Olsson, H. and Wirfalt, E. (2007) A prospective study on dietary fat and incidence of prostate cancer. *Cancer Causes Control*, 18, 1107-1121.

[35] I. Ishii, N. Fukushima, X. Ye and J. Chun (2004) Lysophospholipid receptors:signaling and biology. *Annu. Rev. Biochem.* 73, 321-354.

[36] Fiers, W., Beyaert, R., Declercq, W. and Vandenabeele, P. (1999) More than one way to die: apoptosis, necrosis and reactive oxygen damage. *Oncogene.* 18, 7719-7730.

[37] Nicotera, S., Leist, M. and Ferrando-May, E. (1999) Apoptosis and necrosis: different execution of the same death. Biochem. Soc. Symp. 66, 69-73.

[38] Cui, Z., Houweling, M., Chen, M. H., Record, M., Chap, H., Vance, D. E. and Terce, F. (1996) A genetic defect in phosphatidylcholine biosynthesis triggers apoptosis in Chinese hamster ovary cells. *J. Biol. Chem.* 271, 14668-14671.

[39] Zheng Cuia and Martin Houweling (2002) Phosphatidylcholine and cell death. Biochimica et Biophysica Acta 1585, 87-96.

[40] Anthony, M. L., Zhao, M. and Brindle, K. M. (1999) Inhibition of phosphatidylcholine biosynthesis following induction of apoptosis in HL-60 cells. *J. Biol. Chem.* 274, 19686-19692.

[41] Miquel, K., Pradines, A., Terce, F., Selmi, S. and Favre, G. (1998) Competitive inhibition of choline phosphotransferase by geranylgeraniol and farnesol inhibits phosphatidylcholine synthesis and induces apoptosis in human lung adenocarcinoma A549 cells. *J. Biol. Chem.* 273, 26179-26186.

[42] Lorek, J., Pöggeler, S., Weide, M. R., Breves, R. and Bockmühl, D. P. (2008) Influence of farnesol on the morphogenesis of Aspergillus niger. *Journal of Basic Microbiology,* 48, 99-103.

[43] Adams, T. H., Wieser, J. K. and Yu, J.-H. (1998) Asexual Sporulation in Aspergillus nidulans. *Microbiology and Molecular Biology Review*, 35-54.

Index

A

ABC, 166
abdomen, 355
abnormalities, 11, 173, 328
Aboriginal, 399, 400, 402, 403, 405, 406, 407,
    409, 410, 411, 412, 413, 414, 415, 416, 417,
    418, 419, 420, 421, 422, 423, 424, 425, 426,
    427
abortion, 72, 170, 171, 172
absorption, 168, 202, 203, 213, 265, 279, 363
academic, 167, 232, 273
access, 178, 190
accessibility, 356
accidental, 411
accidents, 63
accommodation, 184, 413
accounting, 381, 382
accuracy, 178, 258
ACE, 18, 67
ACE-inhibitor, 67
acetaminophen, 106, 108, 113, 116
acetate, 106
acetonitrile, 446
acetylation, 236
acetylcholine, 167, 170
acetylcholinesterase, 163, 167, 173, 297
acetylcholinesterase inhibitor, 163
acid, x, 20, 29, 32, 105, 108, 117, 140, 143, 148,
    150, 154, 156, 158, 159, 193, 197, 198, 202,
    217, 219, 221, 222, 224, 225, 226, 228, 231,
    235, 258, 261, 270, 272, 274, 280, 283, 288,
    317, 322, 335, 341, 367, 419, 434, 437, 447,
    450
acidic, xvi, 200, 225, 430

acidification, 200
acidity, 224, 225, 231
acidosis, 224, 225, 231, 232
acquired immunity, 318
actin, 225, 227
action potential, 227
activated receptors, 276
activation, xi, xii, 16, 55, 61, 74, 90, 101, 123,
    165, 166, 167, 173, 193, 195, 227, 239, 242,
    243, 244, 246, 247, 248, 249, 266, 276, 284,
    313, 320, 322, 335, 347, 357, 364, 365, 367,
    402, 404, 409, 411, 414, 418, 425
activators, 167, 327
active oxygen, 285
active smokers, 407
activity level, 311
actuarial, 52, 83
acute, 14, 16, 21, 31, 141, 152, 156, 162, 171,
    225, 259, 267, 273, 275, 285, 322, 335, 398,
    402, 404, 411, 414, 415, 417, 419, 426
acute coronary syndrome, 16
acute infection, 273, 417
acyl transferase, 153
Adams, 90, 129, 452
adaptability, 70, 229, 267, 356, 442
adaptation, xvi, 20, 41, 42, 48, 68, 79, 88, 128,
    183, 223, 256, 259, 263, 266, 267, 268, 269,
    270, 272, 275, 284, 285, 286, 289, 317, 430
adducts, viii, 23, 245, 274
adenine, 140
adenocarcinoma, 159, 452
adenoma, 91
adenosine, 225, 279

adenosine triphosphate, 225
adhesion, 322, 334, 404
adipocyte, 194
adipocytes, 191, 194, 217, 218, 238
adipogenic, 194
adiponectin, xiv, 309, 316
adipose, 13, 29, 91, 124, 169, 187, 194, 200, 208, 213, 214, 215, 216, 217, 218, 219, 220, 221, 222, 233, 236, 314, 327, 331, 414, 424
adipose tissue, 13, 29, 124, 169, 187, 194, 208, 216, 217, 218, 219, 222, 233, 236, 314, 327, 331, 414, 424
adiposity, 29, 187, 190, 192, 194, 214, 215, 220, 244, 328
adjunctive therapy, 426
adjustment, x, 140, 141, 148, 340, 341, 343, 347, 412, 415
administration, 27, 114, 191, 192, 280, 368
adolescence, 360
adolescents, 358, 363
adrenal cortex, 218
adrenal gland, 185
adrenal glands, 185
adult, x, xii, 42, 56, 84, 98, 101, 104, 112, 122, 126, 133, 134, 140, 149, 150, 179, 197, 198, 208, 237, 255, 263, 269, 275, 277, 341, 355, 358, 360, 361, 364, 366, 367, 379, 395
adult organisms, xii, 98, 255
adult population, 341
adult stem cells, 364
adulthood, 42, 230, 235, 270, 279, 362
adults, 27, 102, 157, 251, 289, 340, 349, 358, 363, 364, 407, 414, 415
advanced glycation end products, 191
aerobic, xii, 27, 29, 189, 212, 248, 255, 284
aerobic exercise, 213
aetiology, 59, 410, 414, 425
aflatoxins, 165
Africa, 42, 87, 174, 281, 336, 379
African American, 405, 406, 407
African Americans, 405, 407
agar, 339
agent, 100, 101, 102, 117, 183, 198, 200, 207, 223, 297
agents, 27, 29, 49, 61, 94, 101, 102, 108, 112, 114, 116, 120, 130, 162, 165, 166, 169, 174, 181, 185, 189, 192, 193, 195, 199, 201, 206, 213, 229, 277, 278, 288, 293, 397, 401, 410, 420, 445
age-related macular degeneration, 60, 76, 94

AGEs, viii, 23, 24, 25, 27, 28, 29, 30, 32, 205, 206
aggregates, 296
aggregation, 65, 168, 297
aggressiveness, 361
aging process, ix, xiii, xiv, 10, 13, 25, 26, 97, 98, 99, 101, 102, 105, 109, 116, 118, 122, 125, 145, 180, 181, 231, 239, 256, 278, 293, 303, 304, 309, 312, 316, 317, 321, 326, 328, 362, 373, 383, 388, 430, 437, 442
aging society, vii, 1, 293, 299
aging studies, 117, 371
agonist, 106
agrarian, 399
agricultural, 169, 173, 189
agriculture, x, 42, 161, 162, 163, 169, 336, 398
aid, 29, 203, 204
AIDS, 336
air, x, 43, 84, 161, 207, 268, 272, 273, 360, 431, 434, 441, 449
albumin, 145, 155, 343, 423, 440
albuminuria, 415, 423
alcohol, 84, 142, 143, 144, 147, 148, 149, 150, 153, 154, 159, 292, 298, 343, 399, 418
alcohol consumption, 84, 142, 143, 144, 147, 148, 149, 150, 153, 154, 343, 399
alcoholic liver disease, 85, 158
alcoholism, 67
aldehydes, 206, 248
ALDH2, 153
alien species, 371
alkaline, 231
allele, 11, 15, 16, 39, 80, 118, 120, 126, 298, 312, 315, 318, 320, 321, 322, 324, 382, 393, 402, 403, 404, 406, 425
alleles, 10, 11, 15, 16, 41, 49, 64, 118, 119, 122, 129, 311, 318, 319, 320, 322, 332, 334, 382, 383, 400, 403, 406, 414, 424
allergens, 43, 67
allergic asthma, 67
allergic reaction, 166, 167
allergy, 67, 93, 162, 273
allogeneic, 336
alopecia, 57, 314
alpha, 133, 145, 219, 239, 253, 261, 284, 317, 334, 341
alpha-tocopherol, 341
ALS, 326
alternative, xiii, 70, 195, 211, 226, 303
alternatives, 172

alters, 55, 120, 121, 131, 237, 287
altruism, 86
alveolar macrophage, 266
alveolar macrophages, 266
alveoli, 60
Alzheimer's disease, 60, 67, 93, 200, 296, 310
Amadori, 332
amalgam, 186
ambiguity, 215
amines, 165
amino, viii, 23, 32, 108, 109, 187, 188, 193, 202, 203, 216, 218, 219, 221, 222, 231, 234, 270
amino acids, viii, 23, 109, 187, 188, 193, 203, 216, 218, 219, 221, 222, 231, 270
ammonia, 216, 231
ammonium, 217, 231
amphibians, 387
amputation, 403
amyloid, 92, 93, 197, 235, 295, 296, 297, 298
amyloid beta, 92, 93, 197, 235, 295
amyloid plaques, 296, 297, 298
amyloid precursor protein, 295
amyotrophic lateral sclerosis, 313
anabolic, 181, 182, 222
anaemia, 41
anaerobic, 184
analytical models, 373, 376
anaphylaxis, 410, 422
anatomy, 368, 371
androgen, 170, 175, 452
aneuploid, 112
aneuploidy, 168
angiotensin II, 16, 21, 94, 253
angiotensin-converting enzyme, 94, 298
animal models, 14, 24, 87, 122, 178, 354, 409
animal studies, 27, 106, 268
animal welfare, xv, 373, 386, 387
animals, 270, 362, 364, 398
annealing, 147
annual rate, 293
anorexia, 416
antagonism, 104, 125, 214
antagonist, 234, 399
antagonistic, 28, 53, 217, 311, 317
Antarctic, 258
anterior pituitary, 110
anthracene, 129
anti-apoptotic, 231
anti-atherogenic, 28
antibiotic, 66, 75, 93

antibiotic resistance, 66
antibiotics, 65, 66, 75, 79, 401, 424
antibody, 296, 297, 323, 401, 423
anticancer, 33, 289
anti-cancer, 223
antidiabetic, 30
antigen, 49, 86, 311, 332, 399, 406, 412
antigenicity, 49
antigens, 86, 135
anti-inflammatory drugs, 297
antineoplastic, 272
antioxidant, xi, 13, 14, 25, 28, 31, 32, 33, 107, 111, 115, 121, 130, 132, 134, 136, 150, 177, 180, 181, 187, 189, 191, 202, 204, 210, 213, 229, 235, 238, 240, 257, 259, 267, 274, 277, 341, 350
antioxidants, 180, 189, 199, 213, 229
anti-tumor, 421
antrum, 411
anxiety, 49, 348
aorta, xii, 16, 30, 233, 242, 245, 246
aortic aneurysm, 344
apnea, 421
APO, 10
APOE, 10, 18, 315
Apolipoprotein E, 11, 18
apoptosis, 13, 15, 36, 51, 56, 57, 67, 68, 75, 87, 88, 89, 90, 91, 114, 115, 120, 132, 135, 168, 230, 231, 234, 239, 251, 256, 260, 270, 272, 273, 278, 287, 407, 431, 438, 441, 444, 448, 450, 451, 452
apoptotic, xvi, 11, 31, 62, 91, 100, 118, 230, 231, 283, 430, 432, 441, 444, 450
apoptotic cells, 91
apoptotic effect, 231
APP, 295, 296, 297, 451
appendicitis, 43, 85
appetite, 215, 348
application, 66, 76, 78, 116, 175, 194, 256, 275, 277, 278, 279, 375, 387, 390
arachidonic acid, 322, 335
Arctic, 258
arginine, 269, 280
argument, 41, 76, 186, 260, 304, 305, 306, 346
arousal, 410
arrest, 57, 131, 239
arrhythmia, 43, 277
arrhythmias, 60
arsenic, 170
arterial hypertension, 14, 16, 273

arteries, 145, 269
artery, 243, 288, 333, 412, 421
arthritis, 294, 421
articular cartilage, 91
ascetic, 212, 214
ascorbic, 341
ascorbic acid, 341
asexual, 449
Asia, 397
Asian, 91, 143, 153, 160, 412, 415, 421
aspartate, 297
Aspergillus niger, 449, 452
assaults, 196
assessment, 20, 33, 173, 324, 342, 345, 388, 401,
    411, 414, 418
assimilation, 188, 199, 203, 268, 383
asthma, 67, 93, 251, 273, 274, 276, 284, 289
astigmatism, 43, 47
astrocyte, 237
astrocytes, 184, 287
asymptomatic, 333, 401, 423
asymptotic, 324
atherosclerosis, xi, xiv, 15, 16, 47, 58, 94, 149,
    241, 243, 250, 251, 273, 298, 309, 313, 314,
    317, 318, 320, 322, 323, 325, 333, 335, 336,
    414, 415, 450
atherosclerotic plaque, 322
atherothrombotic, 16, 157
athletes, 288
atmosphere, 267, 272
ATP, 15, 166, 210, 225, 226, 256, 261, 270, 275,
    276, 279, 289, 315, 330
atresia, 261, 263, 269
atrial fibrillation, 67, 94
atrioventricular block, 60
atrophy, 57, 58, 60, 61, 110, 229, 230, 231, 285
attachment, 407
attacks, 9, 278, 336
atypical, 317
auditory hallucinations, 295
Australia, 273, 377, 380, 385, 397, 398, 399, 405,
    406, 407, 410, 411, 416, 419, 420, 421, 423,
    424, 450
Austria, 385
autoimmune, xiv, 67, 273, 309, 319, 324, 334
autoimmune disease, 67, 319, 324, 334
autoimmune diseases, 67, 319, 324, 334
autoimmunity, 323
autonomy, vii, 1, 2

autophagy, 190, 192, 193, 196, 213, 242, 243,
    250, 256, 257, 269, 278, 286
autopsy, 408, 411
autosomal recessive, 317, 332
availability, 49, 103, 182, 184, 192, 215, 221,
    226, 263, 269, 278, 279, 375, 444
average longevity, 374
awareness, 73, 75
azoxymethane, 108
Aβ, 295, 296, 297

B

B cells, 402, 404, 438
babies, 50, 409
Bacillus subtilis, 369
back pain, 43
backlash, 70
bacteria, ix, 16, 35, 48, 66, 67, 74, 93, 194, 306,
    322, 323, 403, 407, 409, 411, 412, 413, 414,
    421, 427, 430
bacterial, 48, 74, 93, 272, 327, 371, 398, 399,
    401, 405, 407, 408, 409, 420, 425, 426, 432,
    437, 450
bacterial infection, 408, 409
baking, 29, 206
Barbados, 155
barley, 28, 29, 31, 32, 33, 189, 201, 204, 206,
    207, 238
barrier, 33, 164, 215, 286, 402
basal metabolic rate, 103, 208, 209, 211, 259
basement membrane, 111
Bayesian, 376, 389
Bayesian analysis, 389
BDNF, 185, 197, 198
beef, 206, 374, 375, 378, 379, 382, 385, 387,
    389, 391, 392, 393, 394
beer, 204
behavior, 117, 122, 142, 151, 160, 197, 199, 281,
    295, 357
behaviours, 50, 51, 73
Belgium, 385
beliefs, 70
beneficial effect, xi, xiv, 8, 13, 120, 150, 196,
    233, 241, 267, 268, 288, 309, 313
benefits, 14, 20, 70, 171, 179, 189, 190, 229, 274,
    279, 297, 370, 372, 452
benign, 91, 204, 258, 290
benign prostatic hyperplasia, 91
benign tumors, 258
benzo(a)pyrene, 106

beta cell, xiv, 219, 275, 309

beta-carotene, 341

beverages, 188

bias, 304, 375

bile, 200, 201

binding, 31, 86, 127, 135, 137, 156, 166, 170, 173, 175, 193, 194, 195, 204, 225, 227, 232, 243, 246, 248, 250, 252, 276, 323, 328, 335, 336, 357, 368, 404, 407, 422

bioavailability, 164, 165, 166

biochemistry, 208, 251, 325

bioenergetics, 236

biogenesis, xvi, 13, 261, 272, 275, 280, 289, 430

biogerontology, xii, 255

biological activity, 404

biological clocks, 99

biological consequences, 157

biological macromolecules, 248

biological processes, 164

biological systems, 128

biomarker, 16, 324, 325

biomarkers, 21, 33, 273, 274, 275, 279, 289, 321, 324

biomass, 306

biomolecules, 172

biomonitoring, 173

biopsies, 266

biorhythm, 286

biosynthesis, 452

biotechnology, 372

biotransformation, 164

Biotransformation, 368

bipolar, 153

bipolar disorder, 153

birds, 121, 132, 258, 284, 358, 374, 387

birth, vii, 1, 2, 4, 110, 170, 171, 174, 258, 293, 374, 383, 387, 389, 391, 399, 409, 416, 417, 420, 424, 426, 442

birth rate, vii, 1, 2

birth weight, 171, 174, 383, 389, 416, 424

births, 8, 77, 408, 409, 410, 417, 420, 423

birthweight, 417, 418, 423

bivalve, 53

black tea, 27

Blacks, 405, 407

bladder, 43, 84, 170

bladder cancer, 84

blindness, 45

blocks, 449

blood flow, 101, 440

blood glucose, 158, 270

blood group, 412, 419

blood monocytes, 406

blood oxygenation level-dependent, 347

blood pressure, x, 44, 85, 140, 141, 144, 148, 150, 153, 244, 268, 343, 344, 415, 421, 440

blood stream, 437, 450

blood vessels, 16, 59, 298

bloodstream, xvi, 191, 221, 225, 430, 438, 439, 440, 444

body composition, 13, 208, 209, 217, 244

body fat, 29, 31, 192, 214, 216, 218, 219, 220, 394

body fluid, 222, 295, 407

Body Mass Index (BMI), 43, 44, 84, 141, 142, 143, 144, 146, 147, 148, 274, 279, 344, 401, 415, 427

body size, 26, 62, 122, 131, 209, 251, 260, 271, 281, 356, 358, 359, 365

body temperature, 210, 244, 258, 259, 281

body weight, 31, 56, 125, 131, 216, 220, 235, 244, 252, 442

Boeing, 23, 31

Bohr, 18

boiling, 188

BOLD, 347

bone density, 105

bone loss, 60, 239

bone marrow, 57, 58, 111, 116, 117, 260, 266, 284

bootstrap, 387

Botswana, 42, 47, 85

bovine, 107, 125, 389, 391, 394, 437

bowel, 92, 276

bradykinesia, 168

brain, 37, 60, 107, 111, 113, 116, 125, 126, 128, 131, 133, 135, 167, 169, 170, 173, 175, 179, 180, 182, 184, 188, 193, 196, 197, 198, 199, 215, 216, 233, 235, 236, 237, 240, 265, 266, 275, 283, 285, 295, 296, 297, 298, 299, 338, 347, 350, 364, 402, 409, 442

brain activity, 338

brain damage, 125, 135, 285

brain development, 170, 196

brain growth, 184

brain tumor, 169

Brassica oleracea, 188

Brazil, 292, 379

breakdown, 39, 225, 243, 407

breast cancer, 166, 201, 444, 452

breast feeding, 169

breast milk, 163, 183

breathing, 273, 360

breeder, 390

breeding, 42, 121, 238, 356, 359, 362, 372, 374, 375, 381, 385, 386, 387, 392, 394

Britain, 410, 412

broad spectrum, 357, 361, 365

broccoli, 188, 201, 207, 239

broccoli sprouts, 207

broilers, 390

bronchial asthma, 284

bronchitis, 43

bronchoalveolar lavage, 406

brothers, 311

bubonic plague, 65

buffer, 101, 147, 183, 265

buildings, 70

bulbs, 70

Bulgaria, 309

burn, 263

burning, 225

burns, 8

butyric, 272, 288

bypass, 270

by-products, 99, 242

C

C reactive protein, 411

C. pneumoniae, 412, 415, 416

Ca^{2+}, 30, 126, 167, 227

cadmium, 103, 105, 107, 109, 112, 113, 134, 170

Caenorhabditis elegans, 10, 12, 18, 19, 102, 123, 124, 126, 128, 130, 131, 132, 133, 134, 136, 137, 194, 239, 287, 326, 327, 354, 356, 358, 367, 368, 370, 371

caffeine, 151, 157, 292

calcium, 43, 144, 226, 227, 256, 340, 372, 416

caloric intake, ix, 8, 13, 25, 97, 99, 105, 108, 126, 178, 199, 210, 211, 217, 235, 236, 362, 369

calorie, xi, xii, 14, 15, 19, 20, 25, 31, 99, 105, 118, 123, 125, 126, 132, 134, 135, 179, 183, 186, 189, 190, 194, 207, 211, 215, 227, 230, 231, 233, 234, 238, 241, 244, 245, 246, 247, 248, 249, 250, 251, 252, 255, 257, 259, 264, 274, 275, 276, 278, 279, 288, 289, 327, 340, 371

calving, 391

campaigns, 408, 410

Canada, 281, 293, 377, 378, 379, 385, 406

cancer cells, 239, 444, 451

cancer stem cells, 452

candidates, 53, 168, 202

capacity, xv, 14, 24, 25, 27, 28, 31, 36, 37, 42, 54, 57, 68, 89, 93, 112, 130, 143, 167, 184, 187, 189, 196, 197, 202, 203, 207, 210, 213, 217, 219, 221, 222, 223, 224, 225, 230, 259, 261, 277, 292, 320, 347, 348, 350, 353, 364, 426

caps, 293

carbohydrate, xiv, 29, 151, 160, 178, 203, 206, 216, 283, 309, 437, 439, 440

carbohydrates, 43, 203, 216, 217, 222, 270, 271, 346

carbon, 217, 270, 285

carbon dioxide, 285

carcinogen, 113, 135, 165

carcinogenesis, 129, 201, 207, 282

carcinogenic, 162, 164, 165, 168, 195, 207

carcinogens, 105, 106, 116, 132, 134, 165, 169, 170, 235, 365

carcinoma, 43, 84, 124, 150, 159, 369

cardiac function, 267

cardiac myocytes, 282

cardiology, 286, 290

cardiomyocytes, 115, 265, 266, 286, 289

cardiovascular disease, xiii, xv, 11, 14, 15, 20, 21, 43, 67, 94, 143, 154, 200, 214, 244, 273, 276, 291, 310, 311, 313, 316, 320, 325, 333, 337, 341, 350, 412, 415, 416, 421, 427, 431, 445

cardiovascular morbidity, 156, 415, 422

cardiovascular risk, 14, 59, 92, 336, 350, 422, 423, 424, 425

cardiovascular system, 314

Caribbean, 331

carotene, 13, 165, 341

carotenoids, 346

carotid arteries, 145

carrier, 166, 402

cartilage, 91

case study, 387

casein, 183, 384, 392

caspase, 235

caspase-12, 235

Caspase-9, 451

cast, 116

CAT, 115

catabolism, 189, 213, 218, 219, 231

catalase, 16, 107, 113, 115, 127, 133, 204, 239, 257, 312, 313
catalyst, 217
catalysts, 184
cataract, 67, 95, 111, 277
cataracts, 58, 61, 108, 314
catechins, 191
cattle, 42, 235, 260, 373, 374, 375, 376, 377, 378, 379, 381, 382, 383, 385, 386, 387, 389, 390, 391, 392, 393, 394, 395, 398, 437
Caucasian, 152, 399, 400, 402, 405, 406, 407, 409, 412, 413, 416, 417, 422, 423, 424, 440
Caucasian population, 406, 412, 423
Caucasians, 315, 400, 405, 414, 417, 427
causal relationship, 119, 170
causation, 85, 422
cavities, 60
CCR, 210, 318, 323
CD95, 451
cDNA, 126
cecum, 134
cell culture, 101, 107, 109, 266, 431, 437, 439, 445
cell cycle, 57, 120, 128, 451
cell death, 15, 31, 51, 56, 90, 100, 107, 112, 114, 123, 167, 168, 230, 282, 283, 448, 450, 452
cell differentiation, 367
cell division, 223, 364
cell fate, 16, 88, 90, 369
cell growth, 170, 175, 189, 448
cell line, 54, 62, 113, 115, 120, 121, 130, 133, 261, 402, 448
cell membranes, 222, 243
cell organelles, 357, 362
cell surface, 234, 335, 404, 407, 434, 441
cellular homeostasis, x, 98, 100, 123
cellular immunity, 265, 279
cellulose, 271
Center for Disease Control and Prevention, 294
central nervous system, 91, 167, 169, 279
cerebellum, 347
cerebral cortex, 198
cerebral ischemia, 43, 59, 71
cerebrospinal fluid, 295, 403, 406, 426
cerebrovascular, x, 140, 141, 152, 200, 294, 299
cerebrovascular disease, x, 140, 141, 200, 294
cerebrovascular diseases, x, 140
certificate, 258
CFA, 406
c-fos, 328

c-Fos, 246
channels, 167, 275, 450
chaperones, 131, 239
check-ups, x, 140, 146
cheese, 206
chelators, 297
chemical industry, 85
chemical properties, 437
chemicals, 49, 67, 162, 164, 166, 168, 173, 187, 188, 195, 206, 207, 214, 434, 445
chemokine, 16, 21, 321, 322, 334, 404
chemokine receptor, 16, 21, 322
chemokines, 16, 422
chemoprevention, 451
chemotherapy, 324, 336, 444, 451
chewing, xiv, 337, 338, 339, 340, 341, 342, 343, 344, 345, 346, 347, 348, 349, 350
chicken, 383, 392, 437
chickens, 84, 374, 390, 437
childhood, 43, 67, 85, 169, 170, 174, 176, 324, 398, 399
children, vii, 2, 43, 50, 167, 169, 273, 284, 299, 336, 358, 399, 403, 407, 415, 419, 424
chimpanzee, 182, 185
China, 77, 273, 292, 299, 450
Chlamydia trachomatis, 417
chloride, 144, 167
chlorination, 170
chlorogenic acid, 150, 151, 158
chlorpyriphos, 175
cholera, 65, 85, 401
cholesterol, xvi, 14, 15, 16, 142, 148, 153, 154, 158, 200, 201, 242, 251, 274, 297, 325, 332, 343, 346, 350, 412, 413, 429, 439, 450
cholesterol-lowering drugs, 297
cholinergic, 175
chondrocytes, 266
Chordata, 182
chromatid, 168
chromatin, 314, 432
chromatography, 437
chromosome, xiv, 11, 40, 82, 93, 135, 293, 310, 311, 317, 324, 331, 336, 364, 391
chromosome 20, 331
chromosomes, 57, 89, 364, 369, 383
chronic disease, 26, 214, 252, 324, 341, 431
chronic hypoxia, 265, 267, 268, 285
chronic obstructive pulmonary disease, 84
chronic renal failure, 33
chronic viral infections, 418

chronobiology, 124

chrysanthemum, 171

cigarette smoke, 293, 405, 407, 408, 417, 421, 425

cigarette smoking, 14, 67, 142, 154, 156, 343, 344

circadian, 32, 238, 271, 409

circadian rhythm, 32, 238, 271, 409

circulation, 59, 168, 184, 297, 299, 348, 439, 442

cirrhosis, xi, 43, 241, 243

citizens, 44, 170

CKD, 416

classes, 10, 15, 164, 323

classical, xv, 386, 397, 408

classification, 10, 69, 72, 169, 170, 390

cleaning, 348

cleavage, 204, 295

clients, 26

clinical symptoms, 324

clinical syndrome, 314

clinical trial, xiii, 291, 296, 297, 298

clinical trials, xiii, 291, 296, 297, 298

clone, 51, 137, 261

cloning, 18, 92, 280, 328

clustering, 326

CML, 206

CMV, 323, 324, 410, 412, 415, 416

CNS, 265, 267, 279

CO2, 257, 259, 266

coagulation, 404, 412

coagulation factor, 412

coagulation factors, 412

coconut, 28

codes, 312, 314, 316

coding, 16, 133, 261, 315

codon, 15, 321

coenzyme, 106, 222, 261

cofactors, 204, 261

coffee, x, 140, 146, 147, 148, 149, 150, 151, 158, 159

cognition, 196, 197, 198

cognitive, xiii, 18, 111, 188, 196, 197, 199, 280, 291, 297, 298, 347

cognitive ability, xiii, 291, 297, 298

cognitive activity, xiii, 291

cognitive capacity, 196, 197

cognitive dysfunction, 280

cognitive function, 199, 297, 347

cognitive impairment, 347

cognitive test, 199

cohort, 31, 154, 157, 159, 160, 173, 209, 315, 331, 333, 338, 342, 345, 346, 350, 423, 424

collaboration, 195

collagen, xi, xii, 27, 30, 31, 32, 90, 111, 126, 191, 233, 241, 242, 243, 244, 245, 246, 248, 250, 252

college students, 49

colon, 43, 92, 108, 117, 129, 159, 213, 344, 431

colon cancer, 159, 431

colon carcinogenesis, 129

colonisation, 408, 409, 411

colonization, 407

colorectal cancer, 150, 159, 200

Columbia, 379

combined effect, 64, 222, 226, 298, 314

combustion, 13, 185, 207

commodities, 188, 196

common findings, 409

Commonwealth of Independent States, 286

communication, 283, 355

communities, 78, 163, 170, 176, 410, 412, 414, 416

community, xiv, 4, 45, 49, 117, 155, 162, 332, 337, 338, 340, 341, 347, 350, 399, 404, 410, 411, 413, 416, 423, 424, 427

compaction, 216

compatibility, 86

compensation, 276

competition, 48, 71, 264

competitiveness, 70

competitor, 70, 71

complement, 184, 204, 207, 240, 324, 335, 336

complement system, 324

complexity, 37, 49, 175, 198, 199, 306, 376

compliance, xi, 178, 274

complications, 43, 47, 61, 145

components, 26, 29, 59, 69, 71, 74, 100, 105, 107, 166, 168, 172, 176, 182, 186, 188, 192, 196, 202, 208, 210, 213, 240, 243, 248, 315, 317, 324, 372, 374, 375, 383, 390, 413, 421, 439, 448

composition, xi, 12, 26, 121, 128, 156, 177, 188, 208, 209, 215, 217, 236, 362, 376, 389, 439

compounds, 13, 24, 27, 28, 29, 30, 32, 108, 111, 120, 151, 163, 165, 166, 167, 168, 169, 171, 173, 185, 188, 201, 206, 231, 234, 237, 238, 244, 409, 433, 445, 446, 448

comprehension, 37, 78, 79, 304

concentrates, 383

concentration, 24, 26, 27, 33, 124, 183, 191, 195, 199, 206, 218, 221, 222, 223, 224, 225, 226, 227, 228, 234, 267, 268, 270, 324, 426, 447, 450

conception, 61, 72, 170, 305

conceptualization, xi, 177

concordance, 166

conditioning, 212

confidence, xiv, 37, 149, 337, 343

confidence interval, xiv, 149, 337, 343

confidence intervals, 149

conflict, 307

confounders, 344, 345, 347

congestive heart failure, 43, 290

conjecture, 198, 199

conjugation, 108, 111, 165

Connecticut, 132

connective tissue, 11, 243, 365

consensus, 107, 180, 297, 305, 317

consent, 146

conservation, 12, 178, 184, 187, 202, 204

constant rate, 293, 442

constipation, 43

Constitution, 392

constraints, 53, 56

construction, 68, 119, 203, 216

consumers, 13, 70, 71

consumption, x, 15, 24, 31, 84, 131, 140, 142, 143, 144, 145, 146, 147, 148, 149, 150, 151, 153, 154, 156, 157, 159, 178, 183, 200, 201, 206, 208, 212, 231, 270, 275, 283, 287, 292, 343, 399, 416, 436, 452

contaminants, 164, 172, 176

contaminated food, 169

contamination, 163

continuity, 162

control group, 10, 25, 178, 208, 220, 223, 274, 275, 297, 412

controlled trials, 94, 349

conversion, 70, 107, 113, 184, 187, 189, 207, 216, 218, 222, 225, 322

cooking, 24, 28, 203

cooling, 239

copper, 103, 372

copulation, 304

corn, 29

coronary artery disease, 288, 333

coronary heart disease, 17, 20, 156, 316, 333, 350, 421, 425, 439, 450

corporations, 2

correlation, 10, 26, 31, 55, 103, 105, 107, 121, 128, 129, 170, 233, 314, 320, 321, 325, 326, 389, 411, 415, 416, 425, 437, 442

correlations, 11, 312, 330, 391, 392, 393, 394

cortex, 198, 218, 296, 347

cortical neurons, 295

corticotropin, 185

cortisol, 184, 217, 218, 219, 328

costs, vii, 1, 2, 69, 71, 75, 162, 171, 295, 370, 386

cotinine, 407

cotton, 169, 170, 171, 175

cough, 49

counseling, 2

couples, 49

coupling, 227, 234

covalent, 173, 237

covering, 168, 316, 383

cows, 374, 376, 378, 381, 382, 385, 387, 388, 391, 392, 393, 394, 437

COX-1, 322

COX-2, 253, 322, 335, 451

CPD, 106

crab, 368

C-reactive protein, xiv, 309, 317, 322, 325, 334, 350, 424, 425

creep, 71

critical points, xiii, 303

criticism, 9

crops, 28, 171, 189

crossbreeding, 373, 381

cross-linking, 30, 233, 435

cross-sectional, 31, 141, 142, 146, 150, 346

cross-sectional study, 141, 142, 146, 346

CRP, 15, 16, 411, 412, 415, 416

crustaceans, xv, 353, 355, 358, 362, 365, 370, 372

cryopreserved, 394

crypt stem cells, 58

crystals, 436

CSF, 295, 403, 409

cues, 328

cultivation, 89, 170

culture, 50, 70, 90, 103, 106, 107, 114, 128, 305, 356, 371, 403, 406, 419, 434

culture media, 114

Curcumin, 451

customers, 71

CVD, xv, 337, 341, 343, 344, 345, 346, 416

cycles, xv, 147, 239, 269, 353, 355, 359, 360, 361, 363, 366

cycling, 103, 288

cyclooxygenase, 335

cyclooxygenase-2, 335

CYP17, 175

cysteine, 121, 131, 231

cystic fibrosis, xi, 241, 243

cytochrome, 164, 173, 237

cytokine, 16, 167, 284, 317, 319, 320, 321, 333, 334, 399, 400, 401, 402, 403, 404, 405, 407, 408, 409, 410, 416, 418, 421, 423, 427

cytokine receptor, 317

cytokine response, 401, 408, 410

cytokines, xi, 16, 91, 241, 243, 247, 250, 253, 317, 320, 322, 333, 399, 400, 401, 403, 404, 405, 408, 409, 410, 411, 412, 414, 420, 422, 424, 425, 426

cytology, 371

cytomegalovirus, 350, 410

cytoplasm, 227, 295, 434, 441

cytoprotective, 249

cytosine, 140, 358

cytosol, 108

cytotoxic, ix, 98, 100, 101, 107, 112, 113, 120, 121, 122, 130, 240, 312, 447

cytotoxic agents, 101, 120, 130

cytotoxicity, 173

Czech Republic, 377, 391

D

daily living, 155, 294, 297, 346, 350

dairy, 373, 374, 375, 376, 377, 378, 382, 383, 385, 386, 387, 388, 389, 390, 391, 392, 393, 394, 395

danger, 75, 401

data analysis, 141

data set, 310, 361

database, 44

DBP, 141

death rate, 17, 293

deaths, 8, 63, 65, 374, 410, 411, 412, 422

decay, 50, 54, 55, 262, 280

decisions, 71, 79

defects, viii, 35, 37, 43, 68, 126, 170, 174, 282, 324

defense, xi, 108, 177, 181, 186, 190, 196, 210, 263, 264, 265, 267, 269, 278, 286, 295, 401

defenses, 12, 13, 112, 115, 116, 134, 136, 207, 240, 401

deficiency, xiv, 15, 41, 49, 57, 59, 85, 114, 115, 125, 195, 270, 272, 285, 309, 324

deficit, 211

deficits, 27, 179, 184, 197, 199, 202, 221, 235, 237

definition, vii, 1, 2, 3, 50, 98, 131, 169, 305, 325, 394, 408, 409, 419

deformability, 450

degenerative disease, 83, 84, 257, 272, 275, 277

degradation, 92, 163, 180, 202, 228, 229, 243, 267

degrading, 92

dehydration, xvii, 430, 431, 432, 433, 435, 436, 439, 442, 443, 445, 447, 448, 449

dehydrogenase, x, 140, 150, 153, 154, 155, 156, 160, 225, 317

delivery, 61, 262

Delphi, 281

delusions, 295

dementia, 18, 59, 93, 200, 294, 295, 297, 298, 299, 320

demographics, 341

demography, vii

denaturation, 147, 191, 203

dendrites, 174, 198

dendritic cell, 322, 404

denervation, 230

Denmark, 377, 385

density, 15, 42, 65, 105, 142, 153, 216, 234, 323, 332, 348, 398, 411

dental caries, 42, 43, 46, 47

dentate gyrus, 123, 134

dentist, 339

denture, 340, 341

dephosphorylation, 328

depolarization, 226, 227

deposition, xi, 29, 192, 194, 195, 214, 217, 218, 219, 220, 241, 245, 295, 297, 298

deposits, 13, 184, 215, 295

depreciation, 181, 183

depressed, 191

depression, 128, 183, 283, 348, 373, 382, 388

deprivation, 24, 123, 130, 178, 183, 185, 192, 194, 195, 199, 217, 233, 240, 276, 282, 371, 416

derivatives, 32, 206, 279

dermatitis, 164

dermis, 59

desert, 8

desiccation, 102, 442, 451

destruction, xiv, 198, 267, 287, 309, 403
detachment, 213, 437
detection, 325, 383, 419
detergents, 67, 445
determinism, xv, 373
detoxification, xi, 120, 163, 164, 165, 176, 177, 181, 187, 188, 189, 200, 201, 205, 207, 213, 256, 363, 365
detoxifying, 31, 162, 164, 207, 217
developed countries, 79, 171, 292, 293, 295, 299
developed nations, 305
developing countries, 67, 171
deviation, 267, 381
dexamethasone, 114
diabetes mellitus, xiv, 15, 61, 67, 94, 156, 289, 309, 310, 314, 316, 329, 427
diabetic nephropathy, xi, 236, 241, 331
diabetic patients, 274, 289
diacylglycerol, 449
dialysis, 415, 416, 425
Diamond, 398, 421
diarrhea, 423
diarrhoea, 49
diastolic blood pressure, 141, 343
dietary, viii, xii, xiv, 13, 15, 19, 23, 24, 25, 26, 27, 29, 32, 43, 46, 85, 98, 105, 108, 109, 122, 124, 126, 127, 129, 130, 132, 135, 136, 137, 176, 178, 182, 183, 185, 186, 187, 196, 198, 199, 200, 202, 206, 208, 211, 217, 218, 233, 235, 236, 237, 238, 239, 240, 242, 248, 249, 257, 274, 288, 310, 312, 327, 335, 341, 348, 349, 362, 368, 371, 439, 452
dietary fat, 452
dietary fiber, 85, 341
dietary habits, xii, 46, 178, 242, 249
dietary intake, 105, 348, 349
dietary supplementation, 257
diets, 14, 25, 33, 46, 105, 107, 118, 201, 205, 224, 244, 249, 298, 324, 440
differentiated cells, 73
differentiation, 91, 110, 194, 197, 198, 223, 261, 263, 312, 367, 402
diffraction, 450
diffusion, 66, 225, 357
digestibility, 203, 287
digestion, 199, 203, 271
digestive enzymes, 202, 363
dioxins, 165
diploid, 82, 89
direct costs, 171

disability, 2, 4, 36, 332, 341, 350
disaster, 65
discipline, 27, 71, 214, 215, 232
discomfort, 304
discordance, 36, 47
discrimination, 9, 99
disease-free survival, 444
disequilibrium, 331
disinfection, 170
disorder, 11, 36, 67, 83, 141, 168, 268
disposition, 166, 186
distress, 267
distribution, 101, 153, 155, 174, 206, 271, 281, 320, 324, 357, 399, 403, 407, 412, 413
divergence, 191, 310, 418
diversification, 370
diversity, 38, 317, 335, 354, 430
diving, 257, 258, 266, 284
division, 223, 306, 307, 363, 364
DNA damage, ix, 11, 33, 97, 99, 106, 111, 115, 116, 132, 136, 168, 202, 231, 275, 311, 362, 443
DNA lesions, 100, 106, 112, 133
DNA polymerase, 54, 147
DNA repair, xii, 12, 18, 99, 106, 107, 113, 115, 130, 134, 136, 170, 181, 251, 256, 271
dogs, 182, 244, 362, 375, 398, 437
domestication, 118, 124, 129, 385, 395
dominance, 119, 359, 361, 381, 390, 393, 394
donor, 89
donors, 17, 54, 94, 269, 328, 406, 408
dopamine, 106, 167, 168
dopamine agonist, 106
dopaminergic, 168
dopaminergic neurons, 168
dosage, 239, 276, 327
Down syndrome, 295
down-regulation, 249
drinking, 141, 142, 143, 144, 146, 147, 149, 150, 151, 153, 159, 170, 298
drinking water, 170
Drosophila, 10, 11, 12, 18, 19, 87, 103, 109, 115, 120, 124, 125, 127, 128, 130, 132, 133, 134, 135, 136, 288, 312, 327, 354, 356, 358, 362, 368, 369, 441, 450
drought, 430
droughts, 271
drug interaction, 166
drug metabolism, 175
drug reactions, 165

drug targets, 336

drugs, 15, 65, 67, 68, 76, 95, 156, 235, 296, 297, 299, 354

drying, 339, 433, 434, 435, 436

duplication, 53, 54, 56, 58

DuPont, 423

duration, 26, 29, 30, 37, 55, 62, 69, 70, 73, 75, 76, 78, 79, 184, 190, 199, 205, 211, 212, 213, 224, 238, 268, 269, 272, 274, 275

dwarfism, 113

dyslipidemia, 30

dyspepsia, 85

dysplasia, 277

dysregulation, 90

E

eating, xiv, 151, 160, 185, 196, 199, 212, 314, 337, 338, 340, 348, 349, 351

eating behavior, 151, 160

eating disorders, 314

ECM, xi, 241, 243

ecological, viii, ix, 2, 4, 35, 36, 41, 42, 43, 45, 46, 47, 48, 53, 62, 64, 65, 66, 67, 68, 72, 73, 75, 79, 162, 176, 182, 239, 257

ecology, 86, 93, 370

economic activity, 294

economic efficiency, 386

ecosystem, 172

education, 249, 325

effusion, 419

egg, 206, 355, 359, 360, 445, 446

eggs, 183

egoism, 78

elaboration, 183, 188, 199

elderly, vii, xiv, 1, 2, 3, 4, 20, 79, 153, 154, 155, 288, 293, 294, 297, 317, 318, 319, 320, 321, 323, 324, 332, 334, 337, 338, 341, 346, 347, 348, 349, 350, 351, 413, 415, 426, 427

elderly population, 155

elders, 293

electrolyte, x, 140, 144, 155

electron, 210, 211, 226, 242, 371, 432

electron microscopy, 371

electrons, 210, 229, 432

elephant, 87

elongation, 90, 223, 432

embryo, 49, 50, 85, 203, 263, 269

embryogenesis, xii, 255, 269, 304, 442

embryology, 366

embryonic development, 267, 355, 357, 363

embryonic stem, 283

embryonic stem cells, 283

embryos, 261, 355, 356, 369

EMF, 275, 276, 279

emission, 432

emotional, xiii, 42, 47, 292, 303, 305, 306

emotional bias, xiii, 303, 307

emotions, 49, 78

emphysema, 43, 60, 84

empirical methods, 385

employees, 2

employment, 2, 69, 192

encapsulated, 258, 278

encapsulation, 365

encoding, xiv, 111, 193, 197, 257, 309, 315, 317, 329, 369

endocrine, xiv, 11, 111, 135, 163, 166, 169, 170, 174, 182, 267, 309, 312, 327

endocrine system, xiv, 111, 166, 182, 267, 309, 312

endocrinological, 111

endocrinology, 129, 132

endometrial cancer, 150, 159, 201

endometrium, 184

endoplasmic reticulum, 112, 133

endosymbionts, 271, 272

endothelial cells, 56, 58, 114, 290, 322, 402

endothelial dysfunction, 15, 59, 84, 268, 426

endothelial progenitor cells, 58, 92

endothelium, 14, 268, 411

endurance, 213, 214, 221, 224, 228, 278, 280, 288

energy density, 216

energy efficiency, 13, 202, 210, 216

engagement, 78

England, 281, 293, 419

engraftment, 284

enlargement, 60, 261

entertainment, 212

enthusiasm, 299

environment, x, 8, 84, 107, 116, 118, 128, 150, 161, 162, 169, 171, 172, 176, 215, 248, 259, 271, 292, 316, 317, 320, 357, 361, 367, 369, 372, 387, 407, 418, 441

environmental chemicals, 174

environmental conditions, xvi, 18, 196, 198, 272, 311, 355, 358, 397, 406, 437, 450

environmental contaminants, 167, 172

environmental effects, xiv, 309

environmental factors, xiv, 4, 6, 8, 10, 12, 140, 242, 298, 309, 313, 314, 319, 354, 361, 401, 414
environmental influences, 374
environmental stimuli, 198
environmental tobacco, 156, 421
enzymatic, 74, 107, 189, 202, 225, 226, 229, 263, 269, 434
enzymatic activity, 202, 226, 229
enzyme, 202, 203, 204, 207, 217, 219, 222, 224, 225, 226, 229, 236
enzyme inhibitors, 94, 203
enzymes, 31, 74, 107, 127, 132, 136, 164, 165, 166, 167, 175, 180, 187, 188, 193, 201, 202, 203, 204, 207, 210, 211, 217, 219, 221, 224, 229, 235, 237, 238, 239, 257, 264, 265, 273, 313, 317, 322, 363, 425, 448
EPA, 169, 170
epidemic, 65, 84, 397, 399, 415
epidemics, 65, 66, 75, 398, 415
epidemiology, 84, 159, 420, 422
epidermis, 59, 67, 365
epigenetic, 201, 357, 358, 366, 367, 370
epigenetic code, 357, 358, 366
epigenetics, 310, 354, 371
epinephrine, 184
epithelial cell, 58, 61, 107, 130, 363, 407, 421, 437
epithelial cells, 58, 61, 107, 130, 132, 363, 407, 421, 437
epithelium, 58, 176
Epstein Barr, 404
Epstein-Barr virus, 422
equality, 2
equilibrium, 28, 39, 40, 41, 80, 81, 82, 208, 209, 265, 311
ERK1, xi, 241, 244, 246
erosion, 364
erythrocyte, 263
erythrocytes, 89, 268
erythrocytosis, 144
erythropoietin, 284
Escherichia coli, 306
ESI, 439, 445, 446, 450
ester, 15, 153, 251
esterases, 166
esters, 171
estimating, 438
estrogen, 183, 201
estrogens, 165

ethanol, 150, 158, 434, 435
ethical issues, 172
Ethiopian, 259
ethnic background, 321
ethnic groups, 154, 405, 407, 409, 410, 414, 440
ethnicity, 144
etiology, 181, 200, 201, 223, 229, 243, 316, 324
etiopathogenesis, 174
eugenics, 72
eukaryotes, 98, 306
eukaryotic cell, 265
Europe, 42, 60, 65, 66, 273, 371, 397, 405
European Union, 387
Europeans, 65, 399, 402, 412, 415, 421
evacuation, 199
evening, 27, 29, 188
evolution, viii, ix, xvi, 6, 7, 17, 35, 54, 66, 70, 82, 83, 86, 87, 88, 93, 105, 122, 157, 183, 184, 224, 232, 233, 239, 260, 269, 273, 282, 306, 307, 310, 311, 312, 367, 418, 430, 442
evolutionary process, 37, 121, 306
examinations, 341, 342, 343, 432
excision, 106, 127, 234
excitation, 227, 234
excitotoxic, 117, 125
exclusion, 184, 206, 408
excretion, 105, 231, 372, 423
execution, 216, 269, 452
exercise, xvi, 15, 20, 26, 29, 30, 83, 134, 186, 188, 212, 213, 214, 221, 222, 223, 224, 225, 226, 228, 229, 236, 252, 267, 275, 278, 288, 290, 310, 429
exertion, 185, 208, 213, 216, 225, 228, 229
exons, 324
exonuclease, 328
exoskeleton, 358
expansions, 282
expenditures, 202
experimental condition, 356
exploitation, 219
extensor, 347
extinction, 182
extracellular matrix, xi, 16, 241, 243
extrachromosomal, 89
extraction, 186, 213, 221, 445
extrapolation, 178
exudate, 28, 189, 406
eyes, 37

F

factor VII, 427

FAD, 295

failure, 37, 38, 43, 53, 57, 60, 61, 104, 112, 163, 213, 375

false positive, 316

familial, 295, 296, 310, 326, 332

family, xi, xiv, 15, 77, 146, 194, 233, 241, 243, 265, 272, 281, 287, 297, 309, 310, 314, 317, 322, 323, 326, 335, 442

family history, 146, 297, 310

family studies, xiv, 309, 310

famine, 14, 214

FAO, 240

farmers, 162, 170, 381, 385

farms, 170, 385, 386

farmworkers, 172

Fas, 451

fasting, x, xi, xiii, 24, 26, 27, 29, 30, 140, 146, 148, 156, 177, 179, 188, 189, 190, 192, 193, 194, 195, 199, 201, 203, 205, 211, 213, 216, 217, 218, 219, 220, 221, 222, 223, 233, 256, 257, 269, 270, 274, 275, 276, 278, 279, 286, 288, 289, 315, 362, 415

fasting glucose, 146, 316

fat, 13, 20, 27, 29, 30, 103, 104, 126, 128, 129, 130, 151, 159, 178, 184, 187, 189, 192, 194, 195, 199, 200, 203, 206, 208, 209, 212, 213, 214, 215, 216, 217, 218, 219, 220, 221, 222, 230, 238, 250, 265, 270, 292, 299, 346, 394, 402, 414

fat reduction, 220

fatigue, 213, 221, 224, 225, 228

fats, 43, 47, 203, 218, 271

fatty acids, 184, 188, 192, 203, 217, 218, 219, 221, 222, 270, 271, 272, 274, 445, 446, 447, 452

faults, 68

fauna, x, 161, 162

FDA, 296

fear, 49

feedback, 160, 269

feeding, 12, 24, 26, 31, 32, 116, 169, 179, 188, 189, 190, 192, 195, 198, 199, 205, 211, 235, 238, 246, 288, 349, 355, 359, 360, 362, 363, 371, 409

females, vii, xiv, 1, 2, 104, 157, 183, 209, 269, 292, 319, 323, 328, 337, 340, 359, 361, 385, 387, 388, 392, 393, 413, 415

fertility, 102, 126, 134, 136, 184, 305, 356, 376, 385, 388, 389, 392, 401, 417

fertilizers, 207

fetal, 86, 107, 170, 171, 173, 259, 263, 395, 418

fetal brain, 173

fetal death, 170, 171, 173

fetus, 170, 286

fever, 49, 273

FGF2, 394

fiber, 85, 225, 227, 238, 341, 346, 348, 363

fibers, 221, 223, 225, 229, 230, 271, 295, 296

fibrinogen, 350, 412, 413, 416, 426, 427

fibrinolysis, 404

fibroblast, xi, 106, 114, 120, 121, 130, 137, 194, 241, 394

fibroblast growth factor, 394

fibroblasts, xi, 59, 89, 107, 108, 112, 121, 127, 137, 194, 239, 241, 250, 253, 282, 328, 402

fibrogenesis, xii, 242, 249, 252

fibronectin, 243

fibrosis, xi, xii, 241, 242, 243, 245, 246, 248, 249, 250, 252, 253

fibrous tissue, 230

filament, 432, 437

filtration, 423, 437, 438, 440

Finland, 380, 385

fish, 49, 88, 206, 342, 354, 358, 362, 367, 369, 371, 387, 445, 446, 452

fish meal, 452

fish oil, 445

fishing, 281

fission, 261

fitness, ix, 35, 36, 37, 48, 49, 50, 51, 52, 53, 54, 57, 58, 61, 62, 64, 122, 126, 261, 346, 347, 348, 349, 350, 351, 385, 387

fixation, 336, 435

flexibility, 167, 214

flight, 103

floating, 432, 440

flora, 67

flow, 101, 283, 339, 340, 345, 349, 416, 440, 442, 444, 446

flow rate, 339, 349, 416, 446

fluctuations, 195, 263, 286

fluid, 155, 295, 403, 406, 426, 434

fluid balance, 155

fluorescence, 30

focusing, xv, 43, 216, 311, 373

folate, 341

folding, 112

follicle, 183, 235, 384

follicle stimulating hormone, 183, 384

follicles, 263

follicular, 261, 269

Food and Drug Administration (FDA), 296

food intake, 122, 211, 362

food poisoning, 401

food production, 162

Ford, 237

forestry, 169

Fox, 330

fracture, 231, 239, 365

fragmentation, 441

France, 293, 381, 385

free radical, 8, 13, 28, 61, 99, 106, 107, 108, 113, 115, 121, 122, 127, 158, 172, 180, 185, 187, 205, 217, 221, 228, 229, 238, 242, 248, 251, 266, 267, 270, 285, 293, 407

free radicals, 8, 13, 99, 107, 108, 180, 185, 217, 228, 229, 242, 267, 270, 293, 407

free will, 79

free-radical, 125, 127

freshwater, 357, 361, 363, 365, 367, 368, 370, 371, 372

fructose, 202

fruit flies, 11, 12, 136, 311, 312

fruits, 78, 341

FTIR, 439

fuel, 68, 207, 213, 214, 218, 228, 237, 260, 263, 264, 270, 445

functional magnetic resonance imaging (fMRI), 347, 350

fungal, 336, 437, 449

fungal infection, 336

fungal spores, 437

fungi, ix, 35, 48, 67, 323, 430, 449

fungicide, 165

fungicides, 162, 165, 167

fungus, 449

fusion, 261, 266

G

G protein, 103

G7 countries, 293

GABA, 167

games, 299

Gamma, 423

gamma globulin, 414

gases, 8, 283

gasoline, 8

gastric, 61, 344, 421, 424, 426

gastric mucosa, 61

gastritis, 61, 411, 426

gastrointestinal, 92, 176, 199, 207, 273, 341, 411

gastrointestinal tract, 199, 207

Gaucher disease, 317

Gaussian, 375, 388

GCC, 321

GDNF, 185, 197, 265

gels, 147

gender, 17, 141, 311, 320, 323, 334, 340, 343, 344, 347, 410, 413, 415, 422

gene expression, xiv, xvi, 8, 12, 62, 128, 130, 132, 173, 181, 189, 201, 220, 250, 251, 263, 265, 283, 309, 313, 314, 320, 321, 324, 333, 335, 357, 367, 368, 369, 370, 374, 429

gene mapping, 120

gene promoter, 333, 414, 421, 422, 423, 426

gene silencing, 187

gene therapy, 72, 73, 76, 78, 95

general knowledge, 98

generation, 13, 14, 29, 38, 78, 80, 107, 113, 124, 125, 133, 134, 172, 180, 185, 187, 200, 210, 228, 229, 256, 261, 266, 267, 285, 297, 345, 355, 356, 382, 385

generativity, 228, 229

genetic alteration, 39, 72, 181, 310

genetic code, 357

genetic control, 293, 312, 317

genetic defect, 452

genetic disease, 57, 68, 71, 72, 73, 76

genetic diversity, 38

genetic endowment, 196

genetic factors, 144, 150, 325, 366, 368

genetic information, viii, 35, 38, 143

genetic instability, 8

genetic linkage, 93

genetic load, 382

genetic marker, 140, 311, 316, 415

genetic mutations, ix, 97, 103, 111, 122

genetic programs, xii, 255

genetics, xv, 8, 10, 18, 82, 88, 91, 117, 130, 133, 156, 163, 176, 289, 310, 311, 315, 328, 329, 332, 334, 354, 368, 373, 374, 375, 386, 388, 410

Geneva, 240, 288

genistein, 451

genome, xiii, xiv, 8, 9, 11, 12, 19, 72, 76, 99, 118, 119, 126, 133, 156, 181, 193, 195, 200, 201, 203, 207, 220, 242, 250, 256, 257, 260,

263, 265, 278, 279, 309, 310, 312, 314, 315, 325, 329, 358, 368, 386, 390

genomic, xi, xiv, 11, 33, 86, 120, 147, 177, 190, 193, 199, 213, 234, 257, 270, 271, 283, 286, 289, 310, 314, 315, 317, 365, 378, 383, 390

genomic instability, 11, 257

genomic regions, 315, 383

genomics, 10, 123, 126, 314, 324, 336, 354

genotoxic, 99, 100, 105, 106, 133, 165, 168, 193

genotoxins, 200

genotype, x, 14, 15, 16, 18, 20, 31, 41, 64, 68, 72, 78, 89, 110, 114, 140, 141, 142, 143, 145, 146, 147, 148, 149, 151, 152, 153, 235, 271, 306, 320, 321, 322, 323, 330, 335, 372, 402, 403, 404, 405, 406, 407, 408, 412, 413, 414, 415, 416, 417, 423, 425

genotypes, 119, 141, 143, 144, 145, 148, 150, 157, 180, 320, 321, 336, 400, 401, 402, 403, 405, 406, 407, 408, 412, 413, 416, 422

geography, 93

geriatric, 155, 157

geriatricians, 325

germ cell tumors, 169

germ cells, 55, 136

germ line, 54

Germany, 86, 89, 189, 293, 353, 355, 377, 380, 385, 387, 391

germination, 28, 189, 203

gerontology, 17, 155, 282, 284, 354, 358

gestation, 374

gestational age, 420

Ghrelin, 234

gingival, 339

ginseng, 27, 29, 30, 31, 33, 188, 191, 201, 206, 213, 229, 233, 239, 240

gland, 185, 223, 371, 372

glass, 434

glaucoma, 154, 155, 277

glia, 170, 174, 198

glial, 90, 174, 197, 265

glial cells, 90, 265

glial fibrillary acidic protein, 174

glioblastoma, 287

globulin, 145, 155, 414, 423

glomerulonephritis, xi, 241, 415

glomerulopathy, 131

glucagon, 217, 219

glucocorticoid receptor, 327

gluconeogenesis, 185, 189, 218, 270

glucose metabolism, 150, 233, 242, 265, 270, 275, 288, 312, 313

glucose tolerance, x, 33, 140, 146, 147, 148, 149, 150, 151, 156, 157, 158, 240, 244, 329

glucose tolerance test, 146, 158

GLUT, 226, 234

glutamate, 235, 237

glutamine, 231

glutathione, 28, 33, 108, 111, 120, 125, 133, 165, 172, 173, 176, 204, 206, 207, 287

glutathione peroxidase, 108, 287

glycation, viii, xi, xii, 23, 24, 26, 27, 28, 29, 30, 31, 32, 33, 177, 180, 181, 190, 205, 206, 213, 233, 236, 237, 238, 256

glycemia, 24, 26, 27, 28, 29, 31, 33, 191, 239, 240

glycerin, 270

glycerol, 192, 217, 218, 449

glycogen, 29, 212, 216, 224, 225, 226, 265, 283

glycolysis, 27, 29, 30, 32, 225, 237, 265, 270

glycosaminoglycans, 243

glycosylated, xvi, 430

goals, 213

God, 78

Gore, 252

government, 293, 294, 299

GPCR, 125

G-protein, 449

grain, 29, 189, 204, 238

grains, 28, 189, 238

Gram-negative, 322, 407, 420

gram-negative bacteria, 16

grants, 249

granules, 372

granulosa cells, 283

granzyme, 118, 135

grapes, 194

graph, 437

grass, 369

gravity, 64, 215, 232

Great Britain, 349

Greece, 371

green tea, 27, 30, 157, 159, 188, 191, 201, 206, 213, 233, 238

green tea extract, 27, 30, 191, 233

Greenland, 20

ground water, 163

groups, viii, 6, 9, 15, 25, 51, 72, 104, 109, 142, 146, 154, 179, 189, 193, 205, 209, 213, 220, 223, 224, 228, 268, 342, 343, 361, 398, 399,

402, 403, 405, 407, 409, 410, 411, 412, 414,
416, 440
growth factor, xi, xiv, 16, 91, 109, 119, 123, 125,
132, 181, 184, 200, 223, 232, 234, 241, 242,
243, 250, 251, 252, 265, 288, 309, 312, 313,
326, 328, 334, 384, 394
growth factors, 16, 91, 243
growth hormone, 14, 20, 110, 113, 118, 123, 124,
125, 126, 127, 137, 182, 217, 221, 222, 242,
265, 279
growth rate, 389, 432
growth spurt, 314
GST, 165
guidance, 143, 151
gums, 340
gustatory, 212
gut, 48, 57, 67, 103, 287

H

H. pylori, 410, 411, 412, 414, 415, 416, 417
haemoglobin, 415
half-life, 438
hallucinations, 295
handling, xv, 353
hands, 67
hanging, 167
haploid, 40, 82
haplotype, 49, 149, 312, 319, 321, 324, 329, 334,
387, 422
haplotypes, 311, 316, 318, 319, 321, 323, 324,
333
HapMap, 329
haptoglobin, 253
harm, 94
harmful effects, 317
harmony, 94
Harvard, 85, 195
harvesting, 204
Hawaii, 290
hazards, 311, 343, 378, 387, 393
HDL, 15, 20, 148, 325, 413
head and neck cancer, 451
healing, 263, 276
health care, 348
health education, 151
health effects, 84, 166, 167
health status, xiv, 4, 337, 341, 350
healthcare, vii, 1, 2, 298
hearing, 43, 84, 294
hearing impairment, 84

hearing loss, 43, 84
heart attack, 9, 336, 419
heart disease, 20, 156, 294, 298, 316, 333, 344,
350, 410, 411, 412, 414, 419, 421, 425, 439,
440
heart failure, 344
heart rate, 362
heat, ix, 25, 28, 29, 31, 97, 101, 103, 105, 107,
108, 111, 115, 128, 131, 132, 134, 205, 210,
214, 256, 258, 269, 284, 287, 313, 326, 327
heat loss, 101, 105
heat shock protein, 31, 108, 111, 115, 128, 132,
134, 269, 313
heating, 25, 205
heavy metal, 103, 107, 109, 111, 112, 123, 312
heavy metals, 103, 111, 312
height, 48, 147, 189
Helicobacter pylori, 85, 350, 410, 419, 420, 421,
423, 424, 425, 426, 427
hematocrit, 144, 268
hematologic, 451
hematological, x, 20, 61, 140, 144, 150, 154
heme, 256, 340
hemodialysis, 420, 427
hemoglobin, 24, 30, 31, 33, 144, 233, 259, 268,
283
hemorrhagic stroke, 21
hepatic stellate cells, 243
hepatitis, xi, 65, 241
Hepatitis A, 398
Hepatitis B, 398
hepatocellular, 150, 159
hepatocellular carcinoma, 150, 159
hepatocyte, 131, 134
hepatocytes, 106, 127, 134, 195, 224, 448
hepatoma, 176
hepatotoxicity, 116
herbicides, 102, 162, 207
herbivores, 270
heredity, 311, 332
heritability, 15, 17, 315, 326, 375, 376, 378, 380
hermaphrodite, 126
heterochromatin, 55
heterogeneity, 169, 252, 357, 376, 378, 382
heterogeneous, 118, 315, 319, 382
heterosis, 373, 381, 382, 393, 402, 422
heterozygosity, 86, 319
heterozygote, 41, 80, 81, 82, 402
heterozygotes, 49, 104, 408
hexachlorobenzene, 166, 171

high blood pressure, 445
high density lipoprotein, 153, 350
high fat, 43, 298
high risk, 156, 406, 407
high temperature, 102, 103, 105
high-density lipoprotein, 15, 142, 332
higher quality, 263
high-fat, 200
high-level, 347, 350
high-risk, 16, 407
high-tech, 273
hip, 150, 160, 231
hip fracture, 150, 160, 231
hippocampal, 31, 135, 234, 237
hippocampus, 105, 117, 123, 188, 197, 198, 199,
    237, 238, 274, 347
histidine, 390
histological, 371
histology, 419
histone, 187, 193, 195, 201, 207, 236, 357
HIV, 65, 66, 336
HIV-1, 336
HK, 86, 130
HLA, 10, 49, 85, 86, 311, 317, 318, 319, 323,
    332, 333, 335, 426
HLA-B, 319
HNE, xii, 242, 243, 245, 246, 248, 252
HNF, 326
holistic, 277
Holland, 91, 125, 176
homebox, 384
homeostasis, xiv, 62, 100, 106, 123, 135, 166,
    167, 239, 268, 310, 312, 315, 401, 448
homeotherms, 129, 158
homogeneity, 2, 169, 439
homogenous, 49
homolog, 135, 137, 327
homozygosity, 15
homozygote, 405
Honda, 103, 128, 267, 285
honey, 28, 189, 354, 370
hormonal control, 357
hormone, 14, 20, 110, 112, 113, 118, 119, 123,
    124, 125, 126, 127, 129, 135, 136, 137, 159,
    165, 167, 174, 182, 183, 185, 188, 217, 218,
    219, 221, 222, 242, 265, 266, 279, 328, 384,
    452
hormones, 16, 110, 113, 114, 175, 182, 183, 184,
    201, 214, 235, 328
horse, 299, 381, 437

horses, 374, 381, 392
hospital, x, 140
hospitalization, 399, 423
host, 48, 49, 64, 67, 90, 166, 260, 273, 401, 411,
    418, 420, 426, 444
House, 121, 285, 421
housing, 110, 113, 357, 366, 387
HPLC, 446
HSCT, 324
HSP, 108, 111
huddling, 287
human brain, 184, 233, 286
human genome, xiv, 309, 325, 329
Human Genome Project, 10
human leukocyte antigen, 332
human milk, 172, 183
human subjects, 332
humidity, 441
Hungary, 385
hunter-gatherers, 42
hunting, 134, 185, 258
hybrid, 110, 119, 381
hybridization, 89, 122, 419
hybrids, 119, 127
hydration, 441
hydro, xvi, 429, 432, 437, 438, 439, 440, 444
hydrogen, 28, 102, 107, 109, 112, 113, 114, 129,
    158, 195, 204, 231, 270, 287
hydrogen peroxide, 28, 102, 107, 109, 112, 113,
    114, 129, 158, 204, 231, 287
hydrolases, 166
hydrolysis, 217, 219, 437, 439
hydrolyzed, 203
hydrophilic, xvi, 429, 432, 437, 438, 439, 440,
    444
hydrophilicity, 435
hygiene, 67, 94, 310, 415
hygienic, 64, 65, 66, 67, 213
hypercapnia, 258, 266, 267, 272, 273, 284
Hypercapnia, 266
hypercholesteremia, 67, 71
hypercholesterolemia, 141, 201
hyperglycemia, 23, 27, 28, 29, 30, 32
hyperlipidemia, 298
hyperlipoproteinemia, 15
hyperopia, 43, 84
hyperplasia, 91, 185, 223
hypersensitivity, 166
hypertension, 15, 42, 43, 45, 47, 67, 84, 141, 150,
    153, 154, 159, 268, 276, 285, 298, 416

hypertensive, 71, 159, 268, 344
hyperthermia, 127, 410
hypertrophic cardiomyopathy, 156
hypertrophy, 43, 57, 60, 223
hyperuricemia, 141, 143, 150, 154
hyperventilation, 266
hypocapnia, 266, 267
hypoglycemia, 26, 27, 185, 188, 192, 270
hypogonadism, 314
hypometabolic, 271
hypothalamic, 127, 183
hypothalamus, 111, 182, 183, 185, 186, 208, 233
hypothermia, 272
hypothesis, 9, 13, 14, 16, 24, 32, 36, 52, 54, 56,
    57, 58, 59, 64, 67, 83, 90, 94, 98, 104, 107,
    116, 158, 181, 185, 237, 250, 267, 272, 295,
    296, 298, 306, 315, 321, 361, 399, 412, 414,
    417, 422
hypoventilation, 271
hypoxia, 134, 258, 259, 263, 264, 265, 266, 267,
    268, 269, 271, 272, 273, 275, 277, 281, 282,
    283, 284, 285, 286, 288, 410
Hypoxia, 266, 268, 279, 283, 285, 286, 288, 289
hypoxia-inducible factor, 284
hypoxia-ischemia, 283
hypoxic, xiii, 256, 257, 259, 268, 269, 272, 273,
    277, 278, 279, 282, 283, 284, 285, 286, 288
hypoxic-ischemic, 284, 285

I

IARC, 169, 170
ICAM, xiv, 309
ICD, 61, 342
ice, 108, 114, 121
id, 287, 297, 320, 340, 343
identical sibling, 357
identification, 72, 156, 439
ideology, 47
IDS, 408
IFN, 16, 318, 320, 402, 405, 407, 413, 418, 425
IgE, 418
IGF, xiv, 11, 109, 112, 113, 114, 115, 116, 119,
    128, 131, 181, 189, 200, 223, 227, 233, 234,
    265, 284, 309, 312, 313, 326, 327, 328
IGF-1, xiv, 11, 119, 128, 265, 309, 312, 313,
    326, 327
IGF-I, 109, 112, 113, 114, 115, 116, 119, 131,
    181, 200, 223, 227, 233, 284, 328
IGF-IR, 110, 114
IgG, 399, 409, 411, 412, 415, 416, 419, 421, 423

IHD, 410, 411, 412, 413, 414
IL-1, 16, 247, 253, 318, 320, 321, 322, 332, 334,
    399, 401, 402, 403, 404, 405, 407, 408, 409,
    413, 415, 416, 417, 418, 419, 421, 422, 424,
    425, 442
IL-10, 16, 253, 318, 320, 321, 322, 334, 399,
    401, 402, 404, 405, 407, 408, 409, 413, 415,
    417, 418, 422, 424, 425
IL-13, 418
IL-2, 318, 320
IL-4, 399, 418
IL-6, 16, 247, 318, 320, 322, 332, 334, 399, 402,
    403, 404, 405, 409, 412, 413, 414, 416, 417,
    418, 419, 421, 426
IL-8, 16, 21, 399, 400, 402, 403, 404, 405, 406,
    407, 421, 422, 425
ILAR, 137
Illinois, 287
images, 214, 433
imaging, 285, 347, 350
imbalances, 63, 316, 324, 418
imbibition, 191, 203
immigrants, 419, 422
immortal, 12, 54, 88, 369
immortality, 7, 63
immune cells, 167, 322
immune function, 166, 201, 323
immune response, xiv, 16, 94, 166, 309, 310,
    311, 312, 317, 319, 323, 333, 365, 399, 402,
    404, 418, 422
immune system, 49, 54, 67, 88, 108, 110, 162,
    166, 167, 173, 176, 317, 322, 335, 362, 365,
    414, 444
immunity, 240, 317, 318, 324, 397, 424
immunization, 297
immunoglobulin, 167, 317, 323, 335, 399, 418
immunoglobulin superfamily, 323
immunoglobulins, 426
immunological, 61
immunology, xv, 373
immunopathology, 423
immunosuppressive, 166
impaired glucose tolerance, 146, 157
impairments, 197
implementation, xiii, 209, 256, 376
imprinting, xiv, 310, 317
in situ, 419
in situ hybridization, 419
in utero, 167, 176, 417

in vitro, xvi, 27, 30, 32, 54, 89, 90, 101, 112, 120, 126, 130, 131, 134, 150, 170, 191, 194, 206, 233, 234, 296, 371, 405, 425, 429, 431, 433, 437, 445

in vivo, ix, 26, 27, 31, 32, 54, 55, 89, 98, 101, 105, 107, 110, 112, 113, 117, 120, 126, 130, 168, 170, 234, 266, 267, 282, 284, 296, 419, 422, 424, 430, 444

inactivation, 165, 203, 448

inactive, 10, 39, 80

inbreeding, 118, 120, 128, 130, 373, 381, 382, 387, 388, 393, 394, 395

incidence, xv, 10, 14, 15, 43, 54, 67, 73, 93, 106, 111, 117, 136, 137, 151, 154, 160, 169, 170, 231, 236, 240, 244, 274, 288, 397, 399, 401, 405, 410, 414, 416, 417, 450, 452

inclusion, 29, 204, 206, 381

income, 3, 412

incompatibility, 215

incubation, 103, 114, 398, 432, 434, 437

incubation period, 398

independence, 2, 294, 349

independent variable, 205

indexing, 164

India, 42, 171, 175, 204, 285, 406, 407

Indian, 27, 171, 331, 403, 423

Indians, 414

indication, 184, 210, 386

indicators, 346, 362

indices, 25, 179, 204, 205, 206, 228, 244, 451

indigenous, 46, 65, 420, 423

Indigenous, xv, 397, 398, 399, 400, 401, 403, 404, 405, 406, 407, 408, 410, 411, 412, 414, 415, 416, 417, 418, 419, 425, 426, 427

indirect effect, 383

individualism, 2

inducer, 222, 253

induction, xi, 33, 107, 112, 114, 134, 166, 173, 179, 192, 217, 222, 225, 234, 241, 243, 250, 269, 275, 289, 402, 452

inductor, 272

industrial, 42, 69, 70, 207, 258, 293, 298

industrial revolution, 42

industrialized countries, 408

industry, 70, 71, 85, 204, 380

inert, 169, 207, 215, 216, 230

inertia, 216

inertness, 216

infant care, 410

infants, 67, 183, 399, 407, 408, 409, 410, 416, 419, 420, 422, 423, 426

Infants, 419

infarction, 16, 17, 141, 157, 277, 419, 426

infection, xv, 49, 75, 94, 120, 128, 335, 345, 397, 398, 399, 401, 402, 403, 404, 405, 407, 408, 409, 410, 411, 412, 415, 416, 417, 418, 419, 421, 422, 425, 426, 427

infections, xv, 16, 49, 63, 64, 66, 67, 167, 273, 278, 318, 324, 336, 397, 399, 401, 403, 404, 407, 408, 409, 410, 413, 414, 415, 416, 417, 418, 420, 424, 425, 426, 427

infectious, xv, 49, 65, 66, 85, 93, 114, 166, 311, 317, 319, 323, 335, 365, 397, 401, 409, 410, 414, 415, 418, 420

infectious disease, xv, 49, 65, 66, 85, 93, 311, 319, 323, 335, 397, 409, 414, 415, 418, 420

infectious diseases, xv, 49, 85, 93, 311, 319, 323, 397, 409, 415, 418, 420

infestations, 66

infinite, 63, 444

inflammation, xi, xiv, xv, 16, 177, 206, 213, 247, 250, 251, 253, 270, 273, 274, 279, 289, 309, 311, 316, 317, 332, 333, 345, 397, 407, 408, 410, 411, 412, 416, 426

inflammatory, 16, 17, 28, 49, 91, 94, 101, 245, 247, 248, 249, 250, 253, 270, 273, 278, 297, 317, 318, 320, 321, 322, 323, 335, 338, 345, 399, 400, 401, 404, 405, 407, 408, 410, 411, 412, 413, 414, 415, 416, 417, 418, 419, 420, 422, 425, 426, 451

inflammatory bowel disease, 94

inflammatory cells, 101, 322

inflammatory disease, 91, 94, 273, 322, 323, 451

inflammatory mediators, 247, 248, 322, 345, 401, 407, 410, 412, 415

inflammatory response, 17, 247, 250, 317, 321, 335, 399, 401, 407, 408, 411, 413, 415, 416, 417, 418, 419, 420, 422, 425

inflammatory responses, 247, 321, 399, 401, 404, 407, 408, 411, 413, 415, 416, 417, 418, 420, 422, 425

influenza, 65, 66, 93, 398, 421

influenza a, 65

informed consent, 146

infusions, 188

ingest, 178, 189, 190, 212, 215

ingestion, x, 25, 28, 29, 43, 132, 161, 164, 171, 185, 204, 205, 207, 208, 221

inhalation, 169, 170, 272

inheritance, 17, 250, 260, 310, 332, 368, 389

inherited, xiv, xvi, 152, 295, 298, 310, 317, 324, 329, 429, 442

inhibition, xi, 16, 27, 29, 90, 94, 165, 166, 167, 168, 177, 180, 190, 192, 194, 201, 205, 220, 229, 237, 247, 266, 448, 450, 452

inhibitor, 15, 106, 127, 168, 234, 266, 285, 297, 384, 435, 441, 442, 449

inhibitors, 94, 163, 165, 174, 203, 206, 297, 434, 441

inhibitory, 28, 152, 191, 194, 195, 225, 297, 323, 335, 404, 447, 448

inhibitory effect, 152, 191, 195, 297

initial state, 209

initiation, 28, 124, 129, 179, 209, 248, 260, 266, 274, 399

injection, 105, 106, 113, 114, 116, 117

injections, 198, 275, 276

injuries, 63

injury, 98, 100, 105, 117, 123, 133, 135, 176, 198, 233, 251, 265, 283, 284, 285, 288, 414

innate immunity, xiv, 310, 312, 317, 322, 370

innervation, 229

innovation, 71

inorganic, 113, 244

inositol, 102

insane, 47

insecticide, 170

insecticides, 162, 170

insects, 358, 362

insertion, 72, 73, 76, 322

insight, 117, 122, 210, 354, 362, 368, 441, 445, 448

inspiration, 268

instability, 8, 54, 57, 99, 168, 250, 329

instinct, 8

insulation, 269

insulin resistance, 11, 14, 31, 151, 160, 276, 286, 314, 315, 331, 332, 414

insulin sensitivity, 24, 29, 30, 187, 205, 236, 244, 314, 315, 328, 415, 421, 426, 427

insulin signaling, 104, 123, 136, 181, 191, 220, 236, 287, 314, 316

insulin-like growth factor, xiv, 109, 119, 123, 125, 132, 181, 200, 223, 232, 234, 242, 309, 312, 313, 328

insulin-like growth factor I, 109, 119, 123, 125, 181, 200, 223, 232, 328

insults, ix, 98, 106, 116, 120, 121, 125, 184, 197, 199, 229, 230, 415

insurance, 2, 299

integrity, vii, xi, 1, 3, 177, 187, 191, 193, 196, 200, 202, 213, 229, 256, 265, 364, 365, 448

intellect, 215

intellectual functioning, 167

intelligence, 199

intensity, 16, 169, 181, 213, 268, 272, 277, 361, 385

interaction, x, xi, xiv, 29, 31, 123, 140, 142, 143, 151, 154, 161, 163, 165, 172, 191, 206, 235, 241, 271, 289, 309, 334, 404, 449

interactions, ix, xvi, 35, 63, 68, 79, 84, 85, 91, 119, 144, 150, 151, 163, 165, 166, 172, 176, 260, 316, 320, 334, 361, 397, 401, 404, 410, 414, 418, 444, 445

interactivity, 223

interference, 72, 244

interferon, 334, 399, 423

interleukin, xiv, 309, 317, 333, 334, 399, 409, 417, 420, 421, 422, 423, 424, 425, 426, 427

interleukin-1, 334, 399, 409, 420, 421, 422, 423, 425, 426

interleukin-6, xiv, 309, 317, 333, 334, 399, 417, 421, 422, 424, 427

interleukin-8, 399, 424

intermediaries, 29

internal clock, 354, 370

International Classification of Diseases, 61

interpretation, 36, 47, 100, 101, 106, 180, 196, 325

interstitial, xi, 241, 243

interval, xv, 25, 26, 29, 50, 179, 191, 196, 211, 226, 278, 284, 288, 290, 337, 378, 379, 380, 381, 385

intervention, 12, 20, 28, 160, 181, 206, 232, 242, 249, 257, 268, 272, 277, 279, 280, 445

interviews, 342

intestinal tract, 24, 164

intestine, 164, 176, 203, 221, 236, 364

intima, 145, 412

intoxication, 168

intracellular signaling, 243, 357

intracerebral, 16, 234

intracerebral hemorrhage, 16

intraindividual variability, 17

intraocular, x, 140, 144, 154, 155

intraocular pressure, x, 140, 144, 154, 155

intrauterine growth retardation, 417, 423

intrinsic, xiv, xv, 37, 53, 62, 79, 102, 242, 304, 309, 362, 368, 373 intron, 334, 423, 425

invasive, 336, 398, 401, 403, 404, 408, 409, 424

inversion, 390

invertebrates, xi, 104, 115, 241, 244, 310, 362, 368

investment, 162, 184, 358

involution, 61, 277

ion channels, 167

ionic, 276, 445, 449

ionization, 439

ionizing radiation, 293

ions, 227, 257, 266, 280, 289, 439

IOP, 144, 150

Iran, 380

Ireland, 331, 385

iron, 49, 85, 197, 235, 251, 266, 372

iron deficiency, 49, 85

irradiation, 104, 106, 117, 248, 267, 277

IRs, 335

IRS, 119, 235

ISC, 87

ischaemic heart disease, 408, 419, 427

ischemia, 43, 59, 71, 114, 116, 137, 263, 266, 267, 283, 285

ischemic, 21, 135, 281, 284, 294, 344

ischemic heart disease, 294, 344

ischium, 365

isoforms, 15, 205, 252

isolation, 397, 399

isoleucine, 317

Israel, 385

Italian population, 320, 322, 332, 412

Italy, 35, 83, 172, 192, 241, 249, 293, 320, 379, 385, 406

IUGR, 417

J

JAMA, 19, 20, 93, 95, 157, 289, 335, 425, 450

Japan, vii, xiv, 1, 2, 3, 4, 20, 139, 143, 147, 149, 151, 159, 160, 273, 291, 292, 293, 294, 299, 337, 339, 340, 342, 350, 426

Japanese, vii, x, 1, 2, 3, 4, 20, 139, 140, 141, 142, 143, 144, 145, 146, 149, 150, 151, 152, 153, 154, 155, 156, 157, 159, 292, 293, 294, 298, 299, 319, 332, 341, 346, 348, 349, 350, 351, 424

Japanese women, 141, 142, 155

Jefferson, 267, 285

JNK, xi, xii, 104, 136, 242, 244, 246, 248, 251

joints, 111, 273

Jordan, 134

judge, 305

judgment, 232

Jun, xi, 104, 113, 241, 244, 246, 250, 290

Jung, 125, 251

justification, 269

juveniles, 355, 363

K

K^+, 289

kainic acid, 105, 117

keratinocytes, 89, 402

ketogenic, 185, 286

ketones, 270

kidney, xv, 23, 43, 91, 106, 107, 108, 111, 113, 126, 127, 170, 231, 243, 246, 271, 277, 397, 408, 415, 416, 422

kidney transplantation, 415

kidneys, 111, 114, 184, 200, 207, 216, 266, 415

killing, x, 63, 161, 294, 324

kin selection, ix, 35, 36, 50, 51, 53

kinase, xi, 102, 104, 113, 114, 127, 136, 174, 241, 244, 283, 312, 313, 328, 383, 435, 442, 449

kinase activity, 114, 442

kinases, 243, 251, 442, 451

kinetics, 87

King, 85, 137, 287, 326

knockout, 19, 114, 118, 123, 126, 235, 272, 367

Korea, 450

Korean, 155

L

labeling, 364, 436

laboratory studies, 167, 271

lactate dehydrogenase, 225

lactation, 183, 382, 392, 393

lactic acid, 225, 226

Langerhans cells, 59

large intestine, 61

large-scale, 146, 325

larva, 133

larvae, 102, 104, 123, 136

laryngeal cancer, 84

larynx, 43

laser, 450

latency, 222, 274, 288

late-onset, 298

late-onset AD, 298

later life, vii, 1, 2
law, 171
laws, 434
LC, 185, 232, 437
L-carnitine, 29, 32, 261
LDL, 15, 16, 153
LEA, 442, 451
leakage, 211
lean body mass, 216, 222
learning, 129, 188, 197, 198, 199, 234, 235, 240, 390
lecithin, 153
lectin, 323, 335, 336, 422
left ventricular, 290
lending, 24
lens, 57, 61, 89, 107, 126, 130, 131
lenses, 258
Leprosy, 398
leptin, xiv, 274, 309
lesions, 106, 111, 116, 133, 281, 322
leucine, x, 140, 317
leucocyte, 332
leukemia, 106, 118, 137, 169
leukocyte, 86, 240, 317, 332, 335, 403, 404
leukocytes, 402, 403, 405, 407, 408, 412, 413, 420
life cycle, 272, 355
life expectancy, vii, xiii, xv, 1, 2, 3, 4, 12, 18, 20, 63, 140, 149, 291, 292, 293, 298, 320, 353, 360, 361, 364, 365, 366, 374, 443
life style, viii, 4, 5, 6, 294, 298, 342
lifecycle, 179
lifestyle, viii, ix, x, 23, 26, 31, 35, 42, 47, 64, 140, 146, 149, 150, 151, 163, 186, 299
lifestyles, 279, 298
life-threatening, xiv, 195, 310, 317, 318
lifetime, 71, 89, 212, 240, 298, 310, 359, 361, 363, 368, 389, 390, 391, 392, 393, 394
ligand, xiv, 15, 125, 167, 309, 323
ligand gene, 323
ligands, 103, 124, 322
likelihood, 183, 232, 311, 390, 398, 404
limitation, ix, 8, 35, 56, 77, 151, 181
limitations, xii, 57, 78, 119, 122, 167, 255, 278, 292, 307
Lincoln, 83, 394
lindane, 171
linear, 375, 376, 378, 379, 380, 381, 387, 388, 389, 393, 394, 439, 446
linear mixed models, 376

linear model, 387, 394
lingual, 61
linkage, 27, 160, 191, 286, 311, 315, 326, 329, 331
links, 111, 206
lipase, 153, 217, 219
lipid, viii, x, 15, 20, 23, 30, 33, 94, 126, 136, 140, 142, 150, 153, 154, 187, 197, 206, 239, 243, 248, 251, 253, 315, 322, 328, 329, 430, 434, 435, 439, 445, 446, 447, 449, 450
lipid peroxidation, 30, 126, 136, 197, 243, 248, 251
lipids, viii, 15, 23, 99, 121, 158, 187, 194, 206, 237, 244, 248, 271, 272, 315, 415, 439, 445, 447, 448, 450
lipofuscin, 267
lipophilic, 164, 165, 166, 171, 214
lipopolysaccharide, 322, 421
lipoprotein, 14, 15, 20, 142, 153, 315, 325, 350
lipoproteins, 15, 153
lipoxygenase, 335
liquidity, 188, 203
literacy, 151
liver, 31, 51, 56, 60, 91, 103, 106, 107, 108, 111, 113, 123, 126, 127, 132, 158, 164, 170, 184, 200, 207, 212, 214, 216, 217, 219, 221, 223, 225, 226, 229, 233, 234, 236, 240, 243, 252, 258, 260, 266, 270, 271, 275, 285
liver cells, 217, 219
liver damage, 106, 108, 113
liver disease, 85, 158
liver enzymes, 219
livestock, xv, 373, 374, 375, 376, 381, 382, 383, 385, 386, 388, 389, 390, 391, 392, 393, 394, 395
living conditions, 259, 416
lobsters, 88, 365, 369
localization, 228, 336
location, 126, 311, 314, 384
locomotion, 111
locus, 49, 86, 110, 119, 126, 130, 134, 315, 319, 326, 336, 382, 383, 389
London, 17, 44, 83, 85, 87, 91, 95, 131, 238, 255, 307, 349, 388, 421, 425
long period, 169, 363, 442
longitudinal study, 298, 332, 336
long-term care insurance, 299
long-term potentiation, 197, 238
losses, 216, 227, 378, 386
love, 87

low birthweight, 417, 420
low risk, 406
low temperatures, 266
low-density, 15, 32, 142
low-density lipoprotein, 15, 32, 142
LPG, 446
LPS, 421
LTD, 288
LTP, 197, 234, 235
lubricants, 68
lumen, 203
lung, xvi, 43, 67, 95, 101, 106, 114, 117, 123, 135, 154, 170, 243, 250, 267, 283, 284, 344, 430, 437, 452
lung cancer, 170
lung function, 67, 95, 154, 267
lungs, 259, 266, 281
lupus erythematosus, 336
luteinizing hormone, 183
lymphocyte, 130, 166, 333, 438
lymphocytes, 17, 106, 126, 403, 437, 438
lymphomas, 277
lysine, 31, 33
lysis, 323

M

machinery, xvi, 430, 442, 443, 445
machines, 70, 260
macromolecules, ix, 13, 97, 99, 180, 192, 203, 248
macronutrients, 178
macrophage, 166, 251, 402
macrophages, 56, 243, 252, 322, 402, 403, 412
macular degeneration, 59, 60, 76, 92, 94
magnetic, 285
magnetic resonance, 285, 347, 350
magnetic resonance imaging, 285, 347, 350
mainstream, 358
maintenance, viii, ix, xi, xv, 12, 19, 35, 36, 53, 68, 90, 98, 99, 123, 177, 183, 193, 196, 197, 202, 213, 216, 218, 224, 230, 257, 260, 265, 273, 278, 282, 337, 347, 358, 359, 364, 365
major histocompatibility complex, 49, 86, 332
malaria, 41, 171, 175
males, vii, xiv, 1, 2, 49, 50, 86, 104, 114, 157, 159, 169, 183, 209, 258, 292, 304, 319, 337, 340, 361, 413
malignancy, 10, 260
malignant, 9, 54, 259, 270, 290, 294
malignant cells, 270

malnutrition, 100, 105, 184, 298, 348, 362, 416, 427
malondialdehyde, 271
mammal, xvi, 53, 129, 281, 378, 430
Mammalian, xvi, 115, 124, 130, 133, 287, 384, 429, 430, 431, 432, 434, 438, 439, 440, 442, 444, 449, 450
mammalian cell, xvi, 125, 236, 260, 395, 429, 431, 437, 439, 450
mammalian stem cells, 364
mammals, xi, xii, 13, 15, 19, 54, 98, 100, 101, 104, 105, 106, 109, 110, 115, 121, 125, 127, 131, 194, 241, 244, 255, 256, 257, 258, 259, 266, 269, 270, 271, 281, 284, 310, 312, 314, 358, 362, 364, 374, 387, 430, 438, 450
management, 32, 78, 150, 375, 382, 387, 390
management practices, 375
manganese, 19, 159
manganese superoxide, 19
manganese superoxide dismutase, 19
manifold, 205
manipulation, 191, 205, 219, 220, 249, 287, 310, 356
man-made, 162
manufacturer, 68, 70, 163
MAPK, xi, 113, 241, 244, 252, 435, 442
MAPKs, 244, 247
mapping, 120, 315, 383, 390, 392
marginalization, 185
market, 69, 71, 164
market structure, 71
marketing, 164
markets, 70
marriage, 78
marrow, 61, 117
Maryland, 23, 350
mass spectrometry, 439, 446
mast cell, 59, 402, 409, 423
mastication, 207, 350
masticatory, xv, 338, 339, 340, 341, 342, 343, 344, 345, 346, 347, 348, 349, 350
mastitis, 391, 392
maternal, 119, 145, 153, 173, 175, 355, 382, 391, 392, 420, 423
maternal inheritance, 153
maternal smoking, 420, 423
matrix, xi, 16, 241, 243, 322, 432, 438
matrix metalloproteinase, 16
maturation, 119, 131, 179, 182, 203, 220, 263, 269, 283, 305, 451

MCP, 252
MCP-1, 252
MDA, 197, 245
meals, 203, 212, 218, 219
mean corpuscular volume, 144
measles, 65, 398
measurement, 131, 136, 210, 283, 325, 347, 357
measures, 9, 68, 73, 75, 77, 79, 103, 111, 119,
    162, 163, 168, 169, 187, 192, 198, 206, 214,
    382, 388, 391, 414
meat, 24, 27, 28, 43, 159, 183, 185, 200, 201,
    206, 231, 232, 234, 440
media, 107, 114, 145, 206, 412, 419
median, 115, 205, 220, 244, 272, 314, 411, 413
mediation, 182, 197, 227
mediators, 104, 168, 234, 239, 242, 243, 247,
    248, 322, 345, 401, 407, 410, 411, 412, 415,
    448
medical services, 9
medical student, 84
Medicare, 295
medication, 273, 275, 298
medicine, 7, 9, 12, 36, 61, 66, 67, 82, 83, 155,
    272, 273, 277, 285, 286, 288, 299, 420
Mediterranean, vii, 5, 6, 13, 14, 19, 20
MEF, 114
meiosis, 134
membranes, 59, 121, 128, 180, 192, 196, 197,
    214, 222, 223, 226, 228, 233, 275, 442, 445,
    448
memory, xiii, 78, 111, 129, 188, 197, 198, 199,
    234, 240, 267, 291, 295, 322, 367
memory formation, 197, 198
memory loss, 267
memory performance, 234
memory processes, 198
men, x, xiii, 2, 14, 15, 42, 45, 47, 49, 65, 78, 86,
    140, 141, 142, 143, 144, 145, 146, 149, 150,
    151, 153, 154, 155, 156, 157, 159, 180, 200,
    201, 270, 288, 291, 292, 293, 294, 299, 331,
    333, 334, 342, 346, 349, 411, 412, 413, 421
menadione, 103
menarche, 184
Mendel, 238
meningitis, 399, 401, 403, 407, 409, 426
menopause, 184
menstruation, 184, 239
mental retardation, 156
mesangial cells, 243
mesenchymal stem cell, 284

mesenchymal stem cells, 284
messenger RNA, 193
messengers, 256
MET, 126
meta-analysis, 94, 336, 345, 421
metabolic acidosis, 231, 232
metabolic changes, 182
metabolic disorder, xiv, 310, 317
metabolic pathways, xiv, 37, 162, 309, 312
metabolic rate, 18, 19, 27, 103, 180, 183, 184,
    185, 208, 210, 211, 235, 259, 281, 362
metabolic syndrome, xiv, 14, 15, 43, 150, 159,
    275, 309, 313, 315, 316, 332, 341, 426
metabolic systems, 218
metabolism, xiv, 13, 120, 123, 124, 132, 150,
    164, 166, 175, 180, 181, 182, 184, 185, 194,
    195, 209, 210, 217, 233, 235, 242, 248, 259,
    263, 265, 270, 274, 275, 286, 287, 288, 310,
    312, 313, 314, 316, 324, 336, 357, 359, 361,
    363, 416, 434, 442, 448
metabolite, 113, 166, 217, 218, 225, 325
metabolites, viii, 23, 103, 163, 165, 166, 174,
    200, 313, 359
metabolizing, 130, 164, 237, 270, 425
metal chelators, 297
metalloproteinase, 16, 250
Metallothionein, 136
metals, 170
metamorphosis, xvi, 429
metastasis, xvi, 430, 444, 452
metastasize, 444
metastatic, 258
metazoan, 259
metazoans, 123
metformin, 30
methanol, 434, 445, 446
methionine, x, 13, 108, 109, 111, 118, 122, 132,
    140, 157, 231
methylation, 357, 358, 360, 366, 367, 370, 448
methylene, 297
methylmercury, 105
Mexican, 332
MHC, 49, 86, 319, 335
MIA, 383
microarray, 122, 178, 374
microbes, 66, 250, 271
microbial, 67, 75, 272, 418, 439
microglia, 59, 60
microglial, 297
micronucleus, 165

micronutrients, 178
microorganisms, 399, 445
microscope, 432
microscopy, 371, 435
microvascular, 283
middle ear infection, 167
middle-aged, x, 14, 71, 111, 140, 144, 146, 149, 151, 153, 154, 155, 157, 159, 179, 227, 229
migration, 16, 334, 404
military, 70, 420
milk, 42, 67, 163, 169, 172, 183, 200, 374, 376, 384, 385, 386, 389, 390, 393, 394, 395
mimicking, 167
mimicry, 49
minerals, 14, 158, 178, 188, 203, 204
Mini-Mental State Examination (MMSE), 347
Ministry of Education, 151
minority, 407
mirror, 8
miscarriage, 49, 170
misfolded, 112
mitochondria, xii, 13, 89, 91, 108, 115, 121, 129, 130, 132, 133, 158, 204, 210, 226, 228, 233, 236, 237, 239, 242, 255, 256, 257, 260, 261, 262, 263, 264, 265, 266, 267, 269, 270, 272, 275, 277, 279, 280, 283
mitochondrial damage, 135, 228, 229, 267
mitochondrial DNA, 113, 133, 140, 145, 149, 152, 153, 154, 155, 156, 158, 242, 251, 275, 279, 280, 282, 311, 316
mitochondrial membrane, 217, 228, 257, 271
mitogen, xi, 217, 241, 244
mitogen activated protein kinase, xi, 241, 244
mitogenic, 132, 223
mitotic, 58, 223, 242, 275
Mitsubishi, 2
MMP, 251
MMS, 106, 112, 113
MMSE, 347
MnSOD, 115, 134, 136
mobility, xvi, 339, 430
modalities, 24, 26, 275
modality, 228, 273
model fitting, 387
model system, 12, 369, 371, 407, 413
modeling, 376, 435
models, ix, xiv, 11, 12, 14, 24, 87, 88, 98, 99, 102, 104, 105, 107, 108, 109, 111, 113, 116, 117, 118, 121, 122, 131, 178, 282, 310, 311, 317, 347, 354, 356, 358, 365, 367, 373, 375,

376, 378, 381, 382, 388, 389, 409, 424, 445, 451
modernity, 207
modulation, ix, 35, 36, 55, 56, 76, 101, 108, 127, 153, 166, 181, 186, 205, 215, 220, 233, 236, 370, 375, 451
modules, 325
moieties, viii, 23, 206, 216, 228
moisture, 204
mold, 122
mole, xii, 112, 121, 133, 255, 257, 258, 279, 280, 281, 287
molecular biology, 304, 354
molecular mechanisms, xv, 117, 178, 186, 210, 217, 238, 253, 267, 283, 363, 364, 373
molecular oxygen, 322
molecules, xii, xvi, 59, 100, 162, 164, 171, 180, 184, 192, 193, 203, 206, 237, 242, 243, 249, 262, 293, 313, 317, 318, 322, 323, 325, 335, 404, 410, 422, 429, 430, 440, 445, 447, 448, 449, 451
mollusks, 53
molting, 355, 357, 358, 363, 366, 370
money, 70
monkeys, 216, 233, 244, 251, 252, 282, 313
monocytes, 16, 402, 404, 406, 407, 412
monogenic, xiv, 95, 310, 317, 324
monomeric, 295
monomers, 439
mononuclear cells, 404, 405
monozygotic twins, 358, 368
mood, 167
morale, 3
morbidity, 16, 37, 73, 75, 79, 156, 176, 232, 244, 258, 320, 415, 422, 444
morning, 27, 29, 49, 212, 276, 279, 299
morphogenesis, 76, 452
morphological, 57, 135, 199, 357
morphology, 198, 223, 314, 437, 441
mortality, xv, 4, 13, 14, 15, 16, 17, 20, 21, 37, 51, 52, 53, 54, 62, 63, 65, 66, 73, 75, 79, 83, 93, 106, 108, 110, 154, 155, 156, 220, 244, 252, 258, 280, 293, 294, 305, 317, 320, 326, 333, 334, 337, 338, 341, 343, 344, 345, 350, 355, 361, 382, 389, 390, 393, 399, 404, 410, 415, 419, 420, 424, 425, 427, 444
mortality rate, 53, 54, 62, 63, 65, 66, 293, 382
mortality risk, 220, 344, 345
Moscow, 288, 289
mother cell, 88

mothers, 169, 171, 410, 417

motor activity, 362

motor area, 347

motor neurons, 229

motorneurons, 18

moulding, 87

mountains, 266

mouse, ix, 11, 16, 18, 19, 31, 88, 90, 98, 110, 112, 115, 116, 117, 118, 120, 121, 122, 124, 125, 126, 127, 129, 130, 131, 133, 134, 137, 165, 175, 211, 233, 235, 236, 237, 288, 354, 356, 364, 365, 367, 370, 437, 445

mouse model, ix, 11, 18, 88, 98, 122, 445

mouth, 339

movement, 216, 299

MRI, 285, 347

mRNA, 107, 111, 113, 165, 275

MRPs, 166

MSC, 266, 279

mtDNA, 152, 256, 257, 260, 261, 262, 263, 266, 267, 279, 283, 285

mucosa, 61

multicellular organisms, xvi, 62, 193, 430, 431

multidimensional, vii

multidrug resistance, 166, 176

multiple factors, 298

multiple myeloma, 336

multiple regression, 346, 347

multiple regression analysis, 346

multiple sclerosis, 67, 94

multiplication, 305

multipotent, 364

multivariate, xiv, 311, 337, 343

murine models, 24

muscle, 19, 21, 24, 29, 31, 56, 60, 89, 90, 91, 105, 107, 108, 114, 115, 130, 135, 184, 187, 193, 200, 206, 208, 210, 212, 213, 216, 217, 218, 220, 221, 222, 223, 224, 225, 226, 227, 228, 229, 230, 231, 233, 234, 235, 236, 237, 238, 239, 243, 265, 266, 275, 280, 284, 285, 286, 289, 322, 369, 416

muscle atrophy, 60, 229, 230, 231

muscle cells, 21, 89, 221, 223, 225, 226, 243, 322

muscle contraction, 223, 224, 225, 226, 227, 228

muscle mass, 216, 227, 229, 230, 231

muscle strength, 227

muscle tissue, 29, 206, 212, 217, 220, 224, 225, 226, 228, 229, 230, 231, 286

muscle weakness, 227

muscles, 134, 187, 210, 214, 221, 223, 224, 225, 226, 227, 228, 229, 230, 265

musculoskeletal, 200, 231, 314

musculoskeletal system, 200

mutagenesis, 103, 152, 271

mutagenic, 111, 117, 164, 165, 170

mutant, ix, 11, 18, 92, 98, 102, 103, 109, 110, 114, 116, 117, 119, 120, 123, 126, 129, 130, 133, 135, 296, 322, 327, 367, 383, 450

mutants, 18, 102, 103, 104, 109, 112, 114, 116, 123, 126, 130, 220, 326

mutation, ix, xiv, 9, 10, 11, 39, 41, 52, 53, 64, 80, 87, 88, 97, 98, 99, 103, 104, 105, 106, 110, 114, 118, 120, 122, 125, 126, 128, 156, 168, 283, 310, 313, 314, 317, 330, 383, 390

mutation rate, 39, 41

mutations, ix, xiv, 11, 16, 41, 52, 97, 99, 102, 103, 104, 109, 110, 111, 112, 114, 117, 118, 121, 122, 125, 126, 128, 130, 133, 145, 168, 201, 257, 260, 261, 262, 295, 310, 311, 312, 314, 317, 324, 329, 336, 444

Mycobacterium, 405, 426

myeloid, 106, 137

myeloma, 336

myocardial infarction, x, 14, 15, 16, 21, 59, 71, 140, 141, 144, 152, 157, 273, 277, 314, 333, 335, 344, 411, 452

myocardium, 266, 284, 286

myocites, 15

myocytes, 56, 60, 221, 223, 224, 266

myofibrillar, 229

myofibroblasts, 243

myoglobin, 265

myopia, 43, 47, 84

myosin, 225, 227, 238

myotonic dystrophy, 91

N

N-acety, 213, 229, 323

NaCl, 435

NAD, 15, 18, 195, 313, 327

NADH, x, 140, 150, 153, 154, 155, 156, 160, 195, 237

NASA, 76, 77, 82

nation, 69, 299

National Academy of Sciences, 124, 125, 126, 127, 130, 134, 135, 137, 190, 233, 234, 235, 236, 238, 240

National Institutes of Health, 85

Native Americans, 405, 415

natural, xii, xvi, 36, 37, 38, 39, 41, 43, 48, 49, 50, 52, 53, 56, 62, 63, 64, 87, 118, 121, 122, 126, 183, 184, 205, 207, 208, 215, 242, 249, 255, 256, 259, 266, 271, 272, 278, 279, 280, 304, 305, 307, 328, 335, 340, 341, 357, 360, 365, 374, 418, 423, 430, 445

natural environment, 118, 259, 278, 418

natural habitats, 259

natural killer, 335

natural killer cell, 335

natural selection, 36, 37, 38, 39, 41, 48, 50, 52, 53, 56, 62, 63, 64, 87, 121, 183, 184, 304, 305, 307

Nebraska, 83, 394

neck, 451

necrosis, xiv, 51, 56, 114, 274, 281, 309, 317, 332, 399, 409, 421, 424, 448, 452

negative selection, 311

neglect, 232, 299, 305

nematicides, 162

nematode, 10, 11, 12, 102, 103, 112, 126, 133, 285, 293, 312, 313, 354, 367, 451

nematodes, 10, 11, 12, 128, 311, 354, 442

neonatal, 383, 419, 424

neonates, 176

neoplasia, 54, 88, 100, 108, 111, 116, 187, 257

neoplasm, 294, 367

neoplastic, 116, 118, 128, 217, 270, 271, 288

neoplastic diseases, 128

nephropathy, 108, 236, 250, 253

nephrotoxicity, 33

nerve, 184, 198, 230, 442

nerve cells, 198, 442

nerves, 185, 299

nervous system, 51, 162, 163, 166, 167, 171, 184, 197, 233

Netherlands, 377, 381, 385, 388

network, vii, xvi, 1, 3, 128, 243, 262, 278, 314, 347, 363, 429, 431, 440, 442

NeuN, 296

neural development, 170

neural function, 196, 197

neural tissue, 184

neurobiological, 251

Neuroblastoma, 451

neurochemistry, 168, 175

neurodegeneration, 105, 117, 126

neurodegenerative, xi, 168, 241, 243, 244, 273, 294, 320

neurodegenerative disease, xi, 241, 243, 273, 294, 320

neurodegenerative diseases, xi, 241, 243, 273, 320

neurodegenerative disorders, 244

neuroendocrine, 103, 135, 327

neuroendocrine cells, 103

neurofibrillary tangles, 295, 296

neurogenesis, 111, 122, 123, 134, 185, 198, 237, 371

neurogenic, 364

neurological disease, 313

neurological disorder, 198

neuronal cells, 296

neuronal loss, 117, 168

neuronal plasticity, 238

neuronal survival, 198

neurons, 31, 56, 60, 86, 168, 184, 196, 197, 198, 218, 229, 230, 237, 265, 266, 274, 282, 283, 287, 296, 364

neurophysiology, 168

neuroprotection, 298

neuroprotective, 199, 236, 297

neuroprotective drugs, 297

neurotoxic, 165, 199

neurotoxicity, 167, 173, 174, 175

neurotransmission, 197

neurotransmitter, 167

neurotransmitters, 167, 197

neurotrophic, 185, 197, 198, 202, 233, 235, 237, 240

neurotrophic factors, 185, 197, 199, 202

neutrophil, 403

neutrophils, 403

New England, 450, 452

New Jersey, 95, 281

New South Wales, 398

New York, 30, 82, 83, 85, 86, 88, 92, 154, 155, 156, 229, 235, 238, 239, 240, 329, 367, 368, 424

New Zealand, 273, 385, 424

Newton, 233, 330

next generation, 260, 385

NF-kB, 247, 322

NF-κB, 370

NHL, 169

Ni, 159

niacin, 340

nickel, 170

nicotinamide, 32

nicotine, 292, 407, 409, 421, 425
Nielsen, 329
NIH, 85
nitric oxide, 269, 280, 402, 408, 411
nitric oxide (NO), 269
nitrogen, 217, 257, 280, 293, 402
NK cells, 16, 322, 323
NMDA, 197, 234, 235, 297
NMDA receptors, 197
N-methyl-D-aspartate, 297
NMR, xii, 255, 256, 257, 258, 259, 260, 263, 270, 271, 272, 280
nociceptive, 49
nodules, 437
noise, 43, 84, 367, 370
non-destructive, 256
non-human, 313
non-human primates, 313
non-invasive, 25
non-linear, 357
nonparametric, 326
non-smokers, 71, 142, 144, 145, 407, 408, 413
non-steroidal anti-inflammatory drugs, 322
nontoxic, 295, 297
normal aging, 11, 277
normal conditions, 56, 208
normocapnia, 257
North America, 27, 188, 414, 416
NSAIDs, 297
N-terminal, xi, 104, 242, 244
nuclear, 11, 61, 67, 95, 165, 167, 174, 243, 247, 256, 260, 261, 263, 276, 280, 314, 320, 369
nuclear genome, 256, 263
nuclease, 74
nuclei, xvi, 204, 223, 230, 429, 441
nucleic acid, 115, 116, 187, 419
nucleotides, 74
nucleus, xi, 18, 54, 222, 241, 243, 306, 441
nurses, 4
nursing, 169, 183, 269, 346, 348
nursing care, 346
nursing home, 348
nutrient, xii, 103, 135, 151, 178, 184, 202, 220, 234, 238, 255, 317, 338, 341, 349, 350
nutrients, 51, 164, 182, 184, 188, 202, 203, 261, 262, 263, 264, 269, 271, 278, 279, 280, 324, 340, 341, 346, 348, 349, 363, 444
nutrition, xv, 12, 46, 127, 235, 257, 261, 262, 270, 279, 312, 314, 315, 316, 324, 336, 338, 340, 346, 348, 349, 351

nutritional deficiencies, 266
nuts, 340

O

oat, 32, 33
obese, 71, 143, 144, 155, 209, 215, 252, 274, 275, 289
obesity, xiv, 23, 31, 42, 43, 44, 47, 67, 84, 156, 200, 201, 208, 215, 298, 310, 314, 315, 316, 317, 328, 332, 336, 414, 415, 416, 417
observations, viii, 5, 6, 13, 91, 263, 275, 402, 408, 410
obsolete, 70, 71
obstruction, 442
obstructive sleep apnea, 265, 268, 280
obstructive sleep apnoea, 285
occasional drinkers, 141, 147
occluding, 339, 340
occlusion, 339, 351
occupational, 175
Oceania, 87
OCs, 165, 166
octopus, 342
odds ratio, x, 140, 142, 149, 343, 402, 404
oedema, 409
oil, 68, 445
old age, xiii, 9, 15, 21, 61, 267, 291, 299, 311, 333
older people, 310, 349, 442
oligomer, 295, 336
oligosaccharides, 323
omission, viii, 5, 6
oncogene, 72, 73, 130, 452
oncogenesis, 72
opportunity costs, 71
optimal health, 26, 199, 201
optimization, 26, 186, 189
oral, xiv, 27, 146, 158, 204, 275, 276, 337, 338, 340, 342, 346, 348, 349, 351, 368
oral cavity, xiv, 337, 338
oral health, 340, 346, 348, 349
organ, xvi, 61, 67, 94, 164, 167, 180, 184, 186, 196, 214, 284, 358, 362, 363, 364, 365, 399, 430, 437
organelle, 227, 228
organelles, 204, 243, 260, 435
organic, 28, 85, 169, 170, 174, 244, 359, 434
organic matter, 170
organic solvent, 434
organic solvents, 434

organism, vii, x, xvi, 12, 13, 38, 40, 45, 47, 48,
    49, 82, 87, 99, 101, 112, 136, 161, 162, 164,
    171, 172, 179, 180, 183, 194, 213, 214, 244,
    259, 260, 263, 277, 285, 286, 307, 317, 371,
    418, 430, 432, 441
organization, 279
Organization for Economic Cooperation and
    Development (OECD), 3
organophosphorous, 173
OSA, 265, 268, 280
oscillations, 257, 259, 263, 264, 269, 286
osmosis, 433
osmotic, 433
osmotic pressure, 433
osteoarthritis, 111, 310
osteocytes, 266
osteoporosis, 43, 57, 60, 231, 277, 294, 310, 314,
    320, 431
otitis media, 419
outpatients, 275, 294
ovarian cancer, 201
ovaries, 261, 363
ovary, 372, 452
overload, 69, 214, 267
overproduction, 243, 269, 295
overweight, 251, 274, 275, 289
overweight adults, 251, 289
oviduct, 282
ovulation, 183, 184
ownership, 163
oxidants, 204, 206
oxidation, ix, 13, 27, 28, 29, 97, 102, 108, 117,
    126, 137, 189, 191, 195, 213, 214, 218, 235,
    239, 251, 270
oxidation products, 251
oxidative damage, xi, xiv, 13, 19, 62, 99, 101,
    108, 112, 113, 115, 116, 121, 122, 124, 125,
    127, 130, 132, 133, 166, 172, 177, 180, 187,
    191, 204, 213, 228, 237, 244, 248, 258, 261,
    266, 271, 309, 312, 316, 362, 367
oxide, 11, 280, 402, 408, 411
oxygen, xii, 8, 11, 13, 103, 107, 112, 123, 131,
    133, 180, 229, 233, 242, 255, 256, 257, 259,
    260, 262, 263, 264, 265, 266, 267, 269, 270,
    275, 277, 278, 279, 282, 283, 285, 286, 287,
    293, 313, 322, 402, 434, 435, 452
oxygen, 263, 282, 283
oxygen absorption, 265, 279
oxygen consumption, 270, 275, 283, 287
oxygen saturation, 277

P

p38, xi, xii, 242, 244, 246, 252, 435
p53, 18, 92, 273, 277, 288, 313, 327
pacemaker, 60
Pacific, 153
PAHs, 165
pain, 43, 49, 333, 340
pancreas, 43, 91, 92, 219, 364, 368
pancreatic, 61, 150, 159, 202, 219, 221, 275, 329,
    344
pancreatic cancer, 150, 159
Pancreatic cancer, 85
pandemic, 66, 93
paper, xii, 53, 180, 198, 204, 255, 256, 273, 293
paradigm shift, 102, 109
paradoxical, ix, 35, 36
Paraguay, 42
paralysis, 66
parameter, 366, 388, 389, 392
parameter estimates, 388, 389
parameter estimation, 392
parasite, 48, 49, 64, 67, 93, 94, 418
parasites, 48, 49, 64, 75, 79, 94, 323, 424
parasitic infection, 75, 418
parasitic worms, ix, 35, 48, 66, 67
parasitosis, 75
parenchyma, 298
parenchymal, 243
parentage, 86
parenteral, 368
parents, 15, 154
Parkinson, 168, 173, 174, 176, 237, 244, 280
Parkinson's disease, 238
particles, 15
passive, 173, 187, 407
pasta, 206
pathogenesis, xiv, xv, 84, 168, 200, 245, 250,
    273, 295, 309, 315, 316, 320, 323, 325, 397,
    400, 411, 422
pathogenic, 48, 120, 407
pathogens, 67, 319, 365, 371, 398, 408, 418, 421
pathology, 100, 111, 115, 118, 141, 166, 256,
    262, 267, 272, 279, 298, 410
pathophysiological, 229, 285, 322
Pathophysiological, 84
pathophysiology, 156, 426
pathways, xi, xii, xiv, 12, 13, 17, 37, 87, 98, 100,
    103, 104, 105, 109, 111, 112, 113, 115, 120,
    121, 122, 162, 166, 167, 210, 241, 244, 256,

257, 265, 269, 270, 271, 273, 277, 278, 279, 293, 309, 310, 312, 316, 320, 324, 345, 354, 370, 402, 404, 440, 441, 445, 447, 448
patterning, 357
PC12 cells, 158
PCBs, 165, 169
PCR, 74, 147
peanuts, 194, 339, 342
pediatric, 93
pedigree, 391, 395
pelvic, 333
pelvic pain, 333
penicillin, 65, 66
pension, vii, 1, 2, 78
peptic ulcer, 43, 85, 411
peptic ulcer disease, 411
peptide, 86, 181, 199, 200, 206, 207, 223, 234, 297, 311, 370
peptides, 103, 188, 221, 222, 295
performance, 130, 167, 175, 234, 272, 280, 288, 292, 339, 346, 349, 357, 374, 381, 387, 389, 390, 393, 408
perinatal, 285, 399
periodic, 299
periodicity, 272
periodontal, 339, 343, 345, 350
periodontal disease, 339, 343, 345
periodontitis, xiv, 337, 338, 339, 345
peripheral, 404, 406
peripheral blood, 284
peripheral nervous system, 167, 197
peritonitis, 134
permeability, 402
permit, ix, 35, 210, 259
Peromyscus maniculatus, 124
peroxidation, 121, 128, 197, 217
peroxide, 28, 104, 107, 114, 133, 204, 231
peroxisomes, 204
peroxynitrite, 266
personal, 27, 67, 232, 294, 305, 355
personal communication, 355
personal values, 294
perturbation, 128
pertussis, 399, 407, 423
pest control, 163
pesticide, x, 161, 162, 163, 164, 166, 168, 169, 171, 172, 173, 174, 175, 176
pesticides, x, 161, 162, 163, 164, 165, 166, 167, 168, 169, 170, 171, 172, 173, 174, 175, 176, 207, 371

pests, 162
pets, 163
P-glycoprotein, 111
pH, 434, 435, 445
phagocytosis, 324, 402
pharmaceutical, 257
pharmacokinetics, 207, 368
pharmacological, xii, 24, 72, 242, 249, 287
pharmacological treatment, 72
phenolic, 32
phenolic compounds, 32
phenotype, xiv, 11, 15, 20, 39, 40, 81, 92, 98, 102, 105, 109, 110, 112, 152, 257, 263, 271, 309, 325, 330, 332, 357, 368, 383
phenotypes, x, 18, 82, 92, 98, 104, 105, 106, 107, 109, 111, 113, 115, 151, 306, 314, 315, 329, 332, 372, 403
phenotypic, 40, 41, 64, 82, 119, 200, 259, 260, 285, 286, 305, 314, 325, 333, 370, 381, 383, 388, 389, 390, 391
phenylalanine, 317
phenylketonuria, 317
Philadelphia, 236
Philippines, 42
philosophical, 29, 212, 215, 386
philosophy, 27, 78
phorbol, 251
phosphate, 29, 217, 218, 225, 226, 265, 449
phosphatidylcholine, 449, 452
phosphatidylethanolamine, 448, 449
phosphatidylserine, 449
phosphocreatine, 225, 226
phospholipids, xvii, 243, 287, 430, 439, 445, 448
phosphorus, 416
phosphorylation, 13, 113, 210, 226, 229, 243, 246, 257, 261, 280, 283
photoreceptor, 59
photoreceptor cells, 59
photoreceptors, 59, 60
phylogenesis, 259
phylogenetic, 109, 178, 182, 232, 371
physical activity, 43, 198, 215, 315
physical environment, 448
physical fitness, 346, 347, 348, 349, 350, 351
physical health, 343
physical properties, 448
physicians, 73, 277, 342
physiological constraints, 56
physiological factors, 25, 208, 222

physiology, x, 37, 117, 161, 163, 201, 221, 223, 224, 231, 251, 286
PI3K, 102, 312
pig, 129, 380, 390, 392, 437
pigs, 374, 383, 387, 388, 391, 398, 437, 438
Pit-1 gene, 123
pituitary, 110, 113, 124, 130, 182, 223, 236
pituitary gland, 182, 223
placebo, 297
placenta, 169
placental, 391
plague, 65
planning, ix, 36
plants, 169, 194, 203, 204, 206, 207, 364, 430, 442
plaque, 146
plaques, 296, 297, 322
plasma, x, 15, 21, 24, 33, 119, 125, 140, 143, 146, 148, 153, 154, 156, 158, 165, 191, 218, 219, 222, 247, 253, 283, 322, 323, 328, 332, 333, 340, 350, 402, 406, 411, 413, 421, 427, 432, 434, 439, 445
plasma levels, 21, 165, 284, 322, 328
plasma membrane, 434, 439, 445
plasma proteins, 219
plasminogen, 116, 131
plasticity, 198, 199, 238, 277, 370
platelet, 144, 402
platelet count, 144
platforms, 374
plausibility, 122
play, xv, xvi, 8, 10, 12, 15, 24, 98, 115, 121, 123, 150, 185, 187, 198, 201, 227, 248, 269, 299, 310, 311, 322, 323, 334, 374, 397, 408, 410, 413, 415, 430, 445, 450
pleasure, 348
pleiotropy, 53, 311, 317
Pleistocene, 233, 239
pleural, 406
Pliocene, 239
pneumoconiosis, xi, 241, 243
pneumonia, 343, 344, 404
point mutation, 283, 295, 329
poisoning, 162, 171, 174, 401
polar ice, 269
polarization, 226
polio, 66
poliovirus, 66
politicians, 70
politics, 78, 79

pollen, 442
pollutant, 407
pollutants, 169, 174, 207, 214, 361, 371, 401
pollution, 43, 84, 162, 248, 298
polygenic, 376, 383
polymer, 212, 224
polymerase, 147
polymerization, 432, 434, 449
polymers, xvi, 216, 430
polymorphonuclear, 402
polypeptides, 203
polysaccharide, 399, 422, 434, 439
polysaccharides, 28, 340, 348, 435, 437, 439
polyunsaturated fat, 452
polyunsaturated fatty acid, 452
pools, 226
poor, xv, 110, 167, 249, 271, 306, 340, 343, 344, 345, 346, 397, 410, 411, 416, 427
population density, 102, 398
population growth, 9
pores, 430, 444
portal vein, 221
portfolio, 71
positive correlation, 169, 415
postmenopausal, 143, 145, 157, 239
postmenopausal women, 143, 145, 157, 239
postmitotic cells, xii, 255, 256, 261, 264, 266
postmortem, 258, 438
postnatal exposure, 170
postural instability, 168
potassium, 144, 275, 315, 330
poultry, 49, 206, 398
poverty, 14
power, 37, 78, 263, 273, 315, 329, 347
practical knowledge, 273
praline, 390
precancerous lesions, 117
precipitation, 432, 434, 450
preconditioning, 233, 256, 259, 268, 269, 282, 283, 284
precursor cells, 198, 199
predators, xv, 48, 50, 257, 359, 366, 373
prediction, ix, 35, 37, 41, 53, 87, 112, 154, 388
predictive models, 424
predictors, 341, 394, 414
preference, 216, 222
prefrontal cortex, 347
pregnancy, 43, 49, 50, 61, 86, 119, 125, 169, 170, 171, 175, 283, 388, 417
pregnant, 49, 269, 283

premature death, 184, 207, 214, 378

prematurity, 417

premenopausal women, 143, 145

premium, 203, 214

presenilin 1, 295

preservative, 180

pressure, x, 70, 85, 100, 122, 140, 141, 144, 148, 150, 153, 154, 155, 244, 263, 268, 299, 333, 343, 344, 415, 421, 434, 435, 440, 445

preterm delivery, 417, 421

prevention, x, xii, 9, 10, 67, 72, 73, 85, 94, 99, 135, 140, 143, 151, 172, 187, 242, 249, 272, 285, 324, 338, 346, 348, 349

preventive, xiii, 9, 65, 73, 75, 79, 146, 150, 246, 291, 299

primary tumor, 444

primate, 53, 182, 183, 220, 237

primates, 8, 32, 199, 216, 238, 244, 251, 327

pro-apoptotic protein, 231

probability, 15, 50, 51, 55, 58, 60, 63, 162, 164, 170, 294, 382

probable cause, 39, 42

proband, 315

procreation, 77

producers, 242, 320

productivity, 162, 199, 386, 391, 393

pro-fibrotic, 245

profit, 162

progenitor cells, 59, 188

progenitors, 122

progeny, 49, 50, 117, 162, 166, 170, 360, 374, 383

prognostic value, 325

program, ix, 35, 36, 38, 79, 83, 89, 112, 249, 279, 280, 304, 306, 341, 445

proinflammatory, 15, 322, 333, 426

pro-inflammatory, 245, 247, 249, 250, 318, 320, 321, 322, 399, 400, 401, 403, 404, 405, 408, 410, 412, 414, 415, 416, 417

pro-inflammatory response, 399, 401, 403, 404, 408, 414, 416, 417

prolactin, 110, 183

proliferation, 12, 90, 91, 123, 130, 181, 184, 189, 198, 199, 202, 207, 217, 223, 256, 261, 263, 322, 327, 364, 401, 402

proliferation potential, 90

promote, xvii, 11, 13, 15, 24, 29, 141, 179, 187, 198, 200, 201, 202, 213, 216, 220, 222, 231, 349, 417, 430

promoter, 194, 195, 251, 322, 324, 333, 334, 335, 336, 404, 414, 421, 422, 423, 425, 426, 427

promoter region, 322, 425

propagation, 28, 49, 118, 260, 437

property, 149, 191

prophylactic, 162, 256

prophylaxis, 288, 316

proposition, 30, 306

prosperity, 3

prostaglandin, 322, 402

prostaglandins, 269

prostanoids, 411

prostate, 91, 170, 175, 201, 234, 445, 452

prostate cancer, 170, 175, 201, 234, 452

prostatectomy, 451

prostatitis, 333

proteases, 324, 407

protection, xi, 12, 14, 15, 20, 67, 94, 106, 108, 111, 121, 184, 193, 207, 217, 229, 231, 241, 248, 250, 265, 268, 401

protective factors, 101, 269

protective mechanisms, xii, 115, 242, 269, 298

protective role, 16, 266, 319

protein aggregation, 168

protein binding, 156

protein denaturation, 191

protein function, xvi, 429

protein kinases, 442

protein oxidation, 126, 235, 239

protein sequence, 439

protein synthesis, 219, 222, 223, 234

proteinuria, 416

proteoglycans, 243

proteolysis, 93

proteome, 213

protocol, xi, 24, 25, 26, 27, 29, 113, 178, 179, 186, 188, 190, 192, 198, 199, 208, 209, 212, 213, 216, 232, 274, 275, 276, 387

protocols, xiii, 25, 178, 189, 190, 256, 268, 269, 272, 273, 276, 279

protons, 225

protozoa, ix, 35, 48

proximal, 183

PRP, 399, 422

PSD, 449

pseudo, 74

psoriasis, 425

psyche, 215

psychiatric disorder, 43

psychiatric disorders, 43

psychological stress, 100
psychology, 78, 151
psychosocial variables, 341
puberty, 304
public, 4, 30, 171, 310, 325, 408, 414
public health, 4, 30, 172, 310, 408, 414
public policy, 325
pulmonary hypertension, 392
pulse, 363
pulses, 364
pumps, 165, 166
purification, 33, 261, 437
Purkinje, 174
pyrene, 106, 174, 368
pyrethroids, 163, 171
pyridoxal, 29
pyridoxine, 29
pyrimidine, 106
pyruvate, 226, 270
pyruvic, 225

Q

QOL, 339, 340, 348, 349
quality control, 261
quality of life, 9, 75, 79, 274, 299, 310, 315, 339
Quantitative trait loci, 384, 390
Quebec, 388
questioning, 273
questionnaire, xiv, 147, 337, 339, 342

R

race, viii, 6, 7, 47
racemization, 258, 280
radiation, xvi, 102, 116, 127, 128, 135, 136, 137,
  251, 293, 430, 443, 444, 451
radiation therapy, 451
radical, 13, 42, 62, 133, 196, 228, 229, 267, 451
radical reactions, 266, 285
radio, 299
rain, 238, 270
rainfall, 163, 270
random, 38, 39, 42, 62, 73, 103, 210, 306, 310,
  381, 437
randomness, 357, 361
range, xiii, 48, 68, 79, 105, 121, 171, 184, 204,
  205, 209, 213, 221, 228, 230, 258, 265, 291,
  292, 295, 299, 303, 304, 323, 330, 356, 359,
  366, 374, 376, 378, 380, 381, 387, 410, 412,
  413, 439, 448

reactants, 27, 29, 322
reactive nitrogen, 280
reactive oxygen, 13, 19, 99, 102, 108, 150, 158,
  172, 233, 242, 280, 293, 312, 402, 452
reactive oxygen species, 13, 19, 99, 102, 108,
  150, 158, 172, 233, 242, 280, 313
reactive oxygen species (ROS), 13, 150, 286
reactivity, 319, 418
reagents, 297
reasoning, 26, 29, 181, 183, 195, 203, 221, 223,
  304
recall, 221, 223, 228
recalling, 80
reception, 197, 199
receptors, xi, 29, 113, 187, 191, 197, 199, 219,
  223, 226, 227, 234, 241, 243, 275, 276, 289,
  297, 313, 323, 335, 404, 441, 442, 452
reciprocal cross, 119, 382
reciprocal translocation, 92
recognition, 187, 197, 240, 323, 335
reconcile, 418
recovery, 90, 167, 198, 265, 275, 278
recreational, 213
recurrence, 444
recycling, 282
red blood cell, 416
Red Cross, 139, 146
red wine, 16, 313
redox, 103, 131, 157, 247, 250, 251, 256, 263,
  265, 286
reducing sugars, viii, 23
reduction, xii, 13, 14, 27, 54, 56, 57, 59, 60, 75,
  100, 103, 109, 110, 112, 116, 119, 122, 136,
  150, 171, 183, 184, 195, 210, 211, 217, 219,
  220, 224, 229, 231, 242, 246, 248, 272, 276,
  279, 293, 313, 320, 339, 343, 345, 348, 362,
  363, 382, 386, 405, 414, 442
redundancy, 49
REE, 208, 209, 210
reflection, 98, 202, 256
reflexes, 171, 176
refractoriness, 126
regenerate, 365
regeneration, xv, 106, 167, 265, 271, 353, 357,
  359, 363, 365, 366, 370
regional, 58, 347, 350
regression, 141, 142, 147, 148, 290, 311, 347
regression analysis, 141, 142, 147, 148, 347
regular, x, 140, 146, 275, 279, 362, 432, 436,
  437, 439

regulation, 15, 19, 20, 55, 56, 91, 98, 102, 109, 115, 116, 117, 118, 122, 134, 135, 136, 164, 198, 208, 234, 245, 249, 250, 251, 253, 256, 277, 279, 320, 325, 327, 333, 367, 368, 369, 383, 391, 404, 424, 451

regulators, 16, 335

rehabilitation, 272

Reimann, 370

relationship, xv, xvi, 25, 48, 50, 75, 86, 89, 98, 104, 108, 109, 120, 143, 144, 157, 159, 167, 169, 170, 171, 180, 185, 191, 192, 195, 214, 238, 244, 259, 267, 336, 340, 341, 343, 349, 353, 354, 366, 372, 387, 389, 390, 393, 395, 418, 424, 430, 437, 438

relationships, 119, 325, 328, 340, 376, 391, 425

relatives, 10, 87, 363, 364, 365, 389, 402

relaxation, 213, 271, 411

relevance, xv, 26, 28, 29, 30, 101, 118, 164, 176, 205, 252, 321, 327, 367, 373, 386

religion, 9, 78, 79

REM, 271

remission, 444

remodeling, 263

remodelling, 90

renal, 23, 25, 33, 43, 60, 84, 132, 154, 415, 420, 423, 424

renal cell carcinoma, 43, 84

renal disease, 154, 415, 420, 423, 424

renal epithelial cells, 132

renal failure, 23

renal function, 60

renin, 94

renin-angiotensin system, 94

reoxygenation, 259, 268

repair, xii, 12, 18, 74, 99, 100, 106, 107, 112, 113, 115, 123, 127, 130, 133, 134, 136, 167, 170, 181, 187, 202, 234, 251, 256, 262, 266, 271, 273, 277, 278, 312, 314, 358, 359, 363, 365

repair interval, 278

repair system, 74

reparation, 8, 189, 213

reperfusion, 114, 268, 284, 285

replacement rate, 394

replication, 54, 56, 57, 61, 115, 250, 252, 262, 315, 330

repression, 55, 228

repressor, 234

reproduction, viii, xv, 5, 6, 8, 19, 36, 37, 53, 72, 86, 102, 117, 170, 183, 240, 262, 306, 326,

353, 355, 357, 358, 359, 360, 362, 363, 366, 370, 373, 388, 390, 391, 393, 394, 401, 417

reproductive age, 417

reptiles, 358, 387

Republic of the Congo, 42

research, vii, xi, xv, 7, 10, 11, 12, 71, 86, 95, 99, 102, 117, 121, 122, 127, 131, 132, 137, 154, 180, 185, 198, 241, 244, 273, 275, 281, 286, 298, 310, 316, 326, 348, 353, 354, 357, 362, 363, 364, 366, 367, 369, 371, 372, 374, 386, 406

research and development, 71

researchers, 25, 27, 109, 140, 145, 178, 189, 191, 192, 195, 198, 258, 273, 277, 293, 296, 297, 298, 304, 383

reservation, 115, 221, 235

reserves, 184, 265, 277, 278, 359, 363

reservoir, 94, 187, 195, 216, 231, 398

residential, 4, 413

residues, 111, 149, 157, 163, 314, 316

resistin, xiv, 309, 316

resource allocation, 19

resources, 50, 53, 71, 73, 133, 180, 183, 196, 262, 278, 304, 310, 326, 358, 359, 366

respiration, 213, 242, 283, 284

respiratory, 43, 101, 117, 143, 150, 162, 164, 261, 267, 273, 281, 336, 399, 407, 409, 421, 422

respiratory arrest, 101

respiratory syncytial virus, 422

responsiveness, 217, 221

restaurants, 299

restriction enzyme, 74, 147

resuscitation, 409

Resveratrol, 194, 313

retardation, 181, 238, 240, 314

retention, 201, 216

reticulum, 112, 133, 227

retina, 59, 60

retinol, 340

retinopathy, 277

retirees, 2

retirement age, 2, 3

revenue, 71

reverse transcriptase, 120, 364

rewards, 71, 212

Reynolds, 31, 32, 235, 358, 359, 370, 450

rheumatoid arthritis, 32, 250, 284, 324, 336, 422

rhythms, 32, 238, 287

ribosomal, 89

ribosomal RNA, 89

rice, 342

rigidity, 168

risk factors, xv, 14, 67, 68, 73, 84, 85, 94, 144, 145, 154, 160, 298, 311, 336, 345, 350, 397, 405, 408, 409, 410, 411, 412, 416, 417, 418, 420, 422, 423, 425

risk management, 150

risk profile, 20, 317

risks, xiv, 21, 73, 150, 170, 309, 312, 341, 382, 393, 415, 422, 424

Rita, 171, 175

RNA, 74, 193, 222

roasted coffee, 158

rodent, ix, 25, 32, 98, 99, 105, 109, 112, 117, 121, 122, 205, 237, 281

rodenticides, 162

rodents, 99, 105, 106, 107, 108, 120, 121, 123, 130, 179, 197, 198, 199, 219, 244, 287, 362, 365

rods, 59

Rome, 387

room temperature, 434

ROS, xii, 13, 150, 242, 243, 248, 255, 256, 257, 260, 261, 262, 263, 264, 265, 266, 269, 270, 273, 277, 280, 283

roseola, 451

rotifer, 354

Royal Society, 17, 238, 389

rural, 174, 411, 416, 427

rural communities, 416

rural population, 174, 427

Russia, 273

Russian, 286, 288, 289, 297

S

Saccharomyces cerevisiae, 51, 88, 282, 327

sacrifice, 202

safety, 75, 273, 294, 324

sales, 71, 299

saline, 434

saliva, 340

salivary glands, 61

salt, 14, 20, 43, 45, 47, 84, 434, 436

sample, 110, 115, 151, 167, 326, 331, 341, 366, 370, 423, 439

sanitation, 310

sarcopenia, 60, 229, 231

SAS, 147

satellite, 90, 223, 363

satellite cells, 90, 223, 363

satisfaction, 3, 4

saturated fat, 151, 160, 346

saturation, 277

SBP, 141

scarcity, 51, 184, 195, 365

scattering, 432

scavenger, 32

school, 299

Schwerin, 390

scientific knowledge, 186

scientists, vii, 5, 6, 178, 180, 195, 297, 304, 310, 314, 378

scleroderma, 253

sclerosis, 243, 245, 250, 276

scores, 387

scrotal, 393

sea level, 261

search, 244, 270, 310, 315, 335

searches, 442

searching, 7

seawater, 270

Second World War, 164, 292

secrete, 67

secretion, 110, 184, 192, 200, 201, 202, 221, 222, 223, 234, 275, 297, 320, 331, 404, 407, 420

security, 162, 294

sedentary, 208, 210, 223, 298

sedentary lifestyle, 298

seed, 451

seedlings, 28, 32, 33, 238

seeds, 188, 203, 442

segregation, 317

seizures, 198

selecting, 385, 390

selective synergism, xi, 177, 199, 205, 232

selectivity, 216, 221, 448

self-assessment, 346

self-destruction, 56, 261

self-esteem, 3

self-help, xiii, 256

self-interest, 305

self-repair, 262

self-report, 4, 157

SEM, 433, 435

seminal vesicle, 451

seminiferous epithelium, 176

senescence, ix, 12, 17, 24, 36, 51, 52, 53, 55, 56, 57, 59, 60, 61, 62, 63, 70, 83, 87, 88, 90, 108, 120, 131, 135, 136, 179, 186, 205, 229, 242,

252, 261, 262, 277, 279, 290, 304, 305, 306,
307, 317, 319, 326, 354, 362, 363, 364, 366,
368, 369, 370
senile, 51, 57, 295
senile plaques, 295
senility, 61, 83
sensation, 212, 224, 225
sensing, 256, 283
sensitivity, 14, 24, 29, 30, 112, 113, 121, 150,
187, 205, 223, 236, 244, 272, 275, 276, 277,
314, 316, 328, 415, 421, 426, 427, 448
sensors, 441
sentences, viii, 5, 6
separation, 366, 434
sepsis, 420, 424
septic shock, 404, 420
Serbia, 5
series, viii, 23, 49, 269, 284, 409, 415
serine, 166, 243, 324, 442
serum, x, 14, 16, 24, 25, 26, 27, 30, 107, 140,
142, 143, 144, 145, 148, 149, 150, 153, 154,
155, 156, 158, 159, 171, 191, 207, 221, 232,
252, 274, 323, 336, 341, 343, 344, 348, 350,
399, 404, 415, 423, 426, 432, 440
serum albumin, 343, 348
severity, xv, 75, 77, 111, 211, 230, 231, 397, 399,
401, 402, 404, 411, 419, 423
sex, 26, 33, 91, 103, 111, 113, 183, 201, 209,
311, 332, 411, 412
sex hormones, 183, 201
sex steroid, 91
sexual development, 220
SGP, 92
shape, 18, 354, 372, 434, 442
shares, 356
sharing, 49
sheep, 375, 378, 380, 381, 383, 387, 388, 389,
393, 394, 395, 437
Shell, 422
shelter, 360
shock, 31, 108, 111, 115, 128, 131, 132, 134,
269, 273, 284, 287, 313, 326, 327, 401, 403,
404, 410, 420, 422, 425
shores, 258
short period, 363
shortage, 3
short-term, xiii, 154, 190, 198, 240, 256, 267,
275, 282, 289, 291, 354
short-term memory, xiii, 267, 291
shrimp, 369, 372

shrinking work forces, vii, 1, 2
sialic acid, 156
siblings, 20, 129, 311, 326, 357
sick sinus syndrome, 344
sickle cell, 41
side effects, x, 161
sign, 59
signal transduction, 12, 166, 167
signaling, xiv, 13, 16, 102, 103, 109, 113, 114,
115, 123, 124, 132, 135, 136, 166, 181, 189,
191, 195, 220, 227, 233, 236, 242, 243, 287,
309, 313, 316, 370, 441, 448, 449, 451, 452
signaling pathway, 13, 16, 102, 104, 109, 114,
115, 233, 314, 441, 449, 451
signaling pathways, 13, 102, 115, 451
signalling, 128, 167, 251, 252, 322
signals, 104, 135, 230, 327, 347, 368, 441, 442
signs, 61, 279, 305
similarity, 275
Singapore, 84
single nucleotide polymorphism, 315, 316, 334,
374, 384, 399, 423, 425
single-nucleotide polymorphism, 160
sinus, 60
sites, 103, 194, 196, 252, 261, 276, 403, 444
skeletal muscle, 24, 31, 90, 105, 107, 108, 115,
130, 135, 184, 187, 208, 210, 216, 227, 229,
230, 231, 233, 234, 235, 237, 238, 239, 265,
266, 275, 284, 285
skeleton, 91
skills, 3, 167
skin, 31, 32, 48, 56, 57, 58, 106, 107, 108, 116,
121, 124, 137, 164, 169, 170, 243, 314, 415
SLE, 324
sleep, 100, 222, 265, 268, 271, 280
small intestine, 58, 92, 203, 221, 236, 364
smallpox, 65
smoke, 156, 407, 409, 410, 421, 425
smokers, 71, 142, 143, 144, 145, 147, 148, 343,
405, 407, 408, 413
smoking, 14, 43, 67, 84, 85, 141, 142, 143, 144,
145, 146, 147, 148, 149, 150, 153, 154, 156,
160, 248, 298, 341, 343, 344, 405, 407, 408,
410, 411, 412, 413, 417, 420, 423, 427
smoking cessation, 143, 160
smooth muscle cells, 21, 243, 322
snakes, 158, 257
SNP, 314, 320, 322, 334, 399, 400, 402, 403,
404, 405, 406, 413, 416, 417

SNPs, 315, 321, 322, 324, 331, 390, 392, 405, 418
social activities, 299
social assistance, 79
social behavior, 86, 357, 361
social class, 340, 412
social costs, 172
social environment, 354
social factors, 298
social influence, 93
social influences, 93
social life, 295
social network, vii, 1, 3, 298
social roles, 347
social security, 294
social stress, 361, 366
socioeconomic, xv, 310, 345, 397, 411, 416, 424
socioeconomic background, 411
socioeconomic conditions, xv, 397, 411
socioeconomic status, 310, 424
sociology, 78
SOD, 132, 257, 275, 280
SOD1, 18, 326
sodium, 144, 171, 434
software, 70, 147, 299
soil, 162, 354
soleus, 134
solubility, 163
solvent, 435
somatic cell, 57, 62, 134, 202, 257, 260, 261, 263
somatic cells, 57, 62, 134, 202, 257, 263
somatic mutations, 125
somatotropin, 182, 221, 223
sores, 415
sounds, 215
South Africa, 174, 258, 281, 379, 394
South America, 136, 336
South Asia, 412, 414, 415, 421, 423
Soviet Union, 286
soy, 28, 208, 234
soybeans, 28, 189, 201, 204, 207
Spain, 161, 255, 303, 373, 377, 380, 381, 385
Spanish flu, 65
spatial, 188, 199, 234, 357
spatial learning, 188, 199, 234
spawning, 355
specialization, 193
specificity, 166, 217, 319, 326
spectrum, 85, 170, 232, 238, 356, 357, 361, 365
speculation, 202

speed, xiii, 69, 167, 291, 433
spermatogenesis, 183
spermatogonia, 117
SPF, 118
spinal cord, 229
spine, 234
spiritual, 279, 294
spleen, 277
spontaneous abortion, 170, 171, 172
spontaneous recovery, 290
sporadic, 298
spore, xvi, 429, 430, 431, 432, 434, 437, 439, 442, 444, 449
spouse, 26
Sprague-Dawley rats, 237
St. Louis, 238
stability, xiii, 7, 12, 17, 88, 120, 171, 199, 234, 256, 257, 271, 278, 279, 365
stabilization, 266
stabilize, 209
stages, 185, 203, 355, 356, 357, 358, 362, 371, 372, 374, 393, 401, 407, 415, 431, 441
standards, 41, 305, 387
staphylococcal, 424
staphylococci, 407, 424
Staphylococcus, 401, 424, 427
Staphylococcus aureus, 401, 424, 427
starch, 238, 340, 348
starch polysaccharides, 340, 348
starvation, vii, 5, 6, 8, 218, 270
statin, 94, 297
statins, 11, 18, 67
statistical analysis, 110
statistics, 63, 93, 273, 425
staurosporine, 114
steel, 28, 188
stellate cells, 243
sem cell, 367, 370
stem cell transplantation, 336
stem cells, 55, 56, 57, 58, 59, 72, 73, 92, 223, 257, 266, 279, 280, 284, 363, 364, 369, 370,
sterile, 401
steroid, 256, 261
steroid hormones, 261
steroids, 91
stillbirth, 421
stochastic, 90, 242, 252, 306, 357, 370
Stochastic, 353, 357, 368
stock, 118, 119, 120, 121
stockpile, 224

stomach, 43, 117, 166, 266
storage, 103, 189, 197, 214, 217, 218, 219, 256, 269, 278, 363
strain, 2, 103, 110, 113, 119, 129, 211, 213, 219, 236
strains, ix, 89, 98, 103, 109, 110, 116, 117, 118, 119, 120, 121, 122, 124, 125, 127, 133, 135, 360
strategies, xii, xiii, 11, 37, 143, 151, 249, 255, 256, 263, 265, 278, 291, 296, 297, 315, 324, 386, 389, 390, 415
strength, 188, 198, 213, 227, 347
stress level, 437
stressors, ix, xiii, 13, 16, 97, 100, 101, 102, 112, 113, 121, 128, 256, 269, 278, 362, 417
stretching, 213, 223
striatum, 198
stroke, 15, 21, 144, 273, 277, 294, 298, 332, 413
strokes, 9, 344
stromal, 266, 334
stromal cell-derived factor-1, 334
structural changes, 451
structural gene, 336
structural modifications, 193
subarachnoid hemorrhage, 16
sbcellular, 285
subcutaneous tissue, 58
subgroups, viii, 5, 6, 146
subjective, 2, 212, 214, 216, 224
subjective well-being, 2
sub-Saharan Africa, 42
subsistence, 25, 28, 204
substances, 43, 66, 67, 164, 165, 166, 193, 219, 228, 229, 434
substantia nigra, 168
substitutes, 73
substitution, 57, 73, 74, 76, 317
substrates, 164, 165, 166, 184, 187, 192, 203, 212, 226
successful aging, 150, 152, 318, 320
sudden infant death syndrome, 419, 420, 421, 422, 423, 424, 425, 426
Sudden Infant Death Syndrome (SIDS), 399, 407, 408, 409, 410, 419, 420, 422, 423, 427
suffering, 36, 60, 294
sugar, viii, 13, 23, 43, 224, 274, 292, 442
sugars, viii, 23, 203, 205
suicide, 78, 171, 230
sulfonylurea, 330
sulfur, 231

sulfuric acid, 231
summer, 269, 270, 299
Sun, 32, 105, 111, 115, 123, 130, 134, 136, 240, 283, 335, 452
superiority, 378
superoxide, 101, 103, 107, 112, 116, 127, 128, 134, 159, 204, 228, 240, 313, 402
superoxide dismutase, 107, 116, 127, 128, 134, 159, 204, 240, 313
supplemental, 188, 203
supplements, 13
supply, 14, 29, 102, 184, 203, 226, 230, 261, 262, 264, 271, 272, 283
suppression, xiv, 166, 179, 180, 183, 186, 190, 202, 205, 208, 217, 220, 223, 230, 260, 309, 314, 407
suppressor, 72, 73, 313, 404
surface area, 440
surfactant, 336
surveillance, 260
survivability, 383, 389
surviving, 162, 164, 182
survivors, 52, 62, 318, 332, 343, 411
susceptibility, x, xiv, xv, 23, 49, 98, 121, 135, 150, 151, 160, 162, 177, 181, 186, 309, 311, 315, 320, 324, 331, 335, 357, 392, 397, 399, 401, 404, 405, 407, 408, 420, 422, 424, 426
sustainability, 212
swallowing, xiv, 337, 338, 348
swamps, 292
Sweden, 293, 298, 378, 380, 385
swelling, 339, 340
switching, 19, 265
Switzerland, 3, 288, 377, 378, 385, 394
sympathetic, 185, 232
symptom, 295
symptoms, 9, 61, 167, 168, 274, 294, 296, 297, 324, 364
synapse, 188, 234
synapses, 196, 198
synaptic strength, 198
synaptogenesis, 198
synaptophysin, 196
synchronization, 196
syndrome, xiv, 11, 16, 18, 56, 57, 61, 62, 68, 92, 129, 137, 273, 276, 284, 310, 314, 317, 325, 328, 329, 330, 333, 392, 419, 420, 422, 424, 425, 426, 427
synergistic, 186, 218, 276, 277, 278, 279
synergistic effect, 218

synthesis, xi, 89, 106, 135, 164, 167, 186, 189, 192, 194, 196, 202, 203, 214, 217, 219, 221, 222, 223, 231, 234, 236, 242, 243, 244, 247, 269, 314, 363, 441, 448, 449, 452

Syphilis, 398

systemic circulation, 184, 297

systemic lupus erythematosus, 336

systems, x, 11, 18, 36, 83, 125, 133, 161, 162, 163, 164, 165, 167, 172, 184, 201, 218, 219, 265, 278, 285, 294, 312, 323, 329, 357, 363, 364, 365, 374, 386, 387, 400, 416

systolic blood pressure, 141, 333, 343

T

T cell, 16, 132, 319, 333, 402, 404

T lymphocyte, 128, 332

Taiwan, 167

tangles, 298

tannins, 191

Tanzania, 42

targets, 75, 76, 123, 165, 174, 287, 316, 322, 336, 445, 451

taste, 53, 61, 348

tau, 296, 297, 298

taxa, 49, 121, 361

T-cell, 106, 111, 114, 332

tea, 27, 29, 30, 188, 189, 191, 240

technology, 70, 272, 273

teeth, 43, 46, 339, 340, 341, 343, 344, 345, 346

telomerase, 54, 55, 56, 57, 61, 88, 90, 91, 92, 120, 127, 130, 133, 293, 316, 364, 365, 369

telomere, ix, 35, 36, 53, 54, 55, 56, 57, 61, 62, 75, 76, 89, 90, 120, 122, 124, 130, 242, 252, 261, 354, 364, 365, 370

telomere shortening, 54, 55, 56, 242, 364

telomeres, 54, 55, 56, 57, 89, 90, 93, 120, 127, 261, 282, 316, 362, 364

TEM, 433, 435

temperature, xv, 25, 100, 102, 103, 105, 204, 210, 244, 258, 259, 281, 287, 361, 373, 448

temporal, xi, 24, 25, 26, 177, 179, 186, 189, 199, 211, 224, 232, 359, 362, 366

tendon, 32, 238

tension, 227, 259, 263, 265, 266, 269, 282, 286

teratogen, 49

teratogenic, 371

terminals, 235

testicular cancer, 108, 169

testosterone, 124, 174, 183, 201, 371

Texas, 97

TGF, xi, xii, 241, 242, 243, 245, 246, 248, 250, 251, 321

TGFβ, 250

thalamus, 117, 347

thapsigargin, 112

theory, viii, ix, xiii, 13, 19, 20, 35, 38, 41, 52, 53, 64, 82, 83, 88, 89, 93, 98, 99, 116, 127, 158, 172, 175, 180, 181, 202, 232, 233, 242, 244, 248, 251, 260, 277, 282, 292, 303, 304, 306, 311, 358, 367, 382, 430

therapeutic agents, 94, 445

therapeutic targets, 445, 451

therapy, xiii, 67, 72, 73, 85, 94, 95, 166, 256, 272, 276, 279, 289, 298, 452

thermodynamics, 434

theta, 133, 176

thinking, 83, 88, 167, 213, 295, 305, 307

thiobarbituric acid, 228

thioredoxin, 115, 117, 125, 131, 135

Thomson, 32, 330, 397, 422

threat, 24

threatening, 442

threats, 162, 278

threonine, 243, 442

threshold, 192, 263, 315, 375, 376, 378, 379, 380, 394, 444

thrombosis, 411, 442

thromboxane, 322

thymus, 277

thyroid, 91, 110, 113, 167, 175, 182, 261, 281

thyroid stimulating hormone, 110

thyrotropin, 183

Tibet, 285

timing, 12, 32, 277, 278, 359

TLR, xiv, 309, 318

TLR4, 16, 322

TNF, 16, 247, 253, 317, 318, 320, 333, 334, 399, 400, 401, 402, 403, 404, 408, 409, 412, 417, 418, 425, 442

TNF-alpha, 253, 334

TNF-α, 401, 402, 403, 425

tobacco, 84, 145, 156, 298, 399, 418, 421

tobacco smoke, 145

Tokyo, 1, 3, 139, 147, 347

tolerance, x, 33, 57, 136, 140, 146, 147, 148, 149, 150, 151, 156, 157, 158, 240, 244, 266, 268, 283, 284, 285, 288, 329, 356

Toll-like, 317, 321, 335

tomato, 340

total cholesterol, 142, 325, 343, 439

toxic, 49, 99, 101, 113, 120, 158, 165, 169, 181, 184, 187, 195, 198, 200, 201, 206, 213, 214, 216, 230, 297, 401, 410, 422, 425
toxic effect, 165, 200
toxic products, 99
toxic shock syndrome, 401, 422, 425
toxicity, 103, 105, 113, 116, 124, 125, 134, 164, 166, 167, 168, 173, 174, 214, 236, 283, 325
toxicology, 129, 168
toxin, 85, 106, 135, 200, 274, 422, 425
toxins, 105, 128, 158, 168, 187, 195, 197, 200, 206, 214, 292, 401, 405, 407, 409, 420, 425, 427
Toyota, 156
trade, 18, 36, 53, 54, 70, 355, 358, 398, 401, 417
trade union, 70
trade-off, 18, 36, 53, 54, 358
training, xiii, 221, 256, 269, 272, 278, 279, 280, 284, 290, 299
traits, xiv, xv, 10, 119, 122, 131, 204, 307, 310, 315, 317, 324, 329, 330, 357, 368, 373, 376, 382, 385, 386, 387, 389, 390, 392, 393, 394
transcript, 165, 210
transcriptase, 120, 364
transcription, xi, xii, 16, 21, 103, 110, 125, 128, 165, 187, 193, 222, 239, 242, 243, 246, 251, 293, 312, 313, 315, 320, 330, 331, 421, 422
transcription factor, xi, 16, 21, 103, 110, 125, 239, 242, 243, 251, 293, 312, 313, 315, 330, 331
transcription factors, 16, 21, 251, 293
transcriptional, 16, 55, 193, 244, 333
transcripts, 102
transduction, 224, 287
transfer, 15, 38, 153, 173, 284, 398
transferrin, 266
transformation, xvi, 70, 73, 259, 271, 306, 429, 430, 431, 432, 433, 434, 441, 445
transformations, 448
transforming growth factor, xi, 241, 243, 250, 251, 252, 288
transgene, 134
transgenerational, 366
transgenic, 11, 30, 115, 116, 117, 125, 131, 134, 135, 250, 296, 297, 354, 367, 451
transgenic mice, 11, 30, 116, 117, 125, 131, 135, 296, 297, 367, 451
transition, 449
transitions, 282
translation, 193

translational, 100, 193
translocation, 226
translocations, 11, 92
transmembrane, 103, 256, 295
trans-membrane, 132
transmission, viii, 35, 197, 256, 329, 336, 371, 420
transplantation, 90, 336, 415
transport, xiv, 15, 103, 166, 173, 202, 203, 210, 219, 222, 226, 234, 235, 236, 242, 265, 275, 310, 317, 444
transportation, 265, 279
transpose, xii, 242
trauma, 48, 78, 100, 273
travel, 172, 398
trees, 53
tremor, 168
trend, 99, 293, 385
trial, xiii, 14, 94, 158, 289, 291, 297, 315
tribal, 398
tribes, 47, 398
tricarboxylic acid, 224
trichloroacetic acid, 434
triggers, 51, 261, 401, 418, 433, 448, 452
triglyceride, 142, 149, 153, 218, 219, 220, 274, 329
triiodothyronine, 244
tripeptide, 206
trisomy, 295
trout, 54, 364
Trp, 151
tryptophan, 13
Tsuga, 349
tuberculosis, 65, 398, 403, 405, 406, 420, 423, 424, 425, 426
tubers, 271
tubular, xvi, 91, 342, 429, 431, 432, 434, 437, 441, 450
tumor, xiv, 130, 179, 236, 258, 274, 288, 309, 313, 314, 317, 332, 364, 365, 421, 424, 442, 444, 445
tumor cells, 364, 444
tumor metastasis, 442
tumor necrosis factor, xiv, 274, 309, 317, 332, 421, 424
tumorigenesis, 129
Tumorigenic, 132
tumors, 30, 106, 108, 113, 116, 135, 169, 240, 258, 260, 274, 277, 278, 288, 365, 366, 444
tumour, 399, 409

tumours, 372

turnover, ix, xii, 35, 36, 53, 56, 57, 58, 59, 60, 61, 62, 67, 68, 72, 73, 76, 78, 91, 110, 256, 275, 364, 365

turtles, 53, 62

Twin studies, 310

twins, 10, 310, 311, 326, 358

type 1 diabetes, xiv, 309, 331

type 2 diabetes, 32, 145, 146, 153, 156, 157, 158, 159, 239, 253, 313, 314, 315, 316, 317, 320, 329, 330, 331, 414, 415, 423, 425, 426, 427

type 2 diabetes mellitus, 156, 157, 239, 329, 425

type II diabetes, 408

typhus, 65

tyrosine, 102, 311, 314, 316, 328, 331

tyrosine hydroxylase, 311

U

ubiquitin, 132, 168

ubiquitous, 88, 369

UDP-glucuronosyltransferase, 165

Uganda, 87

Ukraine, 255

ulceration, 412

ulcerative colitis, 67

ultrasonography, 145

ultraviolet, 133, 267

ultraviolet irradiation, 267

ultraviolet light, 133

uncertainty, 444

underlying mechanisms, 216, 273, 279, 362

unfolded, 112

unfolded protein response, 112

uniform, 78, 369

uninsured, 295

United Kingdom, 70, 293, 340, 379, 380, 385, 423

United States, 66, 84, 93, 171, 175, 293, 341, 385, 391, 450

univariate, 311

urban areas, 163

urban population, 410, 417

urbanisation, 42, 64

urea, 216

uric acid, x, 140, 143, 154, 159, 274, 317

uric acid levels, x, 140, 154

urinary, 32, 105, 294, 344, 423

urine, xvi, 165, 217, 271, 317, 430, 437

urokinase, 116, 131

uterus, 269, 282, 283, 286

UV, xvi, 103, 106, 107, 109, 112, 113, 114, 116, 132, 147, 266, 277, 430

UV irradiation, 106

UV light, 103, 106, 107, 109, 112, 113, 114, 147, 277

UV radiation, 116

uveitis, 277

V

vaccination, 9, 423

vaccinations, 8

vaccine, 7, 9, 17, 399, 422

validation, 388

validity, 54

valine, 15, 317

values, ix, 2, 35, 36, 41, 50, 147, 148, 206, 266, 283, 294, 305, 315, 325, 358, 374, 376, 378, 379, 381, 382, 387

variability, 17, 49, 374, 376, 378, 382

variable, 119, 205, 307, 324, 342, 369

variables, 215, 220, 232, 341

variance, 315, 375, 381, 394

variation, xv, 50, 66, 86, 90, 101, 119, 121, 124, 125, 133, 160, 204, 314, 317, 323, 325, 357, 359, 367, 368, 369, 372, 373, 375, 381, 383, 421, 426

vascular dementia, 93

vascular disease, 9

vascular wall, 15, 16

vasodilatation, 14

vasodilator, 411

vasospasm, 411

VCAM, xiv, 309

vector, 73, 162

vegetables, 49, 206, 207, 341, 346, 349

vegetarians, 232

vegetation, 199, 200, 201, 203, 205, 206

vehicles, 68, 69, 70

vein, 221

vertebrates, 56, 261, 364

vesicle, 412

Vibrio cholerae, 49, 85

victims, 47, 65

Victoria, 398

village, 342

vimentin, xii, 242, 243, 246, 248, 252

vinegar, 342

vineyard, 169, 171

violent, 48

viral infection, 278, 401, 414, 419, 424, 425

viral meningitis, 403

virulence, 412

virus, 67, 73, 74, 118, 236, 288, 398, 407, 408,
    409, 413, 421, 422, 425

virus infection, 67, 398, 408, 409, 413, 422, 425

viruses, ix, 35, 48, 67, 73, 74, 323

viscosity, xvi, 413, 429, 440, 450

visible, 98, 305, 355

vision, 43, 277, 306

visual attention, 167

vitamin A, 13, 340

vitamin C, 280, 340, 341

vitamin D, 272

vitamin E, 13, 341

vitamins, 14, 33, 178, 188, 203, 222

VLDL, 15

vortex, 435

vulnerability, 54, 55, 57, 135, 238

W

Wales, 281, 398, 419

walking, 299, 366, 368

war, 14, 65, 87

warrants, 25, 151, 184, 199, 202, 219

wastes, 33, 71

water, x, xvi, 28, 65, 107, 144, 161, 162, 163,
    164, 169, 170, 188, 203, 207, 213, 258, 268,
    270, 271, 359, 360, 361, 372, 407, 408, 429,
    432, 434, 437, 441, 442, 449, 450, 451

water quality, 162

water-soluble, 407, 408

weakness, 53, 227, 231

wealth, 78, 311

Weibull, 387, 388, 393

weight gain, 208, 268

weight loss, 187, 220, 268

weight reduction, 220, 224

Weinberg, 39, 81, 82, 90, 365, 370

well-being, 2, 71, 299, 386

wheat, 29, 204, 207

white blood cell count, 427

whole grain, 206

whooping cough, 398

wild animals, 52, 305

wild type, 10, 11, 129, 324, 327

wine, 170

winning, 370

winter, 257, 269, 413, 427

Wisconsin, 252, 394

withdrawal, 287

women, xiii, 2, 14, 15, 86, 141, 143, 145, 154,
    157, 159, 160, 167, 170, 184, 232, 239, 291,
    292, 293, 294, 319, 331, 333, 342, 410, 413,
    417, 421

work environment, 170

workers, vii, 1, 2, 3, 4, 154, 169, 170, 171, 175

workforce, 3, 293

World Economic Forum, 3

World Health Organization, 209, 240, 292

World Health Organization (WHO), 209, 240,
    292

World War I, 65, 171

World War II, 171

worm, 12, 67, 102, 356

worms, ix, 12, 35, 48, 66, 67, 93, 94, 102, 293,
    312

X

X chromosome, 317

xenobiotic, 120, 123, 130, 162, 175, 176, 187,
    201, 363, 425

Y

yeast, 10, 11, 12, 29, 31, 51, 54, 62, 87, 88, 89,
    194, 233, 237, 310, 313, 327, 449

yield, 104, 186, 189, 231, 374, 385, 388, 389,
    393, 394

young adults, 415

Z

zebrafish, 357, 365, 369

zinc, 74, 95, 170, 370

Zn, 11, 127, 132, 134

zooplankton, 270